Antibiotic and Chemotherapy

Lawrence P. Garrod
Emeritus Professor of Bacteriology, University of London
Formerly Bacteriologist, St Bartholomew's Hospital and Hon.
Consultant in Chemotherapy, Royal Postgraduate Medical School

Harold P. Lambert
Professor of Microbial Diseases, University of London
Consultant Physician, St George's Hospital, London

Francis O'Grady
Foundation Professor of Microbiology, University of Nottingham
Formerly Professor of Bacteriology,
St Bartholomew's Hospital, London

Pamela M. Waterworth
Principal Microbiologist, Department of Microbiology,
University College Hospital, London

Antibiotic and Chemotherapy

Lawrence P. Garrod
MD (Camb), Hon LLD (Glasgow), FRCP, Hon FRCPath

Harold P. Lambert
MA, MD (Camb), FRCP

Francis O'Grady
TD, MD (Lond), MSc (Lond), FRCP, FRCPath

With a chapter on Laboratory Methods by
Pamela M. Waterworth
MI Biol, FIMLS

FIFTH EDITION

CHURCHILL LIVINGSTONE
EDINBURGH LONDON MELBOURNE AND NEW YORK 1981

CHURCHILL LIVINGSTONE
Medical Division of Longman Group Limited

Distributed in the United States of America by Churchill Livingstone Inc., 19 West 44th Street, New York, N.Y. 10036, and by associated companies, branches and representatives throughout the world.

First edition 1963
Second edition 1968
Third edition 1971
Fourth edition 1973
Fifth edition 1981

ISBN 0 443 02143 0

British Library Cataloguing in Publication Data
Garrod, Lawrence Paul
Antibiotic and chemotherapy. – 5th ed.
1. Antibiotics
I. Title II. Lambert, Harold P
615'.329 RM267 80–41222

Printed and bound in Great Britain by
William Clowes (Beccles) Limited, Beccles and London

Preface to the Fifth Edition

Lawrence Paul Garrod died on 11th September 1979 at the age of 83. To the end, he continued to write in that marvellously round, yet pungent style, that was so special as to move the Editor of the British Medical Journal to publish a selection from the host of comments, answers and criticisms that flowed apparently so effortlessly from his pen. He would sit with a pad on his knee and after moments of concentration, draft a leader or a paragraph in which he would subsequently seldom change more than a word or two. His part of the book was done, reviewed, revised and ready for the press while his junior authors limped along behind. He encouraged, guided and sometimes, when we lagged behind almost out of sight, bullied us into keeping somewhere near the schedule. We miss him sorely. Many of the quips and characteristic turns of phrase that he wrote in earlier editions of the book remain and if with the passage of time they have to go, we will part with them with great regret.

It has taken a long time to complete the new edition but much has happened since the last, and the whole book has been massively revised. Many chapters hae been totally rewritten and much new material and many new agents introduced. With the proliferation of new agents and more and more detailed information about every aspect of each one of them we have been greatly exercised by the difficulty of keeping the size of the book within bounds. We have had to forego extensive reviews of some individual agents in an attempt to give an overall view of some of the more multi-membered families. We have also had to delete much still valid and valuable material and many references to celebrated and pioneer work especially when, as we have indicated, the subject is extensively treated in previous editions of the book. There are many new illustrations and the whole book has been entirely reset in a new and, we hope, attractive format.

As always, we are greatly indebted to the many who have helped us. Above all, to Miss Pamela Waterworth, author of the last chapter of the book, who has checked and rechecked all the references, prepared the index and, most importantly, sustained us mentally and gastronomically through many long authors' meetings.

Our secretaries, Miss Diana Nisbet, Miss Margaret Newton and Miss Maureen West have uncomplainingly typed and re-typed many versions of almost everything. We are also indebted to Miss Susan Winder, formerly Staff Pharmacist at St George's Hospital, for extensively revising the material on preparations, routes and dosages, now presented in a new format, and to Mr Peter Luton, Electron Microscopist, University College Hospital, for all the new photographs in Miss Waterworth's chapter.

We offer our gratitude to all our publisher's staff concerned with production of the book for all the efforts that they have made to sustain and stimulate us.

This book is a tribute to and a memorial of Paul Garrod: we very much hope that our readers will find it a fitting one.

1981

F.O'G.
H.P.L.

Preface to the First Edition

This book is mainly about antibiotics, but embraces sulphonamides and other synthetic drugs employed in the chemotherapy of the microbic infections of temperate climates. That of malaria and most other protozoal infections, helminthiases and malignant disease is excluded. The first part describes the properties of antibiotics and other drugs, with emphasis on their degree of activity against different bacterial species. The large body of detailed information on this presented in a series of tables, some of it hitherto unpublished, provides one essential basis for rational prescribing, since the first requirement of any drug is an adequate and preferably high degree of activity against the species responsible for the infection.

The second part is concerned with chemotherapy in its practical aspects, in infections which are classified by systems. As professional bacteriologists who have had no clinical responsibilities for many years we are fully conscious of our temerity in invading the sphere of therapeutics. Nevertheless each of us has been so frequently consulted by clinical coleagues about the treatment of individual patients that we can claim a knowledge of this subject in its practical as well as theoretical aspects, and feel justified in writing of what we have learned. The treatment we describe is solely that directed against the microbe. We are well aware that other kinds of treatment, quite outside our sphere, are sometimes an important element in success, and moreover that circumstances may exist, again beyond our ken, which can modify the usual indications for chemotherapy. The clinician must be the ultimate judge: our aim has been to provide him with as much factual information as possible, and accounts of the results achieved by previous competent observers. We believe that this information may be found useful at all levels in the profession; to both junior and senior members of hospital staffs and to consultants as well as general practitioners. We trust also that laboratory workers may find the book helpful.

We are indebted to many colleagues for advice, mainly on clinical matters, among whom we would particularly mention Miss J. Allen, FPS, Professor J. W. Crofton, Mr H. G. Dixon, Dr S. C. Gold, Dr D. A. Mitchison, Dr C. S. Nicol, Professor J. G. Scadding, Mr W. H. Stephenson and Dr J. P. M. Tizard. They have not actually read our text, and should not be held responsible for the views expressed, or for any errors. Our special thanks are due to Miss Pamela M. Waterworth, who has served both of us as a research assistant. She performed most of the experiments on which our original observations are based: among those hitherto unpublished are numerous data in Tables XI and XXII, and the findings illustrated in Figures 6 and 9. Some of her other contributions to the subject are referred to in the text. We are also indebted to her for advice about Chapter XXVII and for preparing the index.

1963

M. B.
L.P.G.

Contents

Drug preparations and dosages

In the tables presented at the end of each chapter, British Approved Names have been used for the pharmaceutical preparations. Where the Proposed or Recommended International Non-Proprietary names (p INN), (r INN), and the United States Adopted Names (USAN) differ significantly, they have been given in the text. When the drug is the subject of a monograph in the United States Pharmocopoeia (USP) and the name differs, this has been given.

The doses given are those suggested by the manufacturers in data sheets, or those stated in the British Pharmacopoeia (BP) or the British Pharmaceutical Codex (BPC), or, when different from these, represent the author's opinions.

A selection of international proprietary preparations have been mentioned where available.

Part I

Introduction

The evolution of anti-microbic drugs

No one recently qualified even with the liveliest imagination, can picture the ravages of bacterial infection which continued until rather less than forty years ago. To take only two examples, lobar pneumonia was a common cause of death even in young and vigorous patients, and puerperal septicaemia and other forms of acute streptococcal sepsis had a high mortality, little affected by any treatment then available. One purpose of this introduction is therefore to place the subject of this book in historical perspective.

This subject is chemotherapy, which may be defined as the administration of a substance with a systemic anti-microbic action. Some would confine the term to synthetic drugs, and the distinction is recognized in the title of this book, but since some all-embracing term is needed, this one might with advantage be understood also to include substances of natural origin. Several antibiotics can now be synthesized, and it would be ludicrous if their use should qualify for description as chemotherapy only because they happened to be prepared in this way. The essence of the term is that the effect must be systemic, the substance being absorbed, whether from the alimentary tract or a site of injection, and reaching the infected area by way of the blood stream. 'Local chemotherapy' is in this sense a contradiction in terms: any application to a surface, even of something capable of exerting a systemic effect, is better described as antisepsis.

THE THREE ERAS OF CHEMOTHERAPY

There are three distinct periods in the history of this subject. In the first, which is of great antiquity, the only substances capable of curing an infection by systemic action were natural plant products. The second was the era of synthesis, and in the third we return to natural plant products, although from plants of a much lower order, the moulds and bacteria forming antibiotics.

1. Alkaloids. This era may be dated from 1619, since it is from this year that the first record is derived of the successful treatment of malaria with an extract of cinchona bark, the patient being the wife of the Spanish governor of Peru. Another South American discovery was the efficacy of ipecacuanha root in amoebic dysentery. Until the early years of this century these extracts, and in more recent times the alkaloids, quinine and emetine, derived from them, provided the only curative chemotherapy known.

2. Synthetic compounds. Therapeutic progress in this field, which initially and for many years after was due almost entirely to research in Germany, dates from the discovery of salvarsan by Ehrlich in 1909. His successors produced germanin for trypanosomiasis and other drugs effective in protozoal infections. A common view at that time was that protozoa were susceptible to chemotherapeutic attack, but that bacteria were not: the treponemata, which had been shown to be susceptible to organic arsenicals, are no ordinary bacteria, and were regarded as a class apart.

The belief that bacteria are by nature insusceptible to any drug which is not also prohibitively toxic to the human body was finally destroyed by the discovery of Prontosil. This, the forerunner of the sulphonamides, was again a product of German research, and its discovery was publicly announced in 1935. All the work with which this book is concerned is subsequent to this year: it saw the beginning of the effective treatment of bacterial infections.

Progress in the synthesis of anti-microbic drugs has continued to the present day. Apart from many new sulphonamides, perhaps the most notable additions have been the synthetic compounds used in the treatment of tuberculosis.

3. Antibiotics. The therapeutic revolution produced by the sulphonamides, which included the conquest of haemolytic streptococcal and pneumococcal infections and of gonorrhoea and cerebrospinal fever, was still in progress and even causing some bewilderment when the first report appeared of a study which was to have even wider consequences. This was not the discovery of penicillin—that had been made by Fleming in 1929—but the demonstration by Florey and his colleagues that it was a chemotherapeutic agent of unexampled potency. The first announcement of this, made in 1940, was the beginning of the antibiotic era, and the unimagined developments from it are still in progress. We little knew at the time that penicillin, besides providing a remedy for infections insusceptible to sulphonamide treatment, was also a necessary second line of defence against those fully susceptible to it. During the early 'forties, resistance to sulphonamides appeared successively in gonococci, haemolytic streptococci and pneumococci: nearly twenty years later it has appeared also in meningococci. But for the advent of the antibiotics, all the benefits stemming from Domagk's discovery might by now have been lost, and bacterial infections have regained their pre-1935 prevalence and mortality.

The earlier history of two of these discoveries calls for further description.

Sulphonamides

Prontosil, or sulphonamido-chrysoidin, was first synthesized by Klarer & Mietzsch in 1932, and was one of a series of azo dyes examined by Domagk for possible effects on haemolytic streptococcal infection. When a curative effect in mice had been demonstrated, cautious trials in erysipelas and other human infections were undertaken, and not until the evidence afforded by these was conclusive did the discoverers make their announcement. Domagk (1935) published the original claims, and the same information was communicated by Hörlein (1935) to a notable meeting in London.

These claims, which initially concerned only the treatment of haemolytic streptococcal infections, were soon confirmed in other countries, and one of the most notable early studies was that of Colebrook & Kenny (1936) in England, who demonstrated the efficacy of the drug in puerperal fever. This infection had until then been taking a steady toll of about 1000 young lives per annum in England and Wales, despite every effort to prevent it by hygienic measures and futile efforts to overcome it by serotherapy. The immediate effect of the adoption of this treatment can be seen in Figure 1: a steep fall in mortality began in 1935, and continued, as the treatment became universal and better understood, and as more potent sulphonamides were introduced, until the present-day low level had almost been reached *before penicillin became generally available*. The effect of penicillin between 1945 and 1950 is perhaps more evident on incidence: its widespread use tends completely to banish haemolytic streptococci from the environment. The apparent rise in incidence after 1950 is due to the redefinition of puerperal pyrexia as any rise of temperature to 38° C, whereas previously the term was only applied when the temperature was maintained for 24 hours or recurred. Needless to say, fever so defined is frequently not of uterine origin.

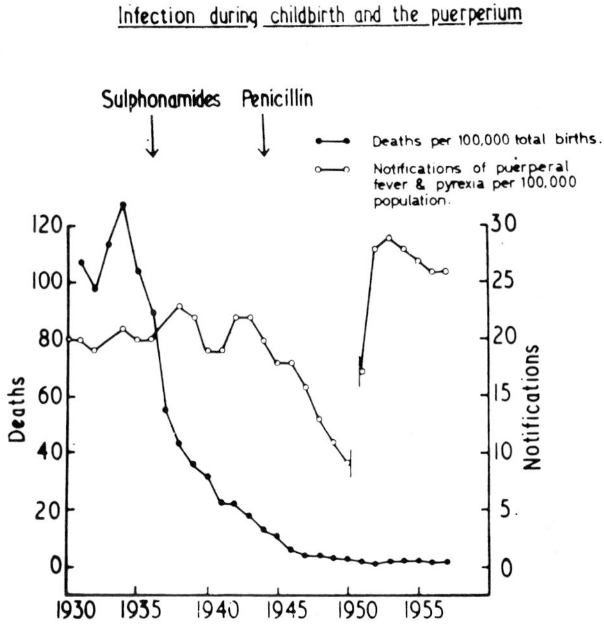

Fig. 1 Puerperal pyrexia. Deaths per 100 000 total births and incidence per 100 000 population in England and Wales, 1930–1957.
N.B. The apparent rise in incidence in 1950 is due to the fact that the definition of puerperal pyrexia was changed in this year (see text).
Reproduced from Barber 1960 Journal of Obstetrics and Gynaecology 67:727 by kind permission of the editor.

Prontosil had no anti-bacterial action *in vitro*, and it was soon suggested by workers in Paris (Tréfouel et al 1935) that it owed its activity to the liberation from it in the body of *p*-amino-benzene sulphonamide (sulphanilamide); that this compound is so formed was subsequently proved by Fuller (1937). Sulphanilamide had a demonstrable inhibitory action on streptococci *in vitro*, much dependent on the medium and particularly on the size of the inoculum, facts which are readily understandable in the light of modern knowledge. This explanation of the therapeutic action of prontosil was hotly contested by Domagk. It must be remembered that it relegated the chrysoidin component to an inert role, whereas the affinity of dyes for bacteria had been a basis of German research since the time of Ehrlich, and was the doctrine underlying the choice of this series of compounds for examination. German workers also took the attitude that there must be something mysterious about the action of a true chemotherapeutic agent: an effect easily demonstrable in a test tube by any tyro was too banal altogether to explain it. Finally, they felt justifiable resentment that sulphanilamide, as a compound which had been described many years earlier, could be freely manufactured by anyone.

Every enterprising pharmaceutical house in the world was soon making this drug, and at one time it was on the market under at least 70 different proprietary names. What was more important, chemists were soon busy modifying the molecule to improve its performance. Early advances so secured were of two kinds, the first being higher activity against a wider range of bacteria: sulphapyridine (M and B 693), discovered in 1938, was the greatest single advance, since it was the first drug to be effective in pneumococcal pneumonia. The next stage, the introduction of sulphathiazole and sulphadiazine, while retaining and enhancing anti-bacterial activity, eliminated the frequent nausea and cyanosis caused by earlier drugs. Further developments, mainly in the direction of altered pharmacokinetic properties, have continued to the present day and are described in Chapter 1.

ANTIBIOTICS

'Out of the earth shall come thy salvation.'

S. A. Waksman

Definition

Of many definitions of the term antibiotic which have been proposed the narrower seem preferable. It is true that the word 'antibiosis' was coined by Vuillemin in 1889 to denote antagonism between living creatures in general, but the noun 'antibiotic' was first used by Waksman in 1942 (Waksman & Lechevalier, 1962), which gives him a right to re-define it, and his definition confines it to substances produced by micro-organisms antagonistic to the growth or life of others in high dilution (the last clause being necessary to exclude such metabolic products as organic acids, hydrogen peroxide and alcohol). To define an antibiotic simply as an anti-bacterial substance from a living source would embrace gastric juice, antibodies and lysozyme from man, essential oils and alkaloids from plants, and such oddities as the substance in the faeces of blowfly larvae which exerts an antiseptic effect in wounds. All substances known as antibiotics which are in clinical use and capable of exerting a systemic effect are in fact products of micro-organisms.

Early history

The study of inter-microbic antagonism is almost as old as microbiology itself: several instances of it were described, one by Pasteur himself, in the seventies of the last century. Therapeutic applications followed, some employing actual living cultures, others extracts of bacteria or moulds which had been found active. One of the best known products was an extract of *Ps. aeruginosa*, first used as a local application by Czech workers, Honl & Bukovsky, in 1899: this was commercially available as 'pyocyanase' on the continent for many years. Other investigators used extracts of species of *Penicillium* and *Aspergillus* which probably or certainly contained antibiotics, but in too low a concentration to exert more than a local and transient effect. Florey (1945) gave a revealing account of these early developments in a lecture with the intriguing title 'The Use of Micro-organisms as Therapeutic Agents': this was amplified in a later publication (Florey, 1949).

The systematic search, by an ingenious method, for an organism which could attack pyogenic cocci, conducted by Dubos (1939) in New York, led to the discovery of tyrothricin (gramicidin + tyrocidine), formed by *Bacillus brevis*, a substance which although too toxic for systemic use in man, had in fact a systemic curative effect in mice. This work exerted a strong influence in inducing Florey and his colleagues to embark on a study of naturally formed anti-bacterial substances, and penicillin was the second on their list.

Penicillin

The present antibiotic era may be said to date from 1940, when the first account of the properties of an extract of cultures of *Penicillium notatum* appeared from Oxford (Chain et al, 1940): a fuller account followed, with impressive clinical evidence (Abraham et al, 1941). It had been necessary to find means of extracting a very labile substance from culture fluids, to examine its action on a wide range of bacteria, to examine its toxicity by a variety of methods, to establish a unit of its activity, to study its distribution and excretion when administered to animals, and finally to prove its systemic efficacy in mouse infections. There then remained the gigantic task, seemingly impossible except on a factory scale, of producing in the School of Pathology at Oxford enough of a substance, which was known to be excreted with unexampled rapidity, for the treatment of human disease. One means of maintaining supplies was extraction from the patients' urine and re-administration.

It was several years before penicillin was fully purified, its structure ascertained, and its large-scale commercial production achieved. That this was of necessity first entrusted to manufacturers in the United States gave them a lead in a highly profitable industry which was not to be overtaken for many years.

Later antibiotics

The dates of discovery and sources of the principal antibiotics are given chronologically in Table 1. This is far from being a complete list, but subsequently discovered antibiotics have been closely related to others already known, such as aminoglycosides and macrolides. A few, including penicillin, were chance discoveries, but 'stretching out suppliant Petri dishes' (Florey, 1945) in the hope of catching a new antibiotic-producing organism was not to lead anywhere. Most further discoveries resulted from soil surveys, a process from which a large annual outlay might or might not be repaid a hundred-fold, a gamble against much longer odds than most oil prospecting. Soil contains a profuse and very mixed flora varying with climate, vegetation, mineral content and other factors, and is a medium in which antibiotic formation may well play a part in the competition for nutriment. A soil survey consists of obtaining samples from as many and as varied sources as possible, cultivating them on plates, subcultivating all colonies of promising organisms such as actinomycetes and examining each for anti-bacterial activity. Alternatively the primary plate culture may be inoculated by spraying or by agar layering with suitable bacteria, the growth of which may then be seen to be inhibited in a zone surrounding some of the original colonies. This is only a beginning: many thousands of successive colonies so examined are found to form an antibiotic already known or useless by reason of toxicity.

Antibiotics have been derived from some odd sources other than soil. Although the original strain of *Penicillium notatum* apparently floated into Fleming's laboratory at St. Mary's from one on another floor of the building in which moulds were being studied, that of *P. chrysogenum* now used for penicillin production was derived from a mouldy Canteloupe melon in the market at Peoria, Illinois. Perhaps the strangest derivation was that of helenine, an antibiotic with some anti-viral activity, isolated by Shope (1953) from *Penicillium funiculosum* growing on 'the isinglass cover of a photograph of my wife, Helen, on Guam, near the end of the war in 1945'. He proceeds to explain that he chose the name because it was non-descriptive, non-committal and not pre-empted, 'but largely out of recognition of the good taste shown by the mould . . . in locating on the picture of my wife'.

Table 1 Date of discovery and source of natural antibiotics

Name	Date of Discovery	Microbe
Penicillin	1929–1940	*Penicillium notatum*
Tyrothricin {Gramicidin, Tyrocidine}	1939	*Bacillus brevis*
Griseofulvin	1939	*Penicillium griseofulvum Dierckx*
	1945	*Penicillium janczewski*
Streptomycin	1944	*Streptomyces griseus*
Bacitracin	1945	*Bacillus licheniformis*
Chloramphenicol	1947	*Streptomyces venezuelae*
Polymyxin	1947	*Bacillus polymyxa*
Framycetin	1947–1953	*Streptomyces lavendulae*
Chlortetracycline	1948	*Streptomyces aureofaciens*
Cephalosporin C, N and P	1948	*Cephalosporium sp.*
Neomycin	1949	*Streptomyces fradiae*
Oxytetracycline	1950	*Streptomyces rimosus*
Nystatin	1950	*Streptomyces noursei*
Erythromycin	1952	*Streptomyces erythreus*
Oleandomycin	1954	*Streptomyces antibioticus*
Spiramycin	1954	*Streptomyces ambofaciens*
Novobiocin	1955	*Streptomyces spheroides*
		Streptomyces niveus
Cycloserine	1955	*Streptomyces orchidaceus*
		Streptomyces gaeryphalus
Vancomycin	1956	*Streptomyces orientalis*
Rifamycin	1957	*Streptomyces mediterranei*
Kanamycin	1957	*Streptomyces kanamyceticus*
Nebramycins	1958	*Streptomyces tenebraeus*
Paromomycin	1959	*Streptomyces rimosus*
Fusidic acid	1960	*Fusidium coccineum*
Spectinomycin	1961–2	*Streptomyces flavopersicus*
Lincomycin	1962	*Streptomyces lincolnensis*
Gentamicin	1963	*Micromonospora purpurea*
Josamycin	1964	*Streptomyces narvonensis* var *josamyceticus*
Tobramycin	1968	*Streptomyces tenebraeus*
Ribostamycin	1970	*Streptomyces ribosidificus*
Butirosin	1970	*Bacillus circulans*
Sissomicin	1970	*Micromonospora myosensis*
Rosaramicin	1972	*Micromonospora rosaria*

Those antibiotics out of thousands now discovered which have qualified for therapeutic use are described in chapters which follow.

FUTURE PROSPECTS

All successful chemotherapeutic agents have certain properties in common. They must exert an anti-microbic action, whether inhibitory or lethal, in high dilution, and in the complex chemical environment which they encounter in the body. Secondly, since they are brought into contact with every tissue in the body, they must so far as possible be without harmful effect on the function of any organ. To these two essential qualities may be added others which are highly desirable, although sometimes lacking in useful drugs: stability, free solubility, a slow rate of excretion, and diffusibility into remote areas.

If a drug is toxic to bacteria but not to mammalian cells the probability is that it interferes with some structure or function peculiar to bacteria. When the mode of action of sulphanilamide was elucidated by Woods & Fildes, and the theory was put forward of bacterial inhibition by metabolite analogues, the way seemed open for devising further anti-bacterial drugs on a rational basis. Immense subsequent advances in knowledge of the anatomy, chemical composition and metabolism of the bacterial cell should have encouraged such hopes still further. This new knowledge has been helpful in explaining what drugs do to bacteria, but not in devising new ones. Discoveries have continued to result only from random trials, purely empirical in the antibiotic field, although sometimes based on reasonable theoretical expectation in the synthetic.

Not only is the action of any new drug on individual bacteria still unpredictable on a theoretical basis, but so are its effects on the body itself. Most of the toxic effects of antibiotics have come to light only after extensive use, and even now no one can explain their affinity for some of the organs attacked. Some new observations in this field have contributed something to the present climate of suspicion about new drugs generally, which is insisting on far more searching tests of toxicity, and delaying the release of drugs for therapeutic use, particularly in the United States.

The present scope of chemotherapy

Successive discoveries have added to the list of infections amenable to chemotherapy until nothing remains altogether untouched except the viruses. On the other hand, however, some of the drugs which it is necessary to use are far from ideal, whether because of toxicity or of unsatisfactory pharmacokinetic properties, and some forms of treatment are consequently less often successful than others. Moreover microbic resistance is a constant threat to the future usefulness of almost any drug. It seems unlikely that any totally new antibiotic remains to be discovered, since those of recent origin have similar properties to others already known. It therefore will be wise to husband our resources, and employ them in such a way as to preserve them. The problems of drug resistance and policies for preventing it are discussed in Chapters 13 and 14.

Adaptation of existing drugs

A line of advance other than the discovery of new drugs is the adaptation of old ones.

An outstanding example of what can be achieved in this way is presented by the sulphonamides. Similar attention has naturally been directed to the antibiotics, with fruitful results of two different kinds. One is simply an alteration for the better in pharmacokinetic properties. Thus procaine penicillin, because less soluble, is longer acting than potassium penicillin: the esterification of macrolides improves absorption: chloramphenicol palmitate is palatable, and other variants so produced are more stable, more soluble and less irritant. Secondly, synthetic modification may also enhance anti-microbic properties. Sometimes both types of change can be achieved together; thus rifampicin is not only well absorbed after oral administration, whereas rifamycin, from which it is derived, is not, but anti-bacterially much more active. The most varied achievements of these kinds have been among the penicillins, overcoming to varying degrees three defects in benzyl penicillin, its susceptibility to destruction by gastric acid and by staphylococcal penicillinase, and the relative insusceptibility to it of many species of Gram-negative bacilli. Similar developments have provided many new derivatives of cephalosporin C, although the majority differ from their prototypes much less than the penicillins.

One effect of these developments, of which it may seem captious to complain, is that a quite bewildering variety of products is now available for the same purposes. There are still many sulphonamides, about 10 tetracyclines, more than 20 semi-synthetic penicillins, and a rapidly extending list of cephalosporins, and a confident choice between them for any given purpose is one which few prescribers are qualified to make—indeed no one may be, since there is often no significant difference between the effects to be expected. Manufacturers whose costly research laboratories have produced some new derivative with a marginal advantage over others are entitled to make the most of their discovery. But if an antibiotic in a new form has a substantial advantage over that from which it was derived and no countervailing disadvantages, could not its predecessor sometimes simply be dropped? This rarely seems to happen, and there are doubtless good reasons for it, but the only foreseeable opportunity for simplifying the prescriber's choice has thus been missed.

References

Abraham E P, Chain E, Fletcher C M, Florey H W, Gardner A D, Heatley N G, Jennings M A 1941 Lancet 2: 177

Chain E, Florey H W, Gardner A D, Heatley N G, Jennings M A, Orr-Ewing J, Sanders A G 1940 Lancet 2: 226

Colebrook L, Kenny M 1936 Lancet 1: 1279

Domagk G 1935 Dtsch Med Wschr 61: 250

Dubos R J 1939 J Exp Med 70: 1, 11

Florey H W 1945 Brit Med J 2: 635

Florey H W 1949 Antibiotics, chap I. Oxford University Press, London

Fuller A T 1937 Lancet 1: 194

Honl J, Bukovsky J 1899 Zbl Bakt, Abt I 26: 305 (See Florey 1949)

Hörlein H 1935 Proc R Soc Med 29: 313

Shope R E 1953 J Exp Med 97: 601, 627, 639

Tréfouel J, Tréfouel J, Nitti F, Bovet D 1935 C R Soc Biol (Paris) 120: 756

Waksman S A, Lechevalier H A 1962 The Actinomycetes, vol 3. Baillière, London

1

Sulphonamides

The discovery and early history of the sulphonamides are described in the introduction. All compounds in this group are derivatives of para-aminobenzene-sulphonamide (sulphanilamide),

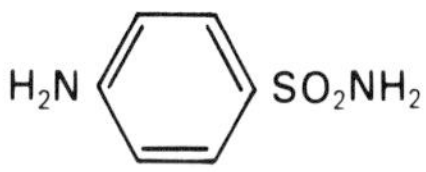

The introduction of further compounds has now continued for over 30 years; advances have been made in the directions of lower toxicity and better tolerance, and of higher antibacterial activity. Compounds of low solubility, which are little absorbed and so act mainly in the bowel, have been developed, as have long-acting preparations which enable the frequency of doses to be reduced. Other sulphonamides have been developed for special purposes, such as the treatment of burns and the management of ulcerative colitis. Combinations of sulphonamides with other compounds, especially trimethoprim, have also become widely used (page 26).

It no longer seems necessary to include a full account of all these numerous drugs in a work of this kind, particularly since the scope of their therapeutic use has been much diminished by the substitution of antibiotics.

ANTIBACTERIAL ACTIVITY

Sulphonamides have what in antibiotics is now called broad spectrum activity. Among Gram-positive organisms, group A streptococci and pneumococci are highly sensitive, staphylococci and *Cl. welchii* moderately so (other clostridia are more resistant), but *Str. faecalis* is resistant. The most sensitive Gram-negative species are the *Neisseria*, but the list includes many enterobacteria, *H. influenzae* and *B. pertussis*; this wide range of possible application has now been much reduced by the development of bacterial resistance. Other less common organisms normally inhibited by sulphonamides include *Yersinia pestis*, *Chlamydia*, *Actinomyces* and *Nocardia*. In combination with other agents which inhibit folic acid synthesis, sulphonamides also show activity against malaria and toxoplasmosis. Thus in the early days sulphonamide treatment was successful in all forms of streptococcal sepsis, pneumococcal pneumonia and other chest infections, gas gangrene, gonorrhoea and cerebrospinal fever, and some enterobacterial infections of both gastro-intestinal and urinary tracts. Of these uses only the last is now common.

All sulphonamides act alike, and an organism sensitive to one will be sensitive in some degree to all others. Much has been written about the relative degrees of activity of different sulphonamides against individual species. Such findings are difficult to evaluate, because comparisons have rarely been made with more than a few other drugs. A greater difficulty is the strong dependence of the result of any *in vitro* test on the composition of the culture medium and on the size of the inoculum (see Fig. 27.2 and page 475). Because of the magnitude of these effects it is impossible to state the minimum inhibitory concentration (MIC) of a sulphonamide for a given organism with anything approaching the precision such as is possible, for instance, with penicillin, which is little affected by either of these factors.

The results of tests of therapeutic activity in mice are also difficult to interpret in comparative terms, since they also are much affected by the conditions of the experiment. As an example, single doses or doses given only twice daily strongly favour long-acting compounds, whereas had they been administered at the usual clinical intervals, a more rapidly eliminated compound might have performed as well or better.

Rather than attempting to review the voluminous and sometimes contradictory literature on the relative *in vitro* activities of different sulphonamides, we felt it necessary to make our own comparison, and the results are given in the previous edition. Noteworthy findings are the comparatively low activity not only of sulphacetamide but of sulphadimidine, the popularity of which in this country may somewhat overrate its merits. The most active among the shorter-acting drugs are sulphadiazine, sulphafurazole and sulphamethoxazole, the last named being of particular interest since it is that with which trimethoprim is combined in co-trimoxazole.

Acquired bacterial resistance

Bacteria can be slowly trained to sulphonamide resistance *in vitro*, and every important pathogenic species has sooner or later been found resistant *in vivo*. This change occurred earliest and most rapidly in gonococci, which nevertheless have reverted to sensitivity during the many years which have elapsed since sulphonamide treatment for gonorrhoea was abandoned. A further quarter-century elapsed before it was seen in the closely related meningococcus (Millar et al., 1963). Sulphonamide resistance among meningococci has become widespread, so that these compounds cannot now be used as primary treatment for meningococcal infection (page 325). Resistant strains of *Str. pyogenes* and pneumococci began to appear in the early 'forties, and but for the advent of the antibiotics there might by now be no effective specific treatment for the important infections caused by these organisms. Resistance in all enterobacteria is now common, and in *Sh. sonnei* almost invariable. Needless to say, resistance to any sulphonamide is accompanied by resistance to all others.

Some mutants owe their sulphonamide resistance to the synthesis of a folic acid synthetase with a lowered affinity for sulphonamide. Some other mutants appear to owe their resistance to changes in the feed-back mechanism. Some overproduce *p*-aminobenzoic acid (Pato & Brown, 1963), an effect which could result from 'switching off' the feed-back control, thereby making the organism insusceptible to sulphonamide interference with enzyme production and function (Richmond, 1966).

Combined action with other antibacterial drugs

Although the effect of sulphonamides is purely bacteristatic, it does not, like that of some similarly acting antibiotics, antagonize the bactericidal effect of penicillin. This is not to say that such a combination is often indicated. With one antibiotic, polymyxin, sulphonamides may act synergically (Herman, 1959; Russell, 1963). By far the most important combination is with trimethoprim, which is so much more effective than a sulphonamide alone that we ventured even in previous editions of this book to say: 'the possibility arises that trimethoprim should also be given whenever sulphonamides are used'. This drug, and its combination with sulphamethoxazole, is described in Chapter 2.

PHARMACOKINETICS

Absorption

Most sulphonamides are well absorbed after oral administration, reaching a peak concentration in the blood after 2–4 hours, which after a dose of 2 g is of the order of 100 μg/ml. Parenteral preparations of some are available, usually sodium salts which are strongly alkaline and can only be given intravenously or, in the case of sodium sulphadimidine, by deep intramuscular injection.

Conjugation

After absorption a proportion of the drug is conjugated, usually with acetate, this proportion, varying considerably with different compounds. The lower this is the better, since the conjugates are inactive therapeutically and the acetyl derivatives are rather more toxic than the free drug. Their solubility in the urine is also a factor to be considered.

Plasma binding

Of sulphonamide in the blood a proportion, varying considerably with different compounds, is contained in the red cells, some is free in the plasma, and another proportion, again varying greatly, is bound to plasma albumin. This bound drug is usually considered to be antibacterially inactive (Newbould & Kirkpatrick, 1960; Anton, 1960), but the findings of Bøe (1966) suggest that this may be an over-simplified view. He compared the effects of adding different amounts of protein on the activity of sulphadiazine and of sulphadimethoxine, which at the same concentration in plasma are respectively 45.1 per cent and 98.7 per cent protein-bound, and found discrepancies inexplicable on this basis.

The extent of protein binding varies with the compound. Sulphanilamide is present mainly in its free diffusible form, and, of the compounds still in use, sulphadiazine is least, and the long-acting sulphonamides most protein-bound. The degree of binding also depends on the serum albumin concentration (Anton, 1968) and on the total drug concentration in the blood, the proportion of protein-bound drug decreasing as the total drug concentration rises.

Protein-bound drug is distributed as protein, and binding consequently affects the concentration of drug entering the tissues from the capillaries. Access to the CSF for example, is normally limited to the unbound drug but with increasing capillary permeability and the passage of protein into the CSF in inflammation, protein-bound sulphonamide enters and the total concentration of sulphonamide in the CSF rises.

The concentration of the short-acting sulphonamides achieved in CSF varies between 30 per cent and 80 per cent of the corresponding plasma concentration. Sulphonamides also enter other body fluids including the eye and, as in the CSF, the drug is present at these sites mainly in its free diffusible form.

Sulphonamides can be displaced from their protein binding sites by a variety of compounds including phenylbutazone and ethyl-bis-coumarin, and simultaneous administration of these substances produces higher concentrations of diffusible sulphonamide (Anton, 1961). This competition for plasma albumin binding sites is also responsible for the effect of sulphonamide in displacing albumin-bound bilirubin (see page 13).

Passage through placenta. Sulphonamides pass readily through the placenta into the fetal circulation and the possible dangers of this to the fetus must be remembered when treating pregnant women with sulphonamides (page 365).

Excretion

The plasma level of free sulphonamide depends on the rate of absorption, the rate and extent of conjugation, and above all, on the rate of excretion. Sulphonamides are excreted mainly in the urine, the free drug and its conjugates being frequently excreted at different rates and by different mechanisms. As a result, the peak plasma concentrations of free drug and conjugate may occur at different times and the proportion of free drug to conjugate may be very different in the plasma and urine.

As with isoniazid (page 395), the capacity to inactivate sulphadimidine is bimodally distributed in the population, those who acetylate most (62–90 per cent) of the drug being clearly different from those who acetylate only 40–53 per cent (Evans & White, 1964). Active acetylators of sulphonamide correspond with rapid inactivators of isoniazid.

Sulphonamides are partly filtered through the glomeruli and partly secreted by the tubules, where some of the excreted drug is reabsorbed. The extent of these processes differs amongst the sulphonamides and may differ markedly for the free drug and its conjugates. As a result, the plasma clearance values vary from <10 to >200 ml/min. Substances with high clearances like sulphafurazole are rapidly eliminated from the plasma and achieve high concentrations in the urine. Substances with low clearances are slowly excreted, plasma levels are maintained for long periods, and low concentrations appear in the urine. If renal function is impaired, excretion may be still further delayed and therapeutic levels may persist for considerably longer. Equally, if such drugs are given repeatedly, high and possibly toxic levels may develop. Naturally no protein-bound drug escapes through the kidney, and therefore highly protein-bound compounds are in general long-acting, but correspondence between the two properties is far from exact because of differences in the degree of tubular re-absorption, which may be a major factor in maintaining the plasma level. The effects of renal impairment on the excretion of sulphonamides is further discussed in Chapter 26.

Excretion in bile. Less than 1 per cent of the dose of the older sulphonamides is excreted in the bile but the proportion is greater (2.4–6.3 per cent) for the new long-acting compounds (Neipp et al, 1964).

TOXICITY

The list of recorded unwanted effects resulting from sulphonamide administration is long and formidable. Some of those caused by the earlier compounds, such as cyanosis and renal blockage from crystalluria, are now rare and side effects from the more recent compounds, given with proper attention to dosage, are relatively uncommon. Some of them are, however, serious, so that, as always, prescribers need to be alert to the possibility of unusual unwanted effects of drugs. All unusual effects of sulphonamide administration recorded in the first 17 years of their use are recorded by Lane et al (1953) and the problem is also extensively reviewed by Weinstein et al (1960).

Renal damage

The first edition of this book (Barber & Garrod, 1963) contained a full page table of the solubilities of 17 sulphonamides and of their conjugates in urine at 4 different ranges of pH. It is now perhaps enough to say that all are more soluble in alkaline than acid urine, that long-acting compounds present little danger because of their slow rate of excretion, and that among others only sulphapyridine (no longer used), sulphathiazole, sulphadiazine and sulphamerazine have dangerously low solubilities. The risk of giving even these and even in maximum doses can be much diminished by giving alkali and enough fluid to ensure a good output of urine, although sulphamerazine may be an exception to this. Triple mixtures containing them render the risk almost negligible. Failing such precautions crystals deposited in the urine may block either the renal tubules or the upper orifice of the ureter. Haematuria is a common early sign. Renal damage during sulphonamide therapy may often, however, be due to a hypersensitivity reaction, rather to tubular blockage, with changes of tubular necrosis or vasculitis. Renal failure has been recorded in several patients after treatment with sulphamethoxazole, as a component of co-trimoxazole (Buchanan, 1978).

Hypersensitivity reactions

Protein-bound sulphonamide can function as a haptene, and the usual result of antibody formation is moderate fever with an urticarial or maculo-erythematous rash occurring on about the ninth day of a course of treatment. Repetition after an interval will elicit the reaction immediately.

Stevens-Johnson syndrome. This fortunately rare but frequently fatal variety of erythema multiforme has been described as an occasional complication of sulphonamide therapy (Salvaggio & Gonzales, 1959). The relative dangers of different sulphonamides cannot be accurately assessed but those which persist in plasma for prolonged periods present a double hazard. They are extensively bound to plasma proteins—and to this extent are more liable to function as haptenes—and their persistence means that toxic manifestations may continue to develop for days after cessation of therapy. A number of reports have described the condition following treatment with long-acting sulphonamides (Beveridge et al, 1964) and the F.D.A. collected 116 cases in which it was believed these drugs were implicated (Carroll et al, 1966). The majority (79) were under the age of 15 and there were 20 deaths. Of the 37 adults, 9 died. The time of onset varied from 2 to 24 days, sometimes as long as 6 days after discontinuing the drug. It was estimated that there had been about 1 or 2 cases per 10 million doses distributed. Toxic epidermal necrolysis (Lyell's syndrome) has also been recorded after administration of long-acting sulphonamides. Other allergic reactions sometimes encountered after sulphonamides are a syndrome more or less identical with serum sickness, with fever, arthropathy, urticaria and eosinophilia, and drug fever without rash. Sulphonamides are among the compounds reported to provoke systemic lupus erythematosus (Alarćon-Segovia, 1969). The earlier compounds were believed to be implicated in the aetiology of polyarteritis nodosa. Myocarditis has also been reported a few times, and some other unwanted effects, described separately below, have their basis in drug hypersensitivity.

Effects of application to the skin. Local treatment of skin conditions with sulphonamides is now recognized as contra-indicated because a very intractable type of sensitization may result, manifested at first by a local dermatitis, later by extension of this to other areas, and sometimes by fever, and persistence of the reaction long after the treatment has been stopped.

Haemolytic anaemia

Sulphonamides, like a number of other drugs, tend to oxidize haemoglobin to methaemoglobin, and this effect is normally combated through the activity of glucose-6-phosphate dehydrogenase. In patients with inherited deficiency of this enzyme, treatment with sulphonamides may cause denatured haemoglobin to accumulate in the red cells in the form of Heinz bodies, and intravascular haemolysis and haemoglobinuria to occur.

Agranulocytosis

The commonest effect of sulphonamides on the bone marrow is a depression of leucopoiesis, and this rarely proceeds to agranulocytosis. Modern sulphonamides seem less liable to have this effect than the earlier (Yow, 1953). Before concluding that a sulphonamide is responsible, the prescription sheet should be reviewed. Discombe (1952), having seen necropsies on three patients from one surgical unit within a month where deaths from agranulocytosis were attributed to sulphapyridine, found that each of them had also been given a proprietary sedative which, unknown to the prescriber, contained amidopyrin. It seems possible here that two marrow depressants had acted synergically. Aplastic anaemia and thrombocytopenia alone are both rare after sulphonamides; eosinophilia can occur alone or as one feature of all allergic syndromes.

Hepatitis

Sulphonamide induced liver injury is rare but well documented. Dujovne et al (1967) collected 106 examples from the literature and added one of their own. The patient described by Tönder et al (1974) developed chronic active hepatitis, with LE cells and positive tests for anti-nuclear factor, after several courses of sulphamethoxypyridazine. A provocation test caused immediate deterioration of liver function tests, and all the changes regressed completely when the drug was withdrawn.

Neonatal jaundice

Bilirubin is transported in the blood bound to plasma albumin and a number of drugs, including some sulphonamides (O'Dell, 1959), compete for the binding sites and so interfere with bilirubin excretion. Sulphonamides administered to pregnant women cross the placenta and may circulate in the fetus for several days or even weeks (Sparr & Pritchard, 1958; Lucey & Driscoll, 1961). Interference with bilirubin transport during this period may increase the free plasma bilirubin level and result in kernicterus. For this reason, sulphonamides should not be given to pregnant women where there is a possibility of rhesus incompatibility, premature delivery, or any history of previous neo-natal jaundice. Sulphonamides should not be given to neonates and this is especially important in premature infants in whom bilirubin conjugation is particularly imperfectly developed.

Lung disease

Respiratory disease in the form of a fibrosing alveolitis has been noted a few times after sulphasalazine (see also p. 21). The changes develop only after several months of drug administration, may progress to severe disability and even death if the association is unrecognized, but tend to abate if the drug is discontinued (Jones & Malone 1972; Davies & MacFarlane, 1974; Thomas et al, 1974).

Embryopathy

There have been several reports of teratogenic activity in experimental animals by some long-acting sulphonamides (Paget & Thorpe, 1964), but in a retrospective study, Cahal (1965) found no evidence of embryopathy in man. *Benign intracranial hypertension* has been reported in two children after receiving sulphamethoxazole (Chi'ien, 1970).

CLINICAL APPLICATIONS

Sulphonamides have a wide antibacterial range, yet they do not produce the troublesome disturbances of gut flora which frequently occur with other broad spectrum agents, notably the tetracyclines. They are active not only against staphylococci, haemolytic streptococci and pneumococci, but also against many enterobacteria including some species resistant to common antibiotics. It has also been claimed—though the evidence for this is not particularly good—that sulphonamides may usefully augment the action of antibiotics in the treatment of a variety of infections.

Although serious toxic manifestations have been described and some authors have condemned sulphonamides on this account, severe reactions are uncommon and treatment for 14 days with conventional doses of current sulphonamides rarely gives rise to trouble. From amongst the thousands that have been synthesized a sulphonamide can be chosen which possesses almost any desirable pharmacological attribute: free absorption from the gut with high blood levels, wide distribution in the body, and ready penetration into the CSF; little or no absorption from the gut; rapid excretion with high urinary concentrations; or very slow excretion with prolonged blood levels. In addition to all this, sulphonamides are cheap and very stable.

In short, except for the fact that they are not bactericidal, sulphonamides approximate closely to the ideal antibacterial agent.

Despite this, absolute indications for their use are very few since the same effect can usually be achieved more rapidly with an antibiotic. Their principal use is for the treatment of urinary tract infection. Their applicability to the treatment of respiratory tract infection is more doubtful, and their value in alimentary tract infection has diminished owing to increasingly frequent resistance in enteropathogenic bacteria. The less soluble compounds continue to be used in combination with neomycin for pre-operative suppression of the bowel flora. Their value in the treatment of meningococcal meningitis is everywhere threatened and in some countries destroyed by the emergence of resistant strains, and few now regard them as a useful adjunct in treating pneumococcal and *H. influenzae* meningitis. Among more exotic uses, sulphonamides appear currently to be the best treatment for nocardiosis, possibly in combination with another drug such as ampicillin (Orfanakis et al, 1972), and, in combination with pyrimethamine, for toxoplasmosis, and perhaps for pyrimethamine-resistant malaria (page 35).

It is a tenable position that except for a few special purposes, such as pre-operative suppression of the gut flora, sulphonamides should no longer be prescribed alone, but only in combination with trimethoprim, a drug which greatly enhances their effect. Its properties, and the wider indications which exist for this combined treatment, are described in the following chapter.

CHOICE OF A SULPHONAMIDE

There is no present need for the existence of so many different sulphonamides, and in our view there is no longer any need to attempt to balance their individual merits by a consideration of all the properties in which they differ. The following brief account only categorizes them and refers to some of the properties of those in commonest use.

Sulphonamides for general use

Among the older compounds, sulphanilamide has been discarded because of its low activity, sulphacetamide for the same reason (except for use as eye drops) and sulphapyridine because of its toxicity. The following remain for consideration.

Sulphathiazole B.P.C. (2-sulphanilamido-thiazole) is highly potent, but peculiarly liable to cause side effects, and is now rarely prescribed alone.

Sulphadiazine B.P.C. (2-sulphanilamido-pyrimidine). This compound has the advantages of high potency, a rate of excretion such that adequate blood concentrations are easily maintained, and low protein binding, facilitating diffusion into the tissues and cerebrospinal fluid. Hence it is often regarded as the best choice for treating meningitis. Renal blockage has to be guarded against.

Sulphadimidine B.P. (2-sulphanilamido-4: 6-methylpyrimidine; sulphamezathine, sulphamethazine). This compound is well absorbed, and excreted moderately slowly. Both the drug and its acetyl derivative are highly soluble, which renders the chance of renal blockage remote, and toxic effects of other kinds and sensitivity reactions are rare. These properties acccount for its high popularity in this country, but in others this does not obtain: in the United States, for instance, consumption is very small and diminishing (Zbinden, 1964). A good reason for this is its low potency: the concentrations required to inhibit many species according to our findings are up to 8-fold higher than those of sulphadiazine, and according to Neipp (1964) some of these differences are much greater. Similar although less extreme differences have been observed in the curative doses for experimental infections. It also suffers by comparison with sulphadiazine in being acetylated to a greater degree and much more highly protein-bound.

Sulphadimidine has evidently given satisfaction in clinical use, and it may seem unjustified to detract from its merits on largely theoretical grounds. It must nevertheless be pointed out that advantage can be taken of the higher potency of other compounds, and some of the risks of using them can be reduced by the use of one of the following combinations.

Triple sulphonamides. The mixture orginally advocated by Lehr contained 37 per cent of each of sulphadiazine and sulphathiazole and 26 per cent of sulphamerazine. Sulphamerazine is more highly protein-bound and less slowly excreted than sulphadiazine and is unsuitable for administration alone in full doses. The main advantage of the mixture is that each drug retains its individual solubility in the urine, and since the dose of each is small, so is the risk of renal blockage: indeed if adequate fluids and alkali are given it may well be negligible. Other advantages claimed are a reduced risk of sensitization reactions and the maintenance of a steadier blood level. Several modifications of the original 'sulphatriad' are now in use.

Highly soluble compounds

The following are highly soluble, even in acid urine, in which they attain high concentrations, and have been largely used for treating urinary tract infections.

Sulphafurazole B.P. (3:4-dimethyl-5-sulphanilamido-isoxazole, sulfisoxazole, U.S.P., Gantrisin). According to our findings this compound is highly active, and if given in sufficiently frequent doses to compensate for its rapid excretion, should serve for treating infection elsewhere as well as in the urinary tract. A curious property, so far unexplained, of this compound is its apparent ability to enhance the bactericidal activity of leucocytes from patients with chronic granulomatous disease (Johnston et al, 1975). The study was made because the authors had noted that some children with this disease showed an improvement too great to be attributed to the direct antibacterial effect of the drug.

Sulphamethizole, B.P. (2-sulphanilamido-5-methyl-1:3: 4-thiodiazole, Urolucosil, Thiosulphil).

Sulphasomidine B.P. (6-sulphanilamido-2:4-dimethylpyrimidine, sulphadimetine, Elkosin). This compound appears rather less active than sulphafurazole. It has also been used as a general purpose sulphonamide.

Compounds of low solubility

Succinylsulphathiazole, B.P (2(p-succinyl-sulphanilamido)-thiazole, sulfasuxidine), and *Phthalylsulphathiazole B.P. (2(p-phthalyl-sulphanilamido)-thiazole, sulphathalidine)* are very little absorbed and owe their activity to the slow liberation of sulphathiazole in the bowel. They may be given together with an antibiotic for pre-operative suppression of the bowel flora. (*Sulphaguanidine B.P.C.* is less suitable for this purpose because less potent and more absorbed.)

Long-acting compounds

These are further divisible into three categories according to their rate of excretion.

'Medium'-long-acting, with half-lives such that two daily doses are given, include the following:

Sulphamethoxazole (5-methyl-3-sulphanilamido-isoxazole, Gantanol) has a high potency and is the compound with which trimethoprim is combined in co-trimoxazole.

The best known long-acting compounds, of which only one daily dose need be given are:

Sulphamethoxypyridazine B.P. (3-sulphanilamido-6-methoxy-pyridazine, Lederkyn, Midicel).

Sulphadimethoxine, B.P.C. (2:4-dimethoxy-6-sulphanilamido-1:3-diazine, Madribon).

Sulphaphenazole B.P.C. (3-sulphanilamido-2-phenylpyrazole, Orisulf).

Sulphamethoxydiazine (2-sulphanilamido-5-methoxypyrimidine, Durenate).

Among these compounds sulphadimethoxine is the most highly protein-bound and sulphamethoxydiazine the least. Various merits have been claimed for each of them and some of these were discussed in previous editions of this book. According to our findings none possesses any outstanding *in vitro* activity, and that of sulphaphenazole is distinctly inferior against all enterobacteria in contrast to the high activity against *Str. pyogenes*. No advantage is clearly discernible in their use except the convenience of a single daily dose, and against this has to be set the possible risk referred to on page 15.

Very long acting compounds include *sulfametopyrazine (2-sulphanilamido-3-methoxypyrazine, Kelfizine)*, for which adequate blood levels can be maintained by giving a dose of 2 g once weekly, and *sulfadoxine* (formerly *sulphormethoxine, 4, p-aminobenzenesulphonamido-5, 6-dimethoxypyrimidine, Fanasil*), given in a dose of 1 g once a week. These compounds have been used in single dose treatment of urinary infections (Gruneberg & Brumfitt, 1967; Williams & Smith, 1970), in chronic bronchitis (Pines, 1967), and in malaria. Reeves (1975) obtained good results using sulfametopyrazine in the treatment of bacteriuria of pregnancy with a cure rate of 67 per cent and 73 per cent from a single 2 g or two 2 g doses respectively, compared with a low 50 per cent success rate for a conventional course of sulphadimidine in a random controlled trial. Quinine followed by a single dose of sulphadoxine-pyrimethamine (Fansidar) has proved a most effective treatment of chloroquine-resistant falciparum malaria (Hall et al, 1975). Long acting sulphonamides have also been recommended for the prophylaxis of rheumatic fever and of meningococcal meningitis.

Sulphonamides for special uses

Mafenide (Marfanil, Sulphamylar). This simple compound, *p*-aminomethylbenzene sulphonamide, now available as the hydrochloride under the name *sulfamylon*, has an interesting history. Synthesized in the U.S.A. where it was soon abandoned as being only feebly active, it was used by the Germans during the war, evidently with great success, as a local application to wounds for the prevention of gas gangrene. Much later it came into its own again as a local preparation for burns (page 315). It is active against *Ps. aeruginosa*. It rapidly diffuses through burned skin and is unusual in that it is not neutralized by *p*-aminobenzoic acid or tissue exudates.

Both the compound and its metabolite, *p*-carboxybenzenesulphonamide, inhibit carbonic anhydrase but White & Asch (1971) while adducing evidence of this effect after administration in man, found no consistent changes in systemic acid-base balance.

Silver sulphadiazine cream has also been widely used in the local treatment of burns and the competing claims of the two compounds are discussed on page 315. Although effective in protecting burns from infection, its value became limited by the emergence of sulphonamide-resistant enterobacteria in a burns unit during its use. Six months after the use of sulphonamides was discontinued most of the gram-negative bacilli had again become sulphonamide-sensitive (Lowbury et al, 1976).

Sulphasalazine (salazopyrine)

This compound is salicylazosulphapyridine. It was found by Baron et al (1962) to be effective in the management of acute attacks of ulcerative colitis and Misiewicz et al (1965) showed that continuation treatment in a dose of 0.5 g q.d.s. reduced the relapse rate in the year following the acute episode. Maintenance treatment was shown to have even more prolonged benefit by Dissanayake and Truelove (1973). They studied 64 patients who had been on the drug for at least one year and whose colitis was quiescent, and found a significant increase in relapse rate in those whose treatment was then changed to a dummy tablet.

Sulphasalazine may also benefit patients with Crohn's disease. Many trials are uncontrolled (BMJ, 1975) but a double blind crossover study by Anthonisen et al (1974) showed a significant reduction of symptoms in the group of patients who had not undergone bowel resection.

The mode of action of sulphasalazine is disputed. The intact compound is absorbed from the upper gastro-intestinal tract, appearing in the blood in 1–2 hours, but cleavage of the azo bond is brought about by colonic bacteria and sulphapyridine is found in the blood 3–5 hours after administration. The other breakdown product, 5-aminosalicylic acid, is partly excreted in the faeces, but its acetyl derivative appears in faeces and urine (Goldman & Peppercorn, 1975).

Antibacterial, anti-inflammatory and immune suppressing effects have all been claimed as the mode of action of sulphasalazine. Early studies noted little effect on the faecal flora but West et al (1974) in a study of 26 patients with proctocolitis or Crohn's disease, demonstrated a decrease, attributable to the drug, in opalescent-negative clostridia, enterobacteria and total non-sporing anaerobes. Sulphasalazine has also been shown to correct the abnormal sodium and water fluxes across diseased bowel mucosa (Harris et al, 1972) and Gould (1975) has postulated that the action of 5-aminosalicylic acid in inhibiting prostaglandin is responsible for the beneficial effect of sulphasalazine, the sulphapyridine component acting merely as a carrier, enabling the active component to reach the colon. This hypothesis has been supported by the work of Azad Khan et al (1977) who showed that retention enemas of sulphasalazine or 5-aminosalicylic acid both caused substantial improvement, whereas no benefit was gained by administration of sulphapyridine enemas. Cowan et al (1977) also showed that, in order to be effective, metabolites of sulphasalazine must reach the lumen of the diseased distal colon.

Unwanted effects common to other sulphonamides are shared by sulphasalazine including a number of rare reactions such as fibrosing alveolitis (page 17) and Lyell's syndrome. Das et al (1973) found that most of their 28 patients with drug toxicity were taking more than 4 g daily and that most of the symptoms could be related to high serum concentration of sulphapyridine itself. The concentration of other metabolites was not related to toxicity. Twenty-four of the 28 patients with unwanted effects were slow inactivators (see page 14) and their mean serum concentration of sulphapyridine was higher (54 μg/ml) than that of the fast inactivators (32 μg/ml). A few patients have developed megaloblastic anaemia after sulphasalazine. One patient with a severe allergic reaction to sulphasalazine was shown to have decreased complement levels and circulating immune complexes. (Mihas et al, 1978.)

References

Alarćon-Segovia D, 1969 Mayo Clin Proc 44: 664
Anthonisen P, Barany F, Folkenborg O, et al 1974 Scand J Gastro 9: 549
Anton A H, 1960 J Pharmacol Exp Ther 129: 282
Anton A H, 1961 J Pharmacol Exp Ther 134: 291
Anton A H, 1968 Clin Pharmacol Ther 9: 561
Azad Khan A K, Piris J, Truelove S C 1977 Lancet 2: 892
Barber M, Garrod L P, 1963 Antibiotic and Chemotherapy. p 26. Livingstone: Edinburgh
Baron J H, Connel A M, Lennard-Jones J E, Avery Jones F 1962 Lancet 1: 1094
Beveridge J, Harris M, Wise G, Stevens L 1964 Lancet 2: 593
Bøe O, 1966 Acta Path Microbiol Scand 68: 81
BMJ 1975 Brit Med J 2: 297
Buchanan N, 1978 Brit Med J 2: 172
Cahal D A, 1965 In Embryopathic Activity of Drugs, ed Robson J M, Sullivan F M, Smith R L. Churchill London
Carroll O M, Bryan P A, Robinson R J 1966 J Amer Med Ass 195: 691
Chi'ien L T, 1970 New Engl J Med 283: 47
Cowan G O, Das K M, Eastwood M A 1977 Brit Med J 2: 1057
Das K M, Eastwood M A, McManus J P A, Sircus W 1973 New Engl J Med 289: 491
Davies D, MacFarlane A 1974 Gut 15: 185
Discombe G, 1952 Brit Med J 1: 1270
Dissanayake A S, Trulove S C 1973 Gut 14: 923
Dujovne C A, Chan C H, Zimmerman H J 1967 New Engl J Med 277: 785
Goldman P, Peppercorn M A 1975 New Engl J Med 293: 20
Gould S R 1975 Lancet 2: 988
Gruñeberg R N, Brumfitt W 1967 Brit Med J 3: 649
Hall A P. Doberstyn E B, Mettaprakong V, Sonkom P 1975 Brit Med J 2: 15
Harris J, Archampong E Q, Clark C G 1972 Gut 13: 855
Herman L G 1959 Antibiotic Ann, 1958–9, p 836
Johnston R B, Wilfert C M, Buckley R H et al 1975 Lancet 1: 824
Jones G R, Malone D N S 1972 Thorax 27: 713
Lane S L, Kutscher A H, Segall R 1953 Ann Allergy 11: 615
Lowbury E J L, Babb J R, Bridges K, Jackson D M 1976 Brit Med J 1: 493
Lucey J F, Driscoll T J 1961 In Symposium on Kernicterus, 1959. Toronto University Press, Toronto
Mihas A A, Goldenburg D J, Slaughter R L J 1978 Amer Med Ass 239: 2590
Millar J W, Siess E E, Feldman H A, Silverman C, Frank P 1963 J Amer Med Ass 186: 139
Misiewicz J L, Lennard-Jones J E, Connel A M, Baron J H, Avery Jones F 1965 Lancet 1: 185
Neipp L, 1964 In Experimental Chemotherapy vol 2, p 169 ed Schnitzer R J, Hawkins F. Academic Press, New York and London
Newbould B B, Kilpatrick R 1960 Lancet 1: 887
O'Dell G B 1959 J Paediat 55: 268
Orfanakis M G, Wilcox H G, Smith C B 1972 Antimicrob Ag Chemother 1: 215
Paget G E, Thorpe E 1964 Brit J Pharmacol 23: 305
Pato M L, Brown G M 1963 Arch Biochem Biophys 103: 443
Pines A 1967 Brit Med J 3: 202
Price Evans D A, White T A 1964 J Lab Clin Med 63: 394
Reeves D S 1975 J Antimicrob Chemother 1: 171
Richmond M H 1966 Symp Soc Gen Microbiol 16: 301
Russell F E 1963 J Clin Path 16: 362

Salvaggio J, Gonzalez F 1959 Ann Intern Med 51: 60
Sparr R A, Pritchard J A 1958 Obstet Gynaec 12: 131
Thomas P, Seaton A, Edwards J 1974 Clin Allergy 4: 41
Tönder M, Nordöy A, Elgjo K 1974 Scand J Gastro 9: 93
Weinstein L, Madoff M A, Samet C M 1960 New Engl J Med 263: 793
West B, Lendrum R, Hill M J, Walker G 1974 Gut 15: 960
White M G, Asch M J 1971 New Engl J Med 284: 1281
Williams J D, Smith E K 1970 Brit Med J 4: 651
Yow E M 1953 Amer Practit 4: 521
Zbinden G 1964 Molecular Modification in Drug Design. Advances in Chemistry Series No 45, p 25. American Chemical Society, Washington DC

Pharmaceutical preparations and dosages are given on page 24.

Sulphonamides. Pharmaceutical preparation and dosage

Name	*Dosage*	*Preparations*	*Common international proprietary names*	
Phthalylsulphathiazole	5–10 g daily in divided doses.	Tablets 500 mg	Thalazole Talidine	(UK) (Fr)
Succinylsulphathiazole	10–20 g daily in divided doses.	Tablets 500 mg	Thiacyl	(Fr)
Sulfametopyrazine	*Adult* 2 g once a week for prolonged treatment. *Children* 30 mg/kg once a week.	Tablets 2 g (soluble) Suspension 500 mg in 5 ml	Kelfizine – W Longum	(UK) (Ger)
Sulphacetamide	For local application to the eyes.	Eye Drops 10%, 20%, 30% Eye Ointment 2.5%, 6%, 10% Ophthalmic solutions (USP)	Albucid Antebor Op-Sulfa, Sulf-10	(UK) (Fr) (USA)
Sulphadiazine	3 g initially, then a maximum of 4 g a day in divided doses.	Tablets 300 mg, 500 mg In combination with Trimethoprim, see Ch. 2	Adiazine	(Fr)
Sulphadimethoxine	*Adults* 1–2 g initially then 500 mg–1 g daily *Children* 30 mg/kg initially then followed by 15 mg/kg daily.	Tablets 500 mg Syrup 250 mg in 5 ml	Madribon	(UK)
Sulphadimidine Sulfamethazine (USP)	*Adult:* 3 g initially, then up to 6 g daily in divided doses. Urinary tract: 2 g initially, then up to 4 g daily in divided doses.	Powder Tablets 500 mg		
Sulphadimidine sodium	*Adults* 1–1.5 g i.v. or i.m. every 6 h; initial dose 6 g.	Injection 1 g in 3 ml	Sulphamethazine	(UK)
Sulphafurazole Sulfisoxazole (USP)	*Adults:* 2 g initially then up to 6 g daily in divided doses.	Tablets 500 mg Syrup 250 mg in 5 ml	Gantrisin Gantrisine Sulfalar, Soxomide	(UK) (Fr) (USA)
Sulphaguanidine	*Adult* Dysentery: 2 g, 4 times a day.	Suspension (also contains dihydrostreptomycin)	Guanimycin Forte Suspension Ganidan Resulfon	(UK) (Fr) (Ger)

Sulphamethizole	*Adult* 100 mg–200 mg every 4–6 hours	Tablets 100 mg Suspension 100 mg in 5 ml	Urolucisol Utrasul, Thiosulfil	(UK) (USA)
Sulphamethoxazole	*Adults* 2 g initially then 1 g every 12 hours *Children* 50–60 mg/kg initially then 25–30 mg/kg every 12 hours	Tablets 500 mg Syrup 500 mg in 5 ml in combination with Trimethoprim, see Ch. 2		
Sulphamethoxydiazine Sulfameter (USAN)	*Adults* 1 g initially then 500 mg daily.	Tablets 500 mg Suspension 500 mg in 5 ml	Kiron Durenat Sulla	(Fr) (Ger) (USA)
Sulphamethoxypyridazine	*Adults* 1–2 g initially then 500 mg daily *Children* 30 mg/kg initially followed by 15 mg/kg daily	Tablets 500 mg	Lederkyn, Midicel Kynex Davosin Sultirene	(UK) (USA) (Ger) (Fr)
Sulphaphenazole	*Adults* 1 g every 12 hours, for 2 days, then 500 mg every 12 hours for 3 days.	Tablets 500 mg Suspension 500 mg in 5 ml	Orisulf Sulfabid	(UK) (USA)
Sulphasalazine Salazosulfapyridine (pINN)	*Adults* 1–2 g every 4–6 hours, then reduce after 3 weeks to a maintenance dose of 500 mg 3 or 4 times a day *Children* 150 mg/kg every 4–6 hours with 20–40 mg/kg as a maintenance dose.	Tablets plain 500 mg Enteric coated 500 mg Suppositories 500 mg	Salazopyrine Sulcolon, Rorasul Salazopyrine	(UK) (USA) (Fr)
Sulphasomidine Sulfisomidine (rINN)	Dose as for Sulphadimidine.		Not available in the UK Elcosine Elkosin	 (Fr) (Ger)
Trisulfapyrimidines (mixed sulphonamides)	Dose varies with preparation and indication.	Tablets Suspension Vaginal preparations	Streptotriad, Sulphatriad, Sultrin, Sulphamagna Streptomagna	 (UK) (other countries)

2

Other synthetic antimicrobial agents

Synthetic agents active against mycobacteria are discussed in Chapter 23, those active against virus infections in Chapter 25, and those used principally or exclusively as topical applications in Chapter 16.

DIAMINOPYRIMIDINES

A group of folate antagonists which owe their importance as antimicrobial agents to an inhibitory effect on the target enzyme in protozoa or bacteria which is enormously greater than that on the corresponding human enzymes. For the best part of a decade the group has been represented by trimethoprim but laboratory and clinical studies on the closely related tetroxaprim have recently been published. (Wise & Reeves, 1979.)

TRIMETHOPRIM

Trimethoprim (Fig. 2.1) was synthesized in the Burroughs Wellcome Laboratories, N.Y. (Hitchings & Bushby, 1961) and was released for general therapeutic use as a mixture with sulphamethoxazole, now called *co-trimoxazole*, in 1969 and for use alone in 1979. It is a weak base with a pKa of about 7.3 soluble to the extent of 4.4 μg/ml water. The lactate is much more soluble: 50 mg/ml water. It is active in concentrations achievable in the plasma, against all the common pathogenic bacteria except Pseudomonas and *M. tuberculosis* (Table 2.1). Co-trimoxazole has been successfully used to treat infection with *Mycobacterium marinum* which is sensitive *in vitro* (Kelly, 1976). There has been a good deal of dispute about the degree to which trimethoprim is bactericidal and Kirven and Thornsberry (1978) found that strains of *H. haemophilus* were clearly divided into those for which the drug was bactericidal and those for which it was not.

Precautions necessary in sensitivity testing are discussed on page 475. Addition of trimethoprim to the medium inhibits the overgrowth of *Proteus* without interfering

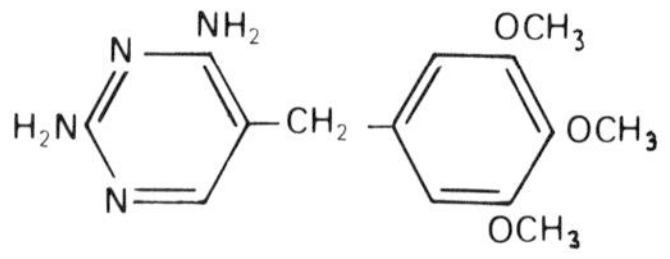

Fig. 2.1 Structure of trimethoprim.

with the recovery of *N. gonorrhoeae* (Seth, 1970), and facilitates the recovery of Group A streptococci from throat cultures (Kurzinski and Meise, 1979).

Table 2.1 Sensitivity of bacteria to trimethoprim

	M.I.C. µg/ml		M.I.C. µg/ml
S. aureus	0.2–1	*N. gonorrhoeae*	8–128
S. pyogenes	0.4–1	*N. meningiditis*	8
S. pneumoniae	0.5–2	*H. influenzae*	0.12–1
S. viridans	0.25	*B. pertussis*	4
S. faecalis	0.25–0.5	*E. coli*	0.01–1
C. diphtheriae	0.4	*K. pneumoniae*	0.5–2
C. perfringens	64	*E. aerogenes*	1–4
M. tuberculosis	R	*Proteus* spp.	1–4
		Salmonella spp.	0.01–0.5
		Shigella spp.	0.5
		P. aeruginosa	12
		B. fragilis	8–16

Bushby S R M 1969 Postgrad med J 45: (Suppl Nov): 10; Waterworth P M 1969 ibid, p 21; Williams et al 1969 ibid, p 71; Phillips I, Warren C 1976 Antimicrob Ag Chemother 9: 736

Synergy

A most important feature of trimethoprim is that it is not only a potent antibacterial agent in its own right, but acts together with sulphonamide in such a way (page 253) that the two agents markedly potentiate each other. Maximum potentiation occurs when the drugs are present in the ratio of their MICs. For example, an organism sensitive to 1 µg/ml trimethoprim and 20 µg/ml sulphonamide, will show maximum inhibition when exposed to a 1:20 mixture. This is the optimum ratio for many organisms, but for others proportionately more trimethoprim is required. Some (of which the *Neisseria* are an important example) are more susceptible to sulphonamide than trimethoprim and for optimum synergy the mixture must contain more trimethoprim than sulphonamide. An idea of the magnitude of increased susceptibility of various organisms to one drug in the presence of subinhibitory concentrations of the other is given in Table 2.2. Many agents exhibit an inhibitory effect on growth at a concentration (the 'minimum antibacterial concentration' or MAC) well below the MIC. The difference between the MAC and the MIC is often due to adaptation of the organism to growth in higher concentrations of the drug during the overnight period of incubation. It appears that mutual suppression by trimethoprim and sulphamethoxazole of adaptive resistance to the other agent is an important component of the synergy observed in conventional MIC titrations (Greenwood & O'Grady, 1976). In addition to lowering the concentration required to inhibit growth the mixture may be bactericidal, where either drug alone is bacteristatic. Daschner (1976) favours the hypothesis that cell wall injury is the final common pathway to bacterial cell death and presents evidence that such injury may be responsible for the bactericidal effect of combinations of trimethoprim and sulphonamide.

In some cases, synergy may be so marked that it can be demonstrated with organisms which would be conventionally regarded as resistant to one or other agent (Bushby, 1969; Lexomboon et al, 1972). In other cases, some degree of sensitivity to both agents must be demonstrable. In a study of over 200 strains of *Sh. sonnei*, all of which were inhibited by 0.23 μg trimethoprim per ml, Jarvis & Scrimgeour (1970) found that only the sulphonamide-sensitive strains showed potentiation. Poe (1976) believes that the reason for synergic activity against sulphonamide resistant organisms is that the primary and synergic effects of sulphonamides are exerted on different enzymes (page 253).

Table 2.2 Degree of potentiation of trimethoprim by sulphonamide

	MIC (μg/ml) Sulphafurazole	Trimethoprim	Mean Potentiation Factor*
Staph. aureus	4–8	0.12–0.5	5.4
Str. pyogenes	1–16	0.25–0.5	7
Str. pneumoniae	2–128	0.5–2	8.4
N. gonorrhoeae	0.5–8	32–64	25
H. influenzae	0.5–64	0.01–.0125	3.5
Esch. coli	4–32	0.12–0.5	5.7
Klebsiella spp.	8–64	0.5–1	4.6
Pr. mirabilis	4–16	0.5–2	26
Pr. vulgaris	4–16	0.5–2	10
Salmonella spp.	16–128	0.06–0.25	2.4
Shigella spp.	4–16	0.03–0.5	6.2

*Factor by which the MIC of trimethoprim is reduced by presence of 9 parts of sulphafurazole (in the case of *N. gonorrhoeae*, 0.3 parts of sulphafurazole): Darrell et al 1968 J clin Path 21: 202

Polymyxin acts synergically both with sulphonamides and trimethoprim against Gram-negative bacilli and the combination of polymyxins and sulphonamide was used as early as 1962 for the successful treatment of proteus septicaemia. Simmons (1970) found that the triple mixture of sulphamethoxazole, trimethoprim and colistin was more active than any pair of these agents against 66 out of 72 enterobacteria. The exceptions were all resistant to sulphamethoxazole. Thomas et al (1976) successfully used this triple therapy in patients infected with multiply-resistant Serratia.

Synergy has also been described between trimethoprim and rifampicin (Kerry et al, 1975) but this has been disputed (Harvey, 1978) and it appears from the degree of interaction that if this combination is to have any therapeutic place, it is likely to be only against more resistant organisms (Grüneberg & Emmerson, 1977; Farrell et al, 1977).

Resistance

Organisms can be rendered resistant to trimethoprim *in vitro* by serial passage in increasing concentrations of the drug, enterobacteria becoming resistant to 500 μg/ml or more, after 12–35 passages (Bushby, 1969). Resistance has emerged in the course of treatment of patients infected with haemophilus (May & Davies, 1972) and with enterobacteria. Resistance may be plasmid-borne or due to chromosomal mutation.

The mechanism of plasmid-borne resistance is unique in that the plasmid codes for the production of an additional dihydrofolate reductase which is about 20 000 times less susceptible to trimethoprim inhibition than is the host enzyme. This enzyme is sufficiently different in its properties from those previously studied for Amyes &

Smith (1976) to suggest that it is not of *Escherichia coli* origin and may well have been derived from a bacteriophage. Plasmid-borne resistance is of particular importance in relation to the possible protective effect of simultaneously administered sulphonamide on the emergence of trimethoprim resistance since the plasmids frequently also carry resistance to sulphonamide (and other agents). Moreover, plasmids may contribute to other resistance mechanisms since Amyes & Smith (1977) found that a plasmid which originally conferred resistance to trimethoprim and sulphamethoxazole, but had lost the ability to transfer trimethoprim resistance, possessed the ability to inspire chromosomal mutation to trimethoprim resistance which was evidently mediated by decreased permeability to the drug. The dihydrofolate reductase of Neisseria is unusual amongst microbial enzymes in showing low affinity for trimethoprim (Averett et al 1979) and this must contribute materially to their natural relative resistance to the drug.

Passage in the presence of trimethoprim is very effective in selecting mutants that are thymine-requiring and hence—since thymine can supply the requirement imposed by trimethoprim (page 252)—trimethoprim resistant. Such organisms have rarely been implicated in infection because tissues generally fail to provide the necessary thymine (Then & Angehrn, 1974). Smith & Tucker (1976) found that thymine-requiring trimethoprim-resistant mutants of Salmonella were less virulent for chickens and mice (particularly when administered orally) than the parent susceptible strain or the thymine-independent revertant. Inability of the organism to multiply in the caecum, where the thymine content was found to be very low, may explain the difference in virulence. Infection with trimethoprim-resistant, thymine- or thymidine-requiring mutants has occasionally been observed in patients treated for prolonged periods with co-trimoxazole. Such organisms do not grow on sensitivity media deficient in thymine or thymidine. Although the concentrations of thymine and thymidine are extremely low in normal human blood or urine, in pathological states sufficient thymine-like compounds (possibly derived from the breakdown of polymorphs) can be detected in the urine of patients infected with such strains (Maskell et al, 1976). Arnold & Kersten (1975) make the interesting suggestion that mutation to the thymine-requiring state is a conservation mechanism since removal of the need for synthesis halts the consumption of tetrafolate (the target of trimethoprim—page 252) making it available for other essential purposes.

Several studies in the U.K. (Correspondence, 1977) indicate that the frequency of acquired resistance remains low despite considerable increase in the use of the drug in recent years, that resistance is substantially more common in *Klebsiella* and *Enterobacter* than it is in *Escherichia* or *Proteus mirabilis* and that it is usually of chromosomal, rather than plasmid, origin. The explanation as far as urinary strains are concerned appears to lie in the remarkable effect of trimethoprim on the faecal and urethral flora. Toivanen et al (1976) confirm the observation, now made several times, that treatment with trimethoprim alone reduces the number of coliform bacilli in the stools without increase in the proportion of resistant strains while similar treatment with co-trimoxazole and particularly with sulphonamide alone, causes an increase in the proportion of strains resistant to sulphonamides.

Stamey et al (1977) have extended their observations on this phenomenon to the vaginal vestibule where co-trimoxazole at full dosage (no doubt because of its special pharmacokinetic properties—page 31) eradicated enterobacteria without producing resistant strains in contrast to oral sulphonamides which carried a high risk of the development of resistance.

Absorption

Trimethoprim is rapidly and near-completely absorbed from the gut, giving peak plasma levels of about 0.9–1.2 μg/ml 1½–3½ hours after a dose of 100 mg, and 2.2–3.2 μg/ml after 250 mg. At these concentrations, 42–46 per cent of the drug is protein-bound. After a single large dose (9 tablets), intended for the treatment of gonorrhoea, Yoshikawa & Guze (1976) found plasma levels after 2 hr of 4–11 μg trimethoprim and 50–150 μg sulphamethoxazole per ml. Mean plasma levels were still 2.16 μg trimethoprim and 31.7 μg sulphamethoxazole after 24 hr. Intravenous infusion of 160 mg trimethoprim and 800 mg sulphamethoxazole over 1 hr every 8 hrs maintained serum levels in excess of 30 μg free sulphamethoxazole and 2 μg trimethoprim per ml (Grose et al, 1979).

In a study of dose regimens in both healthy and sick children, Fowle et al (1975) found that a simple dosage regimen based on fractions of the adult dose according to age produced therapeutically effective plasma concentrations even at the point at which the next dose was due and that the range was no greater than that obtained by others using dosage based on body size. There was a significant increase in plasma levels between the third and sixth days, suggesting that the steady state had not been reached by the third day as it is in adults. Metabolic disposition of sulphamethoxazole in children and adults appeared to be the same. The age-based, 12 hourly dosage regimen they suggest is: 6 weeks–6 months 20 mg trimethoprim + 100 mg sulphamethoxazole with double the dose for those aged 6 months–5 years. The plasma half-life is 6–12 hours (Schwartz & Ziegler, 1969).

Distribution

The volume of distribution of trimethoprim is greater than that of the total body water, indicating concentration at one or more sites, while that of sulphamethoxazole is only about 20 per cent of the body water—a volume corresponding with the extracellular fluid (Fowle, 1973). This difference in distribution accounts for the fact that the ratio of sulphamethoxazole to trimethoprim is 20:1 in plasma while that in the administered mixture is 5:1. If the large volumes reached by trimethoprim but not by sulphonamide include sites of infection this discrepancy plainly has serious significance in relation to the possibility of synergic interaction.

Further evidence of differential distribution is provided by Reid et al (1975) who found the concentrations of trimethoprim in maternal and fetal serum and amniotic fluid to be similar while those of sulphamethoxazole were lower in fetal than in maternal serum and still lower in amniotic fluid. Relative inaccessibility of fetal tissues to the sulphonamide component of the mixture was indicated by a fall in the sulphonamide to trimethoprim ratio from 100:1 in cord blood to 10:1 in liver, 9:1 in placenta and 5:1 in lung.

Trimethoprim fulfils the physicochemical requirements for excretion into the prostatic fluid: high lipid solubility, a pKa that ensures that a large fraction of the molecules in the plasma are uncharged and low protein binding (Stamey et al, 1973). Dabhoiwala et al (1976) measured the concentration of trimethoprim and sulphamethoxazole in washed samples of prostate removed at operation from patients who had received a single dose of 4 tablets about 2–4 hours before operation or had completed a conventional week's course of therapy about nine hours before surgery. In those receiving the single dose they found prostatic levels of 1.7–9.8 μg trimethoprim per g with simultaneous plasma levels of 0.3–5 μg per g, although the difference in the means, 3.6 and 3 μg/g, was not significant. Corresponding levels of free sulphamethoxazole were: in the prostate, less than 1 to 13.3 μg/g and in the plasma, 17.5 to 142 μg/g. In the patients who had completed a week's treatment, the prostatic levels of trimethoprim were 0.8–15.9 with plasma levels of 0.9–6, while the free sulphamethoxazole levels in the prostate were 6.1–27 g with corresponding plasma levels of 15–78 μg/g.

The results strongly confirm previous reports of both the marked difference in partition of the two drugs between the plasma and prostate and delay in reaching equilibrium. The concentrations obtained were adequate in all patients for the treatment of prostatitis due to the common infecting organisms. They question whether non-ionic diffusion can fully explain these findings, but the work of Stamey et al (1973) in the dog excludes the possibility of active transport.

The pH gradient between plasma and vaginal fluid is even greater than that between plasma and prostatic fluid so that substantial concentration of the drug in vaginal secretion might be expected (Stamey et al, 1977). They found vaginal levels of trimethoprim between 0.15 and 2.25 μg per ml in patients receiving low-dose prophylactic therapy and 0.9–10 μg per ml in patients on conventional dosage—in most cases substantially above the corresponding serum levels—while the sulphamethoxazole levels were very low.

In patients undergoing cataract extraction who were given conventional doses of co-trimoxazole on the morning of surgery and on the evening before, Pohjanpelto et al (1974) found concentrations in the aqueous humour of 0.14–0.4 μg trimethoprim per ml and 10–29 μg sulphamethoxazole per ml.

Excretion

Excretion of the drug is almost wholly via the urine giving levels of 50–100 μg/ml of which less than 8 per cent is in conjugated inactive forms. About 70 per cent of the drug is excreted in the first 24 hours, but detectable levels are present in the urine for 4–5 days during which time about 90 per cent of the dose can be recovered.

Sharpstone (1969) found the renal clearance of trimethoprim in the normal subject to be 19–148 ml/min, the wide variation being accounted for to a large extent by the influence of pH. Trimethoprim is a weak base and urinary excretion rises sharply with falling pH as the drug ionises and non-ionic back-diffusion in the tubules decreases. Trimethoprim clearance declines with renal function, but less rapidly than that of creatinine so that at the poorest function levels, trimethoprim clearance exceeds that of creatinine (supporting other evidence that the drug is partly excreted by active tubular secretion) and therapeutic concentrations of the drug are still found in the urine.

In a comprehensive study of the excretion of trimethoprim and sulphamethoxazole in the bile, Rieder et al (1974) found that the biliary level rose from about 50 per cent of the corresponding plasma level at 4 hours to levels approximating to those of the plasma at 24 hours. At 12 hours (that is to say at the usual dose interval) after a single conventional dose the biliary concentration of active sulphamethoxazole was 8–14 μg per ml and that of trimethoprim 0.44–1.03 μg per ml. No evidence was found that the pharmacokinetics of the two compounds modified one another.

Choice of matching sulphonamide. In order to maintain in treated patients a ratio of trimethoprim to sulphonamide as close as possible to the synergic optimum, it was necessary to choose a sulphonamide with pharmacokinetic characteristics as close as possible to those of trimethoprim. Sulphamethoxazole is used in co-trimoxazole and sulphadiazine in co-trimazine.

The available preparations contain 4.5–5 times as much sulphonamide as trimethoprim and this produces a plasma level of sulphonamide about 20 times the simultaneous level of trimethoprim, so achieving the optimum synergic ratio. Against *Neisseria* infections the optimum ratio is markedly different and it may be that for the treatment of infections with these organisms other formulations would be preferable (Garrod, 1969). Similarly, in renal failure differences in handling of the two compounds may disturb the plasma ratio and dosage of the two components may need to be suitably adjusted if treatment of such patients is contemplated (Sharpstone, 1969).

Toxicity and side effects

Nausea, vomiting (occasionally severe enough to require withdrawal of treatment) and skin rashes have occurred in some patients. When the drug was available only as a mixture with sulphamethoxazole, it was not usually immediately plain which component was responsible for any reactions which occurred. Amongst almost thirty thousand patients reviewed by Lawson and Jick (1978) 8% experienced adverse reactions, the frequency in females being twice that in males.

The most serious foreseeable toxic effect of trimethoprim is the induction of folate deficiency. The very low affinity of the drug for the mammalian enzyme and the possibility of by-passing any depressant effect by feeding folate supplements (which cannot be utilized by the parasite—page 253) makes the likelihood of serious haematological disorder seem relatively remote, but it is nevertheless plain that folate metabolism in man does not entirely escape the attentions of trimethoprim (Kahn et al, 1968). In 10 subjects receiving the large dose of 1 g per day, Whitman (1969) found bone marrow abnormalities in 8, and FiGlu excretion in 5, but no abnormality on 200 mg per day. O'Grady et al (1969) found no evidence of folate deficiency in patients treated with small doses (see page 378) for periods up to six years.

Reversible thrombocytopenia and leucopenia, which may have been due to the sulphonamide component, has been recorded several times (Evans & Tell, 1969; Mohan, 1969; Hammett, 1970). Hulme & Reeves (1971) observed leucopenia in four out of 14 patients who received co-trimoxazole together with immunosuppressive agents after renal transplantation.

Chanarin & England (1972) describe four patients with megaloblastic anaemia who responded very poorly to haematinics while receiving co-trimoxazole; and a patient of Jewkes et al (1970), who received 320 mg trimethoprim and 1.6 g sulphamethoxazole daily for a year, is described as having disordered folate metabolism most of the time. By way of convincing confirmation of the site of action of the drug (page 253), folic acid (100 μg/day) was without effect but folinic acid (60 μg/day) restored normoblastic erythropoiesis and banished giant metamyelocytes from the bone marrow. On the other hand, in 10 elderly patients with chronic bronchitis treated for three months, Jenkins et al (1970) found a transient early fall in folate levels with little haematological change except in two patients who were already in poor nutritional state. They were restored to normal by folinic acid supplements.

Stevens (1974) reviews reported haemopoietic complications of co-trimoxazole therapy and describes transient erythroid hypoplasia in a patient who had received co-trimoxazole for 16 months which successfully controlled her previously intractable diarrhoea associated with Crohn's disease. There was no involvement of the white cells. She required several blood transfusions but had recovered fully six months after stopping the drug.

Review of these and other cases so far described leaves no doubt that disordered folate metabolism with attendant haematological changes can occur in patients treated with the drug, but only when other deficiencies, disorders or drugs have already sapped the patient's haematological resilience.

Kalowski et al (1973) describe deterioration of renal function in 16 patients treated with co-trimoxazole; two initially had normal function and in five in whom it was impaired, dosage was appropriately modified. In three of the patients renal function did not recover. They attribute this effect to the sulphonamide component of the mixture and review the mechanisms by which this may occur. In a prospective study of 20 patients with chronic renal failure treated for respiratory or urinary infection, Tasker et al (1975) were unable to confirm that co-trimoxazole may lead to a deterioration of renal function in patients with renal disease. They review the probable reasons for this discrepancy and conclude that co-trimoxazole can be used in patients with chronic renal failure providing the dose is appropriately adjusted (page 455).

Obstruction of the ureter in an elderly man by what is described as a 'metabolite of the combination of sulphamethoxazole and trimethoprim' is described by Siegel (1977).

Sulphamethoxazole occasionally causes hepatic lesions and Colucci & Cicero (1975) describe massive hepatic necrosis in an 80-year-old man treated 10 days before the onset of jaundice with co-trimoxazole for orchitis.

Altogether there is a strong indication that the majority of reported untoward reactions to the combination can be traced to the sulphonamide component (Bernstein, 1975)—a factor of some importance in the debate about the release of trimethoprim for use alone (page 34).

In the rat, doses greater than 200 mg/kg/day were teratogenic, but complete protection was afforded by folinic acid or dietary folate supplements. No abnormalities were produced in the rabbit (Udall, 1969). Williams et al (1969) treated 120 patients with bacteriuria of pregnancy, half of whom were more than half way towards delivery, but 10 were less than 16 weeks pregnant, and in none of their infants was there any abnormality.

Ochoa (1971) reports a patient successfully treated for nocardiasis throughout pregnancy without mishap to mother or baby.

Clinical use

The range of pathogens against which co-trimoxazole is active opened up a wide field of potentially successful therapeutic exploration (Garrod, 1969). The extent to which such exploration has been rewarded is indicated by the successful treatment of infections as diverse as acne, nocardiasis (Beaumont, 1970; Adams et al, 1971; Evans & Benson, 1971), gonorrhoea (page 426), brucellosis (page 302), endocarditis (Fowle & Zorab, 1970; Freeman & Hodgson, 1972) and severe enterobacterial infections including enteric fever (page 337), cholera and generalised infection of childhood (Roy, 1971). The response of *Pneumocystis carinii* infections to co-trimoxazole does not appear to be augmented by the addition of pentamidine (Kluge et al, 1978).

The combination has also been successfully used for the treatment of plague, meningitis (where both components penetrate well into the CSF) and for the prophylaxis and treatment of immunodeficient and immunosuppressed patients. The drug has several times been commended for the control of infection, or febrile episodes of presumed infectious origin, in patients with malignant diseases (Grose et al, 1977).

The principal use of the drug, however, remains in the control, and especially the long term control, of urinary (page 378) and respiratory (page 361) infections.

The virtually identical performance of the mixture containing sulphadiazine in place of sulphamethoxazole is to be expected in view of the considerable doubt about the therapeutic role of the sulphonamide component (Tuomisto et al, 1977).

It was natural to assume that the synergic interaction between the two components of co-trimoxazole that is so easily demonstrable in the laboratory would contribute materially to the therapeutic efficacy of the combination. This assumption has come to be questioned on several grounds. The first is that synergy is by definition demonstrable only when the concentrations of each component is in itself insufficient to exert an antibacterial effect. In this case, the peak concentrations of each agent exceed the MICs of sensitive organisms in the plasma and greatly exceed them in the urine. After a single dose, inhibitory concentrations of trimethoprim can frequently be detected in the urine for several days and as the drug is usually given twice a day it is hard to see a role for synergic enhancement of its effect by the simultaneous presence of sulphamethoxazole. There may be an opportunity for synergic interaction in plasma as the concentration falls, but infected sites are separated from the plasma concentrations by barriers which are not equally permeable to the two components.

Although the plasma profiles of the two drugs show reasonable concordance, their distribution is markedly different (page 30), the trimethoprim reaching many sites relatively inaccessible to the sulphonamide. It remains to be shown whether infections can be identified against which the combination is superior in clinical efficacy to trimethoprim alone. In the meantime, doubt about the general therapeutic importance of synergy and concern about the proportion of patients in whom untoward reactions can be attributed to the sulphonamide component led to pressure to free trimethoprim from the fixed mixture and allow it to be prescribed alone. Resistance to this pressure was based principally on fear that removal of the sulphonamide would allow the ready emergence of organisms resistant to trimethoprim thereby destroying what is generally acknowledged to be a most valuable drug. A glance at the state of trimethoprim resistance (page 28) will confirm that the microbiological situation is complex and on the present evidence we are disinclined to attempt to weigh the hypothetical cost of increased resistance against the likely benefit of reduced untoward effects. Evidence currently available (Towner et al, 1979) does not indicate that removal of the sulphonamide component is likely to increase the prevalence of trimethoprim resistance but predictions about resistance trends are notoriously unreliable and only time will tell whether the scientific grounds for undoing the combination were at least as good as those originally advanced for putting it together.

PYRIMETHAMINE

This agent is principally used as a malaria suppressant, but has also been successfully used to treat leishmaniasis and toxoplasmosis. In effective anti-parasitic doses the drug is more active than trimethoprim against mammalian dihydrofolate reductase, and evidence of folate deficiency is more commonly seen during treatment. Its depressant effect on haemopoiesis disappears on withdrawing the drug and can be reversed during treatment by folinic acid.

Pyrimethamine has been used on the basis of its antifolate effect in man for the successful treatment of CNS leukaemia with some disagreement about the severity of its side effects (Hamers et al, 1974). The drug causes normal stem cells to leave the bone marrow and enter the reproductive cycle, thereby abolishing the selective advantage otherwise enjoyed by normal cells on exposure to antitumour agents, so pyrimethamine (and by analogy, trimethoprim) should not be introduced into courses of cancer chemotherapy (Price & Bondy, 1973). Synergic depression of the bone marrow has not surprisingly also been observed in patients receiving cytotoxic agents who have been treated with pyrimethamine for other reasons, notably toxoplasmosis, or for malaria prophylaxis.

Combinations of sulphonamide with pyrimethamine are at present the treatment of choice for human toxoplasmosis.

References
Adams A R, Jackson J M, Scopa J, Lane G K, Wilson R 1971 Med J Aust 1: 669
Amyes G B, Smith J T 1976 Eur J Biochem 61: 597
Amyes S G B, Smith J T 1977 Genet Res 29: 35
Arnold H H, Kersten H 1975 FEBS Lett 53: 258
Averett D R, Roth B, Burchall, J J, Baccanari D P 1979 Antimicrob Ag Chemother 15: 428
Beaumont R J 1970 Med J Aust 2: 1123
Bernstein L S 1975 Can Med Ass J 112: 96
Bushby S R M 1969 Postgrad Med J 45: (Suppl Nov) 10
Chanarin I, England J M 1972 Brit Med J 1: 651
Colucci C F, Cicero M L 1975 J Amer Med Ass 233: 952
Correspondence 1977 Lancet 2: 926, 774
Dabhoiwala N F, Bye A, Claridge M 1976 Brit J Urol 48: 77
Daschner F 1976 Chemotherapy 22: 12
Evans D I K, Tell R 1969 Brit Med J 1: 578
Evans R A, Benson R E 1971 Med J Aust 1: 684
Farrell W, Wilks M, Drasar F A 1977 J Antimicrob Chemother 3: 459
Fowle A S E 1973 Med J Aust 2: (Suppl June) 26
Fowle A S E, Bye A, Hariri F, Middlemiss D, Naficy K 1975 Eur J Clin Pharm 8: 217
Fowle A S E, Zorab P A 1970 Brit Heart J 32: 127
Freeman R, Hodson M E 1972 Brit Med J 1: 419
Garrod L P 1969 Postgrad Med J 45: (Suppl Nov) 52
Greenwood D, O'Grady F 1976 J Clin Path 29: 162
Grose W E, Bodey G P, Rodriguez V 1977 J Amer Med Assoc 237: 352
Grose W E, Bodey G P, Loo T L 1979 Antimicrob Ag Chemother 15: 447
Grüneberg R N, Emmerson A M 1977 J Antimicrob Chemother 3: 453

Hamers J, van Hove W, Baele G 1974 Lancet 1: 310
Hammett J F 1970 Med J Aust 2: 200
Harvey R J 1978 J Antimicrob Chemother 4: 315
Hitchings G H, Bushby S R M 1961 Proc 5th Int Cong Biochem (Moscow) Sect 7 p 165. Pergamon, London
Hulme B, Reeves D S 1971 Brit Med J 3: 610
Jarvis K J, Scrimgeour G 1970 J Med Microbiol 3: 554
Jenkins G C, Hughes D T D, Hall P C 1970 J Clin Path 23: 392
Jewkes R F, Edwards M S, Grant B J B 1970 Postgrad Med J 46: 723
Kahn S B, Fein S A, Brodsky I 1968 Clin Pharmacol Ther 9: 550
Kalowski S, Nanra R S, Mathew T H, Kincaid-Smith P 1973 Lancet 1: 394
Kelly R 1976 Med J Aust 2: 681
Kerry D W, Hamilton-Miller J M T, Brumfitt W 1975 J Antimicrob Chemother 1: 417
Kirven L A, Thornsberry C 1978 Antimicrob Ag Chemother 14: 731
Kluge R M, Spaulding D M, Spain A J 1978 Antimicrob Ag Chemother 13: 975
Kurzynski T A, Meise C K J 1979 Clin Microbiol 9: 189
Lawson D H, Jick H 1978 Amer J Med Sci 275: 53
Lexomboon U, Mansuwan P, Duangmani C, Benjadol P, M'cMinn M T 1972 Brit Med J 3: 23
Maskell R, Okubadejo O A, Payne R H 1976 Lancet 1: 834
May J R, Davies J 1972 Brit Med J 3: 376
Mohan P 1969 Practitioner 202: 553
Nolan J, Rosen E S 1968 Brit J Ophthal 52: 396
Ochoa A G 1971 J Amer Med Ass 217: 1244
O'Grady F, Chamberlain D A, Stark J E, Cattell W R, Sardeson J M, Fry I K, Spiro F I, Waters A H 1969 Postgrad Med J 45: (Suppl Nov), 61
Poe M 1976 Science 194: 533
Pohjanpelto P E J, Sarmela T J, Raines T 1974 Brit J Ophthal 58: 606
Price L A, Bondy P K 1973 Lancet 1: 727
Reid D W J, Caillé G, Kaufmann N R 1975 Canad Med Ass J 112: 67S
Rieder J, Schwartz D E, Zangaglia O 1974 Chemotherapy 20: 65
Roy L P 1971 Med J Aust 1: 148
Schwartz D E, Ziegler W H 1969 Postgrad Med J 45: (Suppl Nov) 32
Seth A 1970 Brit J Vener Dis 46: 201
Sharpstone P 1969 Postgrad Med J 45: (Suppl Nov) 38
Siegel W H 1977 J Urol 117: 397
Simmons N A 1970 J Clin Path 23: 757
Smith H W, Tucker J F 1976 J Hyg Camb 76: 97
Stamey T A, Bushby S R M, Bragonje J 1973 J Infect Dis 128: (Suppl Nov) S686
Stamey T A, Condy M, Mihara G 1977 New Engl J Med 296: 780
Stevens M E M 1974 Postgrad Med J 50: 235
Tasker P R W, MacGregor G A, de Wardener H E, Thomas R D, Jones N F 1975 Lancet 1: 1216
Then R, Angehrn P 1974 Biochem Pharmacol 23: 2977
Thomas F E, Leonard J M, Alford R H 1976 Antimicrob Ag Chemother 9: 201
Towner K J, Pearson N J, Cattell W R, O'Grady F 1979 J Antimicrob Chemother 5: 45
Towner K J, Pearson N J, Pinn P A, O'Grady F 1980 Brit Med J 1: 517
Toivanen A, Kasanen A, Sundquist H, Toivanen P 1976 Chemotherapy 22: 97
Tuomisto J, Kasanen A, Renkonen O V 1977 Chemotherapy 23: 337
Udall V 1969 Postgrad Med J 45: (Suppl Nov) 42
Whitman E N 1969 Postgrad Med J 45: (Suppl Nov) 46
Williams J D, Brumfitt W, Condie A P, Reeves D S 1969 Postgrad Med J 45: (Suppl Nov) 71
Wise R, Reeves D S 1979 J Antimicrob Chemother 5: Suppl B
Yoshikawa T T, Guze L B 1976 Antimicrob Ag Chemother 10: 462

HEXAMINE (METHENAMINE) AND ITS SALTS

Katul & Frank (1970) review the history of these compounds of which hexamine itself was for many years the only drug capable of killing bacteria in the urine. It has no action *per se*, but in an acid medium is slowly decomposed with the liberation of formaldehyde to which all micro-organisms are susceptible. The odour of sweat is partly due to the action of skin bacteria and hexamine is included in some deodorant preparations where on contact with acid sweat it liberates formalin which inhibits bacterial activity and reduces sweating (evidently by causing keratin occlusion of the sweat glands) to a sufficient degree for local applications to have been used in the control of hyperhydrosis (Cullen, 1975).

It is absorbed from the gut and mainly excreted unchanged in the urine. Because of the effect of acid, formalin will be liberated in the stomach unless the drug is given in enteric-coated tablets. Musher & Griffith (1974) confirm earlier observations that the liberation of formalin in the urine is pH dependent, being greatest at pH 5.5 and absent at pH 7, and relatively slow, but show by means of an *in vitro* system that simulates the hydrokinetic conditions of the urinary bladder that effective levels of formalin are likely to be produced on conventional dosage if the urinary pH is less than 5.8 This means that the treatment is inapplicable to urea-splitting organisms unless the conditions are such that simultaneous administration of acetohydroxamic acid, a potent inhibitor of bacterial urease, can prevent gross alkalinization of the urine (Musher et al, 1974). Some patients on the drug complain of frequent and burning micturition and it is still sometimes recommended that these side-effects be controlled by giving alkali—so guaranteeing an absence of any effect. Prolonged administration or high dosage may produce proteinuria, haematuria and bladder changes.

Hexamine is now generally given in the form of its salts with organic acids which may both exert some antibacterial effect in their own right and serve to reduce the urinary pH to the low levels necessary for the liberation of formaldehyde from hexamine. Mandelic acid is sometimes given alone, usually as the ammonium or calcium salt. Of the two salts generally available, hexamine mandelate and hexamine hippurate, the hippurate appears to give higher urinary formaldehyde levels. The performance of the mandelate may be impaired by its enteric coating.

There is disagreement about the relative action of the salts against different bacterial species *in vitro* but there are suggestions that amongst the most susceptible may be some that are most resistant to antibiotics (Miller & Phillips, 1970; Katul & Frank, 1970). Like hexamine, the salts may produce gastrointestinal intolerance and, in excessive dosage, haemorrhagic cystitis (Ross & Conway, 1970).

Clinical use

There is general accord that if treatment is to be successful excessive fluid intake must be avoided and that fluid restriction may be more important than rigorous acidification of the urine. Possible benefits of diuresis in the treatment of urinary infection which must be waived if this policy is pursued are discussed on page 374. Gibson (1970) used no additional acidifying agents in treating bacteriuria of pregnancy with hexamine hippurate. These agents are not suitable for the treatment of acute urinary tract infection and their value in long-term prophylaxis has been doubted (Vainrub & Musher, 1977) and several times shown to be inferior to co-trimoxazole. Their remaining attraction is that long term antibacterial therapy is constantly threatened by the emergence of resistance and it has generally been accepted that bacteria cannot develop resistance to formalin.

References
Cullen S I 1975 Arch Dermatol 111: 1158
Gibson G R 1970 Med J Aust 1: 167
Katul M J, Frank I N 1970 J Urol (Baltimore) 104: 320
Miller H, Phillips E 1970 Invest Urol 8: 21
Musher D M, Griffith D P 1974 Antimicrob Ag Chemother 6: 708
Musher D M, Griffith D P, Tyler M, Woelfel A 1974 Antimicrob Ag Chemother 5: 101
Ross R R, Conway G F 1970 Amer J Dis Child 119: 86
Vainrub B, Musher D M 1977 Antimicrob Ag Chemother 12: 625

NAPHTHYRIDINE AND RELATED CARBOXYLIC ACIDS

Numerous additions have been made to this group of heterocyclic compounds following the success of nalidixic acid for the treatment of urinary tract infection. The agents closely resemble one another in their properties, although their chemical 'nuclei' are sufficiently different for the family to have been variously described as 'pyridones', 'quinolones' or 'naphthyridines' (Fig. 2.2, p. 43). All have been intended primarily for the treatment of urinary tract infection although there have been excursions into wider therapeutic fields.

NALIDIXIC ACID

Pale yellow crystals slightly soluble in water and soluble in dilute alkali (Lesher et al, 1962). Solutions withstand autoclaving.

Antibacterial activity

It is active principally against Gram-negative organisms, the majority of which, with the exception of *Ps. aeruginosa*, are inhibited by 10 μg per ml or less. Gram-positive organisms are relatively resistant (Table 2.3). Nalidixic acid is bactericidal, although for some organisms concentrations substantially in excess of the MIC are required. The addition of nalidixic acid improves the performance of cetrimide-agar as a selective medium for the isolation of *Ps. aeruginosa* (Lilly & Lowbury, 1972) and its addition to McConkey agar allows the selection of enterobacteria from other Gram-negative rods found in river water which are much less resistant to the drug (Hughes, 1976).

Resistance

Resistance is easily produced by serial passage of organisms in increasing concentrations of the drug and sometimes emerges during the treatment of patients (Atlas et al, 1969). Resistance amongst enterobacteria remains uncommon even in strains resistant to several antibiotics—no doubt because nalidixic acid is not implicated in R factor resistance (Burman, 1977). Chromosomal resistance can develop readily to nalidixic acid in the laboratory yet primary resistance amongst urinary pathogens remains very unusual and the frequency with which the emergence of resistance is responsible for treatment failure has varied widely from one series to another. From their evidence Stamey & Bragonje (1976) argue that resistance is a product of under-dosage and conclude that patients should not be treated with less than 4 g nalidixic acid per day. This conclusion is strongly supported by results in a mechanical model simulating the conditions of bacterial growth in the infected urinary bladder (Greenwood & O'Grady, 1977).

Mutual suppression of the emergence of resistant mutants can be obtained with a mixture of nalidixic acid and rifampicin and Greenwood and Andrew (1978) suggest this as a rational combination for the treatment of urinary infection.

Table 2.3 Sensitivity of bacteria to nalidixic acid and its relatives

	Nalidixic acid	Oxolinic acid	Cinoxacin	Piromidic acid	Pipemedic acid	Flumequine
S. aureus	64	4–16	64–256	256	32–256	16–64
S. pyogenes	R	64–R	R	R	R	
S. pneumoniae	R	64–128	R	R	R	
S. faecalis	R	R	128–R		R	16–R
N. meningitidis	0.5–4	0.06–0.25	2	2	2	
H. influenzae	1–64		1	2	2	
E. coli	4–8	0.25–2	1–4	4–16	2	1–8
Proteus spp.	2–16	0.5–1	1–16	8–64	4–8	1–16
Klebsiella spp.	2–64	0.5–2	2–32			1–16
Salmonella spp.	2–64	1	4	8–16	2–4	
Shigella spp.	2–64	0.5–1	2–4	16	4	
S. marcescens	16		4–8	64	64–R	1–8
P. multocida	2	0.1		1	2	
P. aeruginosa	4–R	64–128	R	R	8–32	2–32
Bacteroides spp.	32–R	64	R	8–R	32–R	4–128

Data based on Deitz W H et al 1964 Antimicrobial Ag Chemother—1963, 583; Feldman H A, Melnyk A 1965 ibid—1964, 440; Turner F H et al 1968 ibid—1967, 475; Wick W E et al 1973 ibid 4: 415; Jones R N, Fuchs P C 1976 ibid, 10: 146; Soussy C J et al 1977 Ann Microbiol (Inst Pasteur) 128B: 19

PHARMACOKINETICS

The drug is readily absorbed from the gut, giving peak plasma levels in normal subjects of about 25 μg/ml following a dose of 1 g but levels may differ greatly from one individual to another (Harrison & Cox, 1970). Nelson et al (1972) found that diarrhoea in infants with acute shigellosis seriously interfered with the absorption of nalidixic acid (and with that of ampicillin). Administration of the drug with alkali can increase both the plasma and urinary levels partly by increasing dissolution (the drug is much more soluble at higher pH) and absorption in the gut, and partly by decreasing its tubular reabsorption. Economou et al (1972) gave the drug without side effects to 50 patients by intravenous infusion of 1 g in at least 500 ml saline 8 hrly for 1–4 days. The plasma half-life is about 1½ hours.

A high proportion of the drug is reversibly bound to plasma albumin from which it may displace other compounds. Nalidixic acid is rapidly metabolized, principally to the hydroxy-acid (which is also microbiologically active) and about 13 per cent of the drug in the urine is in this form. The rest is inactive glucuronides of these two compounds apart from about 4 per cent which appears as dicarboxylic derivatives.

Excretion

About 4 per cent of the drug can be recovered from the faeces and virtually all the administered dose appears in the urine over 24 hours.

Nalidixic acid, like chloramphenicol and nitrofurantoin, is eliminated almost exclusively by the renal route, but before excretion is largely converted to microbiologically inactive metabolites. As a result, in renal failure there is comparatively little accumulation of the active compound since it continues to be metabolized, but the elimination of its inactive derivatives is progressively delayed as renal function declines. This is no doubt why Adam & Dawborn (1971) found that creatinine clearance correlated with clearance of the inactive but not of the active compound.

For the treatment of urinary infection in patients with impaired renal function, therefore, compounds handled in this way have the general disadvantage that breakdown of the drug at a rapid rate relative to its delayed excretion causes accumulation of useless and possibly harmful products and the passage of little active compound into the urine. Plainly such agents should be avoided if possible but if nalidixic acid has to be used justification may be found in the claims that the metabolic products are harmless (Stamey et al, 1969) and adequate concentrations of the active agent still reach the urine. Excretion is impaired in the premature infant.

Excretion products of nalidixic acid interfere with the measurement of urinary 17-ketosteroids and in at least one case have led to mistaken diagnosis of endocrine tumour (Llerena & Pearson, 1968).

Toxicity and side-effects

Nausea, rashes and CNS disturbances, including seizures, have occurred in patients receiving the drug. Amongst 515 reported reactions (Alexander & Forman, 1971) 219 involved visual disturbances, hallucinations or disordered sensory perception. Of 97 skin reactions, 25 were phototoxic (negative lymphocyte transformation tests supported the view that blistered photoreactive eruptions are not of immunological origin), 24 urticarial, 17 'drug rash' erythema and 15 maculopapular. Brauner (1975) reviews the cases of bullous sensitivity so far reported and adds two more. He discusses the possible mechanisms and the contradictory results obtained by various investigators who have attempted to elicit the response by phototesting. Some patients have received very little drug before developing a bullous eruption which requires subsequent, not prior and usually intensive exposure to sunlight.

Several examples of intracranial hypertension in children highly reminiscent of the 'bulging fontanelle syndrome' occasionally seen in infants treated with tetracycline (page 176)—and even less commonly in adults or following other agents (Bhowmick, 1972)—have been reported. In the five-year-old child described by Anderson et al, (1971)—who had received 53.5 g of nalidixic acid over 58 days—papilloedema was accompanied by bilateral 6th nerve palsies which rapidly improved on stopping the drug although strabismus remained. Sellers & Koch-Weser (1970) draw attention to the danger of haemorrhage in patients treated with warfarin and nalidixic acid which can raise the plasma concentration of free anticoagulant by displacing it from its albumin binding sites.

Haemolytic anaemia has several times been ascribed to nalidixic acid in infants, with or without G6PD deficiency, and in adults. Gilbertson & Jones (1972) describe death from autoimmune haemolytic anaemia in a 65-year-old woman who had received several courses of the drug for urinary tract infection, one of which had been followed by jaundice. Arthralgia has been rarely reported (Bailey et al, 1972). Dash & Mills (1976) add a further case of severe metabolic acidosis to the few previously reported. The patient had consumed unknown quantities of nalidixic acid and an assortment of other drugs, including probenecid which in volunteers prolonged the half life of nalidixic acid. The patient's plasma concentrations of nalidixic and hydroxynalidixic acids (297 and 100 μg per ml respectively), though high, were insufficient to account for the low arterial pH which presumably results from some secondary effect, possibly on lactate metabolism.

Clinical use

Nalidixic acid has been successfully used for the oral and rarely parenteral treatment of urinary tract infection and also by instillation into the bladder and for the prophylaxis of transurethral operations to cover the period of catheterization.

Although principally used for its effects on the urinary tract, success has also been described in the treatment of brucellosis and of enteric fever (Hassan et al, 1970).

OXOLINIC ACID

This agent (Figure 2.2), synthesized by Kaminsky & Meltzer (1968) was described by Turner et al (1968) as having greater activity over a similar bacterial range to nalidixic acid, and as being in addition active against *Staph. aureus*. Klein & Matsen (1976) suggest that difficulties in bringing oxolinic acid into solution accounts for major discrepancies in the reported MICs. They, for example, found the majority of their 20 strains of *Pseudomonas aeruginosa* to be inhibited by 1.5–6.3 μg per ml in contrast to the much higher figures generally reported (Table 2.3).

Grüneberg (1974) found about 5 per cent of urinary staphylococci and a few Gram-negative bacilli resistant to nalidixic acid, to be sensitive to oxolinic acid. Organisms passaged in the presence of the drug acquire resistance to both oxolinic and nalidixic acids.

Oxolinic acid is absorbed by mouth and on a regimen of 250 mg 4 times daily d'Alessio et al (1968) obtained mean serum and urine levels of 1.8 and 40 μg/ml. In a comparison of nalidixic and oxolinic acid pharmacokinetics, Mannisto (1976) found very low plasma levels of oxolinic acid (1.4 μg per ml total and 0.7 μg per ml free drug) on the first day of a regimen of 750 mg of the drug b.d. By the third and seventh days the levels had risen 4 to 5 times as high (6.2–6.4 μg per ml total and 3.3–3.6 μg per ml free). Taken with food the peak plasma level was delayed but overall absorption of the drug was not impaired. About 20 per cent of the drug was unbound to plasma protein. The complexity of biotransformation of oxolinic acid contrasts sharply with that of nalidixic acid (DiCarlo et al, 1968). This may be related to the accumulation of what would otherwise be minor biotransformants which results from extensive enterohepatic recycling of the drug. Glucuronides, like those of oxolinic acid, which have a molecular weight above 400, tend to be extensively excreted in bile and enterohepatic recirculation may account for the fact that Mannisto et al (1976) found that the plasma half life of oxolinic acid rose from 4 to 15 hours between the first and seventh days of treatment. The same mechanism probably also accounts for the 20 per cent of oxolinic acid, compared with 4 per cent of nalidixic acid, which can be recovered from the faeces over 48 hours. About half of the drug appears in the urine over the first 24 hours where at least eight metabolites, two with antibacterial activity, have been detected. Of those excreted over the first 6 hours, 43 per cent were oxolinic acid glucuronides and 38 per cent glucuronide and 10 per cent non-glucuronide metabolites.

In patients treated for urinary tract infection side effects were common; amongst those given 750 mg of the drug twice daily by Cox (1970) 27 per cent suffered nausea and vomiting or restlessness and insomnia. In some series the emergence of bacterial resistance was a notable cause of failure. Just as with nalidixic acid (page 38) the major reason for the emergence of resistance as a cause of therapeutic failure is underdosage and Clark et al (1971) recommend that patients should not be treated with less than 2 g per day. An attempt to treat typhoid fever with oxolinic acid (Sanford et al, 1976) was unsuccessful. The experience of Kincaid-Smith and her colleagues of the drug was not a happy one. Although the success rate in urinary tract infection was high, half the failures were due to emergence of resistance (Kalowski et al, 1979) and the high incidence of side effects led them to conclude that the drug is not suitable for general use in urinary tract infection (Kalowski and Kincaid-Smith, 1978).

CINOXACIN

This cinnolinic acid derivative synthesized by Wick et al (1973) has an antibacterial range similar to that of other members of the group (Mårdh et al, 1977) with activity intermediate between that of nalidixic and oxolinic acids (Table 2.5). As with nalidixic acid, activity is greater at acid pH and the activity against *Proteus mirabilis* is antagonized by glucose (Giamarellou & Jackson, 1975). It is bactericidal at concentrations close to the MIC and is less bound to human serum protein than is nalidixic acid. Increasing proportions of serum in the test system from 0–75 per cent had virtually no effect on the activity of cinoxacin while the MIC of nalidixic acid rose 4–8-fold (Giamarellou & Jackson, 1975). As with other agents in the group, resistant mutants are readily produced by passage in the presence of the drug (Holmes et al, 1974). The agent is absorbed by mouth, producing peak serum levels up to 14.8 μg per ml two hours after a dose of 250 mg with median values around 7 μg per ml. Colleen et al (1977) found corresponding values (mean 16.8 μg/ml) after 500 mg but the individual values varied widely. Food causes a 30 per cent reduction in the mean peak serum concentration but the 24 hr urinary recovery is not depressed. Some 60–70 per cent of the drug is bound to plasma protein and about half is excreted in the urine in unchanged form (Black et al, 1979). The drug naturally accumulates in patients with renal failure although the urinary excretion is still sufficient for therapeutic purposes (Szwed et al, 1978). Probenecid significantly reduces the renal clearance of cinoxacin and its rate of extra-renal elimination (possibly by competing for a common metabolic pathway) but does not appear to alter the compartmental distribution of the drug (Rodriguez et al, 1979). In the 2-hour period following the dose urinary concentrations were found by Panwalker et al (1976) to be 88–925 μg per ml. They successfully treated without significant side effects 19 of 20 patients with urinary infection, half of whom had renal involvement. In a larger series, Rous (1978) also obtained a high success rate.

PIPIMEDIC ACID

Both this compound (also known as piparamic acid) and its parent piromidic acid (Figure 2.3) were synthesized by Shimizu et al (1971; 1975) in the Research Laboratories of the Dainnipon Company, Japan. It resembles cinoxacin in being less affected than is nalidixic acid by the presence of serum and like other members of the group it inhibits conjugal transfer of R plasmids during mating (Nakamura et al, 1976). It differs from other members of the group in two respects: it is active against *Pseudomonas aeruginosa* and many strains resistant to nalidixic and piromidic acid are susceptible to pipimedic acid at concentrations of less than 32 μg per ml apparently because resistance to the other drugs is due both to reduced susceptibility of the mutant enzyme and relative impermeability while permeability to pipemidic acid is unaffected (Inoue et el, 1978).

FLUMEQUINE

This compound, discovered in the Riker Laboratories (Rohlfing et al, 1976), has a spectrum which appears on the evidence presently available to resemble that of cinoxacin with additional activity against *Pseudomonas aeruginosa* (Table 2.3). Cross resistance with nalidixic and oxolinic acid is essentially complete. On the basis of results in mice, Rohlfing et al (1977) suggest that the drug may be useful in the treatment of systemic salmonellosis.

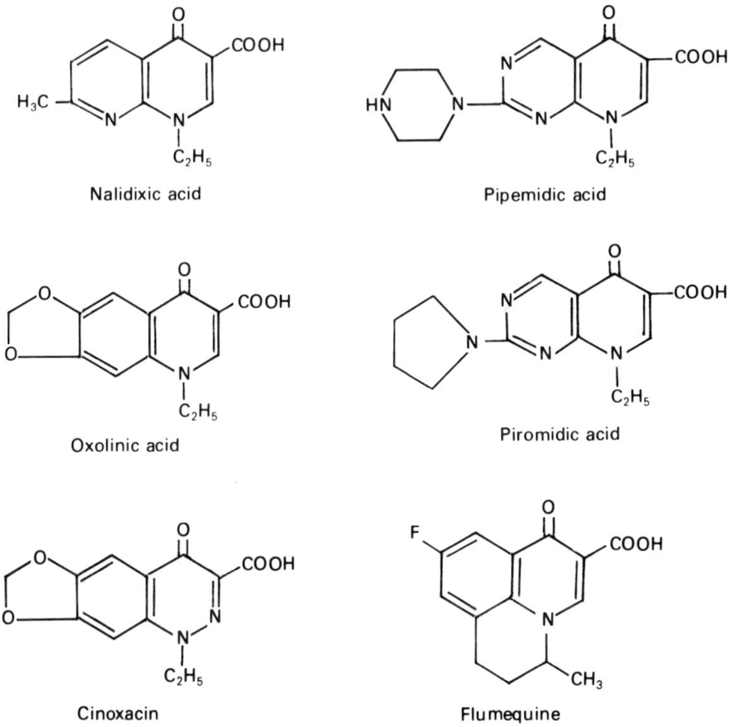

Fig. 2.2 Structures of nalidixic acid and its analogues

References

Adam W R, Dawborn J K (1971) Aust NZ J Med 1: 126
Alexander S, Forman L 1971 Brit J Derm 84: 429
Anderson E E, Anderson B, Nashold B S 1971 J Amer Med Ass 216: 1023
Atlas E, Clark H, Silverblatt F, Turck M 1969 Ann Intern Med 70: 713

Bailey R R, Natale R, Linton A L 1972 Canad Med Ass J 107: 604
Bhowmick B K 1972 Brit Med J 3: 30
Black H R, Israel K S, Wolen, R L et al 1979 Antimicrob Ag Chemother 15: 165
Brauner G J 1975 Amer J Med 58: 576
Burman L G 1977 J Antimicrob Chemother 3: 509
Clark H, Brown N K, Wallace J F, Turck M 1971 Amer J Med Sci 261: 145
Colleen S, Andersson K-E, Mårdh P-A 1977 J Antimicrob Chemother 3: 579
Cox C E 1970 Delaware Med J 42: 327
D'Alessio D J, Olexy V M, Jackson G G 1968 Antimicrob Agents Chemother 1967 p 490
Dash H, Mills J 1976 Ann Int Med 84: 570
Di Carlo F J, Crew M C, Melgar M D, et al 1968 Arch Int Pharmacodyn 174: 413
Economou G, Macis R, Ward-McQuaid N 1972 Brit J Urol 44: 503
Giamarellou H, Jackson G G 1975 Antimicrob Ag Chemother 7: 688
Gilbertson C, Jones D R 1972 Brit Med J 4: 493
Greenwood D, O'Grady F 1977 Brit Med J 2: 665
Greenwood D, Andrew J 1978 J Antimicrob Chemother 4: 533
Grüneberg R 1974 Lancet 2: 1088
Harrison L H, Cox C E 1970 J Urol 104: 908
Hassan A, Wahab M F A, Farid Z, El Rooby A S 1970 J Trop Med Hyg 73: 145
Holmes D H, Ensminger P W, Gordee R S 1974 Antimicrob Ag Chemother 6: 432
Hughes C 1976 J Hyg Camb 77: 23
Inoue S, Ohue T, Yamagishi J et al 1978 Antimicrob Ag Chemother 14: 240
Kalowski S, Kincaid-Smith P, Pavillard R 1979 Med J Aust 1: 345
Kalowski S, Kincaid-Smith P 1978 Clin Exp Pharmacol Physiol 5: 244
Kaminsky D, Meltzer R I 1968 J Med Chem 11: 160
Klein D, Matsen J M 1976 Antimicrob Ag Chemother 9: 649
Lesher G Y, Froelich E J, Gruett M D, et al 1962 J Med Pharm Chem et al 5: 1063
Lilly H A, Lowbury E J L 1972 J Med Microbiol 5: 151
Llerena O, Pearson O H 1968 New Engl J Med 279: 983
Mannisto P T 1976 Clin Pharm Therap 19: 37
Mårdh P-A, Colleen S, Andersson K-E 1977 J Antimicrob Chemother 3: 411
Nakamura S, Inoue S, Shimizu M, Iyobe S, Mitsuhashi S 1976 Antimicrob Ag Chemother 10: 779
Nelson J D, Shelton S, Kusmiesz H T, Haltalin K C 1972 Clin Pharmacol Therap 13: 879
Panwalker A P, Giamarellou H, Jackson G G 1976 Antimicrob Ag Chemother 9: 502
Rodriguez N, Madsen P O, Welling P G 1979 Antimicrob Ag Chemother 15: 465
Rohlfing S R, Gerster J F, Kvam D C 1976 Antimicrob Ag Chemother 10: 20
Rohlfing S R, Gerster J F, Kvam D C 1977 J Antimicrob Chemother 3: 615
Rous S N 1978 J Urol 120: 196
Sanford J P, Linh N N, Kutscher E et al 1976 Antimicrob Ag Chemother 9: 387
Sellers E M, Koch-Weser J 1970 Clin Pharmacol Ther 11: 524
Shimizu M, Nakamura S, Takase Y 1971 Antimicrob Ag Chemother 1970, p 117
Shimizu M, Takase Y, Nakamura S et al 1975 Antimicrob Ag Chemother 8: 132
Stamey T A, Bragonje J 1976 J Am Med Ass 236: 1857
Stamey T A, Nemoy N J, Higgins M 1969 Invest Urol 6: 582
Szwed J J, Brannon D E, Sloan R S, Luft F C 1978 J Antimicrob Chemother 4: 451
Turner F J, Ringel S M, Martin J F et al 1968 Antimicrob Agents Chemother 1967, p 475
Wick W E, Preston D A, White W A, Gordee R S 1973 Antimicrob Ag Chemother 4: 415

NITROFURANS

A group of nitrofurane derivatives (Fig. 2.3) with broad spectrum antimicrobial activity. Since Dodd & Stillman (1944) found that 5-nitro-substitution of a series of 2-substituted furans resulted in remarkable increase in antibacterial activity, several thousand 5-nitrofurans have been synthesized and evaluated as antibacterial and antiprotozoal compounds (Powers, 1976). Some of those which are not commercially available, for example *nitrofuratone* (Matsen, 1971) and *niferpipone* (Massarani et al, 1971) are said to compare favourably with those which are. Of the preparations in current therapeutic use, nitrofurazone and nifuroxime are used locally and are available in preparations suitable for application to the skin, ears, eyes and vagina.

The other agents are given systemically: furazolidone for intestinal infections, nifuratel for vaginitis and nitrofurantoin for urinary infections. Search continues for compounds which surpass nitrofurantoin in antibacterial spectrum, plasma and urine levels, and patient tolerance. The very closely related nifuradine (also called oxafuradine) has had several clinical trials but according to Ronald & Turck (1968) offers no advantages. Chamberlain (1976) has reviewed the properties of the principal members of the group. Figures quoted in the literature for the activity of the agents vary widely – witness the values given by Chamberlain (1976) compared with those in Table 2.4 – but they are unquestionably active against a wide range of bacteria.

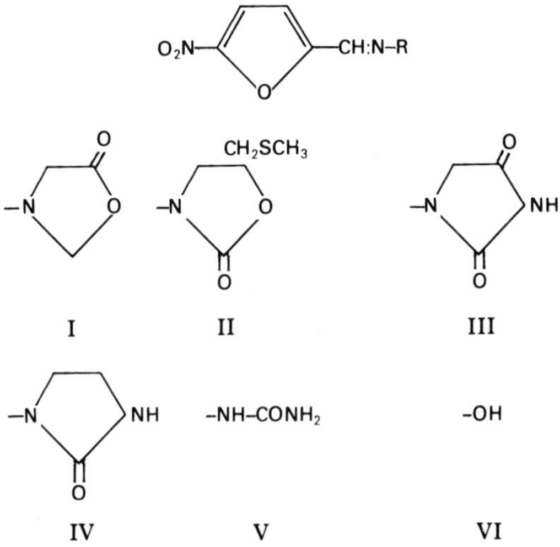

Fig. 2.3 Structures of furazolidone (R = I); nifuratel (R = II); nitrofurantoin (R = III); nifuradene (R = IV); nitrofurazone (R = V) nifuroxime (R = VI).

FURAZOLIDONE

Yellow odourless crystals almost insoluble in water and alcohol, slightly soluble in chloroform. Should be protected from light.

Table 2.4 Antibacterial activity of nitrofurans

	MIC Nitrofurazone μg/ml	MIC Nitrofurantoin μg/ml
Staph. aureus	10	4–30
Str. pyogenes	10	10
Str. viridans	25	8
Str. faecalis	25	4–125
N. gonorrhoeae	10	15
Esch. coli	10	0.4–>250
Proteus spp.	40	7.5–>200
Klebsiella-Aerobacter spp.	10–20	25–>200
Salmonella spp.	5–10	5–15
Shigella spp.	5	5
Ps. aeruginosa	>200	>200

Furazolidone is bactericidal to a wide range of Gram-positive and -negative organisms. Headache, nausea, diarrhoea, rashes and alcohol intolerance may occur. Furazolidone inhibits monoamine oxidase, and Aderhold & Muniz (1970) describe acute toxic psychosis in women given the drug together with amitryptiline similar to that seen on combined treatment with other monoamine oxidase inhibitors and tricyclic antidepressants. It has been successfully used for the treatment of a variety of gastrointestinal infections including enteric fever and other salmonelloses, and shigelloses.

NIFURATEL

This nitrofuran (Fig. 2.3) was first described by Arnold & Delnon (1965), and on the basis of the broad antimicrobial spectrum claimed for it has been promoted for the combined oral and local treatment of vaginitis of mixed aetiology. It has had some successful trials (Aure & Gjønnaess, 1969; Gjønnaess & Aure, 1969) but the consensus of opinion in Britain is that it compares unfavourably with metronidazole for the treatment of vaginal trichomoniasis (Evans & Catterall, 1970). It has also been suggested that its effect relies heavily on the local application and owes little to the systemically administered agent. Its broad antimicrobial spectrum has the advantage that treatment is unlikely to be complicated by the emergence of candidiasis as sometimes occurs with metronidazole (Oller, 1969) and the disadvantage that unrecognized gonorrhoea may be masked (Churcher & Evans, 1969).

NITROFURANTOIN

Yellow odourless crystals discoloured by exposure to light, from which it should be protected. Soluble: 50 μg/ml alcohol; and 60 mg/ml dimethylformamide. Its solubility in water increases markedly with pH (from 220 μg/ml at pH 4.0 to 2.3 mg/ml at pH 7.7), but discoloration occurs in strongly alkaline solutions. The sodium salt is much more soluble and is used to prepare solutions for parenteral administration.

Antibacterial activity

Nitrofurantoin is active against many organisms responsible for urinary infection, particularly *E. coli*, but *Ps. aeruginosa* and some *Klebsiella-Aerobacter* and *Proteus* strains are insensitive (Table 2.4). The MIC may greatly increase with increasing size of inoculum. It is bactericidal in concentrations not much above the MIC but its activity may be reduced as much as 100-fold at pH 8 as compared with pH 5.5, and a bactericidal effect may be obtained only in an acid medium. It is bactericidal to anaerobic bacteria including *Bacteroides fragilis* (Ralph, 1978).

Sensitivity to high concentrations of nitrofurantoin (700 μg/ml) may be used to divide *Nocardia* into two groups (Tanzil & Lintong, 1971).

Resistant variants may be produced by passage in the presence of the drug and have been observed to emerge during the treatment of patients. There is no cross-resistance with other important antibacterial agents but nitrofurantoin antagonises *in vitro* the action of nalidixic acid and the two agents should not be prescribed together (page 485).

As in the case of nitroimidazoles, intracellular reduction of nitrofurans to unstable metabolites that fracture DNA strands plays a key role in antibacterial activity (McCalla, 1977). *Escherichia coli* contains three distinct nitrofuran reductases and loss of one of these is sufficient to confer nitrofuran resistance on some strains (McCalla et al, 1976).

Absorption and excretion

Nitrofurantoin is well absorbed by mouth and rapidly excreted in the urine but very low levels appear in the plasma, partly as the result of rapid tissue breakdown. Marketed preparations composed of macrocrystals are claimed to result in better absorption and consequently less gastrointestinal disturbance. In crossover studies, Meyer et al (1974) found statistically significant differences in the bioavailability of single lots of 14 commercially available nitrofuran products. There was no useful correlation between urinary excretion and disintegration or dissolution characteristics of dosage forms. The two products available as macrocrystals were less bioavailable than the majority of preparations but the levels given were adequate and the differences not significant. Only about a third of the dose can be recovered from the urine. The peak plasma level appears 1–2 hours after an oral dose and has been found by many workers not to exceed 2.5 μg/ml. What little drug is present soon disappears, the plasma half-life being about 20 min. Urine levels are usually in the range 15–46 μg/ml and levels above the MIC for the most sensitive organisms are detectable for about 6 hours.

By the intramuscular route, 180 mg of sodium nitrofurantoin gave peak plasma levels of 1.8–6.4 μg/ml half an hour after injection and peak urine levels of 180–264 μg/ml after one hour (Cox et al, 1971). Following conventional oral doses, the concentrations in milk and amniotic fluid are insignificant and the concentration in cord blood generally less than the maternal level (Perry & LeBlanc, 1967). Since the maternal levels are so low there is little danger of foetal toxicity. Levels in prostatic fluid were only about ¼–½ the plasma level (Dunn & Stamey, 1967).

Nitrofurantoin is excreted by the kidney both in the glomerular filtrate and by tubular secretion. The drug is a weak acid and in alkaline urine about a third is reabsorbed by non-ionic back diffusion in the distal tubule. Calculations suggest that this could result in peri-tubular concentrations of the drug of the order of 12–48 μg/ml—sufficient to exert a useful antibacterial effect. Direct assays of renal lymph (supposed to reflect the composition of renal interstitial fluid) have shown concentrations about twice those of the plasma. In azotaemic patients too little appears in the urine to inhibit sensitive organisms (Felts et al, 1971). At the same time rapid breakdown of the retained drug may allow toxic metabolites to accumulate. Nitrofurantoin is consequently contraindicated in renal failure (Sachs et al, 1968).

Toxicity and side-effects

Through their effects on DNA, nitrofurans produce a variety of changes. They are radiomimetic, mutagenic and can both induce and inhibit experimental oncogenesis (Ebringer et al, 1976). Like metronidazole, nitrofurantoin is toxic for hamster ovarian cells and this toxicity is much increased by reducing the environmental oxygen tension (Mohindra & Rauth, 1976). Nitrofurantoin in a concentration of 20 mg per ml and nitrofurazone at 1 mg per ml immobilize spermatozoa but are not toxic to the epithelium of the vas. Albert et al (1975) suggest that at these concentrations nitrofurans can be used to facilitate sperm disappearance after vasectomy. Nitrofurantoin in concentrations achieved by conventional oral doses inhibits ADP-induced platelet aggregation (Rossi et al, 1975) which may be the immediate cause of thromboembolic phenomena or arterial vascular disease.

In a large series of patients studied by Koch-Weser et al (1971) reactions sufficiently severe to require withdrawal of therapy were seen in 9.2 per cent of those treated with nitrofurantoin. Most were gastrointestinal upsets but skin rashes, eosinophilia and 'drug fever' were seen in 4.1 per cent. Serious reactions were very rare. There have been reports of anaphylaxis following nitrofurantoin, none fatal. Particularly in elderly patients a few days' therapy has been followed by dramatic onset of chills, cough and breathlessness resembling cardiac failure. In the ten years from 1959 about 200 cases of such pleuropneumonic reactions to nitrofurantoin were described (Hailey et al, 1969). The chest signs are often followed by eosinophilia or skin rash. On X-ray there is infiltration especially at the bases with consolidation or effusion.

It is now well established that there are two kinds of pulmonary reaction to nitrofurantoin: the acute variety which is evidently of hypersensitivity origin, and a chronic form in which there is no fever or eosinophilia, but which leads to pulmonary fibrosis with or without interstitial pneumonia. Thirteen cases of pulmonary fibrosis have now been attributed to long term nitrofurantoin treatment. Bone et al (1976) add three more in patients treated for 2–5 years and suggest that it is insufficient simply to stop the drug but with the use of steroids, the prognosis is excellent. All the manifestations disappeared when the drug was withdrawn.

Goldstein et al (1974) add two cases to the six previously reported of hepatotoxicity. Half the patients had fever, rash, jaundice and peripheral eosinophilia. The main biochemical abnormality was a raised serum transaminase which returned to normal on withdrawal of the drug but reappeared when nitrofurantoin was re-administered to one patient. The clinical findings, response to rechallenge and histological changes suggest a hypersensitivity origin but this does not appear to be the mechanism in all cases.

Peripheral neuropathy has developed in a number of patients sometimes following excessive treatment, usually in those with impaired renal function. Onset may be sudden with increasing distal sensory disturbances, severe pain, depressed reflexes, and muscular wasting progressing to severe disablement. As the cases described by Craven (1971) clearly show, neuropathy can develop without renal impairment being sufficiently severe to raise the blood urea. Recovery is usually complete some weeks after stopping treatment but it appears from the observations of Felts et al (1971) that normal nerve conduction cannot regularly be restored simply by reducing the dose.

The neurotoxicity is evidently not simply an exaltation of the effects of uraemia since impaired nerve conduction can be demonstrated in normal subjects treated with conventional doses (Toole et al, 1968). A possible role for folic acid deficiency in neuropathy has been considered since megaloblastic anaemia develops in occasional patients (perhaps as a toxic effect of the hydantoin moiety of nitrofurantoin) but Felts et al (1971) were unable to find any changes supporting this aetiology in their patients. As with a number of other drugs, haemolytic episodes may occur in patients with G 6PD deficiency.

Clinical use

For practical purposes the use of nitrofurantoin is restricted to the prophylaxis and treatment of urinary tract infection (Ch. 21). The low plasma levels achieved make oral treatment useless for systemic infections. Some success has been claimed for treatment of peritonitis and Gram-negative bacteraemia by intravenous infusion of sodium nitrofurantoin.

References

Aderhold R M, Muniz C E 1970 J Amer Med Ass 213: 2080
Albert P S, Mininberg D T, Davis J E 1975 Brit J Urol 47: 459
Arnold M, Delnon J 1965 Ther Umsch Med Biblphie 22: 490
Aure J C, Gjønnaess H 1969 Acta Obstet Gynec Scand 48: 95
Bone R C, Wolfe J, Sobonya R E, et al 1976 Chest 69: Suppl 2 296
Chamberlain R E 1976 J Antimicrob Chemother 2: 325
Churcher G M, Evans A J 1969 Brit J Vener Dis 45: 149
Cox C E, O'Connor F J, Lacy S S 1971 J Urol 105: 113
Craven R S 1971 Aust NZ J Med 1: 246
Dodd M C, Stillman W B 1944 J Pharmacol Exp Ther 82: 11
Dunn B L, Stamey T A 1967 J Urol 97: 505
Ebringer L, Jurasek A, Konicek J, et al 1976 Antimicrob Ag Chemother 9: 682
Evans B A, Catterall R D 1970 Brit Med J 2: 335
Felts J H, Hayes D M, Gergen J A, Toole J F 1971 Amer J Med 51: 331
Gjønnaess H, Aure J C 1969 Acta Obstet Gynec Scand 48: 85
Goldstein L I, Ishak K G, Burns W 1974 Amer J Dig Dis 19: 987
Hailey F J, Glascock H W Jr, Hewitt W F 1969 New Engl J Med 281: 1087
Koch-Weser J, Sidel V W, Dexter M, et al 1971 Arch Intern Med 128: 398
McCalla D R 1977 J Antimicrob Chemother 3: 517
McCalla D R, Olive P, Tu Y, Fan M L 1976 Canad J Microbiol 21: 1484
Massarani E, Nardi D, Degen L, Setnikar I 1971 Experientia 27: 1243
Matsen J M 1971 Antimicrob Agents Chemother 1970, p 260
Meyer M C, Slywka G W A, Dann R E, Whyatt P L 1974 J Pharm Sci 63: 1693
Mohindra J K, Rauth A M 1976 Cancer Res 36: 930
Oller L Z 1969 Brit J Vener Dis 45: 163
Perry J E, LeBlanc A L 1967 Texas Rep Biol Med 25: 265
Powers L J 1976 J Med Chem 19: 57
Ralph E D 1978 J Antimicrob Chemother 4: 177
Ronald A R, Turck M 1968 Antimicrob Agents Chemother 1967, p 506
Rossi E C, Mieyal J J, Strone J M 1975 Molec Pharmacol 11: 751
Sachs J, Geer T, Noell P, Kunin C M 1968 New Engl J Med 278: 1032
Tanzil H O K, Lintong M 1971 Amer Rev Resp Dis 104: 438
Toole J F, Hayes D M, Felts J H 1968 Arch Neurol 18: 680

NITROIMIDAZOLES

A large group of heterocyclic compounds based on a 5-membered nucleus reminiscent of the nitrofurans (page 44). Between them, the compounds exhibit activity against a wide variety of protozoa and bacteria (Bachman et al, 1969; Miller et al, 1970). Few have come into clinical use but it may be taken as an indication of the current interest in the group that seven of the nine compounds listed by Meingassner & Mieth (1976) have achieved trivial names. The outstanding success of metronidazole for the treatment of trichomoniasis (and a growing range of other parasitic disorders) has naturally resulted in a desire by other manufacturers to produce compounds that might participate in this substantial market, but there are in addition two quite different properties of metronidazole that have stimulated a search for related compounds. The first of these properties is activity against anaerobic bacteria, especially the currently fashionable bacteroides, and the second is sensitization of cells to irradiation. This second property is no business of ours except that biochemically metronidazole's antiprotozoal, antibacterial and radiosensitizing activities all hinge on oxygen deprivation.

The cells of solid malignant tumours are poorly oxygenated and because of this, relatively resistant to the lethal effect of irradiation. Attempts to overcome this defect by exposing patients to hyperbaric oxygen have met with mixed success, no doubt due to limited access of oxygen to tumours and its rapid removal. The effect of oxygen can be mimicked by agents which have a high affinity for electrons and nitrofurans, and particularly nitroimidazoles, have been used for this purpose. Such success as metronidazole has enjoyed in this role has been very much dependent on the fact that the drug can be given in large doses without serious untoward effects because it, and related 5-nitroimidazoles, are not particularly avid electron acceptors. On the other hand, 2-nitroimidazoles, which were originally synthesized as potential trichomonacidal agents, are significantly better radio-sensitizers and their potential clinical value is currently being actively explored (Adams et al, 1976). We describe only the best known of the systemic trichomonacides—metronidazole—and its congeners nimorazole, ornidazole and tinidazole (Fig. 2.4)

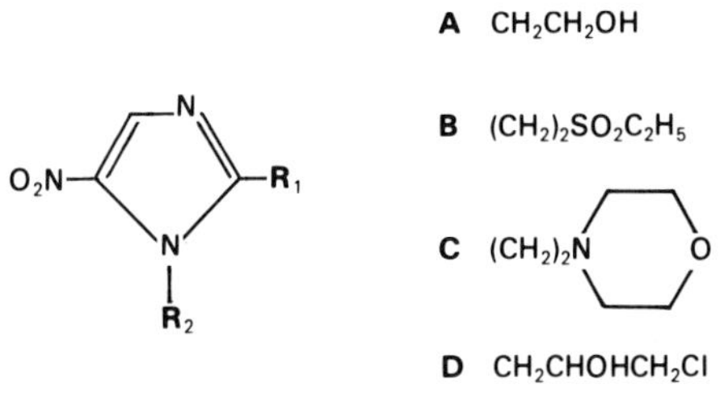

Fig. 2.4 Structures of metronidazole (R_1 = CH_3; R_2 = A); tinidazole (R_1 = CH_3; R_2 = B); nimorazole (R_1 = H; R_2 = C) and ornidazole (R_1 = H; R_2 = D).

METRONIDAZOLE

An almost white crystalline powder, soluble 100 mg/ml water; 5 mg/ml alcohol; and 4 mg/ml chloroform. Metronidazole is a potent trichomonacide, active in concentrations of 1.0–2.5 μg/ml. It is inactive against *Candida*. It is a potent inhibitor of obligate anaerobic bacteria (Table 2.5) and protozoa (*Trichomonas vaginalis*, *Tr. foetus*, and *Entamoeba histolytica*) but not of aerobic bacteria or protozoa—such as trypanosomes. Having enjoyed a long established place as a trichomonacide, the drug has come into prominence again because of its activity against anaerobic bacteria (Brogden et al, 1978; Symposium, 1978).

The precise details of its antimicrobial action are disputed (La Russo et al, 1978) but hinge on interaction of a metabolite, in which the nitro group is reduced, with DNA – events highly reminiscent of the action of nitrofurans (page 47) which metronidazole resembles in being not only a potent microbicide, but a radiosensitiser and mutagen for some bacteria. Its antibacterial activity is accompanied by its inactivation and organisms intrinsically resistant to the drug ordinarily do not degrade it but some aerobic bacteria can inactivate the drug slowly and the possibility has been discussed that the presence of such organisms, for example in the vagina or mixed infections of faecal origin, will interfere with its therapeutic effect (Ralph and Clarke, 1978).

Natural resistant mutants of strictly anaerobic bacteria and protozoa are very rare (Meingassner and Thurner, 1979) but have been produced *in vitro*.

Metronidazole is active against Vincent's organisms, and has been shown to inhibit the Nicols strain of *Tr. pallidum* in a concentration of 3.6–9.5 μg/ml but only when tested aerobically (Meingassner et al, 1978). Similar behaviour was observed in an unequivocally resistant strain of *T. vaginalis* isolated from a patient refractory to treatment. In the *Bacteroides fragilis* mutants studied by Britz and Wilkinson (1979) uptake and metabolism of the drug were depressed. A strain of *T. fetus* rendered stably resistant to metronidazole by 40 successive passages in mice treated with increasing doses of the drug showed 16–64-fold increase in resistance to nine other 5-nitroimidazoles.

It is absorbed by mouth, doses of 200 mg producing serum levels of 2.5–13 μg/ml. Less than 50 per cent is bound to plasma protein (Schwartz & Jeunet, 1976). Wood & Monro (1975) found the peak plasma level 1–2 hours after a 2 g oral dose to be 81 μg per ml when measured microbiologically but only 40 μg per ml when measured chemically, indicating that half the microbiological activity was due to metabolites. The plasma half life has variously been reported to be between 6 and 10 hours. About 60–75 per cent is excreted in the urine (about 70 per cent in the unchanged form) giving levels of 50–390 μg/ml. There are two major metabolites (which can be rapidly and simply measured by high pressure liquid chromatography —Wheeler et al, 1978) of which the hydroxy form has about 30 per cent of the antimicrobial activity of the parent compound. It also appears in the saliva, peak levels up to 9.7 μg/ml being found 3 hours after a 200 mg dose on the third day of treatment. Schwartz & Jeunet (1976) recovered less than 15 per cent of the administered dose from the faeces.

Table 2.5 Antibacterial activity of metronidazole

	MIC μg/ml
B. fragilis	0.5–8
B. melaninogenicus	0.1–1
Bacteroides spp.	0.1–8
F. nucleatum	<0.1–0.5
Fusobacterium spp.	<0.1–1
Peptococcus spp.	0.5–2
Peptostreptococcus spp.	0.1–32
Veillonella spp.	<0.1–16
C. perfringens	0.1–2
Clostridium spp.	<0.1–8
Propionebacterium acnes	R
Enterobacterium spp.	0.5–R
Actinomyces spp.	4–R

Chow A W et al 1977 Proc internat Metronidazole Conf 1976, Excerpta Medica p 286
Fuzi M & Csukas Z 1970 Zentralbl Bakteriol 213: 258
Prince H N et al 1969 Appl Microbiol 18: 728
Sutter V L & Finegold S M 1977 Proc internat Metronidazole Conf 1976 Excerpta Medica, p 279

In human volunteers, Jokipii et al (1977) found that the average CSF levels 90 minutes after an oral dose of 2.4 g were 43 per cent of the corresponding serum level.

Toxicity

Roe (1977) has reviewed the toxicity (and uses) of metronidazole. Nausea, a metallic taste in the mouth, or furry tongue are fairly common. Rashes, paraesthesiae central nervous symptoms, dysuria and dark urine have been occasionally reported. Peripheral neuritis has been reported after long-term therapy. Leucopenia has been described but the changes are generally insignificant (Peterson et al, 1967). Disulfiram-like flushing and hypotension are sufficiently common and severe in those taking alcohol while receiving metronidazole for the drug to have been used in the treatment of chronic alcoholism (Merry & Whitehead, 1968). Artefactual depression of the SGOT may be seen in patients treated with metronidazole because the drug interferes with the assay commonly used (Rissing et al, 1978). By far the most serious accusation levelled against the drug is that it is a carcinogen. This hinges on reported ability of the drug to induce tumours in animals which, coupled with its mutagenic capability, has excited a good deal of speculation about its dangers. Despite the availability of the drug for nearly twenty years during which time it has been administered to huge numbers of women, no human epidemiological evidence has come to light to support the experimental findings. Such evidence is neither easy to obtain nor to interpret but Beard et al (1979) followed up almost 800 women treated with metronidazole for vaginal candidiasis between 1960 and 1969 and found no appreciable increase in cases of cancer.

Clinical use

The principal use of metronidazole is in the treatment of trichomoniasis in which it has been very successful even as short (400 mg 12 hourly to a total of 2 g: Hayward & Roy, 1976) or single dose (Csonka, 1971; Wood & Monro, 1975) courses. Re-treatment, intensive treatment or additional measures are required in some patients. Metronidazole is as effective as penicillin the treatment of Vincent's angina and is being increasingly used for the therapy of bacteroides infection and, in combinations with other appropriate agents, for prophylaxis in surgical and gynaecological procedures likely to be complicated by infections in which non-sporing anaerobic bacteria play a major role (Brogden et al, 1978, Symposium 1978).

Its anti-spirochaetal effect has led to trials of its use in syphilis but it is considered inferior to penicillin. Its only importance in that connection is that it may lead to misdiagnosis since the serum of patients receiving the drug may immobilize treponemes in the T.P.I. test (Wilkinson et al, 1967). Metronidazole is extremely effective in the treatment of amoebic liver abscess (Scragg et al, 1976), but the rapid absorption of the drug from the gut that contributes materially to its success in invasive amoebiasis is a distinct disadvantage when it is directed against intestinal parasites. In the series reported by Spillman et al (1976) *Entamoeba histolytica* cysts reappeared in the stools of 37 per cent of patients within two weeks of treatment with 750 mg metronidazole 8-hourly for five days. Metronidazole is described as the drug of choice in giardiasis (Bassily et al, 1970) and as remarkably effective in dracunculiasis (Antani et al, 1972).

NIMORAZOLE

This nitroimidazole (Fig. 2.4), also known as nitrimidazine, and first described by De Carnieri et al (1970) has had a number of successful trials for the oral treatment of vaginal trichomoniasis (page 431) for which it is held to be just as effective as metronidazole (Wigfield, 1975; Hayward & Roy, 1976). Powell & Elsdon-Dew (1972) found it inadequate for the treatment of intestinal amoebiasis. Tested against fusobacteria and bacteroides it was found to have only a quarter to half the activity of metronidazole or tinidazole (Reynolds et al, 1975).

ORNIDAZOLE

This member of the group (Fig. 2.4) was synthesized by Hoffer & Grunberg (1974) in the laboratory of Hoffman LaRoche. Its properties are summarized by Lean & Vengadasalam (1973). Its solubility is 2.4 per cent in water and more than 50 per cent in ethanol. Aqueous solutions at pH less than 7 lose little activity at 100 °C for one hour. Its antiprotozoal range is evidently similar to that of metronidazole as is its activity against anaerobic bacteria (Goldstein et al, 1978). After a 750 mg dose Schwartz & Jeunet (1976) found mean peak concentrations of 10.9 μg per ml at 2–4 hours. The half-life was 14.4 hours and about 63 per cent of the dose was recovered from the urine and 22 per cent from the faeces. It has been used for the treatment of trichomoniasis, giardiasis and intestinal and hepatic amoebiasis with results evidently identical with those produced by metronidazole (Powell & Elsdon-Dew, 1972; Lean & Vengadasalam, 1973).

TINIDAZOLE

This close congener (Fig. 2.4) of metronidazole was synthesized by Miller et al (1970). Its properties and therapeutic uses are reviewed by Sawyer et al (1976). The concentrations at which it inhibits *Tr. vaginalis* and *Tr. fetus* (2.5 μg/ml) and *Entamoeba histolytica* (40 μg/ml) are similar to those of metronidazole. Howes et al (1970) comment on the difficulty of interpreting the inhibitory activity of antitrichomonal agents after 24 hours' incubation because of spontaneous death of the parasite. Assessed at 6 hours, the concentration of both agents inhibitory to both trichomonads was 10 μg/ml. Tinidazole appeared to be more actively trichomonacidal in that killing of *Tr. vaginalis* by metronidazole required concentrations 4–8 times the effective concentrations of tinidazole. Reynolds et al (1975) found its antibacterial activity against fusobacteria (MIC 0.25–0.5) and bacteroides (MIC less than 0.125–0.5 μg/ml) to be similar to that of metronidazole. The Jokipiis (1977) found it marginally more active.

In a dose of 125 mg, tinidazole produced human plasma levels around 1.5 μg/ml with a half-life of 9.4 hours (Taylor et al, 1970). They found considerably less metronidazole in its active form in the urine than had previous workers, and concluded from their recovery of almost half the dose of tinidazole (and that exclusively in the active form) that it is more resistant to biotransformation. This conclusion is supported by Wood & Munro (1975) who found the peak plasma level of 16 μg per ml 1–2 hours after a 2 g dose to be almost entirely accounted for by unchanged tinidazole. In contrast, half the peak antimicrobial activity of a similar dose of metronidazole was contributed by metabolites. Furthermore, they found the half life to be 12.5 as against 7.3 hours for metronidazole and the plasma concentration 24 hours after a 2 g dose to be three times that of metronidazole. These pharmacokinetic advantages coupled with antitrichomonal activity at least equivalent to that of metronidazole might be expected to be reflected in superior clinical performance, but the results of metronidazole treatment are generally so good that it is not surprising that no distinct advantage has been apparent in practice (Sawyer et al, 1976). Side effects in women successfully treated for trichomoniasis with a single 2 g dose were similar to those following metronidazole (Jones and Enders, 1977).

Tinidazole did not impress Powell & Elsdon-Dew (1972) in the treatment of intestinal amoebiasis, but details of its successful use by Scragg et al (1976) and Ahmed et al (1976) in intestinal amoebiasis in childhood are given on page 339 and its value in both amoebiasis and giardiasis are reviewed by Zaman (1978).

As with metronidazole the drug has been successfully used for the treatment of anaerobic infections (Klastersky et al, 1977) and for prophylaxis in patients undergoing colorectal surgery (Hunt et al, 1979).

References

Adams G E, Dische S, Fowler J F, Thomlinson R H 1976 Lancet 1: 186
Ahmed T, Ali F, Sarwar S G 1976 Arch Dis Child 51: 388
Antani J, Srinivas H V, Krishnamurthy K R, Jahagirdar B R 1970 Amer J Trop Med Hyg 19: 821
Bachmann H J, Shirk R J, Layton H W, Kemp G A 1969 Antimicrob Agents Chemother 1968, p 524
Bassily S, Farid Z, Mikhail J W, Kent D C, Lehmann J S Jr 1970 J Trop Med Hyg 73: 15
Beard C M, Noller K L, O'Fallon W M et al 1979 New Engl J Med 301: 519
Britz M L, Wilkinson R G 1979 Antimicrob Ag Chemother 16: 19
Brogden R N, Heel R C, Speight T M, Avery G S 1978 Drugs 16: 387
Csonka G W 1971 Brit J Vener Dis 47: 456
De Carnieri I, Cantone A, Giraldi P N, et al 1970 Proc 6th Internat Cong Chemother, Tokyo (Progress in Antimicrobial and Anticancer Chemotherapy: I) p 149
Goldstein E J C, Sutter V, Finegold S M 1978 Antimicrob Ag Chemother 14: 609
Hayward M J, Roy R B 1976 Brit J Vener Dis 52: 63
Hoffer M, Grunberg E 1974 J Med Chem 17: 1019
Howes H L Jr, Lynch J E, Kivlin J L 1970 Antimicrob Agents Chemother 1969, p 261
Hunt S, Francis J K, Peck G et al 1979 Med J Aust 1: 107
Jokipii A M, Jokipii L 1977 Chemotherapy 23: 25
Jokipii A M, Myllylä V V, Hokkanen E, Jokipii L 1977 J Antimicrob Chemother 3: 239
Jones R, Enders P 1977 Med J Aust 2: 679
Klastersky J, Husson M, Weerts-Ruhl D, Daneau D 1977 Antimicrob Ag Chemother 12: 563
La Russo N F, Tomasz M, Kaplan D, Muller M 1978 Antimicrob Ag Chemother 13: 19
Lean T H, Vengadasalam 1973 Brit J Vener Dis 49: 69
Meingassner J G, Mieth H 1976 Experientia 32: 183
Meingassner J G, Mieth H, Czok R et al 1978 Antimicrob Ag Chemother 13: 1
Meingassner J G, Thurner J 1979 Antimicrob Ag Chemother 15: 254
Merry J, Whitehead A 1968 Brit J Psychiat 114: 859
Miller M W, Howes H L, English A R 1970 Antimicrob Agents Chemother 1969, p 257
Peterson W F, Hansen F W, Stauch J E, Ryder C D 1967 Amer J Obstet Gynec 97: 472
Powell S J, Elsdon-Dew R 1972 Amer J Trop Med Hyg 21: 518
Ralph E D, Clarke D A 1978 Antimicrob Ag Chemother 14: 377
Reynolds A V, Hamilton-Miller J M T, Brumfitt W 1975 J Clin Path 28: 775
Rissing J P, Newman C, Moore W L Jr 1978 Antimicrob Ag Chemother 14: 636
Roe F J C 1977 J Antimicrob Chemother 3: 205
Sawyer P R, Brogden R N, Pinder R M, Speight T M, Avery G S 1976 Drugs 11: 423
Schwartz D E, Jeunet F 1976 Chemotherapy 22: 19

Scragg J N, Rubidge C J, Proctor E M 1976 Arch Dis Childn 51: 385
Spillman R, Ayala S C, De Sanchez C E 1976 Amer J Trop Med Hyg 25: 549
Symposium 1978 J Antimicrob Chemother 4: Suppl C
Taylor J A Jr, Migliardi J R, von Wittenau M S 1970 Antimicrob Agents Chemother 1969, p 267
Wheeler L A, deMeo M, Halula M et al 1978 Antimicrob Ag Chemother 13: 205
Wigfield A S 1975 Brit J Vener Dis 51: 54
Wilkinson A E, Rodin P, McFadzean J A, Squires S 1967 Brit J Vener Dis 43: 201
Wood B A, Monro A M 1975 Brit J Vener Dis 51: 51
Zaman V (Ed) 1978 Drugs 15 Suppl 1

Pharmaceutical preparations and dosages are given on page 56.

Synthetic antimicrobial agents. Pharmaceutical preparations and dosage

Name	*Dosage*	*Preparations*	*Common international proprietary names*	
Pyrimethamine	*Adult* Oral: 25–50 mg once a week for malaria prophylaxis, 25–50 mg daily for Leishmaniasis and Toxoplasmosis. *Children:* 5–10 yrs, 12.5 mg; 3 mths–5 yrs, 6.25 mg.	Tablets 25 mg	Daraprim Malocide	(UK) (Fr)
Trimethoprim	*Adult* 2 tablets twice a day. *Prophylaxis* 1 tablet at night. *Adult* for Malaria 1.5 g daily for 7 days.	Tablets 100 mg	Ipral Trimopan	(UK)
Co-trimoxazole = Sulphamethoxazole + Trimethoprim in a ratio of 5:1 by weight respectively.	*Adult* Oral: 4 tablets daily, in two divided doses. The maximum daily dose is 6 tablets daily, and the minimum, (for prophylaxis) 2 daily. i.v.: 10–15 ml by infusion every 12 hours. i.m.: 3 ml every 12 hours. *Children* 6–12 yrs: the equivalent of 1 adult tablet twice a day with a maximum of 1½ tablets twice a day. 6 mths–6 yrs: 5 ml of paediatric suspension twice a day. 6 wks–6 mths: 2.5 ml of paediatric suspension twice a day. i.m. i.v.: 30 mg Sulphamethoxazole and 5 mg Trimethoprim per kg body weight daily in 2 divided doses.	Tablets Suspension i.m. injection i.v. injection	Septrin, Bactrim Eusaprim Septra	(UK) (Fr) (USA)
Co-trimazine = Trimethoprim 90 mg + Sulphadiazine 410 mg	*Adult* 1 tablet twice a day. *Children* 6–12 yrs: the equivalent of half a tablet twice a day. 3 mths–5 yrs: the equivalent of a quarter of a tablet twice a day.	Tablets Suspension	Coptin	(UK)
Hexamine Methenamine (rINN)	*Adult* 600 mg–2 g daily.	Tablets	Uritone Unavailable in the UK	(USA)
Hexamine Hippurate	*Adult* 1 g twice a day increasing to 1 g 3–4 times a day in refactory cases. *Children* 6–12 yrs: 500 mg twice a day increasing to 500 mg 3–4 times a day in refactory cases. 1–5 yrs: 250 mg twice a day, increasing to 250 mg 3–4 times a day.	Tablets	Hiprex Urex	(UK) (USA)
Hexamine Mandelate	*Adult* 1 g four times a day.	Tablets	Mandelamine	(UK)

Nalidixic Acid	*Adult* Acute infections: 500 mg–1 g four times a day. *Children* 60 mg/kg body weight, daily in divided doses. For prolonged treatment in chronic infections the above doses may be halved.	Tablets Suspension	Negram NegGram Nogram	(UK) (USA) (Ger)
Furazolidone	*Adult* 100 mg four times a day. *Children* 5 mg/kg body weight daily, in divided doses.	Tablets Suspension (with Kaolin)	Furoxone	(UK)
Nifuratel	*Adult* 200 mg three times a day.	Tablets	Omnes Inimur No longer available in the UK	(Fr) (Ger)
Nitrofurantoin	*Adult* 50–100 mg four times a day. *Children* 1 month and over: 1.25–1.75 mg/kg body weight four times a day. Dose for prophylaxis is less.	Tablets 50 mg 100 mg Capsules 100 mg Suspension 25 mg in 5 ml	Furadantin, Macrodantin Trantoin, Cyantin Fua-Med, Urolong Furadoine	(UK) (USA) (Ger) (Fr)
Oxolinic Acid	*Adult* Oral: 750 mg every 12 hours.	Tablets 750 mg	Utibid No longer available in the UK	(USA)
Cinoxacin	*Adult* Oral: 500 mg twice a day.	Capsules 500 mg	Cinobac	(UK)
Metronidazole	The indications are so varied, that dosages will be found under the uses in various chapters.	Tablets 200 mg 400 mg Suppositories 500 mg 1 g i.v. infusion 500 mg in 100 ml 100 mg in 20 ml	Flagyl Sanatrichom	(UK) (Ger)
Nimorazole	*Adult* 250 mg two or three times a day, depending on the protozoal infection being treated. *Children* a proportion of the adult dose given as a single daily dose.	Tablets 500 mg	Naxogin Acetarol Forte Naxogyn Nulogyl	(UK) (Ger) (Fr) (USA)
Tinidazole	*Adult* for Trichomoniasis, 150 mg twice a day for 7 days, or as a single dose of 2 g to both men and women, or 150 mg three times a day for 5 days. *Children* 50–75 mg/kg body weight as a single dose.	Tablets 150 mg 500 mg	Fasigyn Simplotan Not yet available in the UK	(USA) (Ger)

3

Penicillins

NATURAL

Penicillin, the first of the antibiotics to come into general therapeutic use, is still in many ways the best. Indeed, some of its properties are unique, and it is nothing short of a miracle that so astonishing a substance should have been the first of its kind to be discovered. This is not to say that antibiotics were unknown before that time: many were discovered and used locally for therapeutic purposes much earlier, but this was the first which was suitable for systemic use in man.

The story of the discovery of penicillin by Fleming and of its isolation and systematic study by Florey, Chain and their colleagues in Oxford over ten years later, is now too well known to need re-telling. It took years of hard work to obtain penicillin in the pure state, and the unit of activity by which it had first to be measured, now known to represent 0.6 μg, has persisted to the present day, although all later penicillins are prescribed by weight.

BENZYL PENICILLIN

Physical and Chemical Properties

Penicillin can be prepared in quantity only by the original process of cultivating a mould forming it (a high-yielding mutant of a strain of *P. chrysogenum* is now used) in a suitable liquid medium. In the early stages of large-scale production it was found that four different penicillins were being formed, known as F, G, X and K. Of these G, or benzyl penicillin, had the most desirable properties, and its almost exclusive formation is ensured by adding the appropriate 'precursor', phenylacetic acid, to the medium.

As formed, penicillin is an unstable acid, and in production it is converted to a salt, that of either potassium or sodium, which is more stable. The calcium and

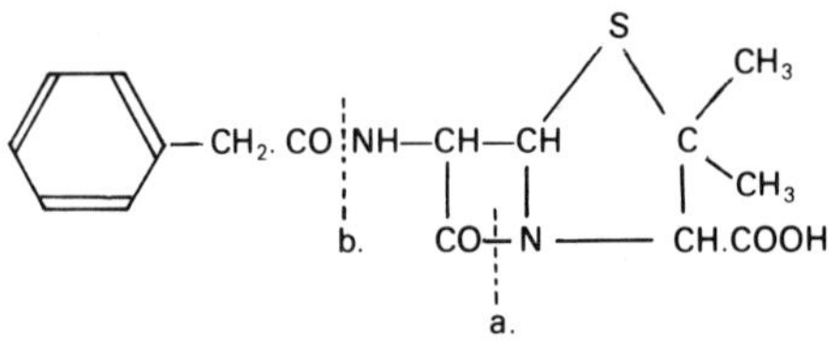

Fig. 3.1 Structure of benzyl penicillin. Sites of action of (a) β-lactamase (b) amidase

ammonium salts have also been prepared, and the former was preferred at one time for certain uses. The structure of benzyl penicillin is shown in Figure 3.1. The potassium or sodium salt is what was commonly known as 'soluble' or 'crystalline' penicillin, both unsatisfactory terms, because they apply to any penicillin, but these salts are distinguishable from other forms of benzyl penicillin introduced later by their high degree of solubility in water and by rapid absorption and excretion.

Stability

Penicillin is stable in the dry state, but deteriorates slowly in solution, this process being accelerated by heat. Among many incompatible chemicals the most important is acid, since the action of gastric acid accounts for the loss of most of a dose of benzyl penicillin if it is swallowed. It is also destroyed by an enzyme, penicillinase, formed by various bacteria, including some staphylococci, various *Bacilli*, some species of *Proteus*, *Ps. aeruginosa*, other coliforms and the tubercle bacillus. Not all these penicillinases are the same. The resistance of staphylococci to penicillin in clinical practice is largely due to this factor: their intrinsic resistance may be comparatively low, but they appear to withstand high concentrations because in fact they destroy it. This can happen in the body, where further injury may be added to insult by interference with the action of the antibiotic on an accompanying sensitive species.

Antibacterial activity

Species susceptibility

At one time bacteria were classed simply as sensitive or resistant to penicillin, but they exhibit degrees of sensitivity over an exceedingly wide range, and the fact that if necessary very large doses can be given enables infections by some moderately resistant species to be treated successfully. Table 3.1 states the concentrations usually required to inhibit the growth of the more sensitive organisms, which include almost all the Gram-positive pathogens and some of the Gram-negative. The least sensitive organisms listed among the latter are included because they can occur in the urine, where high concentrations of penicillin are easily attained.

Abnormal resistance

In some species naturally resistant strains occur, including the following.

Streptococcus viridans. In this very heterogeneous species resistant strains probably exist in every mouth, but they are normally found in any numbers only when sensitive strains have been suppressed by penicillin treatment (Garrod & Waterworth, 1962).

Staphylococcus aureus. Naturally resistant strains owe this property to penicillinase formation. Recently strains have been recognized which although normally sensitive to the inhibitory action of penicillin or its derivatives are not to its bactericidal effect (see below) except in much higher concentrations. These were originally described as 'tolerant' by Best et al (1974), who demonstrated reduced autolysin formation as a possible factor in their resistance. This term is adopted by Sabath et al (1977), who found the concentrations of nafcillin required to exert a bactericidal effect in 24 hours on seven strains to exceed the inhibitory by a factor of 256 to 2000. At 48 hours this difference was much diminished for some strains and unaltered for others. These authors found that of 63 strains isolated from blood cultures in the University of Minnesota Hospitals in the previous year 28 (44 per cent) were tolerant. They do not report the response of their patients to treatment, but Mayhall et al (1976), who also found tolerance common (33 out of 60 recent isolates) achieved a therapeutic effect in three patients with septicaemia due to oxacillin-tolerant strains only when gentamicin was given in addition to oxacillin. This seems to be a new problem the solution of which will not be easy.

Other species do not *acquire* resistance to penicillin, unless to a small extent during very prolonged treatment, and the sensitivity of most susceptible pathogens has remained unchanged despite years of extensive therapeutic use. There are two important exceptions to this.

Neisseria gonorrhoeae. This originally very sensitive species remained so until the late fifties, when somewhat less sensitive strains began to appear, clearly associated with treatment failure from the moderate doses then given. These have steadily and very gradually become more common and more resistant, necessitating much larger doses or the use of alternative drugs. This situation was sharply worsened by the almost simultaneous recognition at two centres in England and one in the United States (Editorial, 1976) of strains which actually form penicillinase, an entirely new development (see Chapter 24).

Streptococcus pneumoniae. Resistance in this species was first observed in an area in New Guinea where monthly injections of procaine penicillin had been given for some years for the prophylaxis of pneumonia, to which the inhabitants are peculiarly subject for climatic reasons. Two strains were also isolated in Australia, but not until several years after this were single isolates reported from elsewhere, including the United States and Great Britain. The degree of resistance is moderate (inhibition by about 0.5 μg/ml), and although this includes some other penicillins and cephalosporins, sensitivity to ampicillin was retained in all but one of 27 strains (Hansman, 1975). In the only case of infection so far reported in this country, a child with meningitis, treatment with ampicillin succeeded after penicillin had failed (Howes & Mitchell, 1976).

A much more formidable type of resistance in this species has appeared in South Africa. A child with pneumonia in the Barangwanath Hospital was the first identified source of this organism, which displayed an exceptional capacity for spread. It was subsequently found in the throats of 75 out of 80 patients in the measles isolation wards (a few of whom developed bacteraemia as well as bronchopneumonia) in 19 per cent of 427 other patients and in 2 per cent of 363 staff. Most of the strains were Danish type 19A (American 57); it is interesting that this type was also the cause of five infections in infants, three fatal, in Durban, but the organism there could not be recovered from any contacts (Appelbaum et al, 1977). The sensitivity pattern of the Johannesburg strains varied, but some were resistant to all penicillins (MIC of penicillin 4 and of ampicillin 2–4 μg/ml) and to cephalothin, chloramphenicol, co-trimoxazole, erythromycin and tetracycline; of the few antibiotics to which they remained sensitive the least toxic were rifampicin and fusidic acid, and these together were extensively used in treatment. This was not entirely successful, some strains becoming resistant to rifampicin despite the second antibiotic. β-lactamase formation could not be demonstrated. A smaller number, apparently only of carrier strains, belonged to type 6A (American 6) which were resistant only to penicillin, tetracycline and chloramphenicol, and not always to all of these, but to no other antibiotics. These events are well described by Jacobs et al (1978).

So far such multiple resistance as that of the major South African type has not been reported in any other country. It may in some way be favoured, as perhaps by malnutrition, in South African children, and have difficulty in establishing itself elsewhere. But the utmost vigilance is called for, and it should no longer be assumed anywhere that a pneumococcal infection will respond to penicillin. It is already being predicted that should multi-resistant strains spread, immunization rather than chemotherapy will have to be relied on for defence against them in future.

Type of anti-bacterial action

In a nutrient medium (i.e. when bacterial growth can occur, but not otherwise) penicillin is bactericidal. About four hours is required to produce a high mortality, and this may proceed to extinction, or there may be a few survivors. This effect is best exerted by a concentration 5–10 times greater than the minimum inhibiting growth, and no increase above this level will accelerate it. Against many strains of two species, *Staph. aureus* and *Str. faecalis*, such an increase actually reduces the death rate, the so-called paradoxical zone phenomenon (Eagle, 1951). This behaviour of penicillin is unique, and no certain explanation for it is known, but one hypothesis is proposed by Eagle in his description of the phenomenon.

Pharmacokinetics

The salts of benzyl penicillin are very freely diffusible: after intramuscular injection absorption occurs within a few minutes to produce a high concentration in the blood. Diffusion takes place into the fetal circulation and into serous cavities: lower concentrations are found in glandular secretions, and still lower in the cerebro-spinal fluid, but these are raised in meningitis owing both to the presence of penicillin in the exudate, and to its more ready diffusibility through the walls of dilated capillaries. Concentrations two to five times that in the blood are found in the bile, but excretion is mainly renal, accounting for about 60 per cent of the dose, some of which is apparently destroyed in the body. This excretion is mainly tubular, and exceedingly rapid—much more so than that of any other drug with an anti-microbic action. Some idea of the wasteful nature of this treatment may be gained from the fact that in an adult with anuria an ample dose for the treatment of a fully sensitive infection would be 2000 units.

The usual way of overcoming this difficulty is simply to give very large doses: the initially very high concentrations thus produced in the body are no bar to this because penicillin is virtually non-toxic. It is important to recognize that doubling the dose does not double the duration of effect. The doses required to maintain a blood level of over 0.1μg/ml for two, four and eight hours have been shown to be respectively 50 000, 235 000 and 1 400 000 units. Thus if *a continuous effect* is expected from penicillin in this form, large and frequent doses are required.

It has often been said that the blood level is not what matters, but that in the lesion: penicillin diffuses into this when the blood level is high and persists there longer. This was long ago shown to be true of wound exudates, and has recently been shown to apply to experimental transudates (Chisholm et al, 1973) but it is not true of inflammation in a vascular area without tissue destruction (Eagle et al, 1953), and it is

Table 3.1 Spectrum of activity of benzyl penicillin (minimum inhibitory concentrations in µg/ml)

	Gram-positive organisms		Gram-negative organisms	
Cocci	*Streptococcus pyogenes* (A)	0.006	*Neisseria gonorrhoeae*	0.003*
	Streptococcus pneumoniae	0.006	*Neisseria meningitidis*	0.012
	Streptococcus viridans	0.012*	*Neisseria catarrhalis*	0.012*
	Streptococcus faecalis	2		
	Staphylococcus aureus	0.012*		
	Staphylococcus albus	0.012*		
	Sarcina lutea	0.0015	*Haemophilus influenzae*	0.25 –1
Bacilli	*Bacillus anthracis*	0.01 –0.04	*Haemophilus pertussis*	0.5 –2
	Clostridium tetani	0.007–0.3	*Haemophilus ducreyi*	0.045–0.15
	Clostridium perfringens	0.06 –0.25	*Bacteroides fragilis*	16*
	Clostridium oedematiens	0.007–0.015	*Bacteroides fusiformis*	0.06 –0.5
	Clostridium septicum	0.03	*Bacteroides melaninogenicum*	0.007–0.06
	Clostridium histolyticum	0.03	*Bacteroides necrophorus*	0.06 –0.12
	Corynebacterium diphtheriae	0.02 –0.6	*Escherichia coli*	20*
	Actinobacillus muris	0.06	*Klebsiella pneumoniae*	2–100
	Erysipelothrix rhusiopathiae	0.04 –0.08	*Proteus mirabilis*	8*
	Listeria monocytogenes	0.2 –0.6	*Salmonella spp.*	2–5
	Actinomyces israeli	0.02 –0.1	*Pasteurella septica*	0.5

*Denotes that some strains are more resistant.

Other sensitive species, the susceptibility of which cannot be measured in this way, are *T. pallidum* and other treponemata and a few of the larger viruses. *Leptospira* spp. are also sensitive to 0.05–0.5 µg/ml.

Resistant species not included in the Table are all organisms of the genera *Brucella, Mycobacterium, Pfeifferella, Pseudomonas, Vibrio, Proteus* (other than *P. mirabilis*). *Klebsiella aerogenes*, all fungi other than *A. israeli*, most viruses, all rickettsias and mycoplasmas.

The concentrations given for commoner species are the approximate mean of many estimations by various authors. Some of the less familiar are derived as follows: From the present writer's own observations *B. anthracis* (Antibiot and Chemother 1952, 2: 689), *A. israeli* (Brit Med J 1952, i: 1263), *Bacteroides* (Brit Med J 1952, ii: 1529), *Clostridia* (J Roy Army Med Corps 1958, 104: 209). For *C. diphtheriae* R Cruickshank et al (Lancet 1948, ii: 517), *E. rhusiopathiae* P H A Sneath et al (Brit Med J. 1951, ii: 1063), *L. monocytogenes* I A Bakulov (Antibiotics 1959, 4: 575), *H. pertussis* E B Wells et al (J Pediat 1950, 36: 752).

(This table also appears in a contribution by one of the authors (LPG) to 'Experimental Chemotherapy', Ed. F Hawking & R J Schnitzer.)

to this category that most acute infections belong. It would certainly appear safer to administer doses calculated to maintain an effective concentration in the blood continuously, and by using forms of penicillin to be described later this is easily achieved.

One way of prolonging the action of each dose of penicillin is also to administer probenecid, which interferes with tubular excretion. It is used not so much for extending the intervals between doses as for maintaining higher blood levels between doses given at usual intervals when such levels are considered necessary, as in the treatment of endocarditis due to less sensitive streptococci.

Long-acting forms of benzyl penicillin

The second possible way of prolonging the effect of a dose is to delay absorption. This was first achieved by suspending the calcium salt in a water-immiscible medium containing oil and beeswax. Much more satisfactory results have since been obtained with penicillin compounds of lesser solubility. The first of these was procaine penicillin, an equimolecular compound of penicillin and procaine, which is administered as a suspension of crystals which dissolve slowly at the site of injection. The 'peak' blood level (which is not a peak but a plateau, and relatively low) is reached in about four hours, and the level falls slowly, being still detectable 24 hours after a moderate dose (Fig. 3.2).

Still less soluble and therefore longer-acting compounds are benethamine penicillin and benzathine penicillin, a single dose of which will provide a low concentration in the blood for four to five days and several weeks respectively. Various mixtures are available, some including the potassium salt for an immediate high level, and procaine penicillin and one of the least soluble compounds to sustain diminishing levels for a long period.

An orally administered form of benzathine penicillin (Penidural) converts the

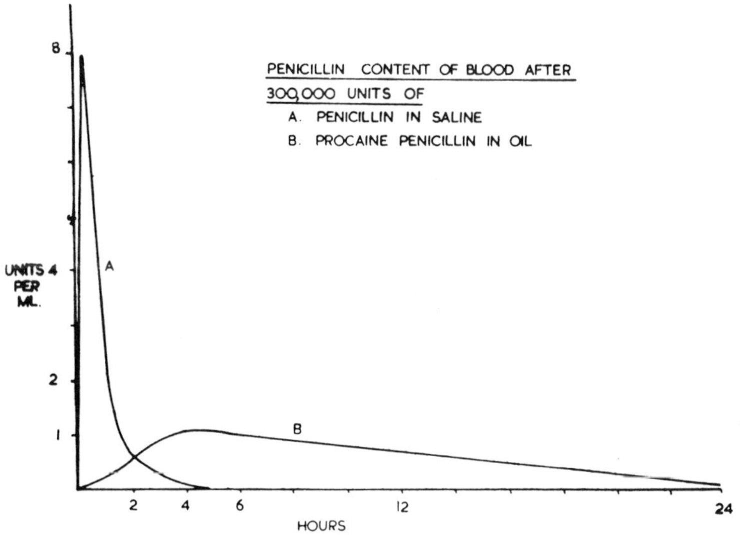

Fig. 3.2 Blood levels produced by the administration of penicillin in two different forms. (Garrod, 1950, reproduced by kind permission of the editor of the British Medical Journal.)

advantage of this compound when injected into a drawback, since, owing to its low solubility, little of a swallowed dose is absorbed. Henry et al, (1957) recovered only 6.7 per cent of an oral dose from the urine, in contrast to 30 per cent of an oral dose of phenoxymethyl penicillin, and over 70 per cent of a dose of either penicillin or procaine penicillin given intramuscularly. Nevertheless the doses usually given to children, particularly neonates, which are larger in relation to body weight, should have an adequate effect, and the preparation has the advantage of palatability.

PHENOXYMETHYL PENICILLIN

The existence of several natural penicillins was recognized in early studies, and many more have been obtained by adding various derivatives of acetic acid to the fermentation medium as 'precursors'. None of these is therapeutically important except phenoxymethyl penicillin, or penicillin V which is obtained when phenoxyacetic acid is the precursor. This substance, originally described in 1948, but without its most important property having been detected, was re-discovered in Austria in 1953, and owes its value to acid stability: it is not destroyed in the stomach, and can therefore be given with confidence by mouth. Absorption is not in fact complete: the proportion of the dose recoverable from the urine is only 25 per cent (Heatley, 1956) but this was a great improvement on the absorption of benzyl penicillin, which is not only on the average much less, but unaccountably variable. Absorption is slower than that after injection, but excretion is equally rapid: hence a moderate dose needs repetition at intervals of four hours. Of different forms of penicillin V, the potassium salt is the best absorbed, the calcium salt next and the free acid least, that being their diminishing order of solubility: absorption is also better from a rapidly disintegrating tablet and after administration in the fasting state (Juncher & Raaschou, 1957). It may seem strange that a second reason, in addition to incomplete absorption, for the apparent bio-availability of less than one third of the dose of penicillin V, should not have been revealed until much later (p. 73).

It was for some time assumed that penicillin V has the same anti-bacterial activity as benzyl penicillin, but this is not so. It is rather *more* active against resistant staphylococci because more slowly destroyed by penicillinase, and slightly *less* active against streptococci, but much less active against Gram-negative species, including the gonococcus, *H. influenzae* and *Proteus* (Garrod, 1960a, b). These differences are exaggerated in the synthetic acid-resistant penicillins described later. Penicillin V therefore affords a very convenient means of treating Gram-positive infections, but is not indicated for gonorrhoea or for Gram-negative infections involving the respiratory or urinary tract.

Therapeutic Applications

These are dealt with individually in the second part of this book, and need only be briefly reviewed here. In the first place, penicillin is almost wholly responsible for the fact that fatal haemolytic streptococcal infection is now almost unheard of: in all serious forms of this infection, whether involving wounds, the air passages or the uterus, it is usually the treatment of choice. The pneumococcus is also invariably susceptible to it (with a hitherto geographically limited exception mentioned on page 60), and its efficacy can therefore be depended on in lobar pneumonia. In staphylococcal infections its value has been reduced by the increasing prevalence of resistant strains, but if the strain is sensitive natural penicillins are preferable to the synthetic.

Among its other principal uses may be mentioned the treatment of both syphilis and gonorrhoea, bacterial endocarditis and actinomycosis. Rarer indications for which it is highly effective are gas gangrene, anthrax and erysipeloid.

Dosage

Because of both the variety of its uses and its lack of toxicity, the dosage of penicillin is remarkably elastic, certainly more so than that of any other drug. The factors determining the necessary dose are, first and foremost, the concentration required to inhibit the growth of the infecting organism, and the accessibility and gravity of the infection. If the inhibitory concentration is known or can be deduced, the aim should be to maintain one exceeding this, preferably several-fold, in the affected tissues. If these are intact and fully vascularized, the concentration in them will be much the same as that in the blood. If there are foci of suppuration or of necrosis, or fibrotic areas with a poor blood supply as in such a condition as actinomycosis, penetration is more difficult. A special indication for high dosage owing to inaccessibility is the attainment of an adequate concentration in the cerebro-spinal fluid in meningitis.

To translate these principles into practical terms, a fully sensitive infection in an area well supplied with blood should respond to 0.5 or even 0.25 g of penicillin V given orally at intervals of four hours or to procaine penicillin given by injection in doses of 300 000 units (180 mg) at intervals of 12 hours. Somewhat higher concentrations can be attained by increasing the dose of either of these preparations, but for maximum effects 'soluble' (i.e. sodium) penicillin must be given either by intramuscular injection at intervals not exceeding six hours or by continuous intravenous infusion: the amount so administered may be anything from four to 20 million units daily or even more.

Toxicity

Penicillin has no toxicity in the ordinary sense except when administered intrathecally: the dose by this route should never exceed 20 000 units, if indeed the route need be used at all, which is doubtful. It is almost impossible to poison a patient with penicillin if he has properly functioning kidneys, but if there is gross renal impairment the antibiotic may accumulate in the blood, in which the level should be estimated, the dose being reduced accordingly. Doses of 25 to 40 mega units of potassium penicillin daily given for presumed or known Gram-negative infections to four elderly patients, all with raised blood ureas, caused partial or complete loss of consciousness with myoclonic movements and sometimes generalized seizures (Bloomer et al, 1967). From a study of 15 patients similarly treated (some with doses of up to 120 mega units daily) in whom the penicillin was assayed in the blood and cerebro-spinal fluid, Smith et al, (1967) conclude that this 'neurotoxicity' results only when a concentration of 10 units per ml is exceeded in the CSF. These patients received either the Na or the K salt, the effects of which are not distinguished. An effect from the cation must be considered whenever large doses of a single salt are given. The disturbances which may follow massive doses of the Na salt are described by Brunner & Frick (1968).

The unique toxicity of penicillin for guinea-pigs, in which a single intramuscular dose is often fatal within a few days, seems finally to have been explained by the work of Farrar & Kent (1965).

Sensitization Reactions

These present a more serious problem with penicillin than with any other antibiotic. Although serious or life-threatening reactions are rare, the possibility of an allergic reaction must be considered on each occasion of penicillin administration and their prevention and management pose many problems.

Types of reaction

The most dangerous form of drug allergy is acute anaphylactic shock, which may develop within a few minutes to 30 minutes after administration. It is characterized by profound collapse, nausea, vomiting, itching, dyspnoea and coma, and may be rapidly fatal. During the 1950s penicillin anaphylaxis had 'replaced foreign sera as the commonest cause of anaphylactic shock' (Kern & Wimberley, 1953) and was said to have caused 500 deaths annually in the U.S.A. alone. Another and distinguishable form of acute reaction is attributed to the accidental intravenous injection of a suspension of procaine penicillin (Tompsett, 1967), is non-allergic in character, and is caused (Bredt, 1965) by blockage of pulmonary capillaries by crystals of the material.

The serum sickness type of penicillin allergy is characterized by urticarial rash and fever. Some patients show other manifestations such as arthritis, lymphadenopathy and eosinophilia. If the tissue oedema affects the larynx, the patient is at risk of respiratory obstruction. In addition to these dramatic syndromes, and of much greater frequency, are a variety of rashes which are usually maculopapular and itchy, but a wide variety of patterns is seen and some patients show a mixture of urticarial and maculopapular elements.

In addition to the generalized allergic reactions, particular organs may be damaged by a variety of immunological mechanisms. Nephritis rarely occurs in patients who have received a long course of large doses of penicillin. Baldwin et al (1968) describe three cases, in one of which persistence with the treatment ended in oliguria and death. The kidneys showed tubular necrosis and dense interstitial infiltration with mononuclears and eosinophiles. Haemolytic anaemia occurs only in patients who have been treated with penicillin before, and again receive a prolonged course of large doses (commonly 20 mega units daily) usually for bacterial endocarditis. The haemolysis is due to the action of IgG antibody on cells which have adsorbed the antibiotic. Rapid recovery ensues when administration is stopped. White et al (1968) describe two cases and review the findings in 12 others. Parker (1975), in a valuable general review of drug allergy, mentions a suggestive association, in two patients, between penicillin therapy and the onset of polymyositis.

Rashes are said to occur in 1–7 per cent of patient courses of penicillin (Levine, 1972). Severe reactions such as acute anaphylaxis are much less common, an estimate of 0.04 per cent being given by Rudolph & Price (1973). Although reactions can occur after any route of administration, the severe forms are much more common after injections than after oral administration.

Pathogenesis of hypersensitivity reactions

Some patients develop allergic reactions only after repeated administration of penicillin, but in others reactions develop on the first occasion penicillin is prescribed. The history of previous antibiotic use is often uncertain but, even when a reliable account is obtainable, non-medical exposure to penicillin may have occurred, for example to aerosols of penicillin in the environment of patients receiving the drug, or by ingestion of penicillin in milk.

The mechanism of penicillin hypersensitivity is that proposed originally by Landsteiner as a general one in drug allergy, that is the combination of a drug or its metabolites, acting as haptens, with endogenous macromolecules to form new antigenic configurations. In the case of penicillin, a variety of metabolites act as haptens. The largest amount of antibody is directed against benzyl penicilloyl determinants, derived from penicillenate, but penicillin itself, penicillenic acid and penicillenate also provoke the production of specific antibody. The important role of the penicilloyl group has led to the development of penicilloyl polylysine (see below) as a skin-testing reagent in the detection of penicillin allergy. Most of the available amino groups are replaced in this compound by penicilloyl residues, so that the risk of inducing antibody by its use as a test reagent is virtually eliminated.

To add to the metabolites of penicillin as allergic determinants, two other sources of penicillin allergy have been defined. All work until very recently has been based on the belief that the sensitizing antigen is a combination of a penicillin derivative with body protein. The subject has now been much complicated by the discovery that a highly reactive pre-formed antigen may exist in penicillin itself (Batchelor et al, 1967; Stewart, 1967). That found by these authors in 6-aminopenicillenic acid, and hence liable to be present in any semi-synthetic penicillin, is believed to be derived from the enzyme used in production, and that in benzyl penicillin from *P. chrysogenum* itself, each existing as a penicilloyl conjugate. These authors also recognized that a reactive substance can be formed in a solution of pure benzyl penicillin, and have since shown that such polymers, to which sensitized animals react, are formed on standing for 8–14 days in solutions not only of benzylpenicillin, but of ampicillin, hetacillin, carbenicillin and cephaloridine. The use of freshly prepared solutions for injection should be a safeguard against the possible effects of this change. Parker & Richmond (1976), in a small group of ten patients, found suggestive evidence that the incidence of ampicillin rash may be reduced by a polymer-free preparation.

The effects of removing protein impurities have been studied. Penicillin freed from the penicilloyl protein impurity (BRL 3000, 'Purapen G') produced no reaction in 11 sensitive volunteers who reacted to ordinary penicillin, but nine reacted to both and one to the purified material only (Knudsen et al, 1967). Similar treatment of ampicillin reduced the incidence of rashes by about one half (Knudsen et al, 1970). De Weck & Schneider (1969) contest the view that these impurities are responsible for reactions, at least to benzyl penicillin, on two grounds: that in animals they have found purified benzyl penicillin to retain its full immunogenicity, and that hydrolyzed crude benzyl penicillin, which owing to the opening of the β-lactam ring cannot form penicilloyl conjugates, does not induce the formation of anti-penicilloyl antibodies.

In general, patients who are allergic to one form of penicillin are allergic to them all, although not perhaps to a uniform extent. A peculiar exception is found in the high prevalence of ampicillin allergy found in infectious mononucleosis, in cytomegalovirus mononucleosis, in lymphatic leukaemia, and in patients with a high serum uric acid (Pullen et al, 1967; Boston Collaborative Drug Survey, 1972). These patients usually show negative skin tests to penicillin components and can often be treated later without further reactions.

Detection and control of penicillin reactions

Penicillin antibodies are easily detected and are commonly present even in normal subjects with no history of allergy. For example Levine et al (1966) using an antigen prepared by coupling penicilloyl groups to red cells in a special suspending medium, obtained enormous titres, and demonstrated agglutinin in almost all of 76 'consecutive' patients, only one of whom had a history of a reaction to penicillin.

More important in the prediction of penicillin reactions are the skin-sensitizing antibodies, and dermal tests for penicillin hypersensitivity have been employed extensively with a variety of antigens. The rationale for the use of penicilloyl polylysine (PPL) has already been discussed and the compound has been licensed for clinical use. Because of the variety of possible haptenic determinants, testing with PPL alone will fail to detect many potential reactors. Green & Rosenblum (1971) found that of 56 patients showing immediate-type penicillin reactions only 26 (46 per cent) gave a positive skin test with PPL. For this reason, other agents must also be used for more complete prediction and Levine & Zolov (1969), testing with PPL and with a 'minor determinant mixture' (containing benzyl penicillin, penicilloate, penilloate and α-benzyl penicilloyl amine), obtained very good results in the prediction and exclusion of penicillin allergy. Scratch tests with each of these were followed if negative by intradermal tests. In 185 patients negative to both and treated with penicillin only one atypical reaction occurred. Of 32 patients positive to one or both, 21 were not treated, and among 11 who were, there were seven accelerated and one immediate urticarial reactions. Similar findings are reported by Adkinson et al (1971), who claim that the application of these tests has much reduced the frequency of penicillin reactions in their unit at the Johns Hopkins Hospital. The phrase 'minor determinant mixture' (MDM) refers to the amount of antibody binding to the components and may be misleading in a clinical context, since anaphylactic reactions tend to be associated with these 'minor' components. Many authors consider that testing with PPL and with benzyl penicillin will predict virtually all reactions (Medical Letter, 1975), since most people who react to MDM also do so to benzyl penicillin. Dermal tests for penicillin allergy are thus of some value in predicting clinical response, although less clear cut results have been obtained by other workers (Vickers & Assem, 1974; Dash, 1975).

A large number of *in vitro* tests has also been developed in an attempt to achieve reliable prediction of clinical reactions while avoiding any potential danger from skin tests: these include lymphocyte transformation (Sakarny, 1967), the radio-allergosorbent test (RAST) to detect IgE antibodies specific for penicillin antigens (Wide & Juhlin, 1971), and bioassays involving the measurement of histamine release on passive sensitization of human tissues (Vickers & Assem 1974).

In summary, at least two reagents must be employed in skin tests. Intradermal tests may result in dangerous reactions and must be preceded by preliminary scratch tests. Even in expert hands, reliable correlation of tests with clinical reactions is not always achieved, and it is uncertain if high standards of testing could be maintained with extensive use of these tests. The *in vitro* tests are as yet too slow or not generally available. We conclude that predictive tests for penicillin allergy cannot yet be widely applied in clinical practice. They may, however, be important in the small number of patients who give a history of penicillin allergy and for whom no other appropriate group of drugs is suitable for treatment. In general the prevention of penicillin allergy must still depend on avoiding its use in patients who say they are allergic to penicillin, although in many of them the evidence for this belief is tenuous and unreliable.

The management of penicillin reactions relies on the use of antihistamines, corticosteroids and, in anaphylaxis or dangerous angio-oedema, adrenaline. Desensitization can sometimes be achieved by careful control of treatment in patients for whom penicillin is strongly indicated (Levine, 1972; Graybill et al, 1974).

Two other methods of controlling penicillin allergy have been proposed. Antigens need multiple combining sites to elicit tissue damage by bridging between antibody molecules. Conjugates with one haptenic group on each carrier molecule can bind anti-penicilloyl antibodies and so prevent allergic reactions. Such a compound RO6-0787 (which is N-ϵ-benzylpenicilloyl-α-formyl-L-lysine, or BPO-FLYS), which has been successfully used with penicillin in allergic patients enabling therapy to be pursued or resumed. Unfortunately 5 per cent of patients allergic to penicillin develop skin reactions to the compound (De Weck, 1975). Another as yet experimental approach has rendered animals specifically tolerant to the BPO determinant by the use of haptens linked to non-immunogenic carrier molecules (Leading article, 1976).

Cross-reactivity with cephalosporins

Contrary to the views expressed soon after the introduction of cephalosporins, a significant minority of patients show cross-reactivity between penicillins and cephalosporins. Dash (1975) reviewing the world literature, found that 5.8–9.0 per cent of patients showing allergic reactions to penicillin also reacted to cephalosporins, (see also Levine, 1973). Since these cross-reactions cannot be easily predicted, cephalosporins should certainly be avoided in patients with a history of immediate-type penicillin reactions, and preferably avoided, if another suitable agent is available, in all patients with a history of penicillin allergy.

References

Adkinson N F, Thompson W L, Maddrey W C, Lichtenstein L M 1971 New Engl J Med 285: 22
Appelbaum P C, Bhamjee A, Scragg J N, Hallett A F, Bowen A J, Cooper R C 1977 Lancet 2: 995
Baldwin D S, Levine B B, McCluskey R T, Gallo G R 1968 New Engl J Med 279: 1245
Batchelor F R, Dewdney J, Feinberg J G, Weston R D 1967 Lancet 1: 1175
Best G K, Best N H, Koval A V 1974 Antimicrob Agents & Chemother 6: 825
Bloomer H A, Barton L J, Maddock R K Jr 1967 J Amer Med Ass 200: 121
Boston Collaborative Drug Surveillance Program 1972 New Engl J Med 286: 505
Bredt J 1965 Dtsch Med Wschr 90: 1602
Brunner F P, Frick P G 1968 Brit Med J 4: 550
Chisholm G D, Waterworth P M, Calnan J S, Garrod L P 1973 Brit Med J 1: 569
Dash C H 1975 J Antimicrob Chemother 1: Suppl 107
De Weck A L, Jeunet F, Schulz K H et al 1975 Ztschr Immunforsch 150: 138
De Weck A L, Schneider C H 1969 Minnesota Med 52: 137
Eagle H 1951 J Bact 62: 663
Eagle H, Fleischman R, Levi Mina 1953 J Lab Clin Med 41: 122

Editorial 1976 Brit Med J 2: 963
Farrar W E Jr, Kent T H 1965 Amer J Path 47: 629
Garrod L P 1950 Brit Med J 2: 453
Garrod L P 1960a Brit Med J 1: 527
Garrod L P 1960b Brit Med J 2: 1695
Garrod L P, Waterworth P M 1962 Brit Heart J 24: 39
Graybill J R, Sande M A, Reinarz J A, Shapiro S R 1974 Southern Med J 67: 62
Green G R, Rosenblum A 1971 J Allerg Clin Immunol 1971 48: 331
Hansman D 1975 Med J Australia 2: 740
Heatley N G 1956 Antibiot Med 2: 33
Hellström K, Rosén A, Swahn Å 1974 Clin Pharmacol Ther 16: 826
Henry L, White G, Meynell M J 1957 Brit Med J 1: 17
Howes V J, Mitchell R G 1976 Brit Med J 1: 996
Jacobs M R, Koornhof H J, Robins-Browne R M et al 1978 New Engl J Med 299: 735
Juncher H, Raaschou F 1957 Antibiot Med 4: 497
Kern R A, Wimberley N A Jr 1953 Amer J Med Sci 226: 357
Knudsen E T, Dewdney J M, Trafford J A P 1970 Brit Med J 1: 469
Knudsen E T, Robinson O P W, Croydon E A P, Tees E C 1967 Lancet 1: 1184
Leading article 1976 Lancet 2: 943
Levine B B 1972 New Engl J Med 286: 42
Levine B B 1973 J Infect Dis 128: S 364
Levine B B, Zolov D M 1969 J Allergy 43: 231
Levine B B, Fellner M J, Levytska V, Franklin E C, Alisberg N 1966 J Immunol 96: 707, 719
Mayhall C G, Medoff G, Marr J J 1976 Antimicrobial Agents & Chemother 10: 707
Medical Letter on Drugs and Therapeutics 1975 17: 54
Parker C W 1975 New Engl J Med 292: 511, 732, 957
Parker A C, Richmond J 1976 Brit Med J 1: 998
Pullen H, Wright N, Murdoch J McC 1967 Lancet 2: 1176
Rudolph A H, Price E V 1973 J Amer Med Ass 223: 499
Sabath L D, Wheeler N, Laverdiere M, Blazevic D, Wilkinson B J 1977 Lancet 1: 443
Sakarny I 1967 Lancet 1: 743
Smith H, Lerner P I, Weinstein L 1967 Arch Intern Med 120: 47
Stewart G T 1967 Lancet 2: 1177
Tompsett R 1967 Arch Intern Med 120: 565
Vickers M R, Assem E S K 1974 Immunology 26: 425
White J M, Brown D L, Hepner G W, Worlledge S M 1968 Brit Med J 3: 26
Wide L, Juhlin L 1971 Clinical Allergy 1: 171

SEMI-SYNTHETIC PENICILLINS

The existence of the penicillin 'nucleus', 6-aminopenicillanic acid, in *Penicillium chrysogenum* fermentations was first detected by discrepancies between the results of chemical and microbiological assays, and more was found to be formed in the absence of added precursor (Batchelor et al, 1959). The second discovery made at this time was that this substance could also be prepared in quantity from benzyl or phenoxymethyl penicillin by the action of an enzyme derived from other micro-organisms: the effect of this amidase is to separate the side chain (for site of action see page 58). The amidase acting on benzyl penicillin is obtainable from numerous enterobacteria (*Escherichia*, *Klebsiella*, etc.) and that attacking phenoxymethyl penicillin is derived from moulds (e.g. *Streptomyces lavendulae* — Batchelor et al, 1961).

Until this discovery different penicillins could only be obtained by adding precursors to the medium, among which only derivatives of acetic acid were effective. The availability of the nucleus itself enabled side chains in a great variety to be attached by a semi-synthetic process. In the Beecham Research Laboratories alone, where these discoveries were made, over 3000 new penicillins have been prepared by this process, and those which have come into therapeutic use possess one or more of the following advantages: (1) resistance to acid, (2) resistance to penicillinase, (3) broader spectrum. These categories will be described in that order.

ACID-RESISTANT PENICILLINS

PHENOXYPENICILLINS

The property of acid resistance, permitting a reliable effect from oral administration, was not new, since it already existed in phenoxymethyl penicillin. Metabolism of this compound has been clarified by the work of Hellström et al (1974), who administered the antibiotic labelled with ^{35}S and determined its concentrations in intestinal contents, blood and urine by both radio- and bio-assay. Levels determined by the former method were everywhere higher, and although it was confirmed that absorption is incomplete (32 per cent of radioactivity remaining in the faeces) it was also proved that some is degraded, both in the bowel and after absorption, mainly to penicilloic acid. Bio-assay confirmed excretion of 30 per cent of the dose unchanged in the urine, radio-assay indicating a content of 49 per cent. Although these studies did not account for the fate of the whole of a dose, their significance seems unquestionable. Similar studies of semi-synthetic phenoxypenicillins have apparently not been made, but the fact that they attain higher blood levels (hitherto attributed simply to better absorption) is the main advantage of phenethicillin and propicillin.

The therapeutic efficacy of these penicillins is the product of three factors, anti-bacterial activity, efficiency of absorption, and extent of protein binding in the blood. The only adequate study taking all these factors into account is that of Bond et al (1963) who assayed not only total but free antibiotic in the blood of volunteers at intervals after a dose, as well as studying the anti-bacterial activity *in vitro* in the presence and absence of serum. This study included phenbenicillin, another such compound, no longer manufactured, which is better absorbed but also much more highly protein-bound than the others (percentages bound were determined as phenoxymethyl penicillin 80, phenethicillin 75, propicillin 89 and phenbenicillin 97). Taking all these factors into account, phenoxymethylpenicillin was judged the most active of the three for streptococcal infections and phenethicillin for staphylococcal.

The anti-bacterial spectrum of phenethicillin and propicillin differs little from that of phenoxymethyl penicillin. Like the latter they are almost as active as benzyl penicillin against sensitive Gram-positive species, but they share and in some instances exaggerate the deficiences of phenoxymethyl penicillin in dealing with various Gram-negative organisms. The reader is referred to Table 10 page 70 in the previous edition of this book for details, but the main facts are clear from Table 3.2 from Rolinson & Sutherland (1973) which we are grateful for permission to reproduce since it is by far the most comprehensive comparison of the activities of a wide range of penicillins to have been carried out in a single laboratory.

A sufficient dose of any of these drugs given at 4-hour intervals should serve any ordinary suitable purpose. If any of them is to be used for a serious and unusual purpose, notably for bacterial endocarditis, its suitability should be verified by an accurate test of the sensitivity of the organism *to the penicillin which it is proposed to use*. It cannot be assumed that the result will be the same as that to be obtained with

Table 3.2 Antibacterial spectra of semisynthetic penicillins[1]

Organism	Minimum inhibitory concentration[2] (μg/ml)						
	Narrow-spectrum penicillins			Penicillinase-stable penicillins		Broad-spectrum penicillins	
	Penicillin G	Penicillin V	Phenethicillin	Methicillin	Cloxacillin	Ampicillin	Carbenicillin
Staphylococcus aureus	0.02	0.05	0.05	1.25	0.1	0.05	1.25
Staphylococcus aureus (penicillinase-producing)	R	R	250	2.5	0.25	R	25
Streptococcus pyogenes	0.01	0.02	0.05	0.25	0.1	0.02	0.5
Streptococcus pneumoniae	0.02	0.02	0.05	0.25	0.25	0.05	1.25
Streptococcus faecalis	2.5	5.0	5.0	25	25	1.25	25
Clostridium welchii	0.05	0.1	0.1	1.0	0.5	0.05	0.5
Neisseria gonorrhoeae	0.01	0.02	0.1	0.1	0.1	0.02	0.05
Neisseria meningitidis	0.02	0.05	0.1	0.25	0.25	0.02	0.05
Haemophilus influenzae	0.5	5.0	5.0	2.5	12.5	0.25	0.25
Escherichia coli[3]	50	125	R	R	R	5.0	5.0
Salmonella typhi	5.0	125	R	R	R	0.5	5.0
Shigella sonnei[3]	50	250	R	R	R	2.5	12.5
Proteus mirabilis[3]	5.0	50	250	250	R	1.25	2.5
Indole-positive *Proteus*[3]	R	R	R	R	R	250	5.0
Klebsiella aerogenes	250	R	R	R	R	250	250
Enterobacter species[3]	R	R	R	R	R	250	12.5
Pseudomonas aeruginosa[3]	R	R	R	R	R	R	50

[1]Beecham Research Laboratories, unpublished data.
[2]Sensitivity of majority of strains. R = MIC > 250 μg/ml.
[3]Resistant strains are encountered.

benzylpenicillin. Likewise when any of them is being assayed in clinical specimens the standard solutions should be of the same compound, and not of benzyl penicillin.

AZIDOCILLIN

Of various other known penicillins distinguished by the property of acid resistance this appears most worthy of description, since it has been much used, mainly in Scandinavia, for the past ten years. Azidocillin was the most promising of a series of α-azido substituted penicillins prepared and studied by Sjöberg et al (1968). Its activity against sensitive Gram-positive cocci is comparable to and indeed in some instances slightly exceeds that of benzyl penicillin, and its curative dose in pneumococcal and penicillin-sensitive staphylococcal infections was lower in some experiments. The notable feature in its spectrum is an activity almost equal to that of ampicillin against *H. influenzae*. Other Gram-negative species are not notably sensitive. Protein binding is 84 per cent. Azidocillin is well absorbed after oral administration, urinary recovery being 58 per cent of the dose; after intravenous injection it was 78 per cent, indicating 74 per cent absorption by the oral route (Simon et al, 1976). In any comparison of therapeutic merits with ampicillin the advantage of better absorption has thus to be weighed against the drawback of greater protein binding. Although azidocillin is evidently used for many purposes, its action on *H. influenzae* has motivated studies of the treatment of otitis media (Bergholz et al, 1973) and of its penetration, which was found to be good, into nasal sinus secretions (Jokinen & Raunio, 1975). Good effects have also been claimed in pertussis (Simon et al, 1976).

Penicillinase-resistant penicillins

Of far greater practical importance than the discovery of the acid-resistant penicillins was the discovery that changes in the side-chain of penicillin can protect the central β-lactam ring from the action of penicillinase without removing anti-bacterial activity. The first of these to be introduced was methicillin, which is acid-labile and thus has to be injected. Others, including the isoxazolyl penicillins, are also acid-stable and can be given orally.

METHICILLIN

Chemistry

Methicillin is 2:6 dimethoxybenzyl penicillin and is supplied as the sodium salt. It is readily soluble in water, but solutions are unstable, particularly at low pH. They must therefore be freshly prepared in distilled water not containing dissolved CO_2.

Anti-bacterial activity

Methicillin is highly resistant to staphylococcal penicillinase, although less so to the penicillinases of many other species. It is, therefore, equally active against penicillin-sensitive and penicillinase-producing strains of *Staph. aureus*. On the other hand, its activity is much less than that of benzyl penicillin against most other penicillin-sensitive species. Methicillin, like benzyl penicillin, is actively bactericidal in optimum concentrations, but, at least against staphylococci, may be less so in higher concentrations. In view of its lack of activity against other species there is no indication for its use except a severe penicillin-resistant staphylococcal infection.

Resistance

Strains of *Staph. aureus* resistant to methicillin, thought at first not to exist and then to be exceedingly rare, came to be encountered more frequently: the percentage resistant among many thousands of strains tested at the Central Public Health Laboratory rose from 0.06 in 1960 to 0.97 in 1964 (Dyke et al, 1966) and to 4.11 per cent in 1969 (Parker & Hewitt, 1970). Since this time there seems to have been no general increase in frequency, but much higher isolation rates have been reported in individual hospitals and particularly from France (Chabbert et al, 1965), Switzerland (Benner & Kayser, 1968; Kayser & Hollinger, 1968) and Denmark (Siboni & Poulsen, 1968). It is now clear that such infections may not respond to treatment with methicillin alone, and the strains concerned are usually resistant to many other antibiotics. An appropriate treatment for serious infections of this nature may be a combination of methicillin or cephalothin with an aminoglycoside which exerts a synergic bactericidal effect (see page 293).

Although these strains form large amounts of penicillinase, they do not destroy methicillin, as has been asserted: their resistance is intrinsic. Only a small minority of the cells in these cultures appears resistant (Sutherland & Rolinson, 1964a)—except on a medium containing an excess of electrolytes, such as 5 per cent NaCl (Barber, 1964)—with the result that a diffusion test of sensitivity with a light inoculum may give a misleading result. Methods for detecting methicillin resistance are discussed in Chapter 27.

Resistance to methicillin is much commoner in *Staph. albus*: Kjellander & Finland (1963) found 10 per cent of clinical isolates resistant. They formed penicillinase, but also possessed intrinsic resistance.

Pharmacokinetics

Methicillin is not acid-resistant and has, therefore, to be administered by intramuscular (or intravenous) injection. Like benzyl penicillin it is rapidly excreted and injections must, therefore, be frequent. The usual regime is 1 g every four hours for the first 24 hours and every six hours thereafter but much larger doses can and may have to be given, and their effect can be reinforced with probenecid. Only about 40 per cent of the drug in the blood is protein-bound, an important fact in assessing its relative merits.

Toxicity

Methicillin has in general the same low toxicity as benzyl penicillin, but has apparently caused bone marrow depression, mainly affecting leucocytes, in a few patients (Levitt et al, 1964). Nephritis has also been described (Brauninger and Remington, 1968) but appears to be little more frequent than that occasionally caused by benzyl penicillin itself (Baldwin et al, 1968). Condemnation because of this very rare complication seems unjustifiable when it is remembered that benzyl penicillin can have the same effect: among patients with penicillin nephritis described by Baldwin et al (1968), three had been treated with methicillin, three with benzyl penicillin, and one with both (see page 66). Patients sensitized to benzyl penicillin will usually, although not always, react to methicillin.

ISOXAZOLYL PENICILLINS

These compounds combine resistance to penicillinase with resistance to acid. The series of 3:5-di-substituted 4-isoxazolyl penicillins was originally described by Doyle et al (1961), and among them cloxacillin was first brought into use in this country and oxacillin in the United States. Their sodium salts are readily soluble in water and neutral solutions are stable at room temperature for 24 hours. They also show a similar degree of resistance to acid to that of phenoxymethyl penicillin. All are highly protein-bound.

CLOXACILLIN

This compound is 3-chlorophenyl-5-methyl-4 isoxazolyl penicillin. The usual inhibitory concentration for all staphylococci is about 0.12–0.25 μg per ml i.e. cloxacillin has fully eight times the *in vitro* activity of methicillin, although still considerably less than that of benzyl penicillin against sensitive strains. It is slightly less resistant than methicillin to staphylococcal penicillinase, with the result that a 2–4-fold higher concentration may be required to inhibit a large inoculum. Activity is diminished even more by protein: in 95 per cent serum this reduction is 8-fold (Barber & Waterworth, 1964). The susceptibility of all other species is less than that to benzyl penicillin, but that of *Str. pyogenes* is noteworthy, since cloxacillin—or oxacillin (Simon & Sakai, 1963)—will eliminate a streptococcal infection complicated by the presence of penicillinase-forming staphylococci when benzyl penicillin has failed because of local inactivation.

Cloxacillin and methicillin exhibit cross-resistance: the position with regard to staphylococci is thus the same for both antibiotics.

Pharmacokinetics.
Cloxacillin should be administered before meals, since food interferes with absorption. Even so this is incomplete: higher blood levels are produced by intramuscular injection, when 30 per cent of the dose is excreted in the urine, compared with 20 per cent after an oral dose (Kislak et al, 1965). About 10 per cent of an oral dose is excreted in the bile (Nayler et al, 1962). The blood levels attained are about twice those given by oxacillin (Report, 1962; Turck et al, 1965) owing both to better absorption and to greater stability, although excretion studies show that some inactivation of both occurs in the body.

OXACILLIN

This compound, 5-methyl-3-phenyl-4-isoxazolyl penicillin, has been extensively used and studied in the United States while similar studies of cloxacillin have been pursued in this country. As would be expected from the fact that only a single chlorine atom distinguishes them, their properties are closely similar and call for no separate description. As already stated, oxacillin is less well absorbed and this difficulty has been overcome in some clinical studies by intramuscular injection for the early stages of severe infections. Its activity against penicillinase-forming staphylococci is also slightly less, and these differences have led some American authors (Sidell et al, 1964) to compare it unfavourably with cloxacillin. The more rapid inactivation of oxacillin in the body (Gravenkemper et al, 1965) is illustrated by the fact that in patients with end-stage kidney disease the blood level fell to nil eight hours after a 1 g dose (Bulger et al, 1964).

DICLOXACILLIN

This more recently introduced compound, which is 3(2,6-dichlorphenyl)-5-methyl-4-isoxazolyl penicillin, furnished as the sodium monohydrate, has interesting properties, well described in comparison with those of cloxacillin and oxacillin by Gravenkemper et al (1965). Its inhibitory concentration for both sensitive and resistant staphylococci is somewhat lower than that of the other two compounds, and it is also highly active against streptococci and pneumococci. The concentrations attained in the blood exceed those of cloxacillin by 2-fold, just as those of cloxacillin exceed those of oxacillin to the same degree, and these concentrations are better sustained. This difference is due not only to better absorption, but to slower excretion: Rosenblatt et al (1968) found the renal clearances of oxacillin, cloxacillin and dicloxacillin to be 226.8, 162.2 and 113.7 ml/min respectively. These authors and Naumann and Kempf (1965) have also shown that >70 per cent of a dose of dicloxacillin is excreted in the urine, the figures for the other compounds being lower (oxacillin 55.5 and cloxacillin 62, according to Rosenblatt et al, 1968). The main defect of dicloxacillin is its very high degree of protein binding: according to these authors the percentages bound are oxacillin 94–96, cloxacillin 93–95 and dicloxacillin 95–97.

FLUCLOXACILLIN

According to the original description (Sutherland et al, 1970) the anti-bacterial activity of this compound now in general clinical use is almost identical with that of cloxacillin, but it is much better absorbed after oral administration, the blood levels attained being about double those produced by the same dose of cloxacillin at all times up to four hours. Protein binding has been determined as 94.7 per cent, in a test showing oxacillin 93.1 and dicloxacillin as 96.9 per cent. Thus better absorption more than compensates for the degree of protein binding. These pharmacokinetic findings have been fully confirmed by others. Nauta & Mattie (1975) not only confirm better absorption than that of cloxacillin but demonstrate slower elimination. Kamme & Ursing (1974) obtained consistently high and well sustained blood levels. Bergeron et al (1976), who determined degrees of protein binding of oxacillin, cloxacillin and flucloxacillin to be 91.5, 93.5 and 94.6 per cent, performed similar experiments to the foregoing and thence calculated concentrations of free antibiotic in the blood, finding those of flucloxacillin to be considerably higher. This study also included tests of anti-bacterial activity, the results of which are given only in terms of bactericidal effect, and show flucloxacillin to have several advantages over the other two compounds. There is now an extensive clinical literature of flucloxacillin, indicating a widespread preference for it, but naturally not including formal proof of superiority by comparative trial, which would have to be on an enormous scale to afford such a result.

OTHER PENICILLINASE-RESISTANT PENICILLINS

NAFEILLIN

The anti-bacterial activity of this compound was studied by Lane (1964) and by Klein & Finland (1963) who also studied absorption, which was irregular and incomplete, although no specific reason for this is adduced. Its *in vitro* antibacterial activity is high, but although acid-resistant it is poorly absorbed after oral administration. Hence in an extensive clinical trial in severe staphylococcal infections Eickhoff et al (1965a) used mainly the parenteral route in a dose of usually 6 but up to 18 g daily, sometimes with probenecid. Results compared favourably with those obtained with methicillin, oxacillin, etc. According to Kind et al (1970) inactivation in the liver reduced the blood levels attainable even after parenteral administration. Its degree of protein binding is reported to be 87 per cent. Reports of the use of this drug, mainly in the United States, continue to appear, but whether there are any special indications for it is uncertain. One remarkable therapeutic success (Ruiz & Warner, 1976) is the recovery of an elderly diabetic with staphylococcal osteomyelitis, septicaemia and meningitis, who was given 3 g intravenously every four hours. Serial blood and cerebrospinal fluid levels were determined after a dose, and the latter rose to 9.5 μg/ml; these are said to be the first observations of the kind.

Others are **Diphenicillin** (**Ancillin**), which is 2-biphenylyl penicillin, similar to oxacillin, but less acid-stable and thus poorly absorbed, and even when given parenterally yielding inferior clinical resluts (Klein et al, 1963), and **Quinacillin**, which is 3-carboxy-2-quinoxalinyl penicillin, described by Richards et al (1963), which has a low activity against organisms other than staphylococci and is very poorly absorbed.

General therapeutic efficacy

All these penicillinase-resistant penicillins have been used mainly for treating severe staphylococcal infections. These are notoriously varied in nature, and many occur in patients with a still greater variety of predisposing conditions, some of these being of the gravest nature in themselves. Hence all extensive clinical studies embrace a mixture of patients with pneumonia, septicaemia, wound infections, etc., with sometimes a few of endocarditis or meningitis, many occurring as a complication of malignant disease, or serious cardiac, hepatic or renal lesions, often in elderly subjects. Such miscellaneous clinical material does not lend itself to an assessment of the relative value of antibiotics which are themselves closely related, and no attempt at such an analysis will be made here.

The main choice lies between methicillin, which has much the lowest intrinsic anti-staphylococcal activity, but of which 60 per cent in the blood is free, and one of the isoxazolyl or other acid-resistant compounds, with higher anti-bacterial activity, but of which perhaps only 5 per cent is free. These contrasting properties are largely self-cancelling, and the probability is that adequate doses of almost any of these penicillins will achieve very similar effects. The possibilities of reducing protein binding by displacement with other drugs which have been explored by Kunin (1966) do not seem hopeful. Initial treatment of a severe staphylococcal infection should always be with one of these penicillins unless or until the strain has been shown to be sensitive to benzylpenicillin.

BROAD SPECTRUM PENICILLINS

AMPICILLIN

This semi-synthetic compound, α-aminobenzyl penicillin, was first described by Rolinson & Stevens (1961). It is administered orally as the free acid, which unlike most other penicillins is soluble only to the extent of about 10 per cent in water.

Anti-bacterial activity

Ampicillin is slightly less active than benzyl penicillin against most Gram-positive bacteria, but slighly more so against *Str. faecalis*. It is destroyed by staphylococcal penicillinase, and is therefore not indicated for resistant staphylococcal infections. *Listeria monocytogenes* is highly sensitive (Seeliger et al, 1967) and several papers (Weingartner & Ortel, 1967; MacNair et al, 1968; Seeliger & Matheis, 1969) commend ampicillin for the treatment of listeriosis.

The outstanding property of ampicillin is an activity four to eight times greater than that of benzyl penicillin against various Gram-negative bacilli, including *H. influenzae*, *Salmonella* and *Shigella* spp., non-penicillinase-forming *Proteus mirabilis*, and most strains of *E. coli* (Sutherland & Rolinson, 1964b; Anderson et al, 1964). *Kl. pneumoniae* may be sensitive, but *Kl. aerogenes*, penicillinase-forming *Proteus*, and *Pseudomonas* spp. are resistant, as are other coliform bacilli forming a penicillinase. *Kl. aerogenes* possesses a high degree of intrinsic resistance, apart from its capacity to destroy ampicillin enzymically (Hamilton-Miller, 1965). The effect of ampicillin, like that of benzyl penicillin, is bactericidal.

Pharmacokinetics

Ampicillin is resistant to acid, and is well absorbed when administered orally, but not completely: 30 per cent of an oral dose is recoverable from the urine, but 60–70 per cent of an intramuscular (Naumann, 1965), for which reason the parenteral route may be preferred for maximal effect. This can also be enhanced with probenecid. When different oral doses are compared, plotting the dose against the blood concentration gives a straight line (Knudsen et al, 1961): i.e. the same proportion of a large dose is absorbed as of a small, whereas the larger the dose of tetracycline, the less the proportion absorbed. The peak concentration is reached in about two hours, and the subsequent fall is gradual, a detectable amount persisting for six hours after a moderate dose (250 mg). Protein binding, about 20 per cent, is the lowest of any penicillin.

Although excretion is mainly renal, fairly high concentrations are attained in the bile. The report by Brown & Acred (1961) of a level in the bile of dogs 300 times that in the blood, does not seem to represent conditions in the human biliary tract, since Ayliffe & Davies (1965) found a mean difference of only 9-fold (extremes 3-48-fold) in a series of patients. There were wide variations in the content among patients with normal biliary tracts: in those with obstructive lesions it was very low or nil. These observations have been confirmed and extended by Mortimer et al (1969). Blecher et al (1966) have shown that ampicillin accumulates and persists in the amniotic fluid, evidently in consequence of renal excretion by the fetus: in most specimens the level exceeded 2.5 μg per ml after three maternal doses of 500 mg.

Ampicillin can also be administered intramuscularly or intravenously, the sodium salt, which behaves identically (Eickhoff et al, 1965b) being more suitable by the latter route. High concentrations are attained in the cerebrospinal fluid in patients with purulent meningitis when 150–200 mg per kg are given intravenously daily (Naumann, 1965) although ampicillin, like benzyl penicillin, traverses the normal blood-brain barrier in very small amounts. Impairment of renal function reduces the rate of excretion, and the dose can be reduced accordingly: renal dialysis will reduce the blood level (Höffler et al, 1966).

Toxic effects

Ampicillin appears to be as free from toxicity as benzyl penicillin. Apart from occasional gastric intolerance, the only significant side effects seen have been rashes, which are decidedly commoner than with other penicillins. A large-scale survey by Shapiro et al (1969) showed that 9.5 per cent of patients treated with ampicillin developed rashes and only 4.5 per cent of those given other penicillins. The route of administration was not a factor, but the effect of dosage was not analysed: it may be significant that a series of patients of whom 20 per cent had rashes were given 6 g daily (Sleet et al, 1964). A rash almost invariably results when ampicillin is given to a patient with glandular fever.

An ampicillin rash is almost always maculo-papular and not urticarial, like that produced by benzylpenicillin. This fact, its much greater frequency, and the usual delay in its onset, strongly suggest that a different mechanism is responsible. Geddes (1973), who confirms that purified ampicillin less often causes it, believes it to be due to impurities and not to true sensitization to the penicillin nucleus. A prospective study on a large scale (Report, 1973) in which a rash occurred in 7.3 per cent of 933 patients, and was more frequent in those suffering from viral infections and in females, confirms the distinct nature of this exanthem. This is important, since an ampicillin rash is then not a contraindication to later penicillin treatment.

Clinical applications

Early reports dealt largely with the treatment of urinary tract infections. Ampicillin is unquestionably the best penicillin for this purpose when the organism is sensitive: it is not only more active than benzyl penicillin (although the same species are moderately sensitive to this) but has the great practical advantage of oral administrability. The phenoxypenicillins, although also administrable by mouth, are insufficiently active against Gram-negative species.

The high hopes originally entertained of efficacy in enteric fever have not altogether been fulfilled. This and other important uses are discussed in the later chapters on the treatment of alimentary tract and respiratory tract infections and meningitis.

ESTERS OF AMPICILLIN

A defect of ampicillin is incomplete absorption after oral administration. This has been overcome by the synthesis of esters, of which three are now available.

PIVAMPICILLIN

The first to be discovered and manufactured by Leo Pharmaceutical Products, is pivaloyloxymethyl-D-α-aminobenzyl penicillinate. This substance is believed to be completely absorbed, and is then rapidly hydrolysed in the blood and tissues with liberation of ampicillin. This process is 99 per cent complete in blood within 15 minutes. The blood levels attained in animals and man are 2–3 times higher than those produced by the same oral dose of ampicillin, and 73 per cent of the dose is excreted in the urine in six hours (von Daehne et al, 1970). These findings with regard to blood and urine levels are confirmed by Jordan et al (1971) and by Foltz et al (1971), who add that administration with food actually improves total absorption although slightly slowing it, whereas it impairs that of ampicillin. They are also confirmed and extended by Roholt et al (1974) and by Simon et al (1974b).

TALAMPICILLIN

This is the phthalidyl thiazolidine carboxylic ester. The pharmacokinetic studies of Leigh et al (1976) indicate identical behaviour to that of pivampicillin, and their clinical observations include that of reduced liability, in comparison with that of ampicillin, to cause diarrhoea, as might be expected from a fully absorbed derivative. This and other ampicillin esters have no anti-bacterial activity *per se*; hence should any be unabsorbed it will have no effect on the gut flora.

BACAMPICILLIN

This compound is described by Bodin et al (1975) and by Rozencweig et al (1976). Here again the findings are those to be expected from complete absorption and rapid hydrolysis by tissue esterases with liberation of ampicillin.

HETACILLIN

This compound, which is converted to ampicillin after oral administration is a condensation product of ampicillin and acetone. It is uncertain whether it has any anti-bacterial action *per se*, but this is difficult to determine, because the rapid liberation of ampicillin from it begins immediately on solution. Unlike ampicillin esters it is no better absorbed than ampicillin itself. It is not available in this country, and in our view has no thereapeutic advantage over ampicillin. The reader is referred to the previous edition of this book for a further account of its properties, which are also more fully described by Rolinson & Sutherland (1973).

EPICILLIN

According to Basch et al (1971) and Gadebusch et al (1971) this closely resembles ampicillin in many properties, but is somewhat more active against *Ps. aeruginosa*. Urinary tract infections were treated with epicillin by Woodruff et al (1971), 11 out of 14 *E. coli* infections responding and four out of seven due to *P. mirabilis*, but only one out of four due to *Ps. aeruginosa*, a discouraging result in view of the activity claimed for it against this species, which is in any case far less than that of carbenicillin and other compounds introduced later. Various other minor advantages over ampicillin have been claimed, but these also have been contested (Basker et al, 1979b). We conclude that their merits are indistinguishable.

AMOXYCILLIN

This compound is not an ester, but a compound absorbed and acting as such. Its antibacterial spectrum is almost identical with that of ampicillin, with which it also shares the properties of acid resistance, low protein binding and susceptibility to penicillinase (Sutherland & Rolinson, 1971). Absorption and excretion were studied by Croydon & Sutherland (1971) and Neu & Winshell (1971a) with very similar results to those reported for pivampicillin, i.e. peak levels in the blood twice those given by ampicillin, and corresponding differences in the amount excreted in the urine. Food does not interfere with absorption. These findings are assembled in a more up-to-date paper by Sutherland et al (1972). In therapeutic tests in mice Acred et al (1971a) found it superior to ampicillin in almost all of 14 infections, in some considerably so, and to some extent after subcutaneous as well as oral administration, a finding which appears to indicate an intrinsically greater activity in addition to its superiority in pharmacological behaviour.

The probable nature of this is revealed by the further therapeutic studies of Hunter et al (1973). When equal doses of ampicillin and amoxycillin were given to mice by injection (thus eliminating the influence of absorption) after intramuscular inoculation with *E. coli*, bacterial counts in the infected muscle were reduced to a much lower level by amoxycillin. The superior bactericidal effect suggested by this observation was confirmed *in vitro*, killing by amoxycillin being more rapid than by ampicillin, although their inhibitory effects were equal. Comber et al (1975) report similar findings in intraperitoneal infection with the same organism.

This is not the place to review clinical results, but it appears from reports on the treatment of a wide variety of infections that amoxycillin has substantial advantages over ampicillin. This is nowhere more evident than in the treatment of typhoid fever, for which ampicillin has unquestionably been disappointing. Amoxycillin, on the other hand, gave results equal and in some ways superior to those of chloramphenicol in extensive studies in children (Scragg & Rubidge, 1975) and in adults (Pillay et al, 1975). Good general reviews of the subject are by Brogden et al (1975) and in Symposium (1974).

CYCLACILLIN

In most features the anti-bacterial activity of this compound is less than that of ampicillin (Yurchenco et al, 1970). An advantage claimed for it is very rapid absorption (Hertz, 1973) but the faster elimination which follows seems to negate this virtue.

ANTIPSEUDOMONAL PENICILLINS

CARBENICILLIN

This compound is disodium α-carboxybenzyl penicillin (Knudsen et al, 1967). It is distinguished by its degree of activity against *Ps. aeruginosa* most strains of which are inhibited *in vitro* by 25 or 50 μg/ml. It is also active against all species of *Proteus* and some other enterobacteria, but inferior to benzyl penicillin against Gram-positive species (Table 3.2). Its action is bactericidal. It is protein-bound to about the same extent as benzyl penicillin, i.e. 47 per cent.

Administration must be parenteral at intervals of four hours, elimination being as rapid as that of benzyl penicillin; probenecid can be given to prolong the effect. It has come to be recognized that although a four-hourly dose of 1 g may suffice for urinary tract infections, systemic infections by *Ps. aeruginosa* demand much larger doses, of the order of 30 g daily. Gentamicin, with which carbenicillin acts synergically, may with advantage be given in addition. In our own experience this combination was effective even in a case of *Pseudomonas* endocarditis, although in a patient whose greatly impaired renal function enabled very high carbenicillin blood levels to be maintained.

An added reason for using this combination is that during treatment with carbenicillin alone *Ps. aeruginosa* may become resistant. Such strains were recovered from 17 patients by Darrell and Waterworth (1969), five of whom had been treated with carbenicillin and ten with other penicillins. Lowbury et al (1969) report the appearance and rapid predominance of highly resistant strains in the Burns Unit at Birmingham. Subsequent study in the Unit by Roe et al (1971) showed that such resistance was transferable to and from other species, both *in vitro* and in experimental burns in mice. These organisms produced a β-lactamase. Further interesting observations made by Ayliffe et al (1972) suggest that resistance transferred to *Ps. aeruginosa* in a burn from a *Klebsiella* or *Proteus* may be latent, only manifesting itself when carbenicillin is administered.

Table 3.3 Antibiotic sensitivities of *Proteus* species

	Ampicillin	*Carbenicillin*	*Cephaloridine*	*Gentamicin*
P. mirabilis	+	+	+	+
P. mirabilis (penicillinase-forming)	0	0	+	+
P. morganii	0	+	0	+
P. rettgeri	0	+	0	+
P. vulgaris	0	+	0	+

+ = sensitive 0 = resistant

The possible usefulness of carbenicillin in *Proteus* infections should not be forgotten. *P. mirabilis*, if penicillinase-forming, is resistant, as it is to ampicillin, but the other three species which are resistant to ampicillin and in general also to the cephalosporin antibiotics, are sensitive, and for infections of the urinary tract or elsewhere caused by these less common species carbenicillin may be the antibiotic of choice. The sensitivities of these organisms to four antibiotics are stated in simplified form in Table 3.3.

Carbenicillin is as free from toxicity as benzyl penicillin except that very high blood levels are liable to cause a coagulation defect manifested by prolonged bleeding time and due to an action on platelets (Brown et al 1975).

Two esters of carbenicillin have been introduced to enable administration to be oral, although only limited effects are so obtainable.

CARINDACILLIN

This is the 5-indanyl ester, carbenicillin indanyl sodium. Laboratory studies are described by English et al (1972) and the principal source of clinical information is in a Symposium (1973). The compound is acid-stable, and after absorption is rapidly hydrolysed to carbenicillin and indanol, the latter being conjugated and excreted in the urine. The peak blood level after a dose of 1 g is only about 10 μg/ml, but high concentrations are attained in the urine. A bitter after-taste and sometimes vomiting are complained of, and doses adequate to achieve a systemic effect would thus be impracticable. The only indication for this drug would appear to be *Pseudomonas* and other urinary infections sensitive only to carbenicillin, in ambulant patients. It should be recognized that this product and carfecillin, unlike esters of ampicillin, are esterified on the side chain, and possess independent anti-bacterial activity. Thus any unabsorbed product can affect the gut flora.

CARFECILLIN

This is the α-carboxyphenyl ester, the hydrolysis of which after absorption yields carbenicillin and phenol, this being conjugated and excreted in the urine. In a study by Wilkinson et al (1975) it was administered in single doses of 500 and 1000 mg to volunteers; blood levels varied widely, but the peak, reached at 90 minutes, averaged rather over 3 and 5 μg/ml respectively from the two doses, with a slow subsequent fall. In some treated patients, mainly owing to reduced renal function, blood levels were higher. In those with good renal function mean urinary levels were about 300 μg/ml, 25 per cent of the dose being so excreted. Urinary infections were treated with 1 g eight-hourly for seven days, successfully in eight out of 12 due to *Ps. aeruginosa* and six out of nine to *E. coli.* Tolerance was good, with no after-taste or nausea, and only occasional mild diarrhoea. This product is thus an improvement on carindacillin, but absolute indications for it appear to be the same (O'Grady, 1979).

It remains to consider several compounds related to carbenicillin which act as such and have to be administered parenterally, but are claimed to possess some advantage over carbenicillin itself.

TICARCILLIN

This product is α-carboxy-3-thienylmethyl penicillin. It was announced as having an activity against *Ps. aeruginosa* exceeding that of carbenicillin by 2- to 4-fold (Sutherland et al, 1971; Neu & Winshell, 1971b) with a correspondingly lower CD_{50} for this infection in mice (Acred et al, 1971b). Its greater *in vitro* activity has been confirmed by all subsequent workers, although with some differences in degree and strain variation. Its spectrum otherwise differs very little, although according to Neu & Garvey (1975) *Enterobacter* and *Serratia* may also be more sensitive to it. Many pharmacokinetic studies have been reported, mainly of the large doses required for treating severe Gram-negative infections in compromised patients. It behaves very similarly to carbenicillin, but according to Simon et al (1974a) although ticarcillin attains higher blood levels and has a rather longer half-life, carbenicillin diffuses better into tissues; this was confirmed by higher relative levels in blister fluid. Neu & Garvey (1975) recovered 95 per cent of the dose of carbenicillin from the urine and 77 per cent of that of ticarcillin, the loss being attributed to conversion to penicilloic acid. The protein binding of ticarcillin is rather higher (65 as against 50 per cent). Haemodialysis reduces its half-life in patients with reduced renal function, but peritoneal dialysis has little effect (Parry & Neu, 1976). Important information on toxicity was obtained by Brown et al (1975) by giving four-hourly intravenous doses of up to 300 mg/kg daily for ten days to 'volunteers obtained through the Texas Department of Corrections' and performing elaborate haematological studies on them. Ticarcillin was no more liable than carbenicillin to cause coagulation disorder, and the lower dose permitted by its higher anti-*Pseudomonas* activity should therefore be safer.

Among studies of therapeutic action that of Rodriguez et al (1973) was conducted in patients with neutropenia following antineoplastic therapy. Various *Ps. aeruginosa* infections responded well, but those due to *Klebsiella* not at all and to *E. coli* (most strains of which were resistant) in only one case out of 11. Ervin and Bullock (1976) treated 28 patients with infections predisposed to in other ways, including 20 with severe pneumonia due to *Ps. aeruginosa* and other Gram-negative species, using doses which although large were less than those of carbenicillin which would have been required, and consider their results encouraging.

UREIDOPENICILLINS

Other derivatives have been described as possessing enhanced anti-Pseudomonas activity, the therapeutic prospects of which nevertheless remain uncertain. Among these are the ureidopenicillins, well reviewed by Rolinson & Sutherland (1973), one of which, *BL-P1654*, was described in our previous edition. Its action on *Ps. aeruginosa* is much affected by inoculum size and it has other disadvantages in relatively low solubility, a very high static : cidal ratio (Sanders & Sanders, 1975), and, according to Bodey et al (1976) in nephrotoxicity. *Sulbenicillin* (α-sulphobenzyl penicillin) is another derivative of which, although it was first described some years ago, little more has been heard. There is still less information on which to assess *PC-904* (Noguchi et al, 1976), which has very high activity but is 96 per cent protein-bound, or *pirbenicillin* (Bodey et al, 1976).

Two further ureidopenicillins have recently been introduced, both Bayer products.

AZLOCILLIN

This compound is distinguished mainly by high activity against *Ps. aeruginosa*: of 100 strains isolated from blood cultures in patients with malignant disease, 75 were inhibited by 12.5 μg/ml (Stewart & Bodey, 1977). Activity was retained against six out of 11 strains resistant to carbenicillin and ticarcillin. Helm et al (1977) treated 30 patients with this infection involving the blood stream, lungs or urinary tract with doses usually of only 4 or 6 g daily, sometimes combined with another antibiotic, with impressive results.

MEZLOCILLIN

This is also highly active against Gram-negative species, but has a broader spectrum. Against *Ps. aeruginosa* its activity is less than that of azlocillin and equal to that of ticarcillin, but *E. coli* (most strains), *Kl. pneumoniae*, *Enterobacter* spp., indole-positive *Proteus* spp. and *S. marcescens* are more sensitive to it than to azlocillin or carbenicillin. A pharmacokinetic study is reported by Issel et al (1978) in which very large doses were tolerated, but no therapeutic results hitherto. In some of these studies a marked inoculum effect was observed in tests with both compounds, and the reason for this emerges from two further reports. Fu & Neu (1978b) determined the rate of hydrolysis of these and three other penicillins by the β-lactamases of Gram-negative species, and found all of them to be unstable to a varying extent; the enzyme from *Ps. aeruginosa*, for instance, hydrolysed both azlocillin and mezlocillin more rapidly than either carbenicillin or ticarcillin. Basker et al (1979a) confirm instability to this enzyme, and add that the β-lactamase of *Kl. pneumoniae* hydrolyses the two new compounds but not cefazolin. These differences are reflected not only in *in vitro* tests with varied inoculum, but in the results of mouse protection tests. The virtue of very high activity in the two new compounds may therefore have to be partly discounted by reason of their β-lactamase instability.

PIPERACILLIN

This was originally synthesized in Japan, but is being manufactured in the United States by Lederle. Its outstanding virtue is very high activity against *Ps. aeruginosa*; Verbist (1978) found the mean MIC for 60 strains to be 3.4 μg/ml, those of carbenicillin and ticarcillin being 37.6 and 16.4 μg/ml. Fu and Neu (1978a) also determined MIC for 14 carbenicillin-resistant strains, the mean being carbenicillin 340, mezlocillin 87, azlocillin 43 and piperacillin 19 μg/ml. Thus there is some degree of all round cross-resistance, but piperacillin remains the most active compound. On the other hand, all authors are agreed that there is a wide divergence between MIC and MBC, some strains examined by Milne and Waterworth (1978) not being killed by piperacillin even at 512 μg/ml. For other species MIC and MBC differ little. Activity is also good against *K. pneumoniae*, *S. marcescens*, *H. influenzae* and *Neisseria* spp. but undistinguished on Gram-positive cocci. Synergy with gentamicin and with amikacin has been demonstrated. Evans et al (1978) studied pharmacokinetics after intravenous injection, confirming that piperacillin behaves much like related compounds and elicits no ill effects.

AMIDINO PENICILLINS

MECILLINAM

Lund & Tybring (1972) of Leo Pharmaceutical Products report a study of 6-βamidinopenicillanic acids, a new group of substances among which the most active was mecillinam. The activity of this substance, compared with that of benzylpenicillin and ampicillin, is low against all Gram-positive species, but remarkably high against *E. coli*, the IC_{50} for four strains varying from 0.016 to 0.1 μg/ml. It is also much greater than that of ampicillin against some strains of *Klebsiella* spp. and of *P. mirabilis* and various other Gram-negative organisms including *Serratia marcescens*. Like other β-lactam antibiotics, mecillinam has bactericidal activity, mitigated by increased osmolality, and induces cell wall changes which lead to the production of spherical osmotically fragile forms. These differ from spheroplasts, however, in that a proportion of them not only survive but actively grow in the presence of the agent without osmotic protection. Such phenotypically resistant variants revert to bacillary form on subculture but retain their resistance to mecillinam for several generations. (Greenwood & O'Grady 1973.)

Tybring (1975) and Tybring & Melchior (1975) give a good account of these and later laboratory studies, mentioning that protein binding is only 5 to 10 per cent, and including observations on the development of resistant variants, on susceptibility to β-lactamase, and on the features of bactericidal action. This was followed in broth inoculated with *E. coli* and containing 1 μg/ml mecillinam, by serial viable counts and by turbidimetry. Turbidity increased while the count fell, owing to the production of swollen forms. The fall in count was slower than that caused by ampicillin and was inoculum-dependent. The extent of lysis varied inversely with the NaCl content of the medium; other salts and sucrose had the same protective effect. According to Neu (1976a) activity is affected not only by osmolality but by conductivity, but this has been disputed. Finally they found the swollen cells highly sensitive to ampicillin, and claimed, not very convincingly, to have demonstrated a synergic effect on *E. coli* and other enterobacteria of mecillinam + ampicillin. This effect has nevertheless been amply confirmed in later studies by Neu (1976b) and by Grunberg et al (1976); it is exerted by mixtures of mecillinam not only with ampicillin but with other penicillins and cephalosporins.

These combinations have not yet been tested clinically at the time of writing. Mecillinam, which has to be given parenterally, or its orally administrable ester, pivmecillinam, the pharmacokinetics of which have been studied by Williams et al (1976) have been used with some success in the treatment of urinary tract infections (Verrier Jones and Asscher, 1975) and of enteric fever (Clarke et al, 1976). Mandal et al (1979) report very disappointing results in 12 patients with enteric fever, only three responding promptly, four more slowly and five not at all. All strains were initiallly sensitive and, so far as could be observed, remained so.

Inhibitors of β-lactamases

As many bacteria owe their resistance to penicillins (and cephalosporins) to the generation of potent β-lactamases, the possibility arises (and this has been pursued intermittently for a long time) that the activity of unstable compounds could be restored by combining them with potent β-lactamase inhibitors. The most recent and most promising of such inhibitors is clavulanic acid.

CLAVULANIC ACID

This is a product of *Streptomyces clavuligerus*, one of several including cephalosporins and penicillin N, and was first detected by workers in the Beecham Pharmaceuticals Research Division; Reading and Cole (1977) describe its production, isolation, chemical structure, which is that of a penicillin, and some of its activities. It has little anti-bacterial activity—indeed none against most species in the concentrations used—but is a very powerful β-lactamase inhibitor. As an example, Jackson et al (1978) tested it against a multi-resistant strain of *Kl. pneumoniae* which had been causing cross-infection for several years in their hospital in Nashville, Tennessee. The mean MIC of cephalothin for strains of this organism was 376 μg/ml, but in the presence of 1, 5 and 10 μg/ml of clavulanic acid this fell to 2, 1.5 and 0.7 μg/ml. Not all differences are as extreme as this, and inoculum size is one of several factors affecting them. The β-lactamases inactivated according, among others, to Wise et al (1978), who made tests with penicillin, amoxycillin and carbenicillin, include that of *Staph. aureus* but not of *B. cereus*, those of *Esch. coli*, *Kl. pneumoniae*, *Pr. mirabilis*, *Bacteroides* spp., *H. influenzae* and *N. gonorrhoeae*, but not those of indole-positive *Proteus*, *Serratia*, most *Enterobacter* spp. or usually *Ps. aeruginosa*. Organisms possessing intrinsic resistance will naturally retain this; likewise sensitivity to cefoxitin, which is resistant to β-lactamases, is unaffected. A fixed ratio combination with amoxycillin is now undergoing extensive clinical trials.

References

Acred P, Hunter P A, Mizen L, Rolinson G N 1971a Antimicrobial Agents and Chemotherapy 1970 p 416

Acred P, Hunter P A, Mizen L, Rolinson G N 1971b Antimicrobial Agents and Chemotherapy 1970 p 396

Anderson K N, Kennedy R P, Plorde J J, et al 1964 J Amer Med Ass 187: 555

Ayliffe G A J, Davies A 1965 Brit J Pharmacol 24: 189

Ayliffe G A J, Lowbury E J L, Roe E 1972 Nature (New Biol) 235: 141

Baldwin D S, Levine B B, McCluskey R T, Gallo G R 1968 New Engl. J. Med 279: 1245

Barber M 1964 J Gen Microbiol 35: 183

Barber M, Waterworth P M 1964 Brit Med J 2: 344

Basch H, Erickson R, Gadebusch H 1971 Infection Immunity 4: 44

Basker M J, Edmondson R A E, Sutherland R 1979a Infection 7: 67

Basker M J, Gwynn M N, White A R 1979b Chemotherapy 25: 170

Batchelor F R, Chain E B, Richards M, Rolinson G N 1961 Proc Roy Soc B 154: 522

Batchelor F R, Doyle F P, Nayler J H C, Rolinson G N 1959 Nature (Lond) 183: 257

Benner E J, Kayser F H 1968 Lancet 2: 741

Bergeron M G, Brusch J L, Barza M, Weinstein L 1976 Amer J Med Sci 271: 13

Bergholtz L, Hallander H, Rudberg R 1973 Scand J Infect Dis 5: 203

Blecher T E, Edgar W M, Melville H A H, Peel K R 1966 Brit Med J 1: 137

Bodey G P, Rodriguez V, Weaver S 1976 Antimicrob Agents Chemother 9: 668

Bodin N O, Ekstrom B, Forsgren U, et al 1975 Antimicrob Ag Chemother 8: 518

Bond J M, Lightbrown J W, Barber M, Waterworth P M 1963 Brit Med J 2: 956

Brauninger G E, Remington J S 1968 J Amer Med Ass 203: 103

Brogden R N, Speight T M, Avery G S 1975 Drugs 9: 88
Brown C H III, Natelson E A, Bradshaw, et al 1975 Antimicrob Agents Chemother 7: 652
Brown D M, Acred P 1961 Brit Med J 2: 197
Bulger R J 1967 Lancet 1: 17
Chabbert Y A, Baudens J G, Acar J F, Gerbaud G R 1965 Rev Franc Clin Biol 10: 495
Clarke P D, Geddes A M, McGhie D, Wall J C Brit Med J 1976 2: 14
Comber K R, Osborne C D, Sutherland R 1975 Antimicrob Agents Chemother 7: 179
Cooper R G, Rice J C, Penfold J L 1969 Med J Aust 1: 517
Croydon E A P, Sutherland R 1971 Antimicrobial Agents and Chemotherapy 1970 p 427
Daehne von W, Frederiksen E, Gundersen E et al 1970 J Med Chem 13: 607
Darrell J H, Waterworth P M 1969 Brit Med J 3: 141
Doyle F P, Long A A W, Nayler J H C, Stove E R 1961 Nature (Lond) 191: 1183
Dyke K G H, Jevons M P, Parker M T 1966 Lancet 1: 835
Eickhoff T C, Kislak J W, Finland M 1965a New Engl J Med 272: 699
Eickhoff T C, Kislak J W, Finland M 1965b Amer J Med Sci 249: 163
English A R, Retsema J A, Ray V A, Lynch J E 1972 Antimicrob Agents Chemother 1: 185
Ervin F R, Bullock W E 1976 Antimicrob Agents Chemother 9: 94
Evans M A L, Wilson P, Leung T, Williams J D 1978 J Antimicrob Chemother 4: 255
Foltz E L, West J W, Breslow I H, Wallik H 1971 Antimicrobial Agents and Chemotherapy 1971 p 442
Fu K P, Neu H C 1978a Antimicrob Agents Chemother 13: 358
Fu K P, Neu H C 1978b Antimicrob Agents Chemother 13: 930
Gadebusch H, Miraglia G, Pansy F, Renz K 1971 Infection Immunity 4: 50
Geddes A M 1973 Current Antibiotic Therapy (ed) A M Geddes, J D Williams. Churchill Livingstone, Edinburgh p 231
Gravenkemper C F, Bennett J V, Brodie J L, Kirby W M M 1965 Arch Intern Med 116: 340
Greenwood D, O'Grady F 1973 J Clin Path 26: 1
Grunberg E, Cleeland R, Beskid G, DeLorenzo W F 1976 Antimicrob Agents Chemother 9: 589
Hamilton-Miller J M T 1965 J Gen Microbiol 41: 175
Hellström K, Rosén A, Swahn Å 1974 Clin Pharmacol Ther 16: 826
Helm E B, Ristow W, Schacht P M, Schacht P, Stille W 1977 Dtsch Med Wschr 102: 1211
Hertz C G 1973 Antimicrob Agents Chemother 4: 361
Höffler D, Stegemann I, Scheler F 1966 Dtsch Med Wschr 91: 206
Hunter P A, Rolinson G N, Witting D A 1973 Antimicrob Agents Chemother 4: 285
Issell B F, Bodey G P, Weaver S 1978 Antimicrob Agents Chemother 13: 180
Jackson R T, Harris L F, Alford R H 1978 Antimicrob Agents Chemother 14: 118
Jokinen K, Raunio V 1975 Acta Otolaryngol 79: 460
Jordan M C, de Maine J B, Kirby W M M 1971 Antimicrobial Agents and Chemotherapy 1970 p 438
Kamme C, Ursing B 1974 Scand J Infect Dis 6: 273
Kayser F H, Hollinger A 1968 Dtsch Med Wschr 93: 1933
Kind A C, Tupasi T E, Standiford H C, Kirby W M M 1970 Arch Intern Med 125: 685
Kislak J W, Eickhoff T C, Finland M 1965 Amer J Med Sci 249: 636
Kjellander J O, Finland M 1963 Proc Soc Exp Biol (NY) 113: 1031
Klein J O, Finland M 1963 Amer J Med Sci 246: 10
Klein J O, Sabath L D, Steinhauer B W, Finland M 1963 Amer J Med Sci 246: 385
Knudsen E T, Rolinson G N, Stevens S 1961 Brit Med J 2: 198
Knudsen E T, Rolinson G N, Sutherland R 1967 Brit Med J 3: 75
Kunin C M 1966 Clin Pharmacol Ther 7: 166
Lane W R 1964 Med J Aust 2: 499
Leigh D A, Reeves D S, Simmons K, Thomas A L, Wilkinson P J 1976 Brit Med J 1: 1378
Levitt B H, Gottlieb A J, Rosenberg I R, Klein J J 1964 Clin Pharmacol Ther 5: 301
Lowbury E J L, Kidson A, Lilly H A, Ayliffe G A J, Jones R J 1969 Lancet 2: 448
Lund F, Tybring L 1972 Nature (New Biol) 236: 135
MacNair D R, White J E, Graham J M 1968 Lancet 1: 16

Mandal B K, Ironside A G, Brennand J 1979 Brit Med J 1: 586
Milne S E, Waterworth P M 1978 J Antimicrob Chemother 4: 247
Mortimer P R, Mackie D B, Haynes S 1969 Brit Med J 3: 88
Naumann P 1965 Dtsch Med Wschr 90: 1085
Naumann P, Kempf B 1965 Arzneimittel Forsch 15: 139
Nauta E H, Mattie H 1975 Brit J Clin Pharmacol 2: 111
Nayler J H C, Long A A W, Brown D N, et al 1962 Nature (Lond) 195: 1264
Neu H C 1976a Antimicrob Agents Chemother 9: 793
Neu H C 1976b Antimicrob Agents Chemother 10: 535
Neu H C, Garvey G J 1975 Antimicrob Agents Chemother 8: 457
Neu H C, Winshell E B 1971a Antimicrobial Agents and Chemotherapy 1970 p 385
Neu H C, Winshell E B 1971b Antimicrobial Agents and Chemotherapy 1970 p 423
Noguchi H, Eda Y, Tobiki H, Nakagome T, Komatsu T 1976 Antimicrob Agents Chemother 9: 262
Parker M T, Hewitt J H 1970 Lancet 1: 800
Parry M F, Neu H C 1976 J Infect Dis 133: 46
Pillay N, Adams E B, North-Coombes D 1975 Lancet 2: 333
Reading C, Cole M 1977 Antimicrob Agents Chemother 11: 852
Report from six hospitals 1962 Lancet 2: 634
Report 1973 Croydon E A P, and 13 others Brit Med J 1: 7
Richards H C, Housley J R, Spooner D F 1963 Nature (Lond) 199: 354
Rodriguez V, Bodey G P, Horikoshi N, et al 1973 Antimicrob Agents Chemother 4: 427
Roe E, Jones R J, Lowbury E J L 1971 Lancet 1: 149
Roholt K, Nielsen B, Kristensen E 1974 Antimicrob Agents Chemother 6: 563
Rolinson G N, Stevens S 1961 Brit Med J 2: 191
Rolinson G N, Sutherland R 1973 In: Advances in Pharmacology and Chemotherapy Vol II. Academic Press Inc, New York & London
Rosenblatt J E, Kind A C, Brodie J L, Kirby W M M 1968 Arch Intern Med 121: 345
Rozencweig M, Staquet M, Klastersky J 1976 Clin Pharmacol Ther 19: 592
Ruiz D E, Warner J F 1976 Antimicrob Agents Chemother 9: 554
Sanders C C, Sanders W E 1975 Antimicrob Agents Chemother 7: 435
Scragg J N, Rubidge C J 1975 Amer J Trop Med Hyg 24: 860
Seeliger H P R, Laymann V, Finger H 1967 Dtsch Med Wschr 92: 1095
Seeliger H, Matheis H 1969 Dtsch Med Wschr 94: 853
Shapiro S, Slone D, Siskind V, Lewis G P, Jick H 1969 Lancet 2: 969
Siboni K, Poulsen E D 1968 Dan Med Bull 15: 161
Sidell S, Bulger R J, Brodie J L, Kirby W M M 1964 Clin Pharmacol Ther 5: 26
Simon C, Junk W, Malerczyk V 1976 Arzneim-Forsch (Drug Res) 26: 424
Simon C, Leuth M, Malerczyk V 1974a Dtsch Med Wschr 99: 2460
Simon C, Nehls R, Malerczyk V, et al 1974b Dtsch Med Wschr 99: 137
Simon H J, Sakai W 1963 Pediatrics 31: 463
Sjoberg B, Ekstrom B, Forsgren U 1968 Antimicrobial Agents & Chemotherapy 1967 p 560
Sleet R A, Sangster G, Murdoch J McC 1964 Brit Med J 1: 148
Stewart D, Bodey G P 1977 Antimicrob Agents Chemother 11: 865
Sutherland R, Croydon E A P, Rolinson G N 1970 Brit Med J 4: 455
Sutherland R, Burnett J, Rolinson G 1971 Antimicrobial Agents & Chemotherapy 1970 p 390
Sutherland R, Croydon E A P, Rolinson G N 1972 Brit Med J 3: 13
Sutherland R, Rolinson G N 1964a J Bact 87: 887
Sutherland R, Rolinson G N 1964b J Clin Path 17: 461
Sutherland R, Rolinson G N 1971 Antimicrobial Agents and Chemotherapy 1970 p 411
Symposium 1973 J Infect Dis 127: Suppl May
Symposium 1974 J Infect Dis 129: Suppl June
Turck M, Ronald A, Petersdorf R G 1965 J Amer Med Ass 192: 961
Tybring L 1975 Antimicrob Agents Chemother 8: 266
Tybring L, Melchior N H 1975 Antimicrob Agents Chemother 8: 271
Verbist L 1978 Antimicrob Agents Chemother 13: 349
Verrier Jones E R, Asscher A W 1975 J Antimicrob Chemother 1: 193
Weingartner L, Ortel S 1967 Dtsch Med Wschr 92: 1098
Wilkinson P J, Reeves D S, Wise R, Allen J T 1975 Brit Med J 2: 250

Williams J D, Andrews J, Mitchard M, Kendall M J 1976 J Antimicrob Chemother 2: 61
Wise R, Andrews J M, Bedford K A 1978 Antimicrob Agents Chemother 13: 389
Woodruff M W, Covert S V, Litinsky S M, Vanneman W M 1971 New York State Med J 71: 1087
Yurchenco J A, Hopper M W, Vince T D, Warren G H 1970 Chemotherapy 15: 209

Penicillins. Pharmaceutical preparations and dosage

Name	*Dosage*	*Preparations*	*Common International proprietary names*
Benzylpenicillin	600 mg are equivalent to 1 000 000 U (1 mega unit) *Adult* i.m. i.v.: 300–600 mg every six hours. In septicaemia and endocarditis much larger doses may be given. Intrathecal injection: the maximum daily dose is 12 mg. Oral: 250–500 mg four times a day. *Children* i.m. i.v.: 15–45 mg/kg body weight daily in divided doses. Intrathecal injection: 1.5–3 mg daily. Oral: 62.5–250 mg four times a day, depending on age.	i.m., i.v., i.t. injection (sodium salt) Tablets 250 mg, Syrup 125 mg, 250 mg in 5 ml (potassium salt)	Crystapen, Crystapen G (UK) Pfizerpen G, QIDpen G (USA) Spécilline G, Nece-Pen (Fr) Pharmacillin (Ger)
Procaine penicillin	*Adult* 300 mg i.m. every 12 or 24 hours. *Children* less than 25 kg body weight, the dose is a proportion of the adult dose.	i.m. injection 300 mg per ml *also* in combination with Benzylpenicillin as Fortified Procaine Penicillin	Depocillin, Penidural AP Bicillin (UK) Crysticillin AS, Pfizerpen-AS (US) Flocilline (Fr)
Benzathine penicillin Benzathine benzyl-penicillin (rINN) Penicillin G benzathine (USP)	*Adults* Oral: 450 mg three to four times a day i.m.: 1.2 mega units every 5–7 days. *Children* Oral: 225 mg three to four times a day or 112.5 mg four to six times a day. i.m.: 0.3–0.6 mega units every 5–7 days.	Suspension 225 mg in 5 ml Oral drops 112.5 mg in 1 ml i.m. injection 225 mg (300 000 U) per ml	Penidural, Penidural LA (UK) Permapen (USA) Extencilline (Fr) Tardocilline (Ger)
Phenoxymethyl penicillin Penicillin V (USP)	*Adults* 250–500 mg every 4–6 hours depending on the severity of the infection. *Children* 125–250 mg every six hours. *Infants* 62.5–125 mg every six hours.	Tablets and Capsules 125 mg 250 mg Syrup 125 mg 250 mg in 5 ml Sachets 125 mg single dose (potassium salt) Suspension 125 mg in 5 ml (calcium salt)	Crystapen V, V-Cil-K, Distaquine V-K (UK) Beromycin, Isocillin (Ger) Paclin V-K, V-Cillin, SK-Penicillin VK (USA) Oracilline, Ospen (Fr)
Phenethicillin	*Adults* 250 mg four times a day. *Children* 2–10 years 125 mg four times a day, under two years, 62.5 mg four times a day.	Tablets, capsules 250 mg Syrup 125 mg in 5 ml (as Potassium salt)	Broxil (UK) Maxipen, Ro-cillin (USA) Pen-200 (Ger) Péniplus, Synthécilline (Fr)

Name	*Dosage*	*Preparations*	*Common International proprietary names*	
Propicillin	*Adults* Oral: 500 mg–1.5 g daily in 4–6 divided doses, before meals. *Children* (under 12 years) 62.5–125 mg every 4–6 hours.	Tablets Syrup	Baycillin, Oricillin Brocilline (No proprietary preparation is available in the UK)	(Ger) (Fr)
Methicillin	*Adult* i.m., i.v.: 1 g every 4–6 hours, the dose may be increased for severe infections. *Children* i.m., i.v.: (2–10 years) 500 mg every 4–6 hours, and under two years, 250 mg every 4–6 hours.	Injection 1 g	Celbenin Azapen Cinopenil Flabelline, Penistaph	(UK) (USA) (Ger) (Fr)
Cloxacillin	*Adult* Oral: 500 mg four times a day, 1 hour before food. i.m.: 250 mg every 4–6 hours, i.v.: 500 mg every 4–6 hours. The dose may be increased for severe infections *Children* 2–10 years, half the adult dose, and under two years, one quarter the adult dose.	Capsules 250 mg 500 mg Syrup 125 mg in 5 ml Injection 250 mg 500 mg	Orbenin Cloxypen, Orbenine Staphobristol Tegopen	(UK) (Fr) (Ger) (USA)
Flucloxacillin Floxacillin (USAN)	*Adult* Oral: 250 mg four times a day. i.m., i.v.: 250–500 mg four times a day. The dose may be increased for severe infections. The dose for children is a proportion of the adult dose, as for cloxacillin.	Capsules 250 mg Syrup 125 mg in 5 ml Injection 250 mg 500 mg	Floxapen Staphlex	(UK) (Ger)
Oxacillin	*Adult* Oral 500 mg–1 g 4–6 times a day. i.m., i.v.: 250 mg–1 g every 4–6 hours. *Children* less than 40 kg: 50–100 mg/kg body weight daily in 4–6 divided doses. Premature infants 25 mg/kg daily in divided doses.	Oral solutions Capsules 250 mg 500 mg Injection	Bactocill Stapenor, Cryptocillin Bristopen Not available in the UK	(USA) (Ger) (Fr)
Ampicillin	*Adult* 1–6 g daily in four divided doses. *Children* The dose is a proportion of the adult dose as for cloxacillin. All oral doses should be taken ½ an hour before food.	Capsules 250 mg 500 mg Injection 100 mg 250 mg 500 mg Syrup 125, 250 mg in 5 ml Paediatric suspension	Penbritin SK Ampicillin, Totacillin Penbritine, Totapen and many other names	(UK) (USA) (Fr)
Amoxycillin	*Adult* oral: 250–500 mg every eight hours. For acute urinary tract infections two single doses of 3 g may be given. i.v.: 1 g every six hours for severe infections. *Children* Oral: 125 mg every eight hours. i.m., i.v.: 50–100 mg/kg body weight, daily in divided doses.	Capsules 250 mg 500 mg Syrup 125 mg 250 mg in 5 ml Injection 250 mg 500 mg 1 g Paediatric suspension Sachets 3 g	Amoxil Clamoxyl Polymox, Larotid	(UK) (Ger) (USA)

Carbenicillin	*Adult* i.m., i.v.: 5g every 4–6 hours. *Children* i.m.: 50–100 mg/kg body weight daily in divided doses. i.v.: 250–500 mg/kg body weight in 4–6 divided doses.	Injection 1g, 5g	Pyopen Microcillin Geopen	(UK) (Ger) (USA)
Carfecillin Carbenicillin phenyl sodium (USAN)	*Adult* Oral: 500 mg–1 g three times a day. *Children* Oral: 30–60 mg/kg daily in three divided doses.	Tablets 500 mg	Uticillin	(UK)
Ticarcillin	*Adult* i.m., i.v.: 15–20 g a day in divided doses every 6–8 hours. *Children* i.m., i.v.: 200–300 mg/kg body weight daily in divided doses every 6–8 hours.	Injection 1 g 5 g	Ticar	(UK) (USA)
Talampicillin	*Adult* Oral: 250–500 mg three times a day depending on the severity of the infection. 1.5–2 g as a single dose for Gonorrhoea.	Tablets 250 mg	Talpen	(UK)
Mecillinam	*Adult* i.m., i.v.: 10 mg/kg every six hours, for severe Gram-negative infections. For urinary tract infections 5 mg/kg every six hours.	Injection 400 mg	Selexidin	(UK)
Pivmecillinam	*Adult* Oral: 600 mg–2.4 g daily in 3–4 divided doses, depending on the severity of the infection.	Tablets 200 mg Sachet 100 mg	Selexid	(UK)
Epicillin	*Adult* Oral: 250–500 mg every six hours. *Children* (less than 20 kg weight) 50–100 mg/kg body weight, daily in divided doses.	Tablets	Dexacillin	(USA)
Carindacillin	(1.4 g Carindacillin is approximately equivalent to 1 g Carbenicillin.) Doses equivalent to 382–764 mg of Carbenicillin every six hours are given.	Tablets	Carindapen Geocillin	(Ger) (USA)
Azlocillin	*Adult* as i.v. bolus or infusion: 2–5 g every 6–8 hours.	Injection 2 g 5 g	Not yet available in the UK	
Mezlocillin	*Adult* i.m., i.v.: 2–5 g every 6–8 hours. *Neonate* 75 mg per kg 12 hourly	Injection 1 g 2 g 5 g	Baypen	(UK)

4

Cephalosporins

The discovery of this group of antibiotics is a much stranger and more complex story than that of penicillin. Moreover, although for rather different reasons, the time which elapsed between the discovery of the organism and final therapeutic application of its purified products was even longer—nearly twenty years. On the other hand the original discoverer had systemic therapeutic use in mind from the beginning, and used a crude product in this way. He was Professor G. Brotzu, of Cagliari, Sardinia, who in 1945 made cultures from sea water at a sewage outfall on the assumption that this might contain organisms antagonistic to intestinal pathogens, and isolated a fungus which he identified as *Cephalosporium acremonium.* Fluid cultures contained a substance active against various pathogens, and crude extracts were administered parenterally with some success for the treatment of typhoid fever and brucellosis. These findings were published in *Lavori dell'Istituto d'Igiene di Cagliari,* a journal not in the World List, and might have remained unknown to the rest of the world had not the late Dr C.O.S. Blyth Brook, who had been public health officer in Sardinia during the war, written to Florey telling him of Brotzu's work. A culture of the cephalosporium was received in Oxford in August, 1948, and the second stage of the work began.

The extraordinary initial findings were well described by Florey (1955) and more fully later by Abraham (1962). They proved that the fungus produced not one antibiotic but seven. These comprised, first, five variants of cephalosporin P, an antibiotic of steroid structure resembling fusidic acid. Cephalosporin N, subsequently named adicillin, is a penicillin with a side chain derived from D-α-aminoadipic acid, less active than benzyl penicillin against Gram-positive organisms, but more so against some Gram-negative species including *S. typhi,* and identical with synnematin B, isolated from a *Tilachlidium* by Gottshall et al (1951). Although it gave promising results in the treatment of typhoid fever (Benavides et al, 1955) adicillin has not been further exploited. Lastly, and at first undetected, was cephalosporin C, and it is from this product that all the present cephalosporins in therapeutic use are derived.

CEPHALOSPORIN C

The existence of this substance among the products of the mould was not even detected for several years, and the yield was at first so small that great difficulty was experienced in obtaining enough for essential laboratory tests. It has the same side chain as cephalosporin N, attached to a nucleus now known as 7-aminocephalosporanic acid, the structure of which is here compared with that of 6-aminopenicillanic acid.

The degree of anti-bacterial activity of cephalosporin C is only moderate, but the property which attracted most attention, at that time unique among antibiotics of this general structure, was a high degree of resistance to staphylococcal penicillinase; moreover it competitively inhibited the action of penicillinase on benzyl penicillin (Abraham & Newton, 1956). It was shown to be therapeutically active in mice and to have a very low toxicity.

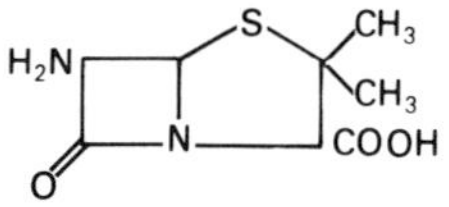

6-amino-penicillanic acid

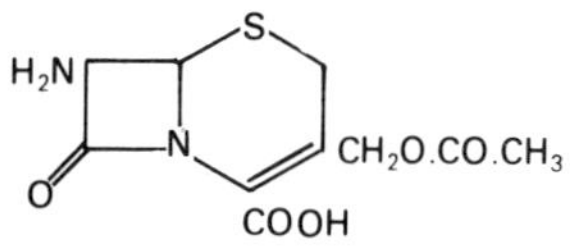

7-amino-cephalosporanic acid

Thanks to the prophetic foresight of its discoverers, determined and prolonged attempts were made to obtain an adequate yield, and when this had been achieved, chemical manipulations, similar to those being applied at the same time to the penicillin nucleus, were undertaken to improve its performance. Whereas the side chain determining the identity of a penicillin is always attached at the same point, substitution in the cephalosporin nucleus can take place at two or even three. In derivatives so obtained anti-bacterial activity is greatly increased, and two of these, cephalothin and cephaloridine, have been in therapeutic use since 1964. Others have followed, and the choice has been widened by the introduction of many new products, the relative merits of which cannot yet be fully assessed. Indeed in very recent times the pace of their discovery has much increased; some have not yet passed the stage of laboratory study, and others, although their therapeutic action has been verified, are still not yet available.

GENERAL PROPERTIES OF CEPHALOSPORINS

As is to be expected from their similarity in chemical structure, cephalosporins have much in common with penicillins. They are bactericidal, and have the same action on the bacterial cell wall. They are in general highly active against staphylococci, and resistant to staphylococcal penicillinase, although it has since proved that the degree of this resistance varies among different members of the group. Their efficacy in staphylococcal infections, and the fact that they could usually be given safely to patients sensitized to penicillin, were leading advantages claimed at an early stage. (Subsequent experience has qualified this claim; according to Dash (1975) nine per cent of penicillin-sensitive patients react to cephalosporins.) Streptococci, except *S. faecalis*, and pneumococci are even more sensitive. Many Gram-negative species are also sensitive, including Neisseria spp., Haemophilus (although only to a moderate degree), *Esch. coli*, *Salmonella* spp., some *Klebsiella* spp. and *Proteus mirabilis*, including penicillinase-forming strains, the latter constituting an advantage over all penicillins. Pseudomonas spp. are highly resistant to all but the latest derivative, cefotaxime. Table 4.1 (p. 102) gives the MIC of 14 cephalosporins for various species. This can only be a rough guide as many species show wide strain variations and some said to be resistant may include sensitive strains. MIC are often much affected by the size of the inoculum, which makes comparisons difficult. Some of the later derivatives are stable to the β-lactamases formed by enterobacteria other than *P. mirabilis* and consequently have a broader spectrum, although this is sometimes partly balanced by reduced activity in other directions.

The cephalosporins share the non-toxicity of penicillin except that renal tubular damage may be caused by some of them, and by one in particular. In their main pharmacokinetic properties they differ little, except as the effect of two factors, their degree of stability and the extent of protein binding, which varies widely. The amount of pain caused by intramuscular injection is another factor which may affect choice of the route of administration or even of the compound to be used. What has been said so far refers to cephalosporins given only by injection, which are not absorbed by the alimentary route. But there are now also several orally administrable products, better absorbed in fact than almost any other antibiotic so administered, which require separate consideration. A general comparison of the pharmacokinetic properties of the principal cephalsporins is given in Table 4.3 (p. 107).

The following account of individual drugs follows mainly the classification proposed by O'Callaghan (1975). The structures of most of these are shown in Figure 4.1, the arrangement of which is adopted from that of Moellering & Swartz (1976).

CEPHALOTHIN

This derivative, one of the first to come into use, was marketed by Lilly in the United States and for a time exclusively used there. It is one of three acetoxymethyl cephalosporins (the others being cephacetrile and cephapirin) retaining the 3-acetoxy group of cephalosporin C (O'Callaghàn, 1975). These compounds have a serious drawback in instability, being reduced by esterases to the corresponding desacetyl compound, which has relatively little anti-bacterial activity. Hence the peak blood level attained is lower and maintenance of an adequate level less prolonged, than those achieved with more stable compounds. In early studies by Kunin & Atuk (1966) it was observed that the half-life of cephalothin even in 'severely oliguric' patients is comparatively short; thus no reduction of dose is indicated on account of renal impairment. The usual dose is 1 g at 6- or 4-hour intervals, and 12 g daily or even more have been given for severe infections. A second drawback is that intramuscular injection causes moderate to severe pain, and intravenous injection is usually resorted to for this reason. About 65 per cent of the drug in the blood is protein-bound. Penetration into the cerebrospinal fluid in meningitis is inferior to that of penicillin, a defect shared with most other cephalosporins. It is even on record that patients being treated with cehaphalothin for infections elsewhere have developed meningitis due to sensitive organisms, some of which were in the blood stream, at an early stage of the treatment (Mangi et al, 1973). Excretion is mainly renal, and tubular.

Just as cephalothin has two drawbacks in comparison with cephaloridine—which for years was its only rival—it has also two advantages. One is a much lesser degree of nephrotoxicity, and the second much greater stability to staphylococcal penicillinase. It thus earned the reputation of being the safer of the two, and for staphylococcal infections the more dependable. It no longer seems necessary to review the earlier literature on its clinical uses, since these are now familiar. A recent change in the method of its use is worth mentioning. Whereas for years it was usually given alone, much more than before it is now administered in combination with a second antibiotic, often gentamicin, either for the treatment of staphylococcal or various Gram-negative infections, or as either preventive or blind treatment in seriously predisposed patients.

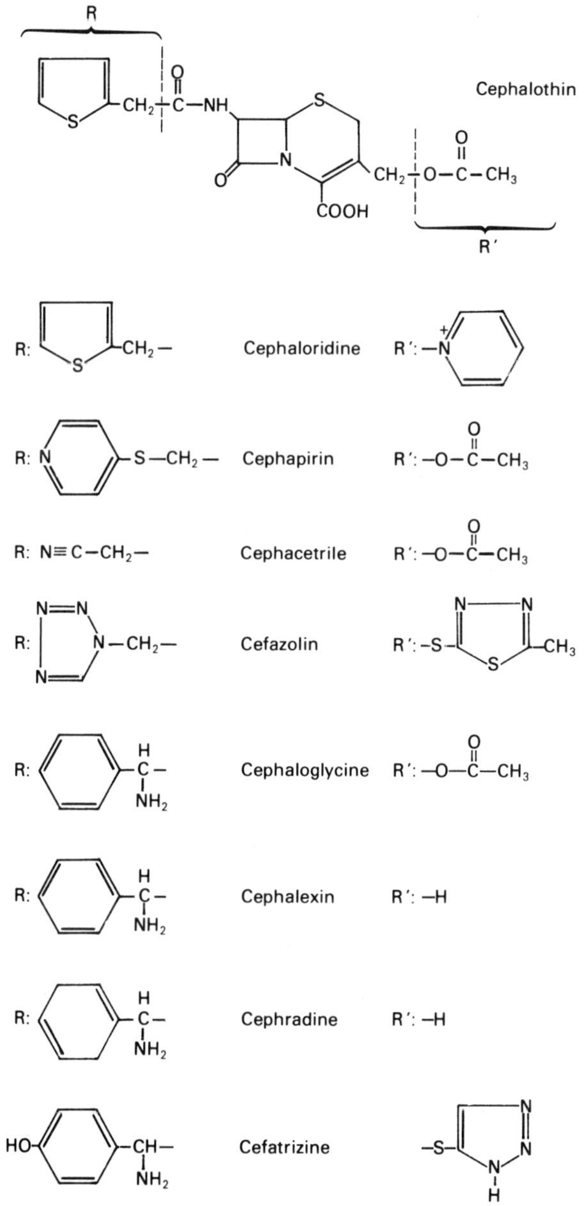

Fig. 4.1 Structure of Cephalosporins.

The following two other derivatives in this class are available only in other countries, and we are thus unable to write from practical experience of them. Both were introduced some years after cephalothin.

CEPHAPIRIN

This has an anti-bacterial spectrum almost identical with that of cephalothin, and has been used in similar doses for the same indications. Its short half-life in the blood suggests a similar degree of instability. The main claim made for this product is better local toleration, both in regard to pain after intramuscular injection and to the incidence of phlebitis after intravenous injection, but even this has not been fully accepted.

CEPHACETRILE

This has been more extensively studied (Maurice et al, 1973: Kradolfer et al, 1974). A profusion of pharmacokinetic data is mainly non-comparative with other derivatives, but many results of assays in blood and urine suggest at least a lesser degree of instability in the body than that of cephalothin. An important claim, substantiated by the findings of Meyer-Brunot et al (1975) is for exceptionally good penetration, for a cephalosporin, into the cerebrospinal fluid, although here again directly comparative data are lacking. In ten patients with acute bacterial meningitis concentrations of 5 to >20 μg/ml were attained on the first day of treatment after an intravenous dose of 3 g, the highest levels being reached after that in the blood was falling. On the fifth day they were much lower, indicating dependence on the inflammatory state of the meninges, although still mostly at 2 to 4 μg/ml.

CEPHALORIDINE

This derivative was introduced by Glaxo in Great Britain at about the same time as cephalothin in the United States, and for five years they were the only such products available. It has several advantages over cephalothin. Its activity against staphylococci, group A streptococci and pneumococci exceeds that of cephalothin by a factor of 2 to 8, although against most Gram-negative species they perform about equally (Barber & Waterworth, 1964; see Table 13, page 69 in the fourth edition of this book). It is stable in the body and therefore attains higher and better sustained blood levels. It is protein-bound only to the extent of 20 per cent. Unlike cephalothin it is excreted via the glomeruli. Finally, intramuscular injections are painless.

To set against these properties are two drawbacks. One is much less resistance to staphylococcal penicillinase than was at first believed. Although earlier observations contain some hint of this, it was first quantified by Ridley & Phillips (1965) and by Benner et al (1965) and dramatically illustrated in a patient of Burgess & Evans (1966) with staphylococcal endocarditis, whose blood cultures remained positive despite the demonstrated presence of high concentrations of the antibiotic in the blood. Subsequent studies embracing as many as eight cephalosporins (Regamey et al, 1975; Fong et al, 1976) have confirmed the high degree of susceptibility of cephaloridine to destruction by staphylococcal penicillinase, exceeded only by that of cefazolin. Bell

(1974) points out that a conventional disc test may fail to reveal this, and strongly criticizes the United States requirement that sensitivity to all cephalosporins be judged by a test performed with cephalothin. He proposes a broth dilution test with a heavy inoculum read after two days as more informative, and Lacey & Stokes (1977) suggest a heavily inoculated plate with a 2-hour period of growth before the antibiotic is introduced. The amount of penicillinase formed by resistant strains of staphylococci varies very widely, and is greatest in strains which are also methicillin-resistant. The suitability of cephaloridine for treating a staphylococcal infection could be assessed by measuring this, but it is clearly safer to use a derivative such as cephalothin which is highly resistant to the enzyme. For treating any life-endangering infection combination with an aminoglycoside is also advisable.

The second drawback of cephaloridine is nephrotoxicity. Although other cephalosporins share this effect, demonstrable by large doses in animals, in which necrosis of the proximal convoluted tubules occurs, smaller doses of cephaloridine produce it, and its consequences have been seen in patients. Like many other antibiotic side effects it was late in being recognized, although suspicion might have been aroused by the fact that only moderate doses produce many hyaline casts in the urine. Larger doses—8 g daily or more—have unquestionably sometimes caused increasing proteinuria with a raised blood urea, going on in some cases to oliguria and renal failure, the lesion responsible being tubular necrosis. We ourselves know of several patients in whom in retrospect it seems that this must have occurred, although the reason for it was unsuspected at the time. In severely ill patients renal failure is not uncommon and may be produced in other ways, but careful observers with extensive experience of the use of this drug (Kaplan et al, 1968; Steigbigel et al, 1968) have satisfied themselves that it has sometimes been responsible for renal damage. It is now recognized that diuretics, which may also be indicated in such patients, enhance the renal toxicity of cephaloridine; this was demonstrated for both frusemide and ethacrynic acid by Dodds & Foord (1970). This is therefore a drug combination to be avoided.

With these two provisos cephaloridine remains a valuable drug for its very high activity, particularly against Gram-positive organisms, its high blood levels, low protein binding and perfect local toleration; it has been successfully used in a wide variety of infections.

CEFAZOLIN

This derivative, originally synthesized in Japan (Nishida et al, 1970) and first made available in this country by Eli Lilly in 1974, has many properties in common with cephaloridine, one being metabolic stability. It is rather less active against staphylococci and at least equally unstable to their penicillinase (Regamey et al, 1975). On the other hand it is rather more active than cephaloridine against *Esch. coli* and some other enterobacteria. Blood levels attained are twice those of cephaloridine and well sustained, but protein binding is about 80 per cent, and when this is allowed for, it may be seen that levels of *free* antibiotic in the blood are lower than those of cephaloridine (Fig. 4.2). This difference is confirmed in an another way by Bergeron et al (1973), who found that the serum of treated patients was less bactericidal than that of those given the same dose of cephaloridine. An outstanding property is the attainment of high concentrations in the bile, shown by Brogard et al (1975) by several methods to exceed those of other cephalosporins. This led Strachan et al (1977) to administer a single dose pre-operatively in biliary surgery, with gratifying results in reducing subsequent wound sepsis. Nephrotoxicity in animals is low and has not been reported in man. Good therapeutic results have been reported in a variety of infections, but without special emphasis (except in the urinary tract) on those caused by enterobacteria, which seem from the spectrum of the drug to indicate its use most clearly.

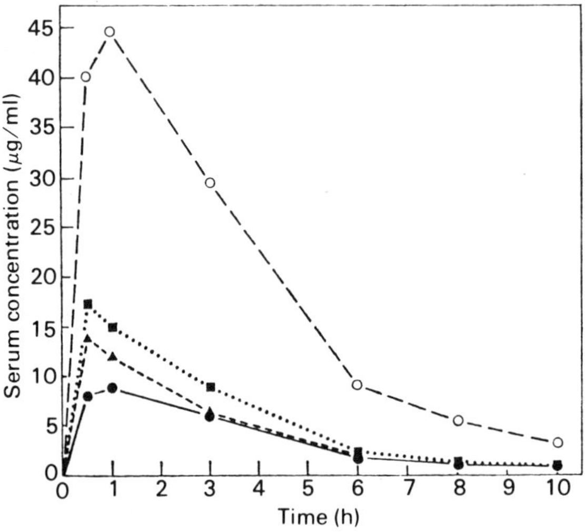

Fig. 4.2 Human serum levels of cephaloridine and cefazolin after one intramuscular dose of 500 mg . . . = total cephaloridine - - - = cephaloridine after allowing for 20 per cent serum binding. — — = total cefazolin; —— = cefazolin after allowing for 80 per cent serum binding. (O'Callaghan, 1975; reproduced with the author's and editor's permission.)

ORALLY ADMINISTRABLE CEPHALOSPORINS

It may be regarded as a drawback of the earlier cephalosporins that they have to be administered several times a day by injection, which virtually confines them to hospital use. This was nevertheless claimed as an advantage of cephalosporin C by early investigators because it promised to ensure discriminating use. Some of the following orally administrable forms are now widely prescribed by practitioners of all kinds, and are understood to have been a great commercial success, although whether the benefits they have conferred are commensurate with their cost seems doubtful. Some of the purposes for which they have been used are often equally well served by one of the penicillins.

CEPHALOGLYCIN

This derivative appears now to be only of historical interest. The first such product to be introduced (Wick & Boniece, 1965) it is in fact very poorly absorbed, only about 10 per cent of a dose being excreted in the urine, and this almost entirely as desacetyl cephaloglycin, but this has most of the anti-bacterial activity of the parent substance (Wick et al, 1971). Blood levels are too low to ensure a dependable systemic effect, and the drug has been used for treating urinary tract infections. Even for this purpose later derivatives are far preferable.

CEPHALEXIN

This derivative, introduced by Glaxo in 1969, has very different properties, and has attained widespread popularity. Its anti-bacterial spectrum is similar to that of earlier cephalosporins, but with a somewhat lower degree of activity against most species, particularly Gram-positive cocci (Thornhill et al, 1969). Usually accepted MIC of cephalothin, cephaloridine and cephalexin for penicillin-sensitive strains of *Staph. aureus* are 0.5, 0.25 and 2.0 μg/ml respectively.

Its action is particularly weak on *H. influenzae*, and the only Gram-negative organisms out of 23 varieties against which its activity was found to exceed that of cephalothin and cephaloridine were ampicillin-resistant strains of *Esch. coli* (Waterworth, 1971). In the light of later work this is evidently due to its stability to β-lactamase of type IIIa.

On the other hand its pharmacokinetic properties are almost ideal. Unlike most orally administered antibiotics it is very well absorbed: mean 1-hour blood levels after doses of 250, 500 and 1000 mg were 5.8, 17.6 and 25 μg/ml, falling to 0.6, 1.5 and 3.1 μg/ml at 4 hours. It is excreted unchanged in the urine, 85 to 96 per cent being recoverable in 6 hours (Perkins et al, 1968). The degree of protein binding is only 11 per cent. Cephalexin sodium is an injectable form, commended by Svensson & Seeberg (1974) for the initial treatment with large doses for severe infections, oral administration being substituted later. It can be argued that if the parenteral route is to be used at all, it would be better to take advantage of the greater anti-bacterial activity of one of the derivatives administrable solely by injection.

Cephalexin has been widely used, mainly for urinary and respiratory infections. Apart from its convenience of administration, which has placed cephalosporin therapy within the reach of all, its merits remain to be fully assessed. A balanced view, in which alternatives for most indications are discussed, is offered by Finland (1972).

CEPHRADINE

This product, introduced in 1973, may be seen from Figure 4.1 to differ very little in structure from cephalexin, and as would be expected from this, their anti-bacterial spectrum and all pharmacokinetic properties are almost identical. Like cephalexin it has been widely used for similar indications. Both an oral and an injectable product are available and this is claimed to be an important advantage, but the argument advanced above with regard to parenteral cephalexin also applies here.

Cephradine has an enthusiastic advocate in Selwyn (1976), who ranks cephalosporins on the basis of seven characters, for all of which cephradine is accorded the highest mark. One of these is resistance to staphylococcal β-lactamase, as demonstrated by a new method (Selwyn, 1977). Basker et al (1980) were unable to obtain consistent results by this technique and using several orthodox methods in a wide-ranging study of the action of the staphylococcal enzyme on penicillins and

Table 4.1 Antibacterial spectra of cephalosporins. R = MIC > 32 μg/ml. Many strains show wide strain variation and considerable inoculum effect

	Cephalo-ridine	Cephalo-thin	Ceface-trile	Cefazo-lin	Cepho-glycin	Cepha-lexin	Cephra-dine	Cefatri-zine	Cefa-droxil	Cefa-chlor	Cefa-mandole	Cefoxi-tin	Cefuro-xime	Cefo-taxime
Staph. aureus	0.25	0.5	1	0.25	2	2	2	0.5	2	4	0.5	4	1	2
Staph. aureus penicillinase positive	4	0.5	2	2	4	2	2	2	4	8	2	4	1	2
Str. pyogenes	0.01	0.12	0.5	0.25	0.12	0.5	0.5	0.12	0.5	0.25	0.12	0.5	0.03	0.06
Str. faecalis	16	32	16	R	R	R	R	R	R	R	32	R	R	2
Str. pneumoniae	0.03	0.06	0.25	0.12	0.25	2	2	0.5	1.0	1.0	0.25	1.0	0.03	
N. gonorrhoeae	0.25	0.25		0.12		0.5	0.5	0.25		0.12		0.25	0.06	0.001
H. influenzae	8	8		8	16	32	32	8	32	2	2	4	0.5	0.03
E. coli	4	8	8	4	2	8	16	8	16	8	4	4	4	0.1
Klebsiella	4	4	8	4	2	8	16	8	16	8	2	4	4	0.1
Enterobacter	R	R	R	R	R	R	R	R	R	R	R	R	8	0.1–R
P. mirabilis	4	4	8	4	2	16	16	8	16	16	2	4	4	0.06
Proteus, indole positive	R	R	R	R	R	R	R	R	R	R	R	8	8	0.2–2
Serratia	R	R	R	R	R	R	R	R	R	R	R	16	8	0.5
Salmonella	2	2	8	2	1	2	8	8	8	2		4	4	0.5
Ps. aeruginosa	R	R	R	R	R	R	R	R	R	R	R	R	R	16–R
Bact. fragilis	32	32			32	R	R			R		4–32	8–64	0.25

Data in Table 4.1 is based on Kradolfer F et al Arzneim-Forsch Drug Res 24: 14–46
Leitner F et al 1975 Antimicrob Agents Chemother 7: 298
Blackwell C C et al 1976 ibid 10: 288
Buck R E, Price K E 1977 ibid 11: 324
Eykyn S et al 1973 ibid 3: 657
Bill N J, Washington J A 1977 ibid 11: 470
Hamilton-Miller J M T et al J Antimicrobial Chemother 4: 437
Finland M et al 1976 J Infect Dis 134: 575
Waterworth P M 1971 Postgrad Med J 47 (Suppl): 25

cephalosporins they showed *inter alia* that the most resistant cephalosporin was cephalothin; cephradine and cephalexin were less resistant to about an equal degree.

CEFATRIZINE

The original announcements (Leitner et al, 1975, a, b) of this product by workers on the staff of Bristol Laboratories, where it was first known as BL-S640, seemed highly encouraging. Comparison of its *in vitro* activity with those of cephalothin, cephaloridine, cefazolin and cephalexin, the latter being included since both are orally administrable, showed it to be highly active against Gram-negative species, particularly against *Esch. coli*, *Klebsiella* and all four *Proteus* spp. It was rather more slowly hydrolysed than the other cephalosporins tested by β-lactamases of types 1a and 1b. Protein binding was found to be 58 per cent. The only adverse finding in the first of these papers is that whereas cefatrizine is fully stable at pH 2.0 its half-life at 7.4 is only 6 hours. The second paper reports favourable pharmacokinetic findings in mice, and very striking therapeutic superiority over all the other four cephalosporins in experimental Gram-negative infections. These findings have not been gainsaid, but later papers are less enthusiastic on other aspects. Blackwell et al, (1976) qualify *in vitro* findings by reporting wide strain variations in sensitivity and dependence on the culture medium used, and Stilwell et al (1975) found also that activity was very inoculum-dependent, particularly in broth. It is generally agreed that most bacteria are more sensitive to cefatrizine than to cephalexin, but according to Actor et al (1976) the peak blood level attained after an oral dose of cefatrizine is much lower than that of cephalexin (e.g., 5.6 and 22.1 μg/ml respectively after 0.5 g) and urinary recoveries in 6 hours were 35 and 68 per cent of the dose. However, the blood level of cefatrizine fell more slowly. Del Busto et al (1976) report similar findings, and add that four daily doses of 0.5 g were given to 33 patients with satisfactory results and no ill effects.

CEFADROXIL

This was compared by Buck & Price (1977) with cephalexin, and in anti-bacterial activity, pharmacokinetic properties including protein binding, and in therapeutic activity in mice only small differences were observed. According to Hartstein et al (1977) cefadroxil (Fig. 4.3) is rather more slowly absorbed and achieves better sustained levels in both blood and urine, which would permit less frequent dosage. Well sustained blood levels in children, little affected by administration with food, were found by Ginsburg et al (1978).

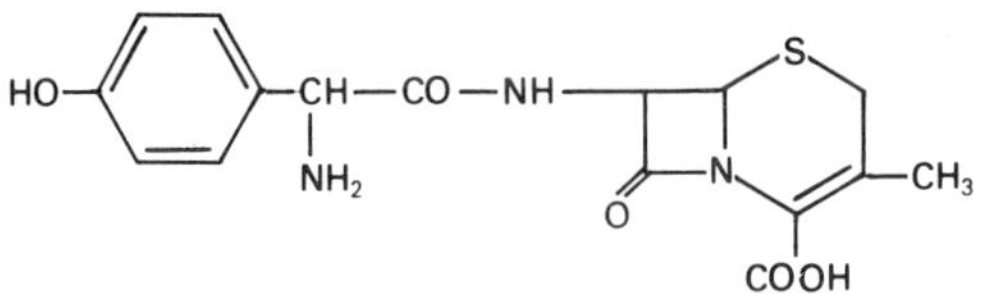

Fig. 4.3 Cephadroxil

CEFACLOR

This has been compared in anti-bacterial activity with cephalexin and cephradine by Bill & Washington (1977), Scheld et al (1977) and by Gillett et al (1979). Cefaclor (Fig. 4.4) is the most active against *E. coli*, *P. mirabilis* and *Kl. pneumoniae*, and notably so against *H. influenzae* and *N. gonorrhoeae*. Its activity is only equal and in some cases inferior against staphylococci and streptococci, and on *Bacteroides fragilis* it is poor. In a study of pharmacokinetics by Korzeniowski et al (1977) the mean peak plasma levels after a 250 mg dose of cefaclor and cephalexin were 6.01 and 9.43 μg/ml, half-lives 0.58 and 0.80 hr and urinary excretion in 6 hour 70.1 and 96.3 per cent of the dose. These differences are now recognized to be due to the instability of cefaclor, which has been found to lose 50 per cent of its activity in broth at 37°C and by Gillet et al (1979) 90 per cent in serum in the same time. This property needs to be taken into account in performing assays; loss is less rapid on the acid side of neutrality. An important question is how far it detracts from the therapeutic merits of cefaclor, and whether it is an indication for rather more frequent dosage.

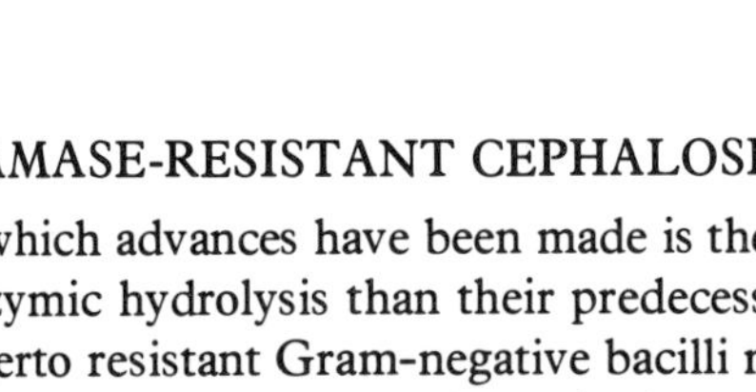

Fig. 4.4 Cefaclor

NEW BETA-LACTAMASE-RESISTANT CEPHALOSPORINS

Another direction in which advances have been made is the synthesis of derivatives less susceptible to enzymic hydrolysis than their predecessors, with the result that infections due to hitherto resistant Gram-negative bacilli may now be amenable to treatment. The β-lactamases formed by such species began to be studied only after the introduction into therapeutic use of ampicillin in 1962, whereas penicillinase formed by Gram-positive species had been recognized up to twenty years earlier. Staphylococcal penicillinase is extracellular and highly inducible. All Gram-negative penicillinases and cephalosporinases are intracellular; only some are inducible and then never to the same degree. The quantitative study of their action therefore requires extraction from cultures and preferably some degree of purification.

These enzymes were classified by Jack & Richmond (1970) into eight types. This list was extended by Richmond & Sykes (1973) to 15, and in a later review by Sykes & Matthew (1976) it has been extended further, while other apparently new enzymes continue to be described. The main basis for their classification is into penicillinases and cephalosporinases, i.e., those acting on both. They are further distinguished by their degree of activity against individual antibiotics in both groups. Some are chromosomally mediated and some by R plasmids. These and other characters have been extensively studied, and the subject has now achieved a high degree of complexity.

It should not be supposed that the resistance of a strain of Gram-negative bacilli to a β-lactam antibiotic depends solely on β-lactamase formation. It varies also with the extent to which the antibiotics can penetrate the outer cell membrane and reach the site of enzyme formation. This property, now known as crypticity, can be measured by comparing the enzyme activity of intact and disrupted cells, and may vary widely. Needless to say, resistance may also be intrinsic.

The question with which we are concerned here is the probable degree of usefulness of these new β-lactamase-resistant cephalosporins. One way in which this can be determined is to measure their rate of hydrolysis by different enzymes. A comparison of this kind was made by Richmond & Wotton (1976) with four representative enzymes. Their main finding is that only cefuroxime and cefoxitin (page 111) are highly resistant to all four. These results are confirmed and extended by the experiments of O'Callaghan detailed in Table 4.2; further reference will be made later to these results. Another method is to determine the sensitivity to these antibiotics of numerous strains of important species. Many comparative studies of this kind have recently been reported; Table 4.1 is based on some of these, but they are difficult to summarize for several reasons, notably strain variation. In the present state of knowledge of this confused subject the only conclusions which can safely be drawn are general: that certain otherwise resistant infections may be amenable to

Table 4.2 Effects of partially purified β-lactamases on some cephalosporin compounds, related to the susceptibility of cephaloridine. (C H O'Callaghan, personal communication, 1979.)

Source of β-lactamase	Type	Rates of hydrolysis relative to CER = 100 CER	CXM	CEM	CET	CEZ	CFX
E. coli R-TEM	III	100	0	63	23	26	0
E. coli R-GN 238	V	100	29	26	93	NT	0
E. coli D31	I	100	0	19	552	78	0
E. coli RP1	II	100	0.6	55	23	25	0
K. aerogenes K1	IV	100	29	150	97	220	0
E. cloacae P99	I	100	0	3	77	94	0
B. fragilis 1600	I	100	13	17	22	22	0
Ps. aeruginosa 1822	I	100	0	0	362	162	0

Key:

CER = cephaloridine
CXM = cefuroxime
CEM = cefamandole

CET = cephalothin
CEZ = cefazolin
CFX = cefoxitin

NT = not tested

treatment with these new products. An *ad hoc* test in a laboratory capable in the first place of fully identifying such bacteria still seems desirable.

Some resistance to Gram-negative β-lactamases has been noted in cephalosporins already described, but this property is a more outstanding feature in those which follow. There is now a considerable literature on three of these, of which only a few items can be quoted here. Their structures are shown in Figure 4.5.

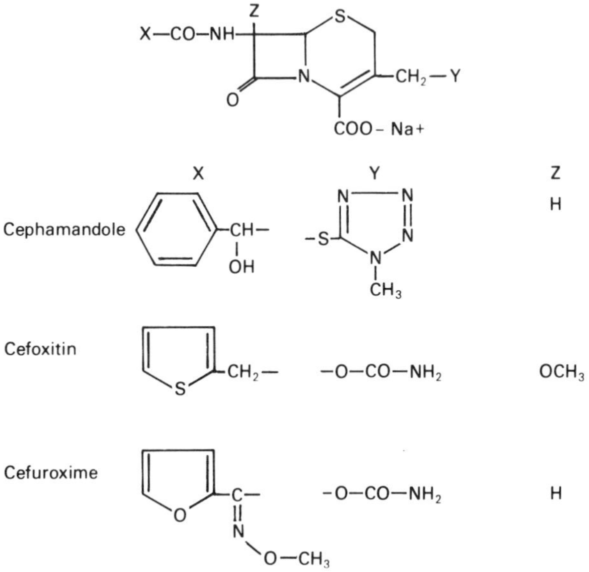

Fig. 4.5 Structures of cephamandole, cefoxitin and cefuroxime. (C. H. O'Callaghan, 1975, reproduced with the authors and editors's permission.)

CEFAMANDOLE

It is interesting that the anti-bacterial activity of this cephalosporin (Fig. 4.5) synthesized by Lilly in the United States, should first have been fully described, and in an American journal, by British authors (Eykyn et al, 1973). From their findings, and those of Neu (1974a), Bodey & Weaver (1976) and Griffith et al 1976) the picture emerges of a drug with full activity against staphylococci and other usually sensitive Gram-positive species, but of particular interest for its action on certain Gram-negatives. One of these is *H. influenzae*; all investigators are agreed that this organism is outstandingly sensitive, most strains being inhibited by 1 μg/ml or less. Among enterobacteria the most notably sensitive species is *Enterobacter cloacae*; the stability of cefamandole to the β-lactamase formed by this organism is fully confirmed in two studies quoted above. *Proteus mirabilis* is also sensitive, but *P. vulgaris* resistant; findings for *P. morgani* and *P. rettgeri* vary. *Esch. coli* resistant to other cephalosporins may or may not be sensitive; in Klebsiella spp. there is no difference. The findings in Table 4.3 show a reduced rate of hydrolysis by several β-lactamases, and emphasize that sensitivity in otherwise resistant species may only be partial. Moreover it is clear from other studies that strain variation plays an important part. Hence the sensitivity of some species is unpredictable and requires confirmation in individual cases.

Table 4.3 Average plasma values for some cephalosporins

	Dose	Plasma peak μg/ml	Half-life hr	Protein bound %
Cefaclor	0.5g	12	0.6–0.8	
Cephalexin	oral	18	0.9–1.2	15
Cephradine		18	0.8–1.3	10
Cephaloridine		40	0.8–1.5	20
Cephalothin		20	0.5–0.8	65
Cefazolin	1g	60	1.4–2.2	80
Cefamandole	i.m.	22	0.5–0.7	70
Cefuroxime		35	1.0–1.2	30
Cefoxitin		20	0.7	70

Administration, either intramuscular or intravenous, is in the form of a more stable ester, cefamandole nafate, which is hydrolysed in the body; its half-life is stated as 13 minutes, but even this delay is unimportant since the ester itself is active. High (although lower than those of cefazolin) and well sustained blood levels are produced; protein binding is about 70 per cent. The unchanged antibiotic is excreted in high concentration in the urine, according to Shemonsky et al (1975) by both glomerular and tubular routes. Among various reports on clinical use two are of particular interest, that by Minor et al (1976) because their study was confined to cases of Gram-negative pneumonia, a hard test in an area to which the drug seems clearly appropriate. Among 17 cases there were only four failures, two being infected by resistant species. A more remarkable finding, although based only on a single case, is the dramatic effect described by Hirschman et al (1977) in severe and neglected typhoid fever. The strain was highly sensitive, as were others despite resistance to chloramphenicol; ampicillin-resistant strains were less so. That *S. typhi* is highly sensitive to cefamandole is also reported by Barros et al (1977).

CEFOXITIN

This is not a cephalosporin but a cephamycin, the most useful of derivatives of cephamycin C synthesized by Merck. This product of the growth of *Streptomyces* spp. is closely similar in structure to cephalosporin C. Accounts of early studies of this and related substances are given by Stapley et al (1972) and Miller et al (1972). It was soon recognized that cefoxitin has a quite unusual anti-bacterial spectrum. It has only about one tenth of the activity of cephalothin against staphylococci (Kosmidis et al, 1973) and other Gram-positive cocci are similarly insensitive, but a high degree of activity against various Gram-negative bacilli, including species resistant to cephalosporins. These authors and Neu (1974b) showed by extracting the enzyme from resistant strains and testing its action on cefoxitin and on cephalosporins that stability to the β-lactamase formed by these organisms is responsible for their sensitivity to cefoxitin. This antibiotic stands alone in not being hydrolysed at all by any of the types of β-lactamase studied in the experiments of O'Callaghan (Table 4.2).

It is nevertheless not possible to compile a definitive table of bacterial sensitivities from these studies and those of Wallick & Hendlin (1974) and Shah et al (1976) because of strain variation and the fact that intrinsic resistance may also play a part. The last-named authors confirm high bactericidal activity, with a 99 per cent kill of *Esch. coli* in $<$60 minutes. Perhaps the most notable activity of cefoxitin is against indole-forming Proteus spp., but activity is retained against various other cephalosporin-resistant enterobacteria, and cefoxitin is also effective against many anaerobic species (see Table 4.1).

Satisfactory pharmacokinetic properties have been demonstrated by Geddes et al (1977), very high concentrations being attained not only in blood and urine but also in bile (but none in cerebrospinal fluid). The half-life is 45 minutes and protein binding only 20 per cent. These authors also treated an impressive series of patients, mainly by the intravenous route, intramuscular injections being painful, including eight patients with septicaemia, six of whom recovered; in one of the failures the infecting organism was a resistant strain of *Enterobacter cloacae*.

CEFUROXIME

The *in vitro* activity of this derivative, synthesized by Glaxo, was first fully described by O'Callaghan et al (1976). It has no special activity against Gram-positive organisms; penicillin-resistant staphylococci are sensitive but methicillin-resistant less so. As compared with cephalothin its activity against Salmonella spp. and Proteus *mirabilis* is about equal, but greater against *Esch. coli* and Klebsiella spp. and much greater against indole-forming Proteus spp. and Enterobacter spp. As may be seen from Table 4.2 it is completely stable to some of the Gram-negative β-lactamases and hydrolysed only slowly by others. Gonococci and *H. influenzae* (including ampicillin-resistant strains) are very sensitive. Eykyn et al (1976) report similar findings, as do Jones et al (1977) from the United States. Greenwood et al (1976), using their own methods, including the 'bladder model' for continuous observation, have confirmed a superior persistent effect in suppressing regrowth of ampicillin-resistant *Esch. coli*.

Ryan et al (1976) report a study of pharmacokinetics in animals and protection tests verifying high therapeutic activity in infections by otherwise resistant Gram-negative species. Protein binding is 33 per cent. Some pharmacokinetic observations in man were made by Norrby et al (1977) during a therapeutic study in 60 patients in Göteborg, Sweden. Treatment was by 8-hourly intramuscular or intravenous injections of doses varying from 0.5 to 2 g. Blood levels 30 minutes after intravenous doses of 1.0, 1.5 and 2 g were 44, 73 and 145 μg/ml; the half-life was about 1½ hours and a mean of 84 per cent of the dose was excreted in the urine in 8 hours. The infections successfully treated were urinary, soft tissue and pulmonary, with ten cases of septicaemia of whom eight recovered. The majority were due to staphylococci or streptococci. Among the enterobacteria isolated, only five out of seven strains of *Esch. coli* were fully sensitive to either cefuroxime or cefoxitin, which was also tested; four of *P. mirabilis* and five of Klebsiella were sensitive to both and one of *P. vulgaris* only to cefoxitin. This series illustrates the difficulty of finding suitable patients in whom to demonstrate the more exclusive virtues of a new antibiotic when these depend on activity against rather uncommon species.

CEFOTAXIME

According to Hamilton-Miller et al (1978) the MIC of this compound (Fig. 4.6) are in a new dimension altogether, lower than those of cefuroxime and cefoxitin by 100-fold

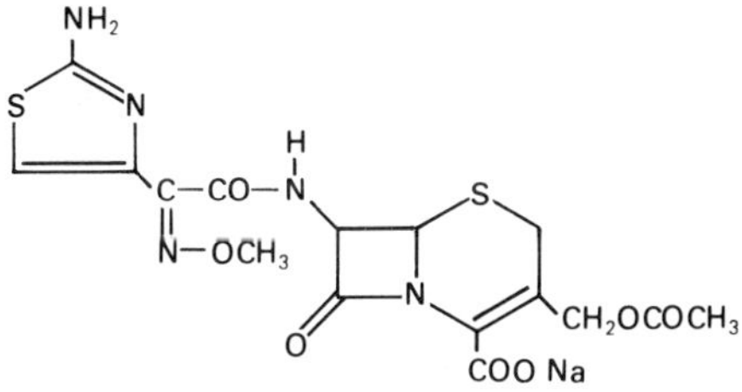

Fig. 4.6 Cefotaxime

or more for many species of Gram-negative bacilli. These include not only those normally cephalosporin-sensitive (geometric mean MIC *E. coli* and *Kl. pneumoniae* 0.063, *P. mirabilis* 0.013) but more resistant organisms (indole-positive *Proteus* 0.048, *Enterobacter* spp. 0.16, *S. marcescens* 0.14, *Citrobacter* spp. 0.13). Other notable MIC are *H. influenzae 0.027 and Ps. aeruginosa* 13.69 μg/ml, four times the activity of carbenicillin for these strains, and a unique property in a cephalosporin. Drasar et al (1978) and other authors report similar findings. The compound is now undergoing extensive clinical trials.

Reference is made on page 476 to the dilemma facing clinical bacteriologists in deciding what tests of sensitivity to perform on the large and growing group of cephalosporins and related compounds.

This is not the end of the list of newly described cephalosporins. They include also ceftezole (Nishida et al, 1976), which seems to differ little from cefazolin, and cefazaflur (Counts et al, 1977), said to be specially active against *Enterobacter* spp., although these authors found wide strain variation and seem somewhat sceptical about its merits. Even some of those which have been much more fully studied during several years are not yet in general use. Difficulties in production may in part account for this, but one may also suspect some hesitation in competing against so many rivals with a product having a limited range of special usefulness.

CLINICAL APPLICATIONS

The wide antibacterial range of the cephalosporins, their favourable pharmacokinetic characteristics and generally low toxicity render them apparently ideal agents in many fields of chemotherapy. As experience in their application has accumulated, however, two paradoxes have emerged. The two chief indications first proposed for them—infection by penicillin resistant staphylococci and infections in penicillin-allergic subjects—are both subject to serious limitations while, despite their favourable properties, there are few identified bacterial infections for which a cephalosporin is the first choice in treatment.

Many patients with penicillin-resistant staphylococcal infections have been successfully treated by cephalosporins, but the relatively poor *in vitro* resistance to β-lactamases of the earlier compounds has been matched by a number of treatment failures in staphylococcal septicaemia and endocarditis, either used alone or in combination with an aminoglycoside. Cephalosporins are also generally unsuitable for the treatment of enterococcal endocarditis. The extent to which these limitations are overcome by the newer cephalosporins and the cephamycins is not yet established. Nor can the general use of cephalosporins be encouraged in penicillin-allergic patients since 9 per cent of patients allergic to penicillin are also allergic to cephalosporins (Dash, 1975). We would be unwilling to use these agents in patients giving a clear history of the more dangerous forms of penicillin allergy, that is, anaphylaxis, angio-oedema, urticaria or severe generalised skin eruptions.

Cephalosporins are widely used in a variety of infections. In the respiratory tract, the oral cephalosporins are an effective alternative to penicillin in streptococcal pharyngitis. Although widely used in bronchitis and pneumonia, they are of course inactive against *M. pneumoniae* and other agents lacking a bacterial cell wall, but the other disadvantage of the earlier compounds, poor activity against *H. influenzae*, is overcome by the newer compounds which show a high degree of *in vitro* activity against this organism.

The wide spectrum of cephalosporins (Table 4.1) has led to their extensive use, often in conjunction with an aminoglycoside, in presumed septicaemias of uncertain cause, although their limitations for this purpose should be noted, namely, those already discussed in relation to staphylococci and enterococci, their lack of activity against Pseudomonas species and against some other species of *Enterobacteriaceae*. Again, these limitations of antibacterial range have been lessened by the development of the newer compounds, e.g. the inhibition of indole-positive Proteus species by cefoxitin. This latter compound is also unusual in its activity against a number of clinically important anaerobes (page 108). In addition to their role in the treatment of Gram-positive and Gram-negative septicaemia, cephalosporins have also been used as agents for short term perioperative prophylaxis in bowel and pelvic surgery (page 343), e.g. Pollock & Evans (1975).

The activity of cephalosporins against the common Gram-negative bacteria associated with urinary tract infections has led to their extensive use for this purpose, reference to which is made in Chapter 21. As regards Gram-negative coccal infections, cephaloridine in a single dose of 2g by intramuscular injections is well established as an alternative treatment for gonorrhoea, and the emergence of penicillinase-producing gonococci has led to the use of the highly β-lactamase resistant compounds in their treatment (page 425).

Cephalosporins should not be used in the treatment of meningitis, with the possible exception of cephaloridine in pneumococcal meningitis (page 327). The potential value of the newer compounds in meningitis caused by penicillin resistant organisms is at present being examined. Cephalosporins generally show poor CSF penetration, so that their use in meningitis can only be justified after very careful pharmacokinetic studies followed by clinical trials.

In spite of their many valuable properties, we seldom find it necessary to use this group of antibiotics, and consider that they are generally too widely employed especially in the forms available for oral administration. The most important positive indications for the use of cephalosporins are first, as a measure of short term perioperative prophylaxis, sometimes in combination with another agent, for selected operations carrying high risk of sepsis (see Chapter 14); and second, as treatment for serious infections caused by specifically identified organisms susceptible to a cephalosporin and resistant to other generally available agents. If the newer agents such as cefuroxime fulfil their promise, they may come to be accepted in another important potential rôle, that of single agent treatment of first choice in presumed septicaemia when circumstances do not indicate Pseudomonas as one of the likely pathogens. Such a policy, if shown effective, would greatly simplify initial treatment of many serious infections by reducing the number of agents administered and especially the need for aminoglycosides.

References

Abraham E P 1962 Pharmacol Rev 14: 473
Abraham E P, Newton G G F 1956 Biochem J 63: 628
Actor P, Pitkin D H, Lucyszyn G et al 1976 Antimicrob Agents Chemother 9: 800
Barber M, Waterworth P M 1964 Brit Med J 2: 344
Barros F, Korzeniowski O M, Sande M A et al 1977 Antimicrob Agents Chemother 11: 1071
Basker M J, Edmondson R A, Sutherland R 1980 J Antimicrob Chemother. In press
Bell S M 1974 Med J Aust 2: 902
Benavides V L, Olson B H, Varelga G, Holt S H 1955 J Amer Med Ass 157: 989
Benner E J, Bennet J V, Brodie J L, Kirkby W M M 1965 J Bact 90: 1599
Bergeron M G, Brusch J L, Barza M, Weinstein L 1973 Antimicrob Agents Chemother 4: 396
Bill N J, Washington J A II 1977 Antimicrob Agents Chemother 11: 470
Blackwell C C, Freimer E H, Tuke G C 1976 Antimicrob Agents Chemother 10: 288
Bodey G P, Weaver S 1976 Antimicrob Agents Chemother 9: 452
Brogard J M, Dorner M, Pinget M, Adloff M, Lavillaureix J 1975 J Infect Dis 131: 625
Buck R E, Price K E 1977 Antimicrob Agents Chemother 11: 324
Burgess H A, Evans R J 1966 Brit Med J 2: 1244
Counts G W, Gregory D, Zeleznik D, Turck M 1977 Antimicrob Agents Chemother 11: 708
Dash C H 1975 J Antimicrob Chemother 1 (Suppl): 107
Del Busto R, Haas E, Madhavan T et al, 1976 Antimicrob Agents Chemother 9: 397
Dodds M G, Foord R D 1970 Brit J Pharmacol 40: 227
Drasar F A, Farrell W, Howard A J et al 1978 J. Antimicrob Chemother 4: 445
Eykyn S, Jenkins C, King A, Phillips I 1973 Antimicrob Agents Chemother 3: 657
Eykyn S, Jenkins C, King A, Phillips I 1976 Antimicrob Agents Chemother 9: 690
Finland M 1972 Drugs 3: 1
Florey H W 1955 Ann Intern Med 43: 480
Fong I W, Engelking E R, Kirkby W M M 1976 Antimicrob Agents Chemother 9: 939
Geddes A M, Schnurr L P, Ball A P et al 1977 Brit Med J 1: 1126
Gillett, A P, Andrews J M, Wise R 1979 Postgrad Med J. 55 (Suppl) 4: 9
Ginsberg C M, McCracken, G H Clahsen J C, Thomas M L 1978 Antimicrob Agents Chemother 13: 845
Gottshall R Y, Roberts J M, Portwood L M, Jennings J C 1951 Proc Soc Exp Biol (NY) 76: 307
Greenwood D, Pearson N J, O'Grady F 1976 J Antimicrob Chemother 2: 337
Griffith R S, Black H R, Brier G L, Wolny J D 1976 Antimicrob Agents Chemother 10: 814
Hamilton-Miller J M T, Brumfitt W, Reynolds A V 1978 J Antimicrob Chemother 4: 437
Hartstein A I, Patrick K E, Jones S R et al 1977 Antimicrob Agents Chemother 12: 93
Hirschman S Z, Meyers B R, Miller A 1977 Antimicrob Agents Chemother 11: 369
Jack G W, Richmond M H 1970 J Gen Microbiol 61: 43
Jones R N, Fuchs P C, Gavan T L et al 1977 Antimicrob Agents Chemother 12: 47
Kaplan K, Reisberg B, Weinstein L 1968 Arch Intern Med 121: 17
Korzeniowski O M, Scheld W M, Sande M A 1977 Antimicrob Agents Chemother 12: 157
Kosmidis J, Hamilton-Miller J M T, Gilchrist J N G, Kerry D W, Brumfitt W 1973 Brit Med J 4: 653
Kradolfer F, Ahrens T, Gelzer J et al 1974 Arzneim-Forsch Drug Res 24: 1446
Kunin C M, Atuk N 1966 New Engl J Med 274: 654
Lacey R W, Stokes A 1977 J Clin Path 30: 35

Leitner F, Buck R E, Misiek M et al 1975a Antimicrob Agents Chemother 7: 298
Leitner F, Chisholm D R, Tsai Y H et al 1975b Antimicrob Agents Chemother 7: 306
Mangi R J, Kundargi R S, Quintiliani R, Andriole V T 1973 Ann Intern Med 78: 347
Maurice P N, Riess W, Welke A, Amson K 1973 Schweiz Med Wschr 103: 718
Meyer-Brunot H G, Schenk C, Schmid K et al 1975 Wien Med Wschr Suppl No 27: 6
Miller A K, Celozzi E, Pelak B A et al 1972 Antimicrob Agents Chemother 2: 281, 287
Miller A K, Celozzi E, Kong Y et al 1974 Antimicrob Agents Chemother 5: 33
Minor M R, Sande M A, Dilworth J A, Mandell G L 1976 J. Antimicrob Chemother 2: 49
Moellering R C Jr, Swartz M N 1976 New Engl J Med 294: 24
Neu H C 1974a Antimicrob Agents Chemother 6: 177
Neu H C 1974b Antimicrob Agents Chemother 6:170
Nishida M, Matsubara T, Murakawa T et al 1970 Antimicrobial Agents and Chemotherapy 1969 p 236
Nishida M, Murakawa T, Kamimura T et al 1976 Antimicrob Agents Chemother 10: 1
Norrby R, Foord R D, Hedlund P 1977 J Antimicrob Chemother 3: 355
O'Callaghan C H 1975 J Antimicrob Chemother 1 Suppl 1
O'Callaghan C H, Sykes R B, Griffiths A, Thornton J E 1976 Antimicrob Agents Chemother 9: 511
Onishi H R, Daoust D R, Zimmerman S B et al 1974 Antimicrob Agents Chemother 5: 38
Perkins R L, Carlisle H N, Saslaw S 1968 Amer J Med Sci 256: 122
Regamey C, Libke R D, Engelking E R, Clarke J T, Kirby W M M 1975 J Infect Dis 131: 291
Richmond M H, Sykes R B 1973 In: Advances in microbial physiology Vol 9 p 31 ed Rose H H, Tempest D W. Academic Press, London, New York
Richmond M H, Wotton S 1976 Antimicrob Agents Chemother 10: 219
Ridley M, Phillips I 1965 Nature Lond 208: 1076
Ryan D M, O'Callaghan, C H, Muggleton P W 1976 Antimicrob Agents Chemother 9: 520
Scheld W M, Korzeniowski O M, Sande M A 1977 Antimicrob Agents Chemother 12: 290
Selwyn S 1976 Lancet 2: 616
Selwyn S 1977 J Antimicrob Chemother 3: 161
Shah P M, Zwischenbrugger H, Stille W 1976 Munch Med Wschr 118: 1469
Shemonsky N K, Carrizosa J, Levison M E 1975 Antimicrob Agents Chemother 8: 679
Stapley E O, Jackson M, Hernandez S et al 1972 Antimicrob Agents Chemother 2: 122
Steigbigel N H, Kislak J W, Tilles J G, Finland M 1968 Arch Intern Med 121: 24
Stilwell G A, Adams H G, Turck M 1975 Antimicrob Agents Chemother 8: 751
Strachan C J L, Black J, Powis S J A et al 1977 Brit Med J 1: 1254
Svensson R, Seeberg S 1974 Scand J Infect Dis 6: 279
Sykes R B, Matthew M 1976 J Antimicrob Chemother 2: 115
Thornhill T S, Levison M, Johnson W W, Kaye D 1969 Appl Microbiol 17: 457
Wallick H, Hendlin D 1974 Antimicrob Agents Chemother 5: 25
Waterworth P M 1971 Postgrad Med J February Suppl: 25
Wick W E, Boniece W S 1965 Appl Microbiol 13: 248
Wick W E, Wright W E, Kuder H V 1971 Appl Microbiol 21: 426

Cephalosporins. Pharmaceutical preparations and dosage

Name	*Dosage*	*Preparations*	*Common international proprietary names*	
Cephaloridine	*Adult* i.m., i.v. 15–30 mg/kg per day in 2 or 3 divided doses. The maximum dose is 40–60 mg/kg daily in 2 to 4 divided doses. The dose varies depending on the severity of the infection being treated. *Children* 20–40 mg/kg daily in divided doses.	Injection 250 mg, 500 mg, 1 g	Ceporin Keflodin Kefspor Loridine	(UK) (Fr) (Ger) (USA)
Cephalothin	*Adults* i.v: 6–12 g daily in 4–6 divided doses. *Children* i.v: 80–160 mg/kg daily in divided doses.	Injection 1 g, 4 g	Keflin Céfalotine Cepovenin	(UK) (Fr) (Ger)
Cephalexin	*Adult* Oral: 1–4 g daily every 6 hours. *Children* Oral: 25–50 mg/kg every 6 hours.	Tablets, Capsules 250 mg, 500 mg Suspension, 125 mg 250 mg, 500 mg in 5 ml	Ceporex, Keflex Ceporexine, Kefcral Oracef	(UK) (Fr) (Ger)
Cephazolin	*Adult* i.m: 500 mg—1 g every 6–12 hours depending on the severity of the infection. The same dose may be given by slow i.v. infusion. *Children* 20–50 mg/kg every 6–8 hours.	Injection 500 mg, 1 g	Kefzol Ancef	(UK) (USA)
Cephradine	*Adult* Oral: 250 mg–500 mg four times a day. i.v., i.m: 2–4 g daily in four divided doses. *Children* Oral: 25–50 mg/kg a day in 2–4 divided doses. i.m., i.v: 50–100 mg/kg a day in four divided doses. The dose may be increased for severe infections.	Capsules 250 mg, 500 mg Syrup 125 mg, 250 mg in 5 ml Injection 250 mg, 500 mg, 1 g	Velosef Auspor Sefril	(UK) (USA) (Ger)
Cefuroxime	*Adults* i.m., i.v: 750 mg every 8 hours, increasing to 1.5 g i.v. every 8 hours, with a maximum dose of 3–6 g daily. *Children* i.m., i.v: 30–100 mg/kg a day in 3–4 divided doses. *Neonates* 30–100 mg/kg daily in 2–3 divided doses.	Injection 250 mg, 750 mg 1.5 g	Zinacef	(UK)

Name	*Dosage*	*Preparations*	*Common international proprietary names*	
Cefoxitin	*Adults* i.m., i.v: 1 g every 8 hours to 2 g every 4 hours depending on the severity of the infection. *Children* (over 2 years) 80–200 mg/kg a day in 3–4 divided doses depending on the severity of the infection.	Injection 1 g, 2 g	Mefoxin	(UK)
Cefamandole	*Adult* i.m., i.v: 500 mg—2 g every 4–8 hours depending on the severity of the infection. *Children* 50–100 mg/kg a day in divided doses every 4–8 hours.	Injection 500 mg, 1 g 2 g.	Kefadol	(UK)
Cefaclor	*Adult* Oral: 250 mg every 8 hours with a maximum of 2 g daily in severe infections. *Children* Oral: 20 mg/kg daily in divided doses every 8 hours. The dose may be increased up to 40 mg/kg daily in severe infections but should not exceed 1 g a day.	Capsules 250 mg Suspension 125 mg, 250 mg in 5 ml	Distaclor	(UK)
Cefapirin	*Adult* i.v., i.m: 500mg—1 g every 4–6 hours, with a maximum of 12 g a day *Children* i.v., i.m: 40–80 mg/kg daily in four divided doses.	Injection	Cefatrexil Bristacef Cefaloject Not available in the UK	(USA) (Ger) (Fr)
Cephacetrile	*Adult* i.v., i.m: 2–4 g daily in mild to moderate infections, increasing to 4–6 g daily if the infection is severe. *Children* i.v., i.m: 50–75 mg/kg daily or 50–75 mg/kg daily for severe infections.	Injection	Celospor Not available in the UK	(Fr, Ger)
Cefotaxime	*Adult* i.m., i.v: 1.5–4 g daily, depending on the severity of the infection. The dose should be given 2, 3, or 4 times daily. *Children* i.m., i.v: 50–150 mg/kg daily in 2–4 divided doses.	Injection	Not yet available in the UK	

5

Aminoglycosides and aminocyclitols

Streptomycin was the first antibiotic to be discovered by means of a systematic examination of soil fungi—a process that was to yield the great majority of subsequently discovered natural antibiotics. Closely related compounds have accumulated over the years but there has recently been a great surge of interest in the whole group for three reasons. Firstly, there was the discovery that a member of the group, gentamicin, is active against the generally very resistant and increasingly important Pseudomonas. Secondly, there was the discovery that the greater part of clinically significant acquired resistance to agents of the group is due to the ability of resistant bacteria to degrade the antibiotics enzymatically. This raised the possibility that chemical modifications of the natural agents might yield a new generation of derivatives resistant to microbial degradation, and hence active against organisms resistant to the parent agent, in the way that semi-synthetic penicillins were made that are resistant to staphylococcal penicillinase. Thirdly, the kind of chemical manipulations required by such modifications and even total synthesis of some agents, were made possible by major advances in the extraordinarily difficult chemistry of the group.

The group is now a large one of which a number are therapeutically important. They are all potent bactericidal agents that share the same general range of antibacterial activity, similar pharmacokinetic behaviour, a tendency to damage one or other branch of the eighth nerve and some tendency to cause renal damage, or at least to impair further the function of an already damaged kidney. The degree of toxicity varies; in some it is such as to preclude systemic use.

Chemistry and pharmacy

The therapeutically important members of the group are typified by the presence of aminosugars glycosidically linked (hence the name 'aminoglycoside') to aminocyclitols. Their structure requires that properly they should be described as 'aminoglycosidic aminocyclitols', but the name 'aminoglycosides' is now too well established to be easily displaced by a more cumbersome title. At the extremes of the group are two compounds that are peculiar, in that one (kasugamycin, Fig. 5.1) contains an aminoglycoside but no aminocyclitol—and is hence a 'pure aminoglycoside'—and the other (spectinomycin, Fig. 5.1) contains an aminocyclitol but no aminoglycoside and is hence a 'pure aminocyclitol'.

The main agents are divided by Rinehart (1969) into two groups according to whether the contained aminocyclitol is streptidine (or a close relative) or deoxystreptamine. The streptidine group includes streptomycin, dihydrostreptomycin and

Kasugamycin

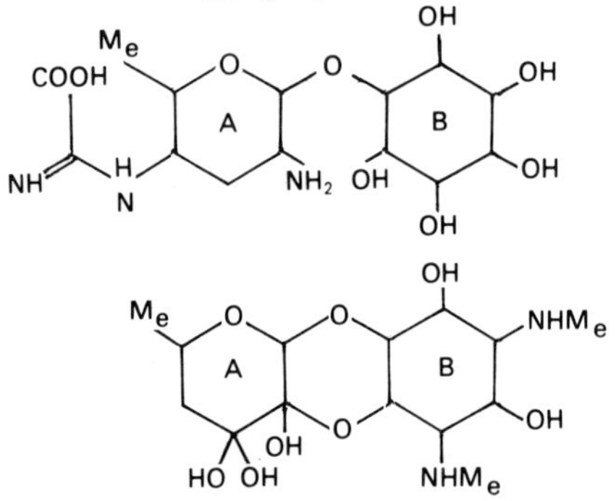

Spectinomycin

Fig. 5.1 Structures of kasugamycin, a 'pure aminoglycoside' (the sugar ring, A, has amino substituents, but the cyclitol ring, B, has none) and spectinomycin, a 'pure aminocyclitol' (the cyclitol ring, B, has amino substituents, but the sugar ring, A, has none)

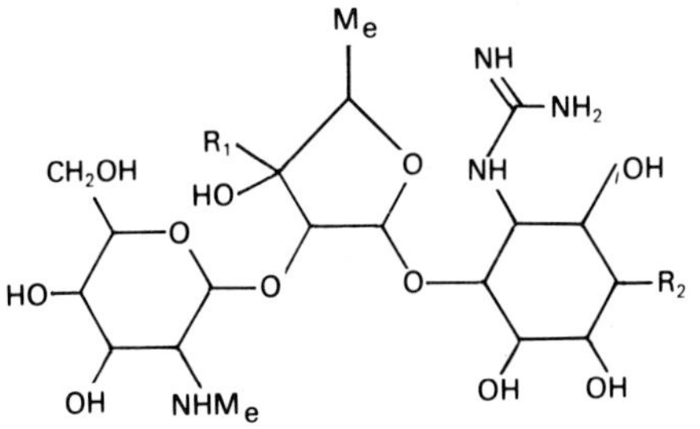

	R_1	R_2
Streptomycin	-CHO	NH-C(=NH)-NH$_2$
Dihydro-streptomycin	-CH$_2$OH	NH-C(=NH)-NH$_2$
Bluensomycin	-CH$_2$OH	-O-C(=O)-NH$_2$

Fig. 5.2 Structures of streptomycin and its relatives

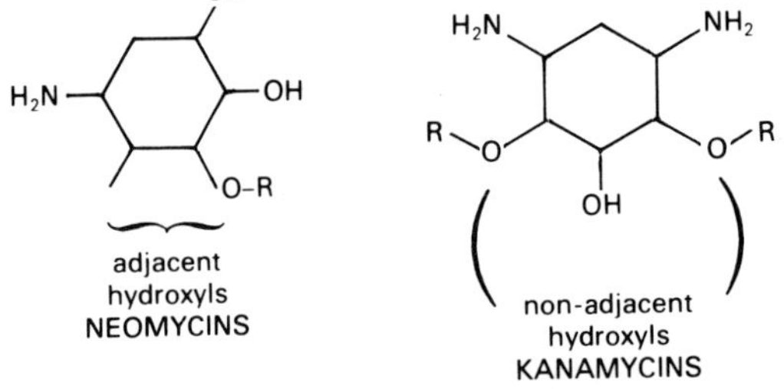

Fig. 5.3 Aminoglycosides are divided into two major groups according to the position of attachment of other rings to the aminocyclitol nucleus. In neomycins (Fig. 5.4), the substituted hydroxyl groups are adjacent and in kanamycins (Fig. 5.5), non-adjacent

bluensomycin (Fig. 5.2). The deoxystreptamine group is more complex and several of the members consist of mixtures of closely related compounds. There are, for example, two neomycins, three kanamycins and numerous gentamicins. Moreover, there are very close relationships between some of the differently named compounds. For example, substitution of an amino- for a hydroxyl group in paromomycin I gives neomycin B (Fig. 5.4) and tobramycin is deoxy-kanamycin B (Fig. 5.5).

The deoxystreptamine group is subdivided into two according to whether the deoxystreptamine nucleus is substituted on adjacent or non-adjacent hydroxyl groups (Fig. 5.3). The 'adjacent' group (conveniently called 'the neomycin group') contains butirosin, the neomycins, paromomycins and ribostamycin. The 'non-adjacent' group contains kanamycin, tobramycin and their semisynthetic derivatives and the important subgroup of gentamicin and its relatives. The chemical differences are important in determining not only the intrinsic activity of the compounds but particularly their resistance to degradation by bacterial enzymes (page 137).

KASUGAMYCIN

The 'pure aminoglycoside', kasugamycin (Fig. 5.1) was discovered by Umezawa et al (1965) during their search for agents active against a fungus disease of rice. The drug shows generally weak antibacterial activity but has a number of interesting features. Therapeutically, attention has been paid to its activity against mycobacteria, pseudomonas (MIC 12–25 μg per ml) and more recently (Kitaoka et al, 1976), leptospira. An interesting feature of its antibacterial activity is that (as with nalidixic acid and some other agents) a plasmid has been found in some strains of *Escherichia coli* that confers not the customary resistance but hypersusceptibility to the drug (Danbara & Yoshikawa, 1975). The most striking contrast with major aminoglycosides is that up to 40 per cent of the drug can be recovered from the urine after oral administration. After a dose of 1 g i.v. peak plasma concentrations are around 100 μg/ml and after the same dose i.m. between 20 and 25 μg/ml at 1–2 hours. The plasma half life is around 3 hours and peak concentrations in the urine exceed 1000 μg/ml. The drug has been used to some effect in the treatment of Pseudomonas urinary infection but anorexia, often severe, is relatively common and this combined with a suggestion (Misiek et al, 1970) of nephrotoxicity, has deprived kasugamycin of the therapeutic interest afforded to the 'pure aminocyclitol', spectinomycin.

SPECTINOMYCIN

Originally called aminospectacin, spectinomycin (Fig. 5.1) was recovered by Mason et al (1961) from the fermentation products of *Streptomyces spectabilis* and subsequently by Oliver et al (1962) from the products of *Streptomyces flavopersicus*. It is not a particularly active compound (Table 5.1) and such activity as it shows is markedly affected by medium composition and enhanced by increased pH. For most organisms the minimum bactericidal concentration is at least four times that of the MIC and the agent is regarded as essentially bacteristatic. In contrast, it is bactericidal for gonococci in concentrations close to the MIC, which is of the order of 2–16 μg per ml for both penicillin-sensitive and resistant strains. Plasma concentrations produced by intramuscular doses have been reported to be 60–80 μg per ml

Table 5.1 Susceptibility of common bacteria to spectinomycin

	MIC μg/ml
Staph. aureus	16–128
Str. pyogenes	2–8
Str. pneumoniae	4
Str. faecalis	16–128
Cl. welchii	64
N. gonorrhoeae	4–16
N. meningitidis	8–32
Esch. coli	8–16
Klebsiella	8–R
Aerobacter	4
Pr. mirabilis	32–64
Proteus, indole +	16–64
Salmonella	4–16
Shigella	4–8
Serratia	16–R
Pseudomonas	32–R

Based on data from:
Levy J et al 1973 Antimicrob Ag Chemother 3: 335
Martin J E Jr et al 1965 Antimicrob Ag Chemother 1964 p 437
Mason D J et al 1962 Antimicrob Ag Chemother 1961 p 965
Washington J A II, Yu P K W 1972 Antimicrob Ag Chemother 2: 427

1 hour after 25 mg per kg (Barry & Koch, 1963) and 40 to 160 μg per ml 1 hour after a dose of 3 g. The plasma half-life is of the order of 2–3 hours. There is a suggestion of nephrotoxicity and treatment of urinary tract infection has not infrequently failed through the emergence of resistance. The therapeutic use of the drug has consequently been restricted to the treatment of penicillin-resistant gonorrhoea for which it has been very successful (page 425).

STREPTIDINE-AMINOGLYCOSIDES

Amongst the members of the streptidine group only streptomycin is important in human therapeutics and with the accumulation of other agents, even it is restricted (with somewhat exotic exceptions, page 124) to a declining use in tuberculosis and the treatment of certain cases of bacterial endocarditis (page 291).

Dihydrostreptomycin is obtained by catalytic reduction of streptomycin but it is also produced naturally by *Streptomyces humidus* (Imamura et al, 1956). Its structure is shown in Figure 5.2 and its properties are described in earlier editions of this book. It closely resembles streptomycin in most respects but as it is much more liable to produce deafness it has no place in clinical use.

Bluensomycin, discovered in the research laboratories of the Upjohn Company as a product of *Streptomyces bluensis* va *bluensi* (Mason et al, 1963) has not been made available for therapeutic use.

STREPTOMYCIN

After more than ten thousand micro-organisms had been examined, Schatz et al (1944) recorded the isolation of streptomycin from a strain of *Streptomyces griseus*, found in a diagnostic culture from a chicken's throat.

Streptomycin (Fig. 5.2) is readily soluble in water and is a strong base, usually supplied as the sulphate which causes the least pain and irritation at the site of injection. Streptomycin sulphate is very soluble in water and almost insoluble in alcohol. Watery solutions are acid, those containing 250 mg/ml having a pH as low as 4.5. Solutions are stable for long periods at a pH between 3 and 7 and a temperature below 18 °C; solutions kept in the cold retain their potency for at least a year.

Antibacterial activity

Streptomycin is particularly active against *Mycobacteria*, Gram-negative bacilli and some strains of staphylococci. Streptococci and pneumococci are relatively resistant, and anaerobic sporing bacilli and fungi almost completely insensitive (Table 5.2).

Table 5.2 Sensitivity of bacteria to streptomycin

Gram-negative Bacteria	MIC μg/ml	Gram-positive Bacteria	MIC μg/ml
E. coli	2– 4	*Staph. aureus*	2
Kl. aerogenes	2	*Str. pyogenes*	32
Kl. pneumoniae	1	*Str. pneumoniae*	64
Proteus spp.	4–>256	*Str. faecalis*	64–>256
Ps. aeruginosa	16–64	*Clostridium* spp.	>128
Salm. typhi	8–16		
Salm. paratyphi	4– 8	*Myco. tuberculosis*	0.5
Salm. spp.	4–16		
Sh. sonnei	2– 4		
Sh. flexneri	2– 8		
N. gonorrhoeae	4		

The antibacterial activity of streptomycin is greatest in a slightly alkaline medium (pH 7.8) and is considerably reduced in media with a pH of 6.0 or less. Streptomycin is so sensitive to the effect of pH that the natural acidity of a solution of streptomycin sulphate may be sufficient to depress its antibacterial activity. Krauss et al (1968) found that 20 μg/ml streptomycin sulphate (pH 7.1) inhibited a strain of pneumococci, while 50 μg/ml (pH 6.8) failed to do so. It is less active under anaerobic conditions, but some strains of anaerobic cocci are inhibited by from 2.0 to 10.0 μg/ml.

Streptomycin is actively bactericidal, a population of 10^7 staphylococci per ml being completely extinguished in eight hours by 20 μg streptomycin per ml, and by 50 and 200 μg/ml in four and two hours respectively. Thus, unlike penicillin, which has a quite low optimum concentration for bactericidal effect, above which no enhancement is obtainable, streptomycin behaves like an ordinary germicide, the velocity of its bactericidal action increasing progressively with rise in concentration.

Acquired resistance

Increase in resistance to streptomycin often occurs after only a few passages in the presence of the antibiotic *in vitro* or within a few days (for the tubercle bacillus a few weeks) of the beginning of streptomycin treatment and resistance of many species is now common. Some streptomycin-resistant strains have a reduced growth-rate and virulence, but many appear to be as virulent as their sensitive parents.

Resistance arises from several distinct mechanisms. High level resistance results from a single step mutation which alters one of the 20 or so proteins which go to make up the ribosomes (page 255) so that binding of streptomycin to the ribosome is reduced (Chang & Flaks, 1970). Low level resistance is due to decreased uptake of the antibiotic (Gundersen, 1967). An important therapeutic consequence of this is seen in enterococci, wild strains of which show two distinct levels of resistance (Standiford et al, 1970). Moderate resistance (MIC 62–500 μg/ml) is due to impermeability of the bacterial cell which prevents the drug reaching its sensitive ribosome. This impermeability can be overcome by simultaneous exposure to agents, such as penicillin, which interfere with synthesis of the bacterial cell wall (page 257) where the permeability barrier is presumably located. As a result strains showing moderate resistance to streptomycin exhibit synergy with penicillin (page 292). In contrast, strains showing high levels of resistance (MIC 1000 μg/ml) have ribosomes which are resistant to streptomycin and hence simultaneous treatment with penicillin is without effect (Zimmermann et al, 1971).

R factor mediated resistance (page 266) is different in that genetic material transferred during conjugation confers on the recipient cell the capacity to synthesize a specific enzyme which destroys streptomycin. All 54 streptomycin-resistant wild strains of *E. coli* examined by Rassekh & Pitton (1971) inactivated streptomycin—even the four strains which did not transfer their resistance. They conclude that resistance in wild strains is generally R factor mediated even when not transferable (Yamada et al, 1968). The ribosomes of these strains are normal. Incubation of susceptible cells in the presence of streptomycin (and other aminoglycosides) induces a general polyamine transport system that can be utilised by streptomycin the uptake of which is thereby greatly enhanced. This enhancement is absent in resistant strains of both ribosomal and plasmid origin. It has been speculated that this element of impaired uptake plays a significant part in plasmid-determined resistance by lowering the concentration of drug presented to the degrading enzyme, but Holtje (1979) showed that in mutants in which he induced the transport system with kanamycin all the transported drug was degraded and no increase in susceptibility to streptomycin occurred.

More than one mechanism of streptomycin resistance also exists in *Staph. aureus* in some strains of which resistance of uncertain mechanism is plasmid borne while in others (Lacey & Chopra, 1972) it is probably due to ribosomal modification resulting from mutation at a single chromosomal locus.

Amongst 200 strains of *Pseudomonas aeruginosa*, Tseng et al (1972) found high level resistance in less than 10 per cent, four-fifths of which was due to ribosomal change and one-fifth to drug inactivation. Low level resistance (up to 200 μg per ml) was due to decreased permeability to the drug.

It is not infrequent to find strains of meningococci, *Staph. aureus*, *E. coli*, *Ps. aeruginosa*, Proteus and *Myco. tuberculosis* which are actually favoured by the presence of the antibiotic or completely dependent on it. Isolated ribosomes from streptomycin-dependent Escherichia will synthesize peptides only in the presence of the drug (Dixon & Polglase, 1969). Mutation to streptomycin dependence in *Escherichia coli* results in a change in the same single ribosomal protein that determines resistance. Whether resistance or dependence develops depends on the parent strain (Wittmann & Apirion, 1975).

Particular attention has been drawn to the possible use of streptomycin-dependent Salmonella as living attenuated vaccines (Vladoianu et al, 1975).

Cross-resistance

There is complete ribosomal cross-resistance between streptomycin and dihydrostreptomycin, and partial cross-resistance between streptomycin and neomycin, kanamycin and paromomycin. This is usually one-way: strains that have developed resistance to neomycin and kanamycin nearly always show a significant increase in resistance to streptomycin (Table 5.3) while streptomycin-resistant bacteria are frequently still sensitive to neomycin and kanamycin. These cross-resistances probably arise from differences in the ribosomal sites of action of the antibiotics.

Table 5.3 Cross-resistance among antibiotics of the neomycin group

	Index* of increase in resistance to:			
Antibiotic to which habituated	Streptomycin	Neomycin	Paromomycin	Kanamycin
Streptomycin	10	5	5	5
Neomycin	6	8	8	8
Paromomycin	6	8	9	9
Kanamycin	6	9	9	10

*e.g. 8 = Increased 2^8 fold (i.e. 256-fold)

Pharmacokinetics

Absorption

Streptomycin is not absorbed in any quantity from the intestinal tract. Its activity in the gut is retained and it is excreted unchanged in the faeces. For systemic treatment streptomycin is usually administered by intramuscular injections which are liable to be painful. The levels obtained are shown in Table 5.4. In patients treated for tuberculosis, Line et al (1970) found considerable variation in the same patient on repeat testing, the peak levels following a dose of 0.75 g sometimes differing by as much as 50 μg/ml.

In premature infants the ability to excrete streptomycin is impaired (Table 5.4) and therapeutic levels (10 μg/ml or more) are still present 4–5 hours after 5 mg/kg (half the adult dose). As renal function declines with age too, so in patients over the age of 40 streptomycin tends to persist longer in the blood and in older adults excretion is commonly incomplete at 24 hours (Line et al 1970).

Distribution

Streptomycin diffuses fairly rapidly into most body tissues but is distributed as if it were present in extracellular fluid only. It appears in the peritoneal fluid in concentrations of about one-quarter to one-half those present in the blood, and in pleural fluid the concentrations may equal those in the blood.

Table 5.4 Plasma levels of streptomycin

	Dose	Peak plasma level		Plasma half-life hours
		Hour	μg/ml	
Adult	0.5G		16–42	2.4–27
	1.0G	½–1½	25–50	
Adult over 40 yrs	0.75G		26–58	up to 9.0
Premature Infant	10 mg per kg	2	17–42	7.0

Adcock J D, Hettig R A 1946 Arch Intern Med 77: 179
Buggs C W et al 1946 J Clin Invest 25: 94
Axline S G, Simon H J 1965 Antimicrob Agents Chemother 1964, p 135
Line D H et al 1970

It does not penetrate into the CSF or thick-walled abscesses but significant amounts are usually present in tuberculous cavities. Levels in cord blood are similar to those in maternal blood.

Excretion

Streptomycin is rapidly excreted from normal kidneys but the amount excreted varies very much. Excretion is by glomerular filtration and is unaffected by agents which block tubular secretion. The renal clearance is 30–70 ml/min and between 30 and 90 per cent of the dose is usually excreted in the first 24 hours, some being destroyed or retained in the body. The concentrations of streptomycin in the urine are often very high: 300–400 μg per ml after doses of 0.5 g and 1000 μg per ml or more after doses of 1 g. In oliguria, the plasma half life is prolonged and dosage must be reduced if toxic levels are to be avoided.

Small amounts of streptomycin, probably less than 1 per cent, are excreted in the bile where levels of from 3 to 12.5 μg/ml have been recorded.

Toxicity and side effects

Pain and irritation at the site of injection of streptomycin are common, but pain can be relieved by giving the antibiotic with procaine. Many patients experience unpleasant symptoms within a few hours of an intramuscular injection of streptomycin, such as paraesthesiae in and around the mouth, vertigo and ataxia, headaches and lassitude and 'muzziness in the head'. These are often trivial, but in ambulant patients in whom blood levels are appreciably higher than in those at rest, they are sometimes sufficient to render the patient unable to work. The most common serious toxic effect of streptomycin is vestibular disturbance.

Effects on eighth nerve

In early clinical trials of streptomycin in tuberculosis, up to 96 per cent of patients treated with 2 g per day developed vertigo. The clinical manifestations of streptomycin-induced vertigo and its marked degree as demonstrated by rotational tests are described by Wilmot (1973). In animal experiments the principal toxic effect of streptomycin is on the sensory epithelia of the labyrinth. Cats treated with

100–200 mg per kg per day eventually have difficulty in standing and although some recovery occurs after cessation of treatment the circling movement characteristic of chronic vestibular damage may remain. Lindeman (1969) concludes that the main injury is to the sensory epithelia of the cristae ampullares. It has been suggested that this results from an inhibitory effect on the ribosomes of these cells analagous to that which is responsible for the antibacterial action of the drug.

The vestibular end-organs are essential to the development of motion sickness, and depression of vestibular function by streptomycin has been utilized in the treatment of patients suffering from Menière's disease.

Vestibular disturbance is related to total dosage and to excessive blood levels so that the age of the patient and the state of renal function must be considered when deciding dosage. In the older patient the risk of damage is higher and when it does occur compensation is less good than in younger patients. Active secretion into the endo-lymph or persistence of the drug in the peri-lymph after the plasma level has fallen may play an important part in its specific ototoxicity. Line et al (1970) studied 27 patients treated with 0.75 g streptomycin daily for tuberculosis, eight of whom became dizzy within six weeks of starting treatment. There was no significant relation between incidence of dizziness and peak streptomycin level, but a highly significant relation with the 24-hour level. Serum levels exceeding 3 μg/ml at 24 hours were found in five out of eight dizzy patients but only two out of 18 unaffected patients, and both of these had had their dosage reduced when it was found that their renal function was impaired.

Deafness

On prolonged follow-up of patients treated with streptomycin for Menière's disease none had developed deafness (Graybiel et al 1967). Nevertheless both man and animals can suffer damage to hearing, sometimes after only a few doses of the drug. Congenital hearing loss or abnormalities in the caloric test or audiogram have several times been described in children born to women treated with streptomycin in pregnancy. There is considerable individual variation in susceptibility to the toxic effects of the drug which may be partly genetically determined (Johnsonbaugh et al, 1974). It may be that such familial susceptibility to streptomycin was implicated in the case of the mother treated in pregnancy and her child, both of whom had audiograms which were abnormal (Conway & Birt, 1965).

Hypersensitivity

In addition to eosinophilia unassociated with other allergic manifestations, skin rashes and drug-fever occur in about 5 per cent of treated patients. They are usually trivial and respond to antihistamine treatment so that in most cases streptomycin therapy can be continued, although this should be done with caution, since occasionally severe and even fatal exfoliative dermatitis may develop.

Skin sensitization is also common in nurses and dispensers who handle streptomycin and may lead to severe dermatitis, sometimes associated with periorbital swelling and conjunctivitis. This can be avoided by exercising care in giving injections, and wearing gloves and, where solution may be ejected, goggles.

Desensitization of those who handle streptomycin is usually possible, but may take several months and quite severe reactions may occur even with the minute doses used. Cover with antihistamines or corticosteroids, together with the use of repeated minute doses, instead of steadily increasing ones, may help to reduce the reactions but will not necessarily eliminate them.

Patients showing hypersensitivity during therapy are generally much more readily desensitized. Reactions most frequently develop between four and six weeks, but may appear after the first dose or after six months' treatment. Desensitization may be achieved by giving 20 mg prednisolone daily plus 10 daily increments from 0.1–1.0 g until by the ninth day normal dosage will usually be tolerated or by giving increased doses of streptomycin every six hours.

Neuromuscular blockade

Streptomycin and its relatives can produce neuromuscular blockade (pages 129 and 212) probably by functioning as membrane stabilizers in the same way as curare. If D-tubocurarine is assigned a blocking value of 1000, neomycin has a value of 2.5, streptomycin 0.7 and kanamycin 0.5. Their effect is, therefore, relatively feeble and it is rare for streptomycin to show any effect in those whose neuromuscular mechanisms are normal. However, antibiotics are customarily given in much larger amounts than curare and patients who are also receiving muscle relaxants or anaesthetics or suffering from myasthenia gravis are at special risk.

A depressant effect on cardiac muscle has been demonstrated in several experimental systems by Cohen et al (1970) who thought that streptomycin toxicity was responsible for persistent hypotension in one of their patients.

Other unusual effects

Occasional cases of aplastic anaemia and agranulocytosis have been reported in patients treated with streptomycin.

Encouraged by evidence of a hypocalcaemic effect in the rat, Roediger et al (1975) gave streptomycin to a patient suffering from malignant hypercalcaemia and achieved a notable fall in serum calcium.

Stenbjerg et al (1975) traced severe bleeding in a patient one week after streptomycin treatment to the transient presence of a circulating factor V antagonist. Of the ten patients so far reported who have developed bleeding from this mechanism, seven had received streptomycin.

Clinical applications

The most important use of streptomycin is in the treatment of tuberculosis (Chapter 23).

Apart from this streptomycin is the most effective antibiotic for the treatment of plague and tularaemia and sometimes also for infections due to otherwise resistant coliform bacilli. In the treatment of such infections, particularly of the urinary tract, large doses should be given for a short period, and combined therapy should be considered, since unless the infection is sterilized within a day or two of the onset of treatment, drug-resistant strains are almost certain to appear.

Streptomycin is a good drug to give in combination with penicillin, since both are bactericidal antibiotics (Chapter 14) and this combination is often useful in the treatment of bacterial endocarditis. Streptomycin in combination with tetracycline has been considered to be the most effective antibiotic treatment for brucellosis (page 302).

DEOXYSTREPTAMINE-AMINOGLYCOSIDES

NEOMYCIN GROUP

The neomycins were first isolated by Waksman & Lechevalier (1949) from strains of *Streptomyces fradiae*. The crude material contains three compounds, Neomycins A, B and C.

In 1947 Decaris noticed a pink mould growing on a damp patch on the wall of his home in Paris which he identified as *Streptomyces lavendulae*. He found that culture filtrates were bactericidal for many species of bacteria (Decaris, 1953). Further

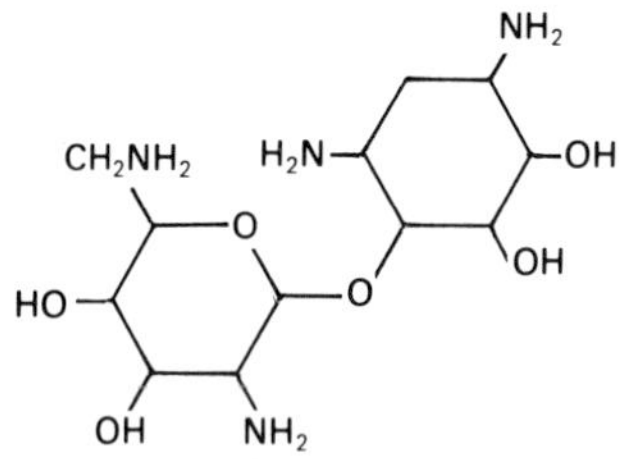

NEAMINE (neomycin A)

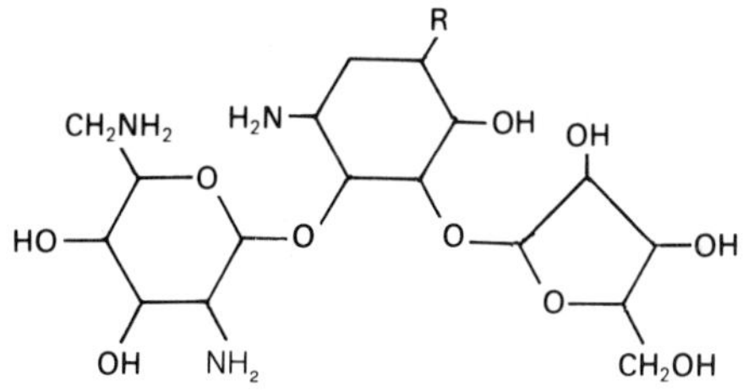

RIBOSTAMYCIN (R = NH_2)
BUTIROSIN (R = $NHCOCH(OH)(CH_2)_2NH_2$)

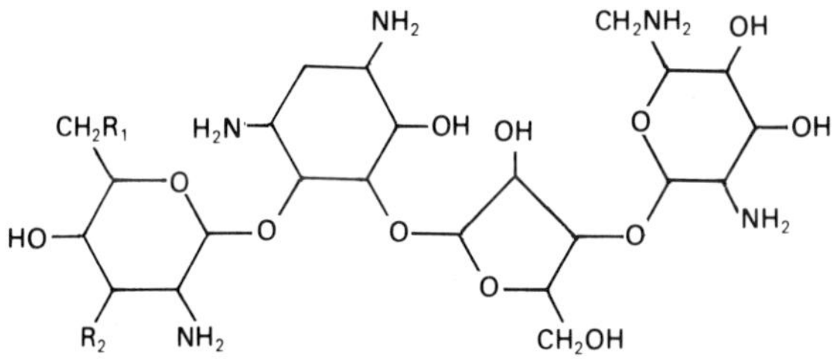

	R_1	R_2
NEOMYCIN B	NH_2	OH
PAROMOMYCIN I	OH	OH
LIVIDOMYCIN B	OH	H

Fig. 5.4 Structures of the neomycins. The family grows by successive ring substitutions of hydroxyl groups. Lividomycin A has a fifth ring

extraction and purification in the research laboratories of Roussel led to the isolation of framycetin, now known to be identical with neomycin B which is also produced by strains of Micromonospora (Wagman et al, 1973)—a genus that first came to attention as the source of gentamicin (page 141).

The neomycins illustrate well the inter-relationships of aminoglycoside families (Fig. 5.4). Neomycin A shows the simplest kind of structure possible in a typical member: an aminoglycoside linked to an aminocyclitol. In ribostamycin a third ring is added and, characteristically for the neomycins as a whole, this replaces the hydroxyl group adjacent to that carrying the aminosugar (Fig. 5.4). In the remaining members of the group (and this includes those used therapeutically) fourth (and even fifth) rings are added. The close relationships of these compounds are shown in Fig. 5.4. Neomycins A and B and paromomycin I and II are stereoisomers. Lividomycin A has a fifth ring.

Compounds not used therapeutically

Neomycin A (neamine) is the least active antibacterially of the three compounds, neomycin B and C are substantially more active but at the same time more toxic (Table 5.6).

Ribostamycin, discovered by Akita et al (1970) in the fermentation products of *Streptomyces ribosidificus* is interesting principally as the parent compound of butirosin which is produced by *Bacillus circulans* (Tsukiura et al, 1973). Ribostamycin is not a very active compound and is susceptible to degradation by several of the enzymes which are usually responsible for resistance to aminoglycosides in clinically important bacteria.

BUTIROSIN

Table 5.5 shows that butirosin is substantially more active against a variety of such resistant organisms (because it is much less susceptible to degradation) and what is just as important, that activity against resistant organisms is not obtained at the cost of loss of activity against sensitive organisms.

Table 5.5 Minimum inhibitory concentration (μg/ml), for selected resistant strains:

		Kanamycin	Ribostamycin	Butirosin	Amikacin
Staph. aureus	A	0.8	1.6	0.8	0.4
	B	100	100	1.6	1.6
E. coli	A	0.8	16	0.8	0.4
	B	>100	>100	0.4	0.4
	C	>100	>100	50	0.2
Ps. aeruginosa	A	25	>100	6	1.6
	B	>100	>100	>100	6.3

Gentamicin (page 142) has generally been used as the index compound when comparing the activities of aminoglycosides and Price et al (1974a) have attempted

Table 5.6 Therapeutic ratios of aminoglycosides

	Toxicity relative to neamine[1]	Activity relative to gentamicin[2]	Ratio toxicity/ activity
Neamine	1	0.13	7
Ribostamycin	1	0.25	4
Butirosin	0.5	0.25	2
Neomycin B	14	0.5	28
Neomycin C	8	0.5	16
Paromomycin	2	0.13	14
Lividomycin A	1.5	0.13	11
Kanamycin A	1	0.25	4
Kanamycin B	2	0.5	4
Tobramycin	3.5	1.0	3.5
Dibekacin	3.5	0.5	7
Gentamicin C	3.5	1.0	3.5
Sissomicin	8	2.0	4

1 LD_{50} compound $\times \frac{\text{molecular weight compound}}{\text{molecular weight neamine}} \times LD_{50}$ neamine

2 MIC gentamicin/MIC compound for *Esch. coli.*
Based on Price et al (1974a)

(Table 5.6) to rank the therapeutic ratios of aminoglycosides by comparing their activities with that of gentamicin and their acute toxicities (allowing for differences in molecular weight) with that of neamine. Butirosin has only one-eighth to one-sixteenth the activity of gentamicin against *Staph. aureus* and a quarter of its activity against *Escherichia coli* but a favourable therapeutic ratio compared with other aminoglycosides.

Keeney & Coodley (1975) found that a dosage of butirosin of 4 mg/kg 8-hourly was sufficient to produce the 12 μg/ml needed therapeutically. The plasma half life of the drug, which was almost completely excreted unchanged in the urine, was two hours. They treated a few patients suffering from urinary infections with satisfactory results and no side effects. Despite this, butirosin has not been actively pursued as a therapeutic antibiotic and its main interest is the peculiar side chain which confers on it the resistance to bacterial degradation that its parent ribostamycin lacks. This side chain has been used in amikacin (page 138) to confer similar resistance on kanamycin A.

Manipulation of butirosin itself (Heifetz et al, 1972) has produced a derivative (AD-BTN) which is as active as gentamicin against gentamicin-sensitive strains of Pseudomonas and almost as active against gentamicin-resistant ones. It has only a third to a half of the acute toxicity of gentamicin for mice.

THERAPEUTIC NEOMYCINS

Neomycin B (commercially available as framycetin) and the isomeric mixture of B and C marketed commercially as 'neomycin' exert a rapid bactericidal effect which, like that of streptomycin, is enhanced at alkaline pH. The activity of streptomycin against *Staph. aureus* increases 512-fold when the pH is raised from 5.5 to 8.5 while that of neomycin increases only 64-fold.

Acquired resistance

The single step mutation to high resistance to streptomycin (page 120) is not seen with other aminoglycosides. Resistance is acquired slowly, although some change may be seen during the treatment of an individual patient. Frequent and long-continued topical use certainly seems liable eventually to generate resistance as in the treatment of nasal staphylococcal carriers or burn sepsis and in some hospitals resistance in staphylococci is now common. The use of Polybactrin spray (neomycin-bacitracin-polymyxin) may well have contributed largely to this as indicated by associated bacitracin resistance in numerous strains resistant to neomycin and kanamycin.

Amongst enterobacteria, Salmonella and Shigella and strains of *E. coli* from infants are now not uncommonly resistant. Resistance has also been seen in enterobacteria from the faeces of patients treated orally: we ourselves have found resistant strains of Proteus in patients given neomycin for pre-operative bowel preparation. The opportunity for the emergence of such resistance is naturally greatly increased on prolonged usage. Oral neomycin has been given for long periods to suppress the gut flora in patients with hepatic encephalopathy (Suh et al, 1979) and to treat familial hypercholesterolaemia because it precipitates ionized fatty and bile acids and so disrupts micelle formation and decreases cholesterol absorption. In 11 of 14 patients so treated for three months to eight years Valtonen et al (1977) found that most of the faecal enterobacteria possessed multiple transferable antibiotic resistance.

Cross-resistance

Most naturally occurring resistant strains, and all those trained to resistance *in vitro*, are almost equally resistant to streptomycin and kanamycin. On the other hand some strains of enterobacteria become resistant, particularly after oral treatment, only to the antibiotic used. Resistant strains of *Staph. aureus* are usually more resistant to kanamycin than to neomycin and the relationship with streptomycin tends to be one-way: i.e. training to resistance to any of the neomycin group produces a substantial increase in resistance to streptomycin, but when streptomycin resistance is induced, the increase in resistance to the neomycin group is much less (Table 5.3). Naturally occurring resistance is even less closely related, or not at all, in that neomycin-resistant bacteria may be fully sensitive to other aminoglycosides.

Pharmacokinetics

Very little neomycin is absorbed after oral administration; the antibiotic retains its activity in the gut and is eliminated unchanged in the faeces. Distribution and excretion after intramuscular injection are as for streptomycin, but the toxicity of neomycin precludes its systemic administration except in the most extreme cases.

Toxicity

Neomycin is the most liable of all aminoglycosides to damage the kidneys and the auditory branch of the eighth nerve (Table 5.7). It was originally welcomed as a second line drug for treating tuberculosis, but deafness so often resulted that this treatment soon fell into disrepute. Since then its use has been almost entirely restricted to topical and oral use.

Table 5.7 Relative toxicity index

	Vestibular	Auditory	Renal
Streptomycin	4	1	<1
Neomycin	1	4	4
Kanamycin	1	3	1
Gentamicin	3	2	2
Tobramycin	2	2	2

Based on Price et al (1974a)

Clinical applications

Topical. Neomycin has been extensively used for the local treatment of superficial infections with staphylococci and many Gram-negative bacilli alone or in combination with bacitracin, chlorhexidine or polymyxin. Neomycin in combination with chlorhexidine or bacitracin is also used in the treatment of staphylococcal nasal carriers but the appearance of neomycin-resistant strains has reduced the value of this proceeding. Prolonged application to the skin may cause sensitization and has proved a particularly fruitful means of facilitating the emergence of resistance.

Intravesical application. Neomycin solution may be introduced into the urinary bladder after instrumentation to kill any bacteria accidentally introduced. If pseudomonas infection is particularly feared, irrigation with a solution containing 40 mg neomycin and 20 mg polymyxin per litre may be preferable. In the test to distinguish infection of the upper from that of the lower urinary tract described by Fairley et al (1967) neomycin (5 mg/l) irrigation is used to free the bladder from bacteria so that any organism appearing in the bladder urine after washing out the neomycin must be derived from the upper urinary tract.

Absorption from topical application

Neomycin aerosol is strongly commended by some authors for the treatment of bronchial infections, particularly bronchiectasis and it has been introduced into the peritoneal cavity at operation for the prevention or treatment of peritonitis. These 'local' applications—like subconjunctival injections—are used with the valid objective of securing high local concentrations of the drug. In fact, neomycin may be absorbed from these sites as readily as it is from intramuscular injection and such administration must be counted as effectively systemic with all its attendant dangers.

The drug has a particular danger in the peritoneum at operation because, like streptomycin, it is liable to produce neuromuscular blockade especially in patients concurrently exposed to anaesthetics and muscle relaxants. As a curariform agent it is three or four times as potent as streptomycin (page 124).

Oral administration

The inefficacy of oral neomycin in the treatment of infections confined to the gut is described on page 338 and utility in infantile gastroenteritis is disputed. Neomycin, usually in combination with other 'unabsorbed' agents, has found considerable use in depressing the gastrointestinal flora in patients prior to abdominal surgery (page 343) or in those of special risk from opportunistic infections with gut bacteria (page

288). The drug has also been very successfully used, generally alone, for a similar purpose in patients at risk from hepatic encephalopathy where the object is to reduce the colonic population of bacteria that generate the ammonia, or other aminotoxins, believed to be responsible for the neurological disorder in these patients (Suh et al, 1979). Large doses so administered for long periods are not without risk of causing deafness (Berk and Chalmers, 1970) and may result in atrophic changes in the intestinal mucosa with malabsorption of fats, carbohydrates and possibly some drugs.

PAROMOMYCIN

This antibiotic (Fig. 5.4) was first described by Haskell et al (1959). The following differently named substances are identical with it (Schillings & Schaffner 1962): aminosidine (marketed in Italy as gabbromycina), catenulin and hydroxymycin. There are two isomeric paromomycins I and II which differ from neomycin only in the substitution of a hydroxy for an amino group. In view of their similarity it is perhaps not surprising that apart from inferior activity against *Ps. aeruginosa* the antibacterial activity of paromomycin is almost identical with that of neomycin.

The importance of apparently trivial differences in the molecule must not be underestimated, however, and paromomycin differs from other aminoglycosides in its activity against *E. histolytica* and apparently some helminths.

In its pharmacokinetic behaviour and liability to produce deafness and intestinal malabsorption it closely resembles neomycin. As an antibacterial agent its uses have been similar to those of neomycin with, as far as can be judged, similar results. The main interest in the agent is in its non-bacterial uses. Excellent results were reported with paromomycin in an extensive study involving treatment of 432 patients with amoebic dysentery in 12 different countries in Asia, Africa and the Americas (Courtney et al 1960). Another peculiar use is as an anthelmintic. In the hands of Wittner & Tanowitz (1971) a single oral dose of 4 g regularly eliminated *T. saginata*, *T. solium* and *D. latum*; repeated doses were often necessary for *H. nana*.

KANAMYCIN GROUP

In addition to the kanamycins and their semi-synthetic derivatives this group contains gentamicin and the closely related nebramycins (of which tobramycin has come into clinical use) netilmicin and sissomicin.

KANAMYCIN

The complex of kanamycin A, B and C (Fig. 5.5) was isolated in Japan from a strain of *Streptomyces kanamyceticus* (Umezawa et al 1957). Kanamycin B has twice the activity and twice the acute toxicity of kanamycin A. Kanamycin C is significantly less active and more toxic than kanamycin A. The commercial preparation is kanamycin A sulphate (the content of kanamycin B being required to be less than 3 per cent in the United Kingdom and less than 5 per cent in the U.S.A.) which is soluble in water (8 g per l) but almost insoluble in alcohol and non-polar solvents. It is very stable, losing less than 10 per cent of its activity on autoclaving at 120 °C for one hour.

Antibacterial activity

Kanamycin differs little from neomycin in antibacterial activity (Table 5.8) but that against all species of *Proteus* is noteworthy. *Mycobacterium tuberculosis* is inhibited by 2–8 μg per ml. Pneumococci, streptococci and anaerobic bacteria are all resistant. Like its relatives, kanamycin is more active at alkaline pH and exerts a rapid bactericidal effect at concentrations a little above the MIC.

Resistance

Kanamycin resistance became common in staphylococci when there was a vogue for its use in the treatment of severe staphylococcal sepsis and many enterobacteria are also now resistant. Mutants which owe their resistance to a ribosomal change analagous to that seen with streptomycin (page 120) occur, but they are of little clinical significance. Such mutants show complete cross-resistance with agents of the neomycin group and partial cross-resistance with streptomycin (Table 5.3). Clinically significant resistance is commonly multiple, plasmid-borne and due to enzymic degradation of the drug. It is to remedy this defect that semi-synthetic derivatives of kanamycin resistant to bacterial degradation have been developed. The classification and properties of aminoglycoside degrading enzymes are discussed on page

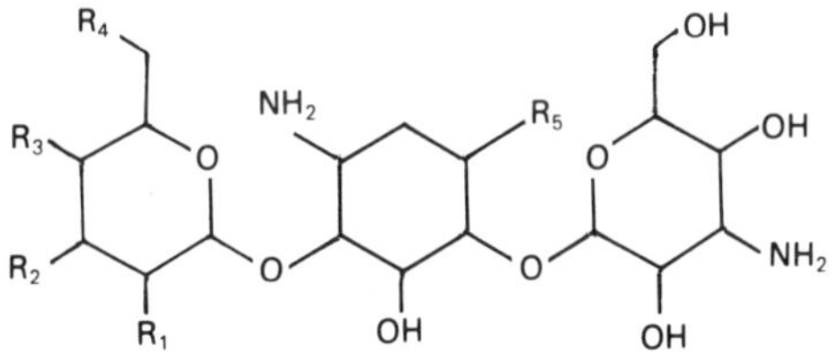

	R_1	R_2	R_3	R_4	R_5
Kanamycin A	OH	OH	OH	NH_2	NH_2
Amikacin	OH	OH	OH	NH_2	HABA
Kanamycin B	NH_2	OH	OH	NH_2	NH_2
Tobramycin	NH_2	H	OH	NH_2	NH_2
Di-deoxy-kanamycin B	NH_2	H	H	NH_2	NH_2
Kanamycin C	NH_2	OH	OH	OH	NH_2

Fig. 5.5 Structures of the kanamycins

Pharmacokinetics

Like other aminoglycosides, kanamycin is barely absorbed from the intestinal tract, as much as 25 mg per g of faeces being recovered after an oral dose of 6 g. Nevertheless, the development of ototoxicity in patients receiving prolonged oral therapy indicates that the hazards of oral neomycin also attend the use of kanamycin and Kunin (1966) has shown that concentrations in urine can reach 12 μg per ml after daily oral doses of 6 g.

The drug is normally given by intramuscular injection when a dose of 500 mg produces peak plasma levels after one hour of about 20 μg per ml. The proportion bound to plasma protein is very low. The plasma half-life is 2.5 hours. The volume of distribution indicates that like its relatives the drug is confined to the extracellular fluid. It does not enter the CSF in therapeutically useful concentrations even in the presence of meningeal inflammation and on the rare occasions that kanamycin is required for the treatment of meningitis it must be given intrathecally, the usual single daily dose being 100 mg for adults and 50 or 25 mg for children over or under 1 yr respectively.

The traditional dosage for neonates (7.5 mg/kg 12-hourly) has several times been shown to produce plasma concentrations less than the 15–25 μg per ml believed to be therapeutically necessary. Using doses of 5 and 10 mg per kg, Hieber & Nelson (1976) showed that the peak plasma concentration in the neonate is dose related and the concentration 1 hour after 10 mg per kg was 8.4–30 μg per ml (mean 17.6 μg per ml). They support the view that the standard dose for the neonate should be 10 mg per kg 12-hourly.

Excretion

Kanamycin is excreted almost entirely by the kidneys and almost exclusively in the glomerular filtrate so that probenecid has no effect on its plasma level. Renal clearance is about 80 ml per minute. Most of the administered dose appears unchanged in the urine over the first 4–6 hours producing concentrations of several hundred μg per ml and over the first 24 hours up to 80 per cent of the dose is eliminated. Less than 1 per cent of the dose appears in the bile and the fate of the remaining 20 per cent or so has not been established. Such dependence for excretion on the renal route means that the drug is retained in proportion to reduction in renal function and because of its potential toxicity the appropriate dosage must be determined (page 453) if it is essential to treat patients at the extremes of life or suffering from known renal disorders.

Toxicity

Intramuscular injections are moderately painful and minor side effects similar to those encountered with streptomycin (page 122) have been described. Eosinophilia in the absence of other manifestations of allergy occurs in up to 10 per cent of patients. As with other aminoglycosides the most important toxic effects are on the eighth nerve and much less frequently, but more importantly, on the kidney. Nephrotoxicity is seen principally in patients with pre-existing renal disease or treated concurrently or sequentially with other potentially nephrotoxic agents. The resulting renal impairment usually resolves on stopping the drug but may take months to do so.

Less dramatic deterioration of renal function, particularly exaggeration of the potential nephrotoxicity of other drugs or of existing renal disease, is principally important because it increases the likelihood of ototoxicity. Vestibular damage is uncommon but may be severe and prolonged. Hearing damage is usually bilateral and fortunately typically affects frequencies above the conversational range. If the tinnitus which usually heralds the onset of auditory injury is heeded, further damage can be prevented by withdrawing therapy—providing, of course, that the patient's renal function is sufficient to allow prompt elimination of the remaining drug.

Clinical use

Kanamycin has been used topically and orally in much the same way, for much the same purposes and with much the same strictures as neomycin (page 129). It enjoyed a vogue for the treatment of severe staphylococcal sepsis and as a second-line agent for tuberculosis, but its importance in both those connections has been almost completely overtaken by other agents. With the realization that the key to success in severe sepsis is effective therapy from the earliest possible moment, kanamycin with its broad spectrum of bactericidal activity against Gram-negative organisms became standard treatment in combination with an agent providing complementary activity against Gram-positive organisms for patients with severe but unidentified bacterial infection. That place has been to a large extent usurped by gentamicin because of the growing participation of *Pseudomonas* in hospital-acquired infections. Where *Pseudomonas* is unlikely, kanamycin offers a better therapeutic ratio against the majority of organisms. It remains a valuable agent in the treatment of intractable *Proteus* urinary infections (page 377) and may prove on laboratory testing (page 485) to be the aminoglycoside of choice in combination therapy of bacterial endocarditis.

IMPROVED KANAMYCINS

It is plain that while kanamycin has a number of desirable properties, there is room for extension to its antibacterial activity and reduction in its toxicity. Antibacterial advantage has been sought principally in activity against *Pseudomonas* and against strains of naturally sensitive species with acquired resistance to kanamycin. Activity would also be welcomed against organisms responsible for severe infections which are naturally resistant to kanamycin, notably streptococci, and anaerobic bacteria. Relatives of kanamycin with improved activity have been obtained from natural sources and by chemical manipulation of the kanamycin molecules.

The natural compound chemically closest to kanamycin is a deoxykanamycin, now marketed under the name of tobramycin, which was extracted from the complex family of the nebramycins.

NEBRAMYCINS

The nebramycins are a family of aminoglycosides isolated from the fermentation products of *Streptomyces tenebraeus* (so named because of its sensitivity to light) by Stark et al (1968) in the Research Laboratories of Eli Lilly. The original complex was found to contain at least seven components (Thompson & Presti, 1968) of which factors 2, 4, 5 and 6 were isolated and their antibacterial activity and animal toxicity evaluated (Wick & Wells, 1968). All the factors were active against staphylococci and a variety of enterobacteria and factors 2 and 6 were also active against *Pseudomonas*. All the factors were less toxic to mice than neomycin or gentamicin. In its toxicity for rats, factor 2 (given the trivial name apramycin) was similar to kanamycin and factors 4, 5 and 6 were more toxic. In both *in vitro* tests and in animal protection studies factor 6 was the most active of the components (Black & Griffiths 1971) and has been developed under the name of tobramycin. Apramycin which has a unique chemical structure (O'Connor et al, 1976) apparently associated with a number of novel properties, is being evaluated for use as an oral preparation for the treatment of animal infections. Walton (1978) describes its action against enterobacteria and the properties of resistant strains.

TOBRAMYCIN

Purified nebramycin factor 6 (Fig. 5.5) is supplied as the sulphate.

Antibacterial activity

The loss of a single oxygen atom from the large molecule of kanamycin B which resulted in the formation of tobramycin exerts a beneficial effect on antibacterial activity of three kinds: tobramycin is substantially more active than is kanamycin against the majority of susceptible bacteria; it is very much more active against Pseudomonas, surpassing up to four-fold the activity of the earlier discovered gentamicin (Table 5.8) and it is active against a number of strains with acquired resistance to gentamicin; against this it is significantly less active against a number of other organisms including Proteus and Serratia.

The analogue of tobramycin in kanamycin A (3′-deoxykanamycin A) is as active as kanamycin A against *Staph. aureus* and *Esch. coli* and 20 times more active against Pseudomonas—almost as active as tobramycin (Price et al, 1974a).

Table 5.8 Minimum inhibitory concentrations of aminoglycosides for important pathogenic bacteria

	Gentamicin	Kanamycin	Tobramycin	Amikacin	Sissomicin
Staph. aureus	0.03–0.12	0.5–4	0.12–0.25	0.1–2	0.25–2
Str. pyogenes	4–8	64–128	16	16–R	
Str. pneumoniae	8–16	64–128	16–32	64–R	
Str. faecalis	2–4	32–R	2–8	16–R	
Cl. welchii	R	R	R	R	
N. gonorrhoeae	2	8			
N. meningitidis	2	8			
H. influenzae	0.5	0.5–1	0.5	2	
Esch. coli	0.25–1	2–8	0.25–1	0.5–8	0.1–8
Klebsiella	0.25–1	0.5–4	0.12–1	0.1–4	0.1–8
Enterobacter			0.25–4	0.25–4	
Pr. mirabilis	0.25–2	1–4	1–4	0.5–8	
Proteus, indole +	0.25–2	1–4	0.25–2	0.25–4	0.25–4
Serratia marcescens	0.25–0.5	2–8	1–4	0.25–8	0.25–0.5
Salmonella spp.	0.12–0.25	0.5–2	0.12–1	1–8	0.25–1
Shigella spp.	0.12–1	1–4	0.12–2	2–8	
Ps. aeruginosa	0.25–2	32–256	0.12–2	0.1–8	
Bacteroides spp.	R	R			

Based on

Crowe C C & Sanders E 1973 Antimicrobial Agents and Chemotherapy 3: 24
Hyams P J et al 1973 Antimicrobial Agents and Chemotherapy 3: 87
Kluge R M et al 1974 Antimicrobial Agents and Chemotherapy 6: 442
Waitz J A et al 1972 Antimicrobial Agents and Chemotherapy 2: 431

Interaction

Like other aminoglycosides, tobramycin exhibits bactericidal synergy when combined with penicillins or cephalosporins, but such mixtures must not be used in infusion fluids because of mutual inactivation analagous to that seen with gentamicin (page 142). Anderson et al (1975) found the proportion of strains which showed *in vitro* synergy with carbenicillin against Pseudomonas or with penicillin against streptococci to be in each case less with tobramycin than with gentamicin.

Acquired resistance

A major advantage claimed for tobramycin is activity against gentamicin resistant organisms. Of the strains examined by Waitz et al (1972) about 30 per cent were sensitive to both gentamicin and tobramycin and of the gentamicin resistant strains about half were sensitive to tobramycin. Strains resistant to tobramycin but sensitive to gentamicin also occur. Cross-resistance is probably due to reduction in aminoglycoside transport into the cells but independent resistance to gentamicin depends on the resistance of tobramycin to a gentamicin degrading enzyme elaborated by the resistant strains (page 137).

Pharmacokinetics

Like other aminoglycosides, tobramycin is not absorbed from the gut and its pharmacokinetic behaviour after systemic administration closely resembles that of gentamicin. Mean peak plasma concentrations of 3.7 μg per ml were found 30 minutes after intramuscular injection of 80 mg by Simon et al (1973). Thirty minutes after intravenous injections of 1 mg per kg, Naber et al (1973) found serum concentrations of 6–7.5 μg per ml. The half-life has been variously reported to lie between 1.5 and 3 hours. Continuous intravenous infusion of 6.6 μg per ml produced steady state levels around 1 μg per ml. Higher levels of 10–11 μg per ml were obtained by Stratford et al (1974) by bolus injections given over about 3 minutes.

Excretion

Tobramycin is eliminated in the glomerular filtrate and is unaffected by probenecid. After a dose of 80 mg, urinary concentrations of 90 to 500 μg per ml were obtained during the first three hours. Renal clearance at 88 ml per min is not significantly different from that of gentamicin. Sixty per cent of the administered dose has been recovered from the urine over the first ten hours. The nature of the extra-renal disposal of the remaining 40 per cent of the drug has not been established. Tobramycin is said to be up to 30 per cent bound to plasma protein. The volume of distribution (16.9 litres) slightly exceeds the extracellular water volume. In patients with impaired renal function, urinary concentrations of the drug are depressed and its plasma half-life is expectedly prolonged in proportion to the rise in serum creatinine, reaching 6–8 hours at a creatinine level of 350 μmol/l. In view of the virtual identity and behaviour of the two drugs, modification of tobramycin dosage in patients with impaired renal function may be based on the procedures used for gentamicin (page 453). About 70 per cent of the drug is removed by haemodialysis over 12 hours (Lockwood & Bower, 1973).

Similarity in behaviour to gentamicin extends to the neonate where peak serum concentrations of 4–6 micrograms per ml half to one hour after doses of 2 mg per kg were obtained by Kaplan et al (1973). Mean plasma half lives of 4.6–8.7 hours were inversely proportional to the birth weight and creatinine clearance. The half-life was initially extremely variable (3.5–17.1 hours) in infants weighing 2.5 kg at birth but considerably more stable (3.9–8.5 hours) at the end of therapy 6–9 days later. Concentrations in the urine after doses of 2 mg per kg ranged around 10–100 μg per ml over the first 8 hours but the total urinary recovery varied widely. Published evidence indicates that tobramycin also resembles gentamicin in its poor capacity to reach the bronchial lumen or the CSF.

Toxicity

Previous experience with aminoglycosides leads to the expectation that any toxic manifestation of tobramycin will be exhibited principally against the eighth nerve and the kidneys. Anticipated enhancement of renal toxicity by concurrent or sequential administration of cephalothin has been demonstrated (Klasterksy et al, 1975) and by analogy similar interaction is likely to be seen with frusemide. Comparison of the effects of tobramycin and gentamicin on cochlear electrophysiology and histology (Brummett et al, 1972) indicated that comparable degrees of damage were produced by doses of gentamicin about half those of tobramycin. The possibility that the difference in toxicity for the ear resides not in the effect on the target organ but on access of the drug to the middle ear appears to be excluded by the observations of Federspil et al (1976) who show that levels of both drugs in the perilymph and subsequently in the endolymph of the inner ear of the guinea pig are very similar, are related to the dose, and persist for many hours after the plasma levels have fallen below detectable limits. Guinea pigs receiving the drugs exhibited a dose-related failure to gain weight. Again, the dose required to reduce the normal weight gain by 25 per cent was about 100 mg per kg in the case of tobramycin but only 60 mg per kg in the case of gentamicin.

Electrocochleography showed an immediate dramatic reduction in the cochlear activity of three patients when the serum tobramycin concentration exceeded 8–10 μg per ml (Wilson & Ramsden, 1977). There were no associated symptoms and function recovered fully as the drug was eliminated. The speed of onset suggested a metabolic block but the relation of this very prompt change to long term ototoxicity is not yet known.

Clinical use

Tobramycin is for practical purposes identical with gentamicin except in its superior activity against Pseudomonas (offset by its inferior activity against some other organisms), its activity against some strains resistant to gentamicin (offset by the reverse situation in other strains) and its lower toxicity for the guinea pig. Accepting that it is generally twice as active against sensitive strains of Pseudomonas and half as toxic, it exhibits a four-fold advantage in its therapeutic ratio over gentamicin for the treatment of proven Pseudomonas infection. Because of its lower activity against other possibly implicated organisms there is no good reason to substitute tobramycin for gentamicin in the speculative treatment of severe undiagnosed infection.

DIBEKACIN

Tobramycin is naturally occurring deoxykanamycin B. Removal of two hydroxyl groups produces dideoxykanamycin B (Umezawa et al, 1971) originally called DKB and now developed under the name dibekacin. The drug has about half the activity of gentamicin against most sensitive strains but was found by Paradelis et al (1978) to be the most active aminoglycoside tested against *Ps. aeruginosa* and it is resistant to degradation by some enzymes that attack gentamicin (Table 5.9). Deoxygenation increases toxicity and dibekacin, like tobramycin, has about twice the acute toxicity for mice of the parent kanamycin (Table 5.6). The corresponding dideoxy compound in kanamycin A is similar to the 3′-deoxy compound (page 134) which resembles tobramycin closely but is slightly inferior in activity.

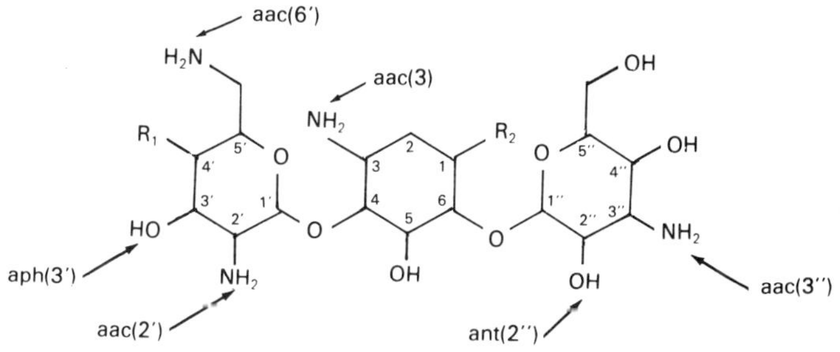

Fig. 5.6 Sites of action and nomenclature of bacterial enzymes destroying kanamycin and its relatives

AMINOGLYCOSIDE DEGRADING ENZYMES

Reference has already been made several times to the elaboration by bacteria of enzymes which destroy aminoglycosides to which the bacteria are resistant. This mechanism of resistance shares many features with β-lactamase production by organisms resistant to penicillins or cephalosporins (page 109) in that the cells remain intrinsically sensitive to the agent (and owe their survival to its destruction) and that a considerable (and growing) number of enzymes has been identified from different bacterial species and strains. These enzymes differ in the way they attack aminoglycosides and in the aminoglycosides they will attack. Since a substantial part of the effort to develop new aminoglycosides has been devoted to producing agents resistant to degradation by these enzymes it may be helpful to say something about their properties before reviewing the remaining aminoglycosides.

A rational nomenclature for these enzymes has been proposed by Mitsuhashi (1975). The enzymes are of three types. The first, aminoglycoside acetyltransferases (abbreviated to *aac*) attack amino groups and the others—aminoglycoside phosphotransferases (abbreviated to *aph*) and what were originally called aminoglycoside adenyltransferases (abbreviated to *aad*) attack hydroxyl groups. The adenyltransferases have now been renamed aminoglycoside nucleotidyltransferases (abbreviated to *ant*) because although adenylated antibiotic is the major product, guanylate and inosinate can also be found (Price et al 1976). The sites of attack of these enzymes are shown in Fig. 5.6. The position of the group attacked and the ring that carries it is shown by the number of the enzyme: thus *aac*(3) is the acetyltransferase which attacks the amino group in the 3-position on the central aminocyclitol ring and *aac*(2′) and *ant*(2″) enzymes which attack groups at the 2-positions on the rings attached to the left and right of the aminocyclitol (Fig. 5.6). Where two enzymes act at the same position but differ in the aminoglycosides they can degrade, they are distinguished by numerals: for example *aph*(3′)1 and *aph*(3′)2. The resistance of systemically administered aminoglycosides to some enzymes so far characterized is shown in Table 5.9.

As far as the origins of these enzymes are concerned, *aac*(2′) is more common in *Proteus rettgeri* and *stuartii*, *ant*(2′) is found in Escherichia and Klebsiella and *aph*(3′) and *aac*(3) found in Pseudomonas and Klebsiella. Some of the enzymes, for example *aac*(3)2 from Pseudomonas and *aac*(2′) from Proteus, have not been shown to be plasmid-borne. The most prevalent patterns of resistance encountered in clinical isolates by Price et al (1976) were associated with the presence of *aph*(3′)1 and 2. The common combination of resistance to kanamycin, gentamicin and tobramycin with susceptibility to amikacin could be due to a mixture of enzymes.

The prevalence of these enzymes is naturally greatly affected by local differences in the availability of organisms receptive to the plasmids which code for them, by anti-

Table 5.9 Range of activity of bacterial enzymes destroying kanamycin and its relatives

	KMA	KMB	DKB	AK	GM	TM	SMi	NMi
aph(3′)1	+	+						
aph(3′)2	+	+						
aac(2′)1					+	+	+	+
(2′)2		+	+		+	+	+	
aac(3)1					+		+	(+)
2	+	+	+		+	+	+	
3		+			+	+	+	(+)
aac(6′)1	+	+						
2		+			+	+	+	
3		+	+		+	+	+	
4		+	+	+	+	+	+	+
ant(2″)	+	+	+		+	+	+	

aph: aminoglycoside phosphotransferase; aac: aminoglycoside acetyltransferase; ant: aminoglycoside nucleotidyltransferase
KMA: kanamycin A; KMB: kanamycin B; DKB: dideoxykanamycin B; AK: amikacin; GMi: gentamicin; TM: tobramycin; SMi: sissomicin; NMi: netilmicin.

biotic prescribing habits and by opportunities for resistant organisms to spread. Reports in the literature on the prevalence of organisms resistant to older but susceptible to newer aminoglycosides consequently differ a good deal and have questionable general applicability. The prevalence of strains resistant to some aminoglycosides but susceptible to others must be established locally.

AMIKACIN

Amongst chemically modified kanamycins, most attention has been given to the derivative of kanamycin A synthesized by Kawaguchi et al (1972) and originally called BBK8 which has been marketed under the name amikacin (Fig. 5.5) It is supplied as the sulphate. Its properties have several times been reviewed (Finland et al, 1976; Symposium, 1977).

Antibacterial activity

Broadly, it is more active than kanamycin (Table 5.8) even to exhibiting activity against *Pseudomonas* although it is less active in this respect than gentamicin or tobramycin. It has about a quarter of the activity of gentamicin against *Staph. aureus* and half the activity against Escherichia and Pseudomonas. Various mycobacteria and *Nocardia asteroides* are susceptible. It otherwise exhibits typical aminoglycoside characteristics including synergic activity with β-lactam agents (Klastersky et al 1974) and an effect of divalent cations on its activity against *Pseudomonas aeruginosa* (Kelly & Matsen 1976) analagous to that seen with gentamicin (page 466).

Its particular interest is that it is little or not affected by the great majority of enzymes that degrade gentamicin and tobramycin (Table 5.9) and is consequently active against strains that owe their resistance to the elaboration of those enzymes. Price et al (1974b) collected 152 strains of various organisms, mostly Gram-negative rods, resistant to a number of aminoglycosides, and determined their sensitivity to the average peak plasma concentrations produced by conventional doses of kanamycin (20 μg per ml), gentamicin (8 μg per ml), tobramycin (8 μg per ml) and amikacin (20 μg per ml). On this basis they found the commonest resistance patterns amongst the 152 strains to be: kanamycin plus gentamicin plus tobramycin (49 strains), kanamycin alone (28), kanamycin plus gentamicin (19, mostly *Pseudomonas*), gentamicin plus tobramycin (17, mostly *P. stuartii*) and kanamycin plus tobramycin (12, mostly Serratia). Amikacin resistance was not found alone or in any combination except with resistance to kanamycin, gentamicin and tobramycin in 12 strains of various species.

In the U.K. Drasar et al (1976) examined Gram-negative rods resistant to 8 μg gentamicin per ml and found amikacin at a level of 16 μg per ml (allowing for the higher plasma levels obtained on conventional dosage) to be active against 85 per cent of the strains of *Pseudomonas aeruginosa*, all the indole-positive *Proteus* and Enterobacteria (also resistant to tobramycin and sissomicin) and the great majority of Providence and Klebsiella (which were all resistant to sissomicin and half to tobramycin). Against other species the activity of amikacin was comparable with that of tobramycin and much superior to that of sissomicin.

Pharmacokinetics

The pharmacokinetic behaviour of amikacin is virtually identical with that of its parent, kanamycin. Bodey et al (1974) found mean peak plasma concentrations of 25.4 μg per ml after an intramuscular dose of 300 mg/m^2 and 52.4 μg per ml at the end of a 15 minute intravenous infusion of a similar dose. Kanamycin given similarly produced a concentration of 45 μg per ml. The half-life of kanamycin of 1.9 hours compared with 2 hours for amikacin by the intravenous and 2.8 hours by the intramuscular routes. Meyer et al (1975) found that an intramuscular dose of 7.5 mg/kg produced a mean peak plasma concentration of 27.6 μg/ml. Clarke et al (1974) found that in volunteers intravenous infusion of 3.33 mg per kg for 6 hours followed by 1 mg per kg produced a steady state concentration of 12 μg per ml. Yates et al (1978) found that after rapid intravenous injection the period for which the serum level exceeded 10 μg/ml was only about 30 min after a 125 mg dose but 3 hr after 500 mg. The pharmacokinetic behaviour of amikacin appears to be considerably more predictable than that of gentamicin, serum levels of which differ considerably in individuals receiving similar doses (Walker et al, 1979).

Howard & McCracken (1975) found plasma levels of 17–20 μg per ml in infants receiving 7.5 mg/kg intravenously and no accumulation after doses of 12 mg/kg for 5–7 days. Intravenous infusion of the same dose over 20 minutes produced very low levels. They recommend an initial dose of 10 mg/kg followed by 7.5 mg/kg twice daily (Howard et al 1976). The plasma half-life was longer in babies of lower birth weight and was still 5–5.5 hours in babies a week or more old. There was little change in the plasma concentration (18.3 and 20.6 μg per ml) or the half-life (1.7 and 1.9 hours) on the third and seventh days of a period over which 150 mg/m^2 was infused over 30 minutes 6-hourly. When the dose was raised to 200 mg per m^2 the concentration of the drug between infusions never fell below 8 μg per ml.

Distribution and excretion

The apparent volume of distribution (23–28 per cent) indicates distribution of the drug through the extracellular water. Amikacin does not appear to be bound to plasma protein. CSF levels in adult volunteers receiving 7.5 mg/kg i.m. were less than 0.5 μg/ml (Briedis and Robson, 1978).

Elimination is by the renal route although there may be some extrarenal elimination in anephric patients (Regeur et al 1977) and urinary recovery has been variously reported to be between 65 and 85 per cent over 24 hours with urinary concentrations of 170–2900 μg per ml. Renal clearance values, variously given as 70–84 ml/min, suggests the drug is filtered and the ratio of amikacin to creatinine clearance (0.65–0.7) indicates that, just as with the parent kanamycin, tubular reabsorption is insignificant.

The drug naturally accumulates in patients with impaired renal function and should it be necessary to treat such patients, the virtual identity of pharmacokinetic behaviour means that the dosage could be modified as suggested for kanamycin (page 453).

Madhavan et al (1976) found the mean plasma half-life in patients on, or recently off, haemodialysis to be 3.75 hours, while that on peritoneal dialysis was 28 hours. Evidently the drug is removed reasonably effectively by haemodialysis but will certainly accumulate in patients managed by peritoneal dialysis. This is confirmed by Regeur et al (1977) who make recommendations for the treatment of patients undergoing intermittent dialysis.

Toxicity

The acute toxicity of amikacin for mice is equal to that of kanamycin and about a quarter that of gentamicin. Amongst 1098 patients reviewed by Gooding et al (1976) neurosensory hearing loss (mainly high tone deafness) was detected by audiometry in 16 patients in only one of whom it was found to be severe. Coloric testing revealed labyrinthine injury in 11 patients, in nine of whom it was reversible. Impairment of renal function was observed in 37 patients, in 28 of whom it was mild or transient. Of 77 patients treated by Black et al (1976) with 7.5 or more mg per kg 8-hourly, three developed tinitus but none vertigo or nystagmus. High frequency (but not conversational) hearing loss was found in almost a quarter of the patients monitored audiometrically. Hearing remained abnormal in 10 out of 13 patients and in one, cochlear damage appeared after cessation of treatment. Patients with high tone hearing loss had generally received more drug (average total dose 24 as against 9.6 g) for longer (19 as against 9 days) than patients without. Over half the patients with peak serum levels exceeding 32 or trough levels exceeding 10 μg per ml developed cochlear damage. Both in this series and in that reported by Gooding et al (1976) the main contributory factor was previous treatment with other aminoglycosides.

Clinical use

The properties and clinical uses of amikacin have been extensively reviewed (Finland et al 1976). Amikacin is generally less active and less toxic by a factor of 2 or 4 than are gentamicin or tobramycin, a difference which is almost exactly offset by the greater peak plasma levels attained on conventional dosage. The place of amikacin (certainly at its present cost) is in the treatment of infections due to organisms resistant to other aminoglycosides because of the ability to degrade them. Amikacin may show no advantage against strains that owe their resistance to reduced permeability to aminoglycosides (page 143).

GENTAMICIN GROUP

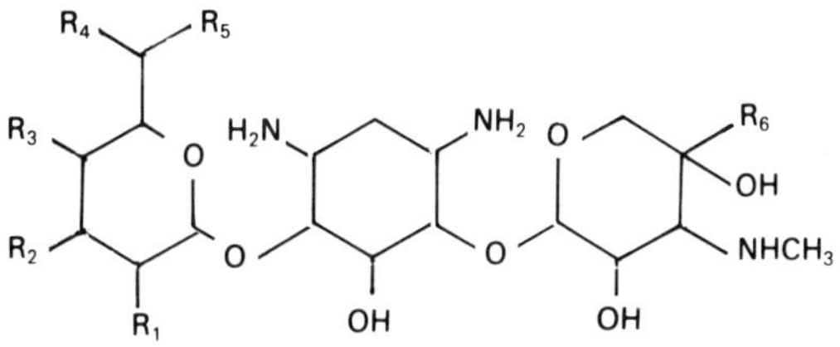

		R_1	R_2	R_3	R_4	R_5	R_6
GENTAMICIN	A	NH_2	OH	OH	H	OH	H
	B	OH	OH	OH	H	NH_2	CH_3
	C_1	NH_2	H	H	CH_3	$NHCH_3$	CH_3
	C_{1a}	NH_2	H	H	H	NH_2	CH_3
	C_2	NH_2	H	H	CH_3	NH_2	CH_3
	B_1	OH	OH	OH	CH_3	NH_2	CH_3
	X	NH_2	OH	OH	H	OH	CH_3

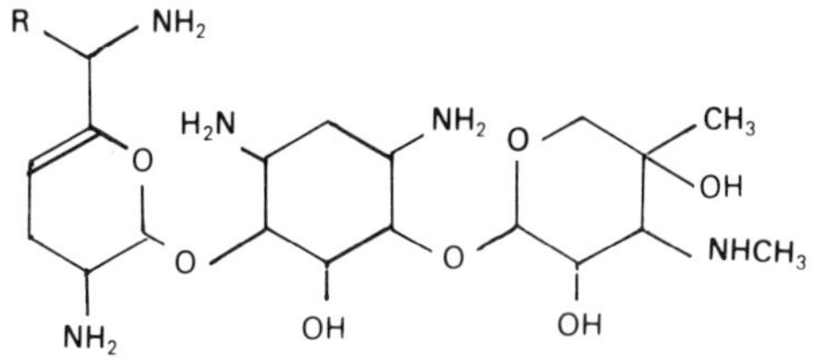

SISSOMICIN (R = H) and VERDAMICIN (R = CH_3)

Fig. 5.7 Structures of the gentamicins and their relatives

The gentamicin family has seen several additions since the original complex was discovered as the product of a strain of *Micromonospora purpurea* in the Schering Research Laboratories (Weinstein et al 1964). Its name is so spelt because the termination 'mycin' should be considered to denote derivation from a Streptomyces. Naturally formed gentamicin contains several components (Fig. 5.7) of which those designated C_1, C_1A and C_2 are required to be present in the commercial product in certain proportions.

Isolation, identification and further manipulation of minor components A, B, B_1 and X have been reported (Lee et al 1976). Gentamicin A has one-quarter to one eighth the activity of the gentamicin C complex against *Staphylococcus aureus* and *Escherichia coli* and virtually no antipseudomonal activity. Gentamicin X is similar. The overall activities of gentamicin B and B_1 are somewhat greater but their toxicity is similar to that of gentamicin X. Gentamicin A and X are 20–50 times more inhibitory to *Trichomonas vaginalis* than is gentamicin C. Gentamicin X is also active against *Entamoeba histolytica.*

GENTAMICIN

Commercial preparations of the gentamicin C complex are supplied as the sulphate. It is freely soluble in water but virtually insoluble in ethyl alcohol and non-polar solvents. β-lactam antibiotics (penicillins and cephalosporins) are commonly prescribed in combination with gentamicin (or other aminoglycosides) and the two agents frequently inactivate one another if mixed together in infusion fluids. Depending on the identity and concentration of the agents, the composition, the pH and temperature of the fluid, amongst other factors, the β-lactam agent or the aminoglycoside may be the more severely affected. For example, McLaughlin & Reeves (1971) have shown that when carbenicillin and gentamicin are mixed in an intravenous fluid and the concentration of carbenecillin is much the higher, the gentamicin is progressively inactivated, while in a mixture of methicillin and kanamycin it is the penicillin and not the aminoglycoside which suffers. The process, which is believed to be due to the opening of the β-lactam ring with inactivation of the penicillin and reaction with the methylamino group of gentamicin to form an inactive amine (Ervin et al 1976) takes several hours and is seen in clinical practice only if the agents are mixed in a bottle for slow parenteral infusion—a practice which is any case to be deprecated since it produces inadequate levels of gentamicin.

Antibacterial activity

As will be evident from Table 5.8 gentamicin is more active than other aminoglycosides against most of the species listed. The most significant activity is against *Pseudomonas aeruginosa* which is 5–10 times greater than that of neomycin or kanamycin. The actual MIC of gentamicin for sensitive strains of *Pseudomonas aeruginosa* found by different workers varies considerably. The probable explanation for this has been proposed by Garrod & Waterworth (1969) who found that the result of many such tests can vary as much as 32-fold with the magnesium content of the medium. Magnesium ions, which are essential for the growth of this species and enhance its pigment production, also, with increasing concentration, reduce apparent sensitivity to this antibiotic. This is a factor very difficult to control and the test is better conducted by direct comparison with a number of strains of the same organism having a known normal sensitivity. Calcium ions and excessive concentrations of NaCl also affect its activity. As with other aminoglycosides, activity is diminished under anaerobic (Harrell and Evans, 1978) or hypercapnic conditions (Reynolds et al 1976).

Since gentamicin is commonly relied on for the speculative treatment of severe undiagnosed infection it is important to note that activity against streptococci is only moderate, although again exceeding that of kanamycin, and that clostridia and other anaerobic bacteria are resistant. Because of its wide antibacterial spectrum of activity (in higher concentrations) against mycoplasma, gentamicin has been successfully used to control contamination of tissue cultures not only of viruses but of chlamidia and rickettsiae which are themselves susceptible to the standard mixture of penicillin and streptomycin (White et al 1976). The action of gentamicin is bactericidal and influenced in the usual way by pH but to different degrees according to bacterial species.

Bactericidal synergy with a wide variety of β-lactam agents can be demonstrated *in vitro* against many Gram-negative rods, notably *Pseudomonas aeruginosa* but not all combinations are equally effective. Amongst those tested against Pseudomonas infections in the rat, Andriole (1974) found that of gentamicin with carbenicillin to be markedly superior to those with either cephalothin or cefaclor and amongst many aminoglycoside-β-lactam combinations tested against a number of Gram-negative rods *in vitro* Klastersky et al (1974) found combinations with carbenicillin to be those most frequently synergic against Pseudomonas and those with cephalothin against Klebsiella.

Resistance

Strains of staphylococci, enterobacteria and Pseudomonas resistant to gentamicin have now been reported from many centres but apart from localized outbreaks remain, in this country at least, relatively uncommon. There seems nevertheless no doubt that they have increased in frequency—for example, Richmond et al (1975) in Manhattan isolated 29, 24, 10, 136 and 468 resistant strains of various Gram-negative rods over the period 1970–4. There are numerous examples in the literature of hospital outbreaks of infection similar to that described by Bint et al (1977) involving a strain of *Staphylococcus aureus* or that described by Rennie & Duncan (1977) in which a klebsiella acquired an R factor which conferred on it resistance to gentamicin and tobramycin.

Until comparatively recently resistance of this kind (in which acquisition of R factors confers on previously sensitive strains the ability to synthesize enzymes which destroy aminoglycosides) was held to be the only resistance of clinical significance. Indeed, this belief was the basis of much of the stimulus to synthesize new aminoglycosides and most of the strains so affected are sensitive, for example, to amikacin.

It has several times been noted that gentamicin-resistant organisms are most frequently isolated from urine and more often in patients who have received the drug (Baird et al 1976) and it is now clear that another variety of resistance to aminoglycosides which is not due to antibiotic degradation by R factor specified enzymes may be clinically significant. This resistance is probably due to reduced cell permeability and while peculiar to aminoglycosides affects them all to a greater or lesser degree. This type of resistance usually results from exposure to the drug (notably topical) but may be conferred, together with the ability to synthesize aminoglycoside degrading enzymes, by some plasmids. Its clinical significance is that newer aminoglycosides which are active against strains resistant to older members of the group by virtue of their insusceptibility to degrading enzymes may show no advantage against relatively impermeable strains—in fact even the reverse. It is generally held that natural impermeability of the cell plays an important part in the resistance of *Pseudomonas aeruginosa* to a variety of antibiotics and as further evidence of this, Mills and Holloway (1976) were able to isolate mutants of Pseudomonas with modified permeability characteristics which were hypersusceptible to gentamicin.

Pharmacokinetics

Like other aminoglycosides, gentamicin is almost unabsorbed from the alimentary tract and must be administered parenterally. The plasma level of gentamicin produced by a great variety of administration schedules has been the subject of exhaustive investigation since the introduction of the drug. This intense activity was stimulated initially by concern that dangerously high levels might occur and subsequently because it was recognized that fear of toxicity might result in therapeutically ineffective dosage. If gentamicin had been introduced before penicillin we might well now know much more about optimum antibiotic dosage schedules.

In normal subjects there are wide variations between individuals in the peak plasma concentrations and half-lives of the drug observed after similar doses, but in the large study of Siber et al (1975) individual patients tended to behave consistently. The peak plasma level is achieved 1.5 to 2 hours after intramuscular injection and the average peak concentration resulting from a dose of 1 mg per kg in adults with normal renal function has been generally found to be about 4 μg per ml. The peak plasma concentration increases proportionally with dose. It is now generally held that concentrations above 5 μg per ml are necessary for adequate therapeutic effect and Noone & Rogers (1976) present evidence that in the case of pulmonary infection 8 μg per ml may be required. The plasma half-life has been held to about 2 hr, but more sensitive methods of assay have now revealed that while the bulk of the drug is excreted relatively rapidly a significant proportion is eliminated much more slowly, the terminal half-life being of the order of 12 days (Kahlmeter et al, 1978).

There is a marked effect of age: in children up to 5 years the peak plasma concentration is about half and for children between 5 and 10 about two-thirds of the level produced by the same dose in adults. According to Siber et al (1975) this difference can be eliminated to a large extent by calculating dosage not on the basis of weight but on surface area—which is much more closely related to the volume of the extracellular fluid in which gentamicin is distributed. They found that the peak plasma concentrations of 4–6 μg per ml generally thought to be therapeutically necessary could be produced in all age groups by a dosage of 60 mg per metre^2 or 2.5 mg per kg in patients between the ages of 6 months and 5 years, 2 mg per kg in those of 5–10 years and 1.5 mg per kg in those over 10 years.

After intravenous injection or infusion over a period up to one hour the concentration and elimination of the drug after the second hour are similar to those seen after corresponding intramuscular injection, but the immediate concentrations produced by very rapid infusion are, of course, substantially higher. Some patients with normal renal function develop unexpectedly high and some unexpectedly low peak values on conventional doses of gentamicin. Fever appears to be a significant factor in reducing the peak concentration (Pennington et al 1975) and anaemia has been found by some workers (Barza et al 1975) to be a significant factor in raising it. The mechanisms involved in these effects have not been elucidated but it suggested that haemodynamic changes associated with fever and anaemia might facilitate mobilization of the drug from intramuscular injection sites to raise the peak concentration or to modify drug distribution and renal handling in such a way as to lower it. Whatever the mechanism, the frequent simultaneous presence of fever, anaemia and renal impairment in severely infected patients emphasizes the uncertainty of the plasma concentration likely to be obtained and the need to monitor the plasma level in severely ill patients.

Distribution

Gentamicin is distributed in the extracellular fluid and since fat contains less extracellular fluid than other tissues, obesity should be an indication to reduce the dose per kg body weight unless some of the drug is taken up by fat. On the basis of pharmacokinetic comparisons in obese and normal subjects, Schwartz et al (1978) conclude that the volume of distribution in obese subjects closely approximates to the lean body mass plus 40 per cent of the adipose mass. Gentamicin traverses the placenta producing a concentration in the fetal blood about one-third of that in the maternal. Access to the lower respiratory tract is limited and Pennington & Reynolds (1975) suggest that in treating pulmonary infection the dosage regimen should take into account the MIC of the infecting organism and the fact that in their dog experiments rapid intravenous infusion produced the highest but shortest-lived intrabronchial concentrations while intramuscular injection produced lower but more sustained levels. As some indication of the concentration to be expected in inflammatory exudate MacGregor (1977) found the maximum concentration in saline-induced peritoneal exudate in the rabbit to be about a third of the peak plasma concentration but to persist very much longer. The drug does not reach the CSF in useful concentrations after systematic administration (Chang et al, 1975).

Excretion

After the first day of therapy, when some retention occurs, gentamicin is almost quantitatively excreted unchanged in the urine, principally by glomerular filtration but since some 20–30 per cent of the drug is bound to plasma protein there is probably an element of tubular secretion. In severely oliguric patients some extrarenal elimination by unidentified routes evidently occurs. Riff & Jackson (1971) found urinary levels of 16–125 μg per ml in patients with normal renal function who were receiving 1.5 mg per kg per day as maintenance therapy. In the presence of severe renal impairment with persistence of the drug in the circulation, urinary levels as high as 1 mg per ml may be found.

The clearance of the drug is linearly related to that of creatinine and this relationship is used as the basis of the modified dosage schedules which are required in patients with impaired renal function in order to avoid accumulation of the drug. In view of the great variation reported by many workers in the plasma levels produced by the same dose of the drug in different patients (page 144) it comes as no surprise that predictions of appropriate dosage for individual patients based on formulae, nomograms or even computer programs are not particularly reliable (Kaye et al 1974). This is not to say, however, that imperfect performance means that such guides to dosage are valueless since the need to take into account the patient's size, age and renal function when initiating therapy is not in doubt; rather it is a warning against over-elaboration of the mathematical basis of dosage prediction in an area where the biological basis of variation is still only partly elucidated.

Haemodialysis removes the drug at about 60 per cent of the rate at which creatinine is cleared while peritoneal dialysis removes only about 20 per cent of the administered dose over 36 hours—a rate which does not add materially to normal elimination (Gary 1971). The efficacy of haemodialysis differs amongst dialysers. Halpren et al (1976) found plasma half-lives reduced from about 50 hours to 7.4–11.3 hours in patients dialysed on four different machines in all of which the rate of clearance increased with flow rate.

Toxicity

Gentamicin is ototoxic, vestibular function being that usually affected. To what extent it is also nephrotoxic is disputed but at least this effect is rare. Where it occurs, it is presumably related to the high concentrations of gentamicin that develop in the kidney (Edwards et al 1976). It has several times been reported that dose related impairment of renal function is not uncommon in those receiving gentamicin but this is mild and reversible. Where more severe and less readily reversible nephrotoxicity occurs it is almost invariably seen in patients with pre-existing renal disorders (Bygbjerg & Moller 1976). Autoradiographic localisation indicates that gentamicin is very selectively localised in the proximal convoluted tubules (Kuhar et al 1979) and Mitchell et al (1977) describe a specific effect on potassium excretion which may both indicate the site of toxicity and provide an early indication of renal damage. Because of the frequency with which gentamicin is used in combination, potentiation of its toxicity by other agents has received considerable attention. There have been a number of reports describing augmented nephrotoxicity in patients treated with combinations of gentamicin and cephalosporins and this has been regarded as an example of 'synergic toxicity' where each of the agents exerts a detrimental effect on the same target organ which is generally clinically insignificant when the agents are given alone but notable when they are given together. Allegations that these drug combinations are unusually nephrotoxic have, however, been criticized on the grounds that the patients affected were suffering from severe sepsis associated with shock or disseminated intravascular coagulopathy, or from other disorders that are themselves associated with renal failure. Attempts to resolve this therapeutically important issue by functional and structural studies of the kidneys of treated animals have so far added more complication than clarification. Far from adding to the renal toxicity of gentamicin, cephazolin, cephalothin and even cephaloridine, generally regarded as the most nephrotoxic of the cephalosporins in current use (page 99), actually protected the rat kidney from gentamicin nephrotoxicity (Luft et al 1976a; Dellinger et al 1976). To what extent these and other experimental findings are peculiar to the animal models used cannot at present be judged but pending further clarification it appears prudent to avoid where possible the simultaneous or sequential administration of potentially nephrotoxic or ototoxic agents. In rats given prolonged courses, Luft et al (1978a) found that the initial tubular necrosis resolved and the regenerated renal epithelium was resistant to further gentamicin damage.

It seems originally to have been assumed that the enhanced antibacterial activity of gentamicin in comparison with other aminoglycosides is paralleled by equal enhancement of ototoxicity and a lower scale of dosage was decided on accordingly. The original scales suggested carried caution too far. In our experience and that of many others the present normal dosage has never proved ototoxic in patients with good renal function. Toxicity assumes importance in patients with renal impairment (including that occurring naturally in the very young or not-so-old) or treated previously or concurrently with other potentially ototoxic drugs—not forgetting previous treatment or excessive dosage of gentamicin itself. The subject is placed in proper perspective by the extensive study of Jackson & Arcieri (1971) who found the overall incidence of ototoxicity to have been 2 per cent. Vestibular damage occurred in 66 per cent, auditory in 15 per cent and both in 18 per cent. Analysis of 913 courses of treatment, in 70 of which damage occurred, showed the main determinant to be impaired renal function.

Clinical applications

These are referred to elsewhere in the book but they may be briefly summarized here. The principal field for gentamicin treatment which has clearly increased in scope and popularity in the last few years is serious coliform infections in various sites. In the urinary tract it is particularly indicated for *Pseudomonas aeruginosa* infections. In Gram-negative septiciaemia many workers now regard gentamicin as the antibiotic of choice. In severe sepsis of unknown origin it is usually combined with an agent active against Gram-positive organisms and, where they are thought likely to be implicated (for example, in severe sepsis following abdominal surgery), an agent active against anaerobes. In systemic *Pseudomonas aeruginosa* infection it is advisable to combine gentamicin with large doses of carbenicillin. A noteworthy feature has been success in treating severe infection in neonates, including septicaemia and meningitis, for which intrathecal or intraventricular injections may be necessary. *Pseudomonas aeruginosa* meningitis and Gram-negative pneumonia have been successfully treated in adults. It should be remembered that another organism highly sensitive to gentamicin is *Staph. aureus*, and Richards et al (1971) report success in various staphylococcal infections, some severe. Various forms of local application have been successful particularly in eliminating the highly sensitive staphylococcus from burns, bed sores, various sorts of dermatitis and nasal carriage sites, but as with other local applications of antibiotics this practice has in many cases been complicated by the emergence of gentamicin-resistant strains. Oral administration for pre-operative suppression of the bowel flora is said to be successful with much smaller doses than those of neomycin used for this purpose.

SISSOMICIN

This naturally occurring dehydro derivative of gentamicin C_1a (Fig. 5.7) was recovered in the Research Laboratories of the Schering Corporation from the fermentation products of *Micromonospora myosensis* (Weinstein et al 1970). Verdamycin, the corresponding dehydro-gentamicin C_2 is less active than is sissomicin. There is conflicting information about its *in vitro* activity compared with that of gentamicin and tobramycin but Scheer et al (1979) found superior activity against many enterobacteria and Pseudomonas strains. Activity against *Staph. aureus* is equal. Against Enterobacter spp., Habwe and Shadomy (1979) found it more active than amikacin, gentamicin, netilmicin or tobramaycin. It is active against some strains resistant to gentamicin and tobramycin but its advantage in this respect seems unlikely to be great since its susceptibility to the aminoglycoside degrading enzymes listed in Table 5.9 is identical with that of gentamicin. In the treatment of experimental infections its margin of superiority is sometimes greater (Waitz & Miller, 1979). Like other aminoglycosides it has been shown to act synergically with β-

lactam antibiotics, but the observations of Klastersky et al (1973) do not suggest any particular advantage over other aminoglycosides in this direction. Its pharmacokinetic behaviour is virtually identical with that of gentamicin (Rodriguez et al, 1975) but specific dosage recommendations for the treatment of patients with impaired renal function have been proposed (Pechère et al, 1976).

Its acute toxicity exceeds that of gentamicin but in nephrotoxicity they do not differ and sissomicin takes longer to produce deafness in animals than does gentamicin although gentamicin has slightly less effect on vestibular function (Hoffmann & Luckhaus, 1979). Studies in man accord generally with these findings: Gruenwaltd et al (1976) in a review of 1561 patients treated with sissomicin and 1484 with gentamicin record otovestibular toxicity in 2.1 per cent and 4.5 per cent respectively. These include probable, possible and doubtful effects, the percentages of probable were 0.6 and 2.

Most of the claims even for marginal superiority in antibacterial activity over gentamicin against naturally susceptible strains have been disputed and in its pharmacokinetic behaviour and susceptibility to bacterial degradation sissomicin closely resembles gentamicin. Any claim for preference over the better established agent must rest therefore almost entirely on the claimed differences in toxicity. There may be a special place for its use that we have not identified but looking at the other competitors in the race against gentamicin, sissomicin at the moment can only be listed as 'also ran'. A derivative, 5-episissomycin (Waitz et al 1978), is more active against several species and resistant to a number of aminoglycoside-degrading enzymes (Watanakunakorn, 1978).

Netilmicin

It was found in the laboratories of the Schering Corporation that 1-*N*-alkylation of certain aminoglycosides produces derivatives that are active against many aminoglycoside-resistant bacteria. The *N*-ethyl derivative of sissomicin appears particularly promising and has been developed under the name netilmicin (Wright, 1976). Against normally susceptible strains it has been found generally to be similar in activity to gentamicin but less active against Serratia, Pseudomonas (Kantor & Norden 1977) and Providencia (Briedis & Robson 1976). It is active against many gentamicin-resistant strains, particularly (Miller et al 1976) those which elaborate ant(2″) (page 137), but even amongst the publications which have already appeared there have inevitably been disagreements about the proportion of strains and even species from various sources which are resistant to other aminoglycosides but accessible to netilmicin.

It exhibits such typical aminoglycoside properties as bactericidal activity at or close to the MIC, greater activity at alkaline pH, depression of activity against Pseudomonas by divalent cations and synergy with β-lactam antibiotics, although the experience of Fu & Neu (1976) does not suggest that it is particularly active in this respect. After intramuscular administration of 2 or 3 mg/kg to normal subjects Humbert et al (1978) found mean peak serum concentrations around 5 and 9 μg/ml and after similar intravenous infusions terminal levels around 12 and 16 μg/ml. The serum half life was 2.2 hr in normal subjects and linearly inversely related to creatinine clearance. Dialyser clearance is similar to that reported for gentamicin (Luft et al 1978b).

The special interest of the compound, apart from its activity against resistant strains, is that in the rat at least, as judged by functional and microscopical studies, the drug is distinctly less nephrotoxic than is gentamicin (Luft et al 1976b) and its experimental otoxicity, both vestibular and cochlear appears to be particularly low (Symonds, 1978). Igarashi et al (1978) found the drug to be less ototoxic than gentamicin for squirrel monkeys. Nephrotoxicity observed in 4 of 25 patients treated by Panwalker et al (1978) could, in two cases, have been related to host factors. The drug has been used successfully to treat severe Gram-negative bacillary infection (Edelstein and Meyer, 1978) and complicated urinary infections (Maigaard et al 1978).

References on page 150.

Pharmaceutical preparations and dosages on p. 153

References

Akita E, Tsuruoka T, Ezaki N, Niida T 1970, J Antibiot (Tokyo) 23:173
Anderson E L, Gramling P K, Vestal P R, Farrar W E 1975 Antimicrob Ag Chemother 8: 300
Andriole V T 1974 J Infect Dis 129: 124
Baird I M, Slepack J M, Kauffman C A, Phair J P 1976 Antimicrob Ag Chemother 10: 626
Barry J M, Koch R 1963 Antimicrob Ag Chemother 1962 p. 538
Barza M, Brown R B, Shen D, Gibaldi M, Weinstein L 1975 J Infect Dis 132: 165
Berk D P, Chalmers T 1970 Ann Intern Med 73: 393
Bint A J, George R H, Healing D E et al 1977 J Clin Path 30: 165
Black H R, Griffith R S 1971 Antimicrob Ag Chemother 1970 p. 314
Black R E, Lau W K, Weinstein R J, Young L S, Hewitt W L 1976 Antimicrob Ag Chemother 9: 956
Bodey G P, Valdivieso M, Feld R, Rodriguez V 1974 Antimicrob Ag Chemother 5: 508
Briedis D J, Robson H G 1976 Antimicrob Ag Chemother 10: 592
Briedis D J, Robson H G 1978 Antimicrob Ag Chemother 13: 1042
Brummett R E, Himes D, Saine B, Vernon J 1972 Arch Otolaryngol 96: 505
Bygbjerg I C, Moller R 1976 Scand J Infect Dis 8: 203
Chang F N, Flaks J G 1970 Proc Nat Acad Sci US 67: 1321
Chang M J, Escobedo M, Anderson D C et al 1975 Pediatrics 56: 695
Clarke J T, Libke R D, Regamey C, Kirby W M M 1974 Clin Pharmacol Ther 15: 610
Cohen L S, Wechsler A S, Mitchell J H, Glick G 1970 Amer J Cardiol 26: 505
Conway N, Birt B D 1965 Brit Med J 2: 260
Courtney K O, Thompson P E, Hodgkinson R, Fitzsimmons JR 1960 Antibiot Ann 1959–60 p. 304
Danbara H, Yoshikawa M 1975 Antimicrob Ag Chemother 8: 243
Decaris L J 1953 Ann Pharmacol Franc 2: 44
Dellinger P, Murphy T, Barza M et al 1976 Antimicrob Ag Chemother 9: 587
Dixon H, Polglase W J 1969 J Bact 100: 247
Drasar F A, Farrell W, Maskell J, Williams J D 1976 Brit Med J 2: 1284
Edelstein P H, Meyer R O 1978 J Antimicrob Chemother 4: 495
Edwards C Q, Smith C R, Baughman K L et al 1976 Antimicrob Ag Chemother 9: 925
Ervin F R, Bullock W E Jr, Nuttall C E 1976 Antimicrob Ag Chemother 9: 1004
Fairley K F, Bond A G, Brown B, Habersberger P 1967 Lancet 2: 427
Federspil P, Schätzle W, Tiesler E 1976 J Infect Dis 134: (Suppl) S200
Finland M, Brumfitt W, Kass E H (eds) 1976 J Infect Dis 134: Suppl Nov S235
Fu K P, Neu H C 1976 Antimicrob Ag Chemother 10: 526
Garrod L P, Waterworth P M 1969 J Clin Path 22: 534
Gary N E 1971 J Infect Dis 124: (Suppl) S96
Gooding P G, Berman E, Lane A Z, Agre K 1976 J Infect Dis 134: Suppl Nov S441
Graybiel A, Schuknecht H F, Fregly A R et al 1967 Arch Otolargyngol (Chicago) 85: 156
Gruenwaltd G, Arcieri G, Conti A 1976 Infection 4: Suppl 4: 505
Gundersen W B 1967 Acta Path Microbiol Scand 69: 214
Habwe V, Shadomy S 1979 J Antimicrob Chemother 5: 73
Halpren B A, Axline S G, Coplon N S, Brown D M 1976 J Infect Dis 133: 627
Harrell L J, Evans J B 1978 Antimicrob Ag Chemother 14: 927
Haskell T H, French J C, Bartz Q R 1959 J Amer Chem Soc 81: 3480
Heifetz C L, Fisher M W, Chodubski J A, DeCarlo M O 1972 Antimicrob Ag Chemother 2: 89
Hieber J P, Nelson J D 1976 Antimicrob Ag Chemother 9: 899
Hoffmann K, Luckhaus G 1979 Infection 7 Suppl 3: 252
Höltje J-V 1979 Antimicrob Ag Chemother 15: 177
Howard J B, McCracken G H 1975 Antimicrob Ag Chemother 8: 86
Howard J B, McCracken G H, Trujillo H, Mohs E 1976 Antimicrob Ag Chemother 10: 205
Humbert G, Leroy A, Fillastre J P, Oksenhendler G 1978 Antimicrob Ag Chemother 14: 40
Igarashi M, Levy J K, Jerger J 1978 J Infect Dis 137: 476
Imamura A, Hori M, Nakazawa K et al 1956 Proc Imp Acad (Japan) 32: 648
Jackson G G, Arcieri G 1971 J Infect Dis 124: (Suppl) 130
Johnsonbaugh R E, Drexler H G, Light I J, Sutherland J M 1974 Amer J Dis Child 127: 245
Kahlmeter G, Jonsson S, Kamme C 1978 J Antimicrob Chemother 4: 143
Kantor R J, Norden C W 1977 Antimicrob Ag Chemother 11: 126
Kaplan J M, McCracken G H Jr, Thomas M L et al 1973 Amer J Dis Child 125: 656
Kawaguchi H T, Naito T, Nakagawa S, Fujisawa K 1972 J Antibiot 25: 695
Kaye D, Levison M E, Labovitz E D 1974 J Infect Dis 130: 150
Keeney R E, Coodley E L 1975 J Clin Pharmacol 15: 695

Kelly M T, Matsen J M 1976 Antimicrob Ag Chemother 9: 440
Kitaoka M, Mori M, Arimitsu Y 1976 Jap J Med Sci Biol 28: 285
Klastersky J, Hensgens C, Debusscher L 1973 Antimicrob Ag Chemother 7: 640
Klastersky J, Hensgens C, Henri A, Daneau D 1975 Antimicrob Ag Chemother 5: 133
Klastersky J, Nyamubeya B, Vandenborre L 1974 J Med Microbiol 7: 465
Krauss M R, King J C, Cox R P 1968 J Bact 95: 2413
Kuhar M J, Mak L L, Lietman P S 1979 Antimicrob Ag Chemother 15: 131
Kunin C M 1966 Ann N Y Acad Sci 132: 811
Lacey R W, Chopra I 1972 J Gen Microbiol 73: 175
Lee B K, Condon R G, Wagman G H, Katz E 1976 Antimicrob Ag Chemother 9: 151
Lindeman H H 1969 Acta Otolaryngol (Stockh) 67: 177
Line D H, Poole G W, Waterworth P M 1970 Tubercle (Lond) 51: 76
Lockwood W R, Bower J D 1973 Antimicrob Ag Chemother 3: 125
Luft F C, Patel, V, Yum M N, Kleit S A 1976a Antimicrob Ag Chemother 9: 831
Luft F C, Yum M N, Kleit S A 1976b Antimicrob Ag Chemother 10: 845
Luft F C, Rankin L I, Sloan R S, Yum M N 1978a Antimicrob Ag Chemother 14: 284
Luft F C, Brannon D R, Stropes L L et al 1978b Antimicrob Ag Chemother 14: 403
MacGregor R R 1977 Antimicrob Ag Chemother 11: 110
Madhavan T, Yaremchuk K, Levin N et al 1976 Antimicrob Ag Chemother 10: 464
Maigaard S, Frimodt-Möller N, Madsen P O 1978 Antimicrob Ag Chemother 14: 544
Mason D J, Smith R M, Dietz A 1961 Antibiot Chemother 11: 118
Mason D J, Dietz A, Hanka L J 1963 Antimicrob Ag Chemother 1962 p. 607
McLaughlin J E, Reeves D S 1971 Lancet 1: 261
Meyer R D, Lewis R P, Carmalt E D, Finegold S M 1975 Ann Intern Med 83: 790
Miller G H, Arcieri G, Weinstein M J, Waitz J A 1976 Antimicrob Ag Chemother 10: 827
Mills B J, Holloway B W 1976 Antimicrob Ag Chemother 10: 411
Misiek M, Chisholm D R, Leitner F, Price K E 1970 Antimicrob Ag Chemother 1969, p. 225
Mitchell C J, Bullock S, Ross B D 1977 J Antimicrob Chemother 3: 593
Mitsuhashi S 1972 In: 'Drug Inactivating Enzymes and Antibiotic Resistance' ed. Mitsuhashi S et al Prague Avicenum p. 115
Naber K G, Westenfelder S R, Madsen P O 1973 Antimicrob Ag Chemother 3: 469
Noone P, Rogers B T 1976 J Clin Path 29: 652
O'Connor S, Lam L K, Jones N D, Chaney M O 1976 J Org Chem 41: 2087
Oliver T J, Goldstein A, Bower R R et al 1962 Antimicrob Ag Chemother 1961, p. 495
Panwalker A P, Malow J B, Zimelis V M, Jackson G G 1978 Antimicrob Ag Chemother 13: 170
Paradelis A G, Douboyas J, Stathopoulos G et al 1978 Antimicrob Ag Chemother 14: 514
Pechère J-C, Pechère M M, Dugal R 1976 Antimicrob Ag Chemother 9: 761
Pennington J E, Dale D C, Reynolds H Y, MacLowry J D 1975 J Infect Dis 132: 270
Pennington J E, Reynolds H Y 1975 J Infect Dis 131: 158
Price K E, De Furia M D, Pursiano T A 1976 J Infect Dis 134: Suppl Nov S249
Price K E, Godfrey J C, Kawaguchi H 1974a Adv Appl Microbiol 18: 191
Price K E, Pursiano T A, DeFuria M D, Wright G E 1974b Antimicrob Ag Chemother 5: 143
Rassekh M, Pitton J S 1971 Chemotherapy 16: 239
Regeur L, Colding H, Jensen H, Kampmann J P 1977 Antimicrob Ag Chemother 11: 214
Rennie R P, Duncan I B R 1977 Antimicrob Ag Chemother 11: 179
Reynolds A V, Hamilton-Miller J M T, Brumfitt W 1976 Lancet 1: 447
Richards F, McCall C, Cox C 1971 J Amer Med Assoc 215: 1297
Richmond A S, Simberkoff M S, Rahal J J, Schaefler S 1975 Lancet 2: 1176
Riff L T, Jackson G G 1971 J Infect Dis 124: (Suppl) 98
Rinehart K L Jr 1969 J Infect Dis 119: 345
Rodriguez V, Bodey G P, Valdivieso M, Feld R 1975 Antimicrob Ag Chemother 7: 38
Roediger W E W, Ludwin D, Hinder R A 1975 Postgrad Med J 51: 399
Schatz A, Bugie E, Waksman S A 1944 Proc Soc Exp Biol (NY) 55: 66
Scheer M, Weinstein M J, Waitz J A 1979 Infection 7 Suppl 3: 241
Schillings R T, Schaffner C P 1962 Antimicrob Ag Chemother 1961, p. 274
Schwartz S N, Pazin G J, Lyon J A et al 1978 J Infect Dis 138: 499
Siber G R, Echeverria P, Smith A L et al 1975 J Infect Dis 132: 637
Simon V K, Mösinger E U, Malerczy V 1973 Antimicrob Ag Chemother 3: 445
Standiford H D, de Maine J B, Kirby W M M 1970 Arch Int Med 126: 255
Stark W M, Hoehn M M, Knox N G 1968 Antimicrob Ag Chemother 1967, p. 314
Stenbjerg S, Husted S, Mygind K 1975 Scand J Haemat 14: 280
Stratford B C, Dixson S, Cobcroft A J 1974 Lancet 1: 378

Suh B, Stephens J L, Kunin C M 1979 Antimicrob Ag Chemother 16: 519
Symonds J M 1978 J Antimicrob Chemother 4: 199
Symposium 1977 Amer J Med 62: 863
Thompson R Q, Presti E A 1968 Antimicrob Ag Chemother 1967, p. 332
Tseng J T, Bryan L E, Van den Elzen H M 1972 Antimicrob Ag Chemother 2: 136
Tsukiura H, Fujisawa K, Konishi M et al 1973 J Antibiot (Tokyo) 26: 351
Umezawa H, Okamj Y, Hashimoto T et al 1965 J Antibiot 18: 101
Umezawa H, Ueda M, Maeda K et al 1957 J Antibiot Series A 10: 181
Umezawa H, Umezawa S, Tsuchiya T, Okazaki Y 1971 J Antibiot 24: 485
Valtonen M V, Suomalainen R J, Ylikahri R H, Valtonen V V 1977 Brit Med J 1: 683
Vladoianu I R, Dubini F, Bolloli A 1975 J Hyg (Camb) 75: 203
Wagman G H, Marquez J A, Watkins P D et al 1973 J Antibiot 26: 732
Waitz J A, Moss E L Jr, Drube C G, Weinstein M J 1972 Antimicrob Ag Chemother 2: 431
Waitz J A, Miller G H, Moss E Jr, Chiu P J S 1978 Antimicrob Ag Chemother 13: 41
Waitz J A, Miller G H 1979 Infection 7 Suppl 3: 259
Waksman S A, Lechevalier H A 1949 Science 109: 305
Walker J M, Wise R, Mitchard M 1979 J Antimicrob Chemother 5: 95
Walton J R 1978 J Antimicrob Chemother 4: 309
Watanakunakorn C 1978 J Antimicrob Chemother 4: 474
Weinstein M, Luedemann G M, Oden E M, Wagman G H 1964 Antimicrob Ag Chemother 1963, p. 1
Weinstein M J, Marquez J A, Testa R T et al 1970 J Antibiot 23: 551
White L A, Hall H E, Tzianabos T, Chappell W A 1976 Antimicrob Ag Chemother 10: 344
Wick W E, Welles J S 1968 Antimicrob Ag Chemother 1967, p. 341
Wilmot T J 1973 J Laryngol Otol 87: 235
Wilson P, Ramsden R T 1977 Brit Med J 1: 259
Wittman H G, Apirion D 1975 Mol Gen Genet 141: 331
Wittner M, Tanowitz H 1971 Amer J Trop Med Hyg 20: 433
Wright J J 1975 J Chem Soc Chem Commun 6: 206
Yamada T, Tipper D, Davies J 1968 Nature (Lond) 219: 288
Yates R A, Mitchard M, Wise R 1978 J Antimicrob Chemother 4: 335
Zimmermann R A, Moellering R C Jr, Weinberg A N 1971 J Bact 105: 873

Aminoglycosides. Pharmaceutical preparations and dosage

Name	*Dosage*	*Preparations*	*Common international proprietary names*	
Streptomycin	*Adult* i.m.: 750 mg–1 g daily, or at longer intervals. *Children* i.m.: 20–40 mg/kg daily in divided doses. *Premature and Full-term infants* 20–30 mg/kg body weight daily, for no longer than 10 days.	Injection 1 g	Streptomycin Sulphate	
Neomycin	*Adult* Oral: The dosage varies up to a maximum of 1 g every four hours.	Tablets 500 mg Ophthalmic preparations Aural preparations Topical preparations In combination with various antibiotics in the above forms	Mycifradin, Nivemycin Neobiotic, Otobiotic Bykomycin, Myacyne	(UK) (USA) (Ger)
Kanamycin*	*Adult* i.m.: 15 mg/kg daily in divided doses, with a maximum dose of 1.5 g a day. For severe infections the drug can be given by slow i.v. infusion at a dose of 15 mg/kg daily in two divided doses. *Children* 15 mg/kg a day in 2 divided doses. *Premature Infants* 7.5–10 mg/kg a day in divided doses.	Injection 1 g in 3 ml Capsules 250 mg	Kantrex Kamycine, Otokalixan Kanabristol	(UK) (Fr) (Ger)
Framycetin	*Adult* Oral: 2–4 g daily. *Children* Maximum 50 mg/kg body weight daily.	Ophthalmic and aural preparations. Topical applications. Tablets, sterile powder.	Soframycin	(UK)

Name	*Dosage*	*Preparations*	*Common international proprietary names*	
Paromomycin	*Adult* Oral: 2–4 g daily in divided doses		Grabbomycin No proprietary preparation is available in the UK	(Ger)
Gentamicin*	*Adult* 60 kg body weight and over: i.m., i.v. 80–160 mg every 8 hours *Children* up to 2 weeks old i.m., i.v.: 3 mg/kg 12 hourly. 2 weeks–12 years 2 mg/kg every 8 hours.	Injection Topical, Ophthalmic and Aural preparations	Cidomycin, Genticin Garamycin Gentalline Refobacin, Sulmycin	(UK) (USA) (Fr) (Ger)
Tobramycin*	*Adults* i.m., i.v.: 3–5 mg/kg body weight over 24 hours. It should be given every 8 hours. *Neonates* 4 mg/kg daily in 2 divided doses.	Injection	Nebcin	(UK)
Amikacin*	*Adults and Children* 15 mg/kg a day in 2 divided doses, with a maximum of 1.5 g a day for adults. *Neonates and Premature Infants* 10 mg/kg as an initial loading dose then 15 mg/kg a day in 2 divided doses.	Injection	Amikin	(UK)
Sissomicin	0.5–1.25 mg/kg up to 3 times a day.	Injection	Not yet available in the UK	
Spectinomycin	*Adult* i.m.: Males a single dose of 2 g Females a single dose of 4 g	Injection	Trobcin Stanilo	(UK) (Ger)

*See also Chapter 26

6

Chloramphenicol

Chloramphenicol was the first broad spectrum antibiotic to be discovered. It was isolated independently by Ehrlich et al (1947) from a streptomycete (*S. venezuelae*) from soil in Venezuela and by Carter et al (1948) from a similar organism found in a sample of soil from a compost heap in Illinois. A method of synthesizing chloramphenicol from *p*-nitroacetophenone has proved practicable on a large scale, and alone among clinically important antibiotics chloramphenicol is manufactured synthetically.

Chemical properties
Chloramphenicol consists of yellowish-white crystals with an intensely bitter taste. Its solubility is about 2.5 mg/ml water and about 400 mg/ml alcohol. Aqueous solutions have a pH of about 5.5 and are extremely stable. They keep indenfinitely at ordinary room temperature if protected from light, and will withstand boiling. Some hydrolysis occurs on autoclaving.

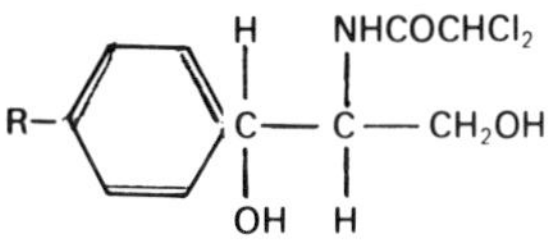

Fig 6.1 Structures of chloramphenicol (R = NO_2) and thiamphenicol (R = CH_2SO_2)

There are four isomers of chloramphenicol, all of which have been synthesized, but none has greater activity than natural chloramphenicol. Because the antibacterial activity (and toxicity) of chloramphenicol might be due to metabolic intermediates in which the nitro group is reduced, a series of such compounds was synthesized by Corbett and Chipko (1978) but all were less active than the parent compound.

One derivative, thiamphenicol (page 165) in which the nitro group of chloramphenicol is replaced by a sulphomethyl group (Cutler et al 1952) has received renewed attention in recent years because of potentially advantageous pharmacokinetic behaviour, but particularly because it is claimed that thiamphenicol does not induce the potentially fatal aplastic anaemia that rarely mars the otherwise excellent performance of chloramphenicol (page 161).

Table 6.1 Sensitivity of bacteria to chloramphenicol

	MIC μg/ml		MIC μg/ml
C. diphtheriae	0.5–3.0	*H. influenzae*	0.2–0.5
Str. pneumoniae	1.0–4.0	*Pasteurella* spp	0.2–10
Actino. israeli	1.0–4.0	*B. pertussis*	0.2–12.5
Clostridium spp	1.5–>500	*N. meningitidis*	0.5–1.5
Str. pyogenes	2.0–4.0	*N. gonorrhoeae*	0.5–1.5
B. anthracis	2.5–5.0	*Kl. pneumoniae*	0.5–2.0
Str. faecalis	4.0–12	*Salmonella* spp.	0.5–10
Staph. aureus	4.0–12	*Kl. aerogenes*	0.5–30
Myco. tuberculosis	12–25	*Brucella* spp.	0.8–2.5
		Esch. coli	0.8–8.0
		Bacteroides spp.	1.0–8.0
		Salm. typhi.	2.0–4.0
		Sh. sonnei	2.5–6.0
		Proteus spp.	2.5–64
		Ps. aeruginosa	50–125

Based on
McLean I W et al 1949 J Clin Invest 28: 953
Chen C H et al 1949 South Med J 42: 986
Garrod L P 1952 Antibiot Chemother 2: 689
Garrod L P 1952 Brit Med J 1: 1263
Garrod L P 1955 Brit Med J 2: 1529
Welch H et al 1952 Antibiot Chemother 2: 693

Antimicrobial activity

Chloramphenicol is active against a wide range of Gram-positive and Gram-negative bacteria (Table 6.1), and chlamydia (page 428). *Salm. typhi*, *H. influenzae* and *B. pertussis* are more susceptible to chloramphenicol than to almost any other antibiotic, a fact to be remembered in considering indications for clinical use. Chloramphenicol is strictly bacteristatic against almost all bacterial species including *Brucella*, Escherichia, Streptococci, and Salmonella. It exerts a bactericidal effect against some strains of Gram-positive cocci and against *H. influenzae* (Turk, 1977) and Neisseria (Rahal and Simberkoff, 1979). A good deal has been made of the bacteristatic effect of chloramphenicol because of its capacity, when given in combination, to inhibit the action of penicillins which rely for their action on the continuing growth of the bacterial cell (page 258). This has been held to be specially important in meningitis (page 325) and Carrizosa et al (1975) in experimental rabbit endocarditis showed that chloramphenicol antagonized the bactericidal effect of penicillin on *Streptococcus viridans*. No antagonism between empicillin and chloramphenicol was observed by Cole et al (1979) against either ampicillin-sensitive or -resistant strains of *H. influenzae*. Anyone who might still be tempted to make general rules about interactions between bacteristatic and bactericidal agents should note that inducible enzymes are inhibited by concentrations of chloramphenicol lower than those required to interrupt total protein synthesis and hence bacterial growth (Michel et al, 1977). As a result, subinhibitory concentrations of chloramphenicol prevent the production of β-lactamase by a variety of bacterial strains and far from preventing the bactericidal action of simultaneously administered penicillin, facilitate it.

Acquired resistance

Resistant strains of various bacterial species have been isolated by serial passage *in vitro* (Reeve & Suttie, 1968). As the concentration of chloramphenicol is increased, mutants resistant at successive genetic loci emerge, and resistance increases in a stepwise fashion. These mutants commonly grow less rapidly than the sensitive parent strain and show antigenic and morphological changes including loss of flagella. Similar stepwise resistance to chloramphenicol, tetracycline and penicillin due to the additive effect of several genes has been transferred to *Neisseria gonorrhoeae* by transformation.

Resistance has been seen in many wild strains of both Gram-positive and Gram-negative organisms and the prevalence of resistant strains has often followed faithfully the frequency of usage of the drug.

The chloramphenicol molecule can be attacked at a number of different points by bacteria, and the degradation products have no antibacterial activity. Naturally occurring chloramphenicol-resistant *Staph. aureus* owe their resistance to inactivation of the agent by an inducible acetylase (Shaw & Brodsky, 1968). Such resistance can be spontaneously lost, or 'cured' by acridines, indicating a plasmid location for the responsible gene (page 267). An analogous situation exists in many enterobacteria. In Escherichia, where the capacity to acetylate chloramphenicol accounts for the resistance of many clinical isolates, three types of chloramphenicol acetyl transferase occur (Zaidenzaig & Shaw, 1976), the codes for which are carried by different R factors (page 266). Chloramphenicol resistance has now been encountered in *Haemophilus influenzae* and *Bacteroides fragilis* (Britz and Wilkinson, 1978) where it appears to be due to synthesis of an acetyl transferase with such similar properties to those observed in Escherichia as to suggest its transfer from that organism. The nature of the enzyme and the genetic background to such a transfer are discussed by Shaw et al (1978). Inevitably plasmid-borne resistance is likely to be linked to others and the therapeutically feared combination of resistance to both chloramphenicol and ampicillin has already been seen (Bryan, 1978).

Spontaneous chromosomal mutation to high resistance in *Proteus mirabilis* is similarly accompanied by enzyme synthesis. Transfer to such strains of an R factor conferring resistance to chloramphenicol results in additional synthesis of the same enzyme (Shaw, 1971).

The outstandingly important example of transferable chloramphenicol resistance is in the *Salm. typhi* responsible for an outbreak in Mexico and subsequently imported both into Britain and into the U.S.A. E.S. Anderson has repeatedly drawn attention to the grave threat to the effective therapy of enteric fever posed by such transferable resistance which is now widespread in *Salmonella typhi* in Mexico, India and the Far East (Anderson, 1975).

Resistance of *Pseudomonas aeruginosa* to chloramphenicol (and to some other agents) is partly enzymic and partly due to impermeability of the organism to the drug. Ingram & Hassan (1975) describe a strain which could be cured of chloramphenicol resistance by acridine dyes (page 267) with elimination of both acetyl transferase and the permeability barrier. Intriguingly, the same effect was brought about by the natural phenazine dye, pyocyanin, which this strain of *Pseudomonas* did not produce.

The appearance of strains of *Haemophilus influenzae* resistant to ampicillin (page

328) is threatening the use of that agent for the treatment of severe haemophilus infection, notably meningitis. Most are generally susceptible to chloramphenicol and co-trimoxazole but strains also resistant to chloramphenicol already occur (Uchiyama et al, 1980).

Dependent strains which will not grow, or grow very poorly, in the absence of chloramphenicol have also been described.

PHARMACOKINETICS

Absorption

The usual route of administration is oral, and the peak blood levels obtained are shown in Table 6.2. The dissolution and absorption of poorly soluble compounds like chloramphenicol depends to an important extent on size and aggregation of the primary particles. Direct comparisons show that preparations containing large particles may give blood levels only ¼–½ those arising from small particles (Glazko et al, 1968). Reducing or increasing the dose has a proportionate effect on the level attained. This falls comparatively slowly and since there is some cumulative effect, a level of 4–6 μg per ml can be maintained by giving 0.5 g at six-hour intervals, or a correspondingly higher one by raising the dose.

Table 6.2 Serum levels of chloramphenicol after oral administration in patients of different ages

Age	*Dose mg/kg*	Peak *Hour*	Peak *ug/ml*	*Half-life Hours*
Adult	7(0.5 g)	2–3	8–13	2–5
	30(2 g)		15–25	
1–2 days	50	6–12	30–40	24–28

Glazko et al 1968 Clin Pharmacol Therap 9: 472
Weiss et al 1960 New Engl J Med 262: 787

Children can neither swallow the capsules given to adults nor tolerate the exceedingly bitter taste of the free drug. The alternative for them is a suspension of chloramphenicol palmitate, a tasteless compound which is itself inert, and is not absorbed until it is hydrolysed in the gut, liberating chloramphenicol. Chloramphenicol palmitate (and the same is true of the stearate) exists in two distinct crystalline and an amorphous form. Hydrolysis time in the gut is a major determinant of the efficacy of absorption and as one crystalline form is substantially more rapidly hydrolysed than the other, the blood levels obtained are directly related to the proportion of that form which is present in the preparation (Aguiar et al, 1967). Better plasma levels may be obtained if the drug is dispersed in a freely soluble matrix such as urea (Chiou, 1971).

Parenteral administration

Simple suspensions of finely ground chloramphenicol are available which are suitable only for intramuscular injection. Chloramphenicol sodium succinate, on the other hand, which is freely soluble and undergoes hydrolysis in the tissues with the liberation of chloramphenicol, can be injected in a small volume intramuscularly, intravenously or subcutaneously.

The levels of the drug after administration by these routes are half or less of those following the same dose by the oral route (Snyder et al 1976). The peak level is of course attained immediately after intravenous injection. In contrast to this, the absorption of an intramuscularly injected suspension appears to be slower (peak at 4–5 hours) than that from the bowel, detectable blood levels persisting longer (half-life 4–6 hours).

Distribution

About 60 per cent of the chloramphenicol in the blood is bound to protein. Binding is reduced in cirrhotic patients and neonates with correspondingly elevated concentrations of free drug (Koup et al, 1979b). Studies of organ distribution have shown the diminishing order of concentration to be kidney, liver, lung, heart, spleen, muscle and brain. Free diffusion occurs into serous effusions, and into the fetal circulation. Penetration into all parts of the eye has also been demonstrated, therapeutic levels in the aqueous humour being obtained even after local application of a 0.5 per cent ophthalmic solution (Beasley et al, 1975). Perhaps most important of all, the concentrations attained in the cerebro-spinal fluid are higher than those of any other antibiotic: they amount to 30–50 per cent of those in the blood even in the absence of meningitis. Two hydrocephalic infants with shunt-associated ventriculitis had ventricular fluid concentrations (23 and 57 per cent of serum level) outside this range and Yogev and Williams (1979) suggest that adequate concentrations at this site cannot be relied upon. Glandular secretions also contain some of the antibiotic: its presence in the saliva occasions a bitter taste and accounts for changes in the oral flora but the secretion is too variable to allow salivary levels to be used as a measure of serum concentration (Koup et al, 1979a).

Metabolism

Before excretion, most of the chloramphenicol in the body is inactivated either by conjugation with glucuronic acid or by reduction to inactive aryl amines, and the main site of these processes is the liver. Hill & Struck (1973) identified the microsomal amidase, which cleaves chloramphenicol to its main excretory product by removing the dichloroacetate group, as being probably identical with that which hydrolyses acetanilide, phenacetin and lidocaine. With such dependence on hepatic metabolism, the clearance of the drug in patients with impaired liver function is naturally depressed (Koup et al, 1979b).

Pre-treatment with phenobarbitone, a potent inducer of the liver microsomal enzymes concerned with glucuronide conjugation, results in diminished blood levels of chloramphenicol and increased urinary excretion of the glucuronide. Conversely, chloramphenicol (in common with other drugs including sulphaphenazole, phenylbutazone and dicoumarol) inhibits hepatic microsomal mixed function oxidases so that the levels of some unrelated drugs metabolized by the same pathway may be raised. Toxicity from dicoumarol or diphenylhydantoin and hypoglycaemic collapse from tolbutamide in patients also receiving chloramphenicol have been ascribed to this cause (Christensen and Skovsted, 1969). By the same mechanism, chloramphenicol inhibits the action of cyclophosphamide which depends for its cytotoxicity on transformation into active metabolites by hepatic microsomal enzymes (Faber et al, 1975). Similarly, pre-treatment with chloramphenicol delayed the recovery of experimental animals anaesthetized with pentobarbitone (or other barbiturates eliminated by metabolism) but not of those anaesthetized with barbitone which is largely excreted unchanged in the urine (Adams, 1970). In the fasting rat, Alvin & Dixit (1974) found the glucuronide conjugation of chloramphenicol to be depressed as a result of which the half-life of the active drug was increased and hexobarbitone sleeping time correspondingly prolonged. This effect could be reversed by glucose. The findings of Mehta et al (1975) in malnourished children appear analagous, although their plea for revised dosage schedules in such children based on these findings were editorially held to be premature. Following a single dose of 25 mg chloramphenicol per kg they found the peak plasma levels 2–4 hours later to be 1.5–2 times higher and the plasma half life to be 2½ times longer (30 and 12 hours) in malnourished children as compared with normal children. They attribute this to impaired conjugation of the drug since malnourished children excreted only 35–55 per cent of the drug (as compared with 75–85 per cent in normal children) in the conjugated form.

Excretion

Excretion is mainly renal: 90 per cent of the dose can be detected in the urine by chemical methods, but only about 10 per cent of this amount is unaltered antibiotic. In experimental animals, the microbiologically active drug (but not its conjugates) exerts a potent relaxant effect on the ureter (Benzi et al, 1970). Chloramphenicol itself is excreted by the glomeruli, but excretion of its inactive derivatives is also by active tubular secretion. Excretion diminishes linearly with renal function. At a creatinine clearance of less than 20 ml/min, maximum concentrations of 10–20 μg/ml in urine are found in contrast to 150–200 μg/ml in the normal. Despite this, blood levels of active chloramphenicol are only marginally elevated but microbiologically inactive metabolites accumulate. This may explain both the poor results of treatment of urinary infection plus exalted toxicity found in some (especially elderly) patients (Lindberg et al, 1966).

Very young infants are deficient in the ability to form glucuronides and their glomerular and tubular excretion capabilities are low. The rate of disappearance of chloramphenicol from the blood is consequently greatly prolonged (Table 6.2) and in the new-born the dose and frequency of administration must be reduced (page 449) if toxic quantities of the drug are not to accumulate.

About 3 per cent of the administered dose is excreted in the bile but only about 1 per cent appears in the faeces and that mostly in inactive forms. The idea that high concentrations of chloramphenicol can be demonstrated in the bile appears to have come from studies in the rat, in which, in contrast to man, the bile is a principal route of excretion.

Side effects and toxicity

Chloramphenicol passed the usual toxicity tests in animals, and had been in worldwide use for several years before it was recognized as a potentially highly dangerous bone marrow depressant. More years passed before it was observed to be the cause of the 'grey syndrome' in infants, another usually fatal condition. It thus has the unenviable distinction of exerting lethal toxic effects of two different kinds. Other effects are of only minor importance.

Alimentary tract

Soreness of the mouth is fairly common if a course of treatment exceeds one week. It is attributable to a depression of the normal flora by the antibiotic in the saliva and consequent overgrowth of *Candida albicans*. Mild cases show little change, but in the more severe there is a frank stomatitis: it is possible that vitamin B deficiency or even a direct action of the antibiotic on the epithelium, which in the tongue shows atrophic changes, may also play some part. Nausea, vomiting and diarrhoea, although they may occur, are much less common and less severe than those capable of being caused by tetracyclines.

Contrary to the claim that chloramphenicol intensifies the destruction of G-6-PD-deficient erythrocytes, Chan et al (1971) found that treatment reduced the rate of red cell destruction in Chinese patients with typhoid fever.

Marrow aplasia

A few isolated reports of granulocytopenia and aplastic anaemia following chloramphenicol therapy appearing about 1950 attracted little attention. The storm burst in 1952, when a succession of papers described such effects, not merely in single cases but in series. By the end of 1963 the Registry of Blood Dyscrasias of the American Medical Association had collected 674 cases of drug-induced marrow aplasia in 299 of which chloramphenicol was implicated. Despite unabated publicity given to the relationship between aplasia and chloramphenicol (Dunne et al, 1973) the drug continues to be given for trivial reasons and in extravagant doses.

Simple granulocytopenia is uncommon: the usual effect is a total aplasia of the marrow. The first signs are purpura and pallor, and a blood count reveals a deficiency of all blood cells including platelets. In over 400 cases reviewed by Best (1967) manifestations appeared *during* treatment in only 22 per cent. In 10 per cent there was an interval between the cessation of treatment and onset of dyscrasia of 130 days or more. Cause and effect may thus never be connected. Most patients die despite repeated transfusions. Survival is most likely in those with early onset of dyscrasia in which few cell types are depressed (Best, 1967). A few patients survive with protracted aplasia and in them myeloblastic leukaemia may ultimately supervene. Cohen & Huang (1973) raised the possibility that this results from chloramphenicol induced chromosomal damage because in the cells of one of their patients they observed a large chromosome resembling that described in some other myeloproliferative disorders.

The frequency of marrow aplasia in treated patients is difficult to compute with any accuracy because of the problem of establishing the size of the population at risk. The value of overall figures is also doubtful because some physicians have given very large doses or treated thousands of patients (Lietman et al, 1964; Woodward & Smadel, 1964) without encountering haematological abnormalities, while others have seen several cases of aplastic anaemia over a limited period. One of us saw three cases, two of them fatal, among an estimated number of 1200 patients treated with chloramphenicol at St. Bartholomew's Hospital up to 1952.

From a Statewide survey in California Wallerstein et al (1969) calculated that the overall risk of fatal aplastic anaemia was two cases per million population per annum. In patients treated with an average of 4 g of chloramphenicol the risk was 13 times greater. By comparison, the risk in patients treated with oxyphenylbutazone was increased 4-fold and that in patients treated with mepacrine was increased 10-fold.

The claim (though contested: Letters, 1970) that marrow aplasia is peculiar to patients of Northern European or even those of English stock and that free use of the drug in other populations, for example in Italy, Israel and South America has not resulted in this complication has been disposed of for Israel at least by a nationwide survey (Modan et al, 1975) which revealed a mean annual incidence of aplastic anaemia of 7.1 and 8.7 per million males and females respectively, in 25 per cent of which chloramphenicol was implicated. Survival was inferior in the patients who had received chloramphenicol and ten patients (half of whom had received chloramphenicol and half had not) went on to develop leukaemia.

It has several times been suggested (though there is no direct evidence for this) that the toxic agent is not chloramphenicol itself but some metabolite, and that marked differences in the incidence of aplasia may be explained by some genetic predisposition. This idea is attractive, but as Best (1967) points out, difficult to reconcile with the extreme rarity of aplasia in more than one member of treated families.

Mechanism

It is now established that chloramphenicol exerts a regular dose-related but reversible depressant effect on the marrow of all those treated with the drug, resulting in vacuolization of erythroid and myeloid cells, reticulocytopenia and ferrokinetic changes (increase in serum iron, increased saturation of iron-binding globulin, and reduced plasma-iron clearance and utilization) indicative of decreased erythropoiesis. Despite the highly suggestive nature of these changes, there is no evidence that this common marrow depression is the precursor of potentially fatal aplasia which differs in being (fortunately) rare, late in onset, irreversible and may follow the smallest dose (Carpenter, 1975).

In mammalian cells, protein synthesis in the cytoplasm differs from that in mitochondria where the process closely resembles that seen in bacteria. As a result, mammalian mitochondrial protein synthesis is subject to inhibition by such agents as erythromycin and chloramphenicol which can interfere so severely with mitochondria as to produce visible structural damage (Agam et al, 1976; Skinnider & Ghadially, 1976). Ferrochetalase is a protein of mitochondrial origin and its inhibition, with consequent blockade of the last stages of haem synthesis, may be responsible for the effect of chloramphenicol on the erythroid series. Corresponding inhibition of mitochondrial membrane-bound cytochromes resulting in impairment of mitochondrial respiration may underly the marked, but reversible, reduction in the number and type of cell colonies that chloramphenicol produces in bone marrow cultures (Ratzan et al, 1974).

The relationship between the common dose-dependent reversible marrow depression and the uncommon non-dose-dependent irreversible aplasia is still not clear but there may be a clue in the not altogether surprising fact that dose-dependent marrow depression is more profound if erythropoiesis or leucopoiesis is already abnormal (Schwarz & Firkin, 1976). Morley et al (1976) make the interesting suggestion on the basis of experimental evidence in mice that the few patients in whom chloramphenicol induced bone marrow depression pursues a relentless and irreversible course may have pre-existing marrow deficiency of genetic or environmental origin. By means of busulphan they produced a mild hypoplastic marrow failure in mice which was difficult to detect by standard methods but persisted for long periods. On exposure to concentrations of chloramphenicol in drinking water that were insufficient to produce changes in normal mice, the marrow deficient animals exhibited a progressive fall in pluri-potential cells and granulocytic precursors.

Amongst other explanations, immunological, metabolic and bone-marrow microcirculatory disorders have been postulated.

Chloramphenicol is not ordinarily antigenic for man but some treated patients develop antibodies which might conceivably exalt the drug's toxicity or diminish its antibacterial effect (Orgel & Hamburger, 1971). One effect of such antibodies is that they will react with chloramphenicol used as a preservative in some commercial red cell reagents and produce false positive red cell antibody tests (Beattie et al, 1976).

Chloramphenicol is a phenylalanine analogue, and diverse observations link chloramphenicol with phenylalanine metabolism. Chloramphenicol inhibits the intestinal uptake of phenylalanine, and the morphological abnormalities of red cells which regularly follow administration of the antibiotic resemble those seen in phenylalanine deficiency. There is, however, no good evidence to link phenylalanine metabolism with chloramphenicol toxicity or to support the view that phenylalanine is useful in its prevention or treatment (Hughes, 1973).

Inhibition of mammalian protein synthesis

The ability of chloramphenicol to inhibit mammalian mitochondrial protein synthesis has naturally produced concern about possible detrimental effects on various host responses, notably antibody synthesis and wound healing. There is no good evidence of a depressant effect on the antibody response of treated patients, but chloramphenicol can be shown to impair immunological responses in certain experimental circumstances. Lipsky et al (1976) found that both chloramphenicol and its L-isomer suppressed a graft versus host reaction beneath the renal capsule and abolished lymphocyte proliferation at the graft site. They concluded that this was the mechanism of the rejection since the L-isomer has no effect on mitochondrial protein synthesis.

Neither Bloom & Grillo (1970) nor Donati (1971) found any evidence that treatment with chloramphenicol (or tetracycline) impaired the healing of experimental wounds in the guinea-pig or rat, but Caulfield & Burke (1971) found that wound healing was greatly delayed in rats treated with intravenous chloramphenicol sodium succinate which presumably produced higher peak plasma levels.

Encephalopathy

Delirium in patients treated with chloramphenicol has usually been explained as an effect of toxic bacterial products liberated spontaneously or in response to treatment. Levine et al (1970) challenge this explanation because they observed episodes of asterexis and delirium in three chloramphenicol-treated patients who had no infection (two were treated in an attempt to depress the synthesis of myeloma protein). Interestingly, doses of the drug which were toxic by mouth were innocuous when given intravenously. It is suggested that chloramphenicol which reaches the liver via the portal vein interfers with hepatic function in such a way as to produce a state of phenylalanine deprivation.

The 'grey syndrome' in infants

This grave disorder in which vomiting, refusal to suck and abdominal distension are followed by circulatory collapse with flaccidity, ashen colour and hypothermia (the 'grey' syndrome) is seen in infants given large doses of chloramphenicol who, because of their immature conjugation and excretion mechanisms, develop exceedingly high plasma levels of the drug. Laxdal and Hallgrimsson (1974) describe similar, but reversible, manifestations in older children (2–8 years) given large doses (90–110 mg per kg per day) for the treatment of meningitis—a further warning against the use of the drug in excessive doses or circumstances in which the ability to eliminate it is suspect.

Other side effects

A number of cases have been described of optic neuritis in children with cystic fibrosis of the pancreas, receiving prolonged chloramphenicol treatment for pulmonary infection. Harley et al (1970) describe the development of optic neuritis in 13 out of 98 patients suffering from cystic fibrosis treated for 80–1500 days with 10–100 mg chloramphenicol/kg/day. Of the 13, 11 promptly improved when the drug was discontinued but central visual acuity in three of six patients who again received the drug was permanently impaired. Morizono and Johnstone (1975) found that 10 per cent propylene glycol or 5 per cent chloramphenicol sodium succinate in Ringer's solution produced irreversible deafness when instilled into the middle ear of the guinea pig. They warn against the use of propylene glycol in ear drops and recommend substantially lower concentrations of chloramphenicol.

Clinical applications

There is a great diversity of opinion on this subject, depending on the degree of importance to be attached to the possibility of toxic effects. We believe that this possibility should not be disregarded, and the following principles, which have frequently been enunciated, should therefore be not only assented to but observed.

Chloramphenicol should never be prescribed for minor infections. There have been many tragic fatalities following its use for trivial conditions such as respiratory catarrh.

It is currently still the drug of choice in typhoid fever and other severe salmonella infections. Some authorities take the view that these are the *only* indications. The least contested of other indications are meningitis or severe respiratory infection due to *H. influenzae*. Pertussis may be an indication in severe cases at an early age and if treatment can be begun early enough. It should be prescribed for other serious infections only when these are resistant, or much less sensitive, to other antibiotics.

Both the daily dose (usually not exceeding 2 g) and the duration of the course (e.g. ten days) should be limited. Although patients may show toxic manifestations after receiving very little of the drug, the danger is almost certainly increased by excessive or repeated dosage or by treatment of patients with impaired hepatic or renal function—including those at the extremes of life.

Despite repeated warnings and appeals to restrict its use (Dunne et al, 1973), some clinicians, guided by their own experience, believe chloramphenicol to be a most valuable drug for much wider indications and prescribe it freely. Apparently the profession is divided into those who, perhaps having seen chloramphenicol cause marrow aplasia, fear this effect and rarely use the drug, and a larger number who ignore this possibility because it seems too remote and prescribe chloramphenicol freely. There is no doubt that chloramphenicol can be, and frequently has been, life-saving in the treatment of severe infections. It can also produce a condition which is commonly irreversible and fatal. The onus is on anyone who prescribes it to show that he has excellent reasons for doing so.

THIAMPHENICOL

Considerable effort has been devoted to the possible synthesis of analogues of chloramphenicol that possess its admirable pharmacokinetic and antimicrobial properties without its capacity to induce irreversible bone marrow aplasia. Up to the time of the synthesis of a trifluoro derivative (Hansch et al 1973) which exhibits almost twice the activity of the parent compound, all chloramphenicol analogues have been less active and only one has come into clinical use. This is the compound in which the nitro group of chloramphenicol is replaced by a sulphomethyl group (page 155) and which is marketed under the name thiamphenicol. It is generally less active than chloramphenicol against both Gram-positive and Gram-negative bacteria but there are important exceptions in that the two compounds are equally active against *S. pyogenes*, pneumococci, Haemophilus and meningococci (Table 6.3). Moreover, the bactericidal activity which chloramphenicol exerts against Haemophilus and Neisseria in contrast to other species, is exhibited to an even greater degree by thiamphenicol. There appears to be complete cross resistance with chloramphenicol, thiamphenicol being acetylated by bacteria which carry plasmids coding for chloramphenicol acetyl-transferase, although the affinity of the enzyme for thiamphenicol is lower than that for the parent compound.

Table 6.3 Comparative activities of thiamphenicol and chloramphenicol against some common bacteria.

	MIC (μg/ml)	
	Thiam-phenicol	Chloram-phenicol
Staph. aureus	4–32	2–4
Str. pyogenes	1–2	1–2
Str. pneumoniae	2	2
N. meningitidis	1	0.5–1
H. influenzae	0.1–2	0.1–2
Esch. coli	4–64	1–16
Klebsiella	4–32	1–8
Proteus spp.	2–32	1–8
Ps. aeruginosa	16–128	32–128
Bacteroides	0.5–32	0.5–16

Original observations supplemented by data from Van Beers D et al 1975 Chemotherapy 21: 73.

Thiamphenicol is absorbed by the oral route, a dose of 500 mg producing a peak plasma level of 3–6 μg per ml after about two hours. The plasma half-life has been reported to be 2.6–3.5 hours. This is similar to that of chloramphenicol but disposal of the drug is quite different. Thiamphenicol is not a substrate for hepatic glucuronyl transferase and its elimination, in contrast to its parent (page 159) is not by conjugation, and its half-life is consequently not affected by phenobarbitone induction. Instead, it is excreted in the urine in the active form, about 50 per cent of the dose being recovered after the first eight hours (in contrast to 5 per cent of chloramphenicol) and 70 per cent over 24 hours (in contrast to 10 per cent of chloramphenicol). The drug is correspondingly retained in the presence of renal failure and in anuric patients the plasma half-life has been reported to be nine hours—a value not significantly affected by peritoneal dialysis (Furman et al, 1976). The persistence of the drug in the circulation in an active form as a result of its resistance to conjugation may underlie the claim that it reaches the bronchial lumen in concentrations sufficient to exert a bactericidal effect on Haemophilus (Cambieri et al, 1970).

These differences are interesting, but the therapeutic attention which has been devoted to the drug rests largely on the claim that no case of irreversible bone marrow aplasia has been traced to its use after about 12 million courses of treatment (Symposium, 1974). Reversal in the course of time of such claims—for example the immunity of the Israeli population to chloramphenicol aplasia (page 162)—has taught us to scrutinize such evidence with extreme caution, but it is interesting that there are differences in the detail of the biochemical effects of thiamphenicol and chloramphenicol on mammalian cells which could be consistent with a difference in their haemotoxicity (Yunis, 1974). Notwithstanding any difference that there may be in the capacity to produce irreversible aplasia, however, there is no doubt that thiamphenicol induces dose-dependent reversible depression of haemopoiesis and immunogenesis (page 162) to a greater extent than does chloramphenicol. This has two consequences. The first is that the drug is of interest as an immunosuppressive agent—and may be a particularly solicitous choice in patients in whom its broad spectrum antibacterial activity is also required. The other is that therapeutic doses (1–1.5 g) are likely to depress erythropoiesis especially in the elderly or those with other reasons for having impaired renal function. On the present evidence, therefore, it appears that substitution of thiamphenicol for chloramphenicol would be more likely to produce the common reversible form of bone marrow depression and less likely to cause the uncommon irreversible kind. In Europe the drug has been widely administered to the evident satisfaction of physician and patient for a great variety of conditions suggested by its broad antimicrobial spectrum. Despite this popularity, the low therapeutic ratio of the drug (its MIC for many common pathogens exceeds the plasma levels obtained on doses which do not commonly depress haemopoiesis) suggests that it should be reserved for those conditions where its special properties make it particularly appropriate. First amongst these is severe infection with Haemophilus, for which chloramphenicol is often used but against which thiamphenicol is more actively bactericidal *in vitro*. Thiamphenicol is not available in the UK.

References

Adams H H 1970 J. Amer Vet Med Ass 157: 1908
Agam G, Gasner S, Bessler H, Fishman P, Djaldetti M 1976 Brit J Haemat 33: 53
Aguiar A J, Krc J Jr, Kinkel A W, Samyn J C 1967 J Pharm Sci 56: 847
Alvin J, Dixit B N 1974 Biochem Pharmacol 23: 139.
Anderson E S 1975 J Hyg (Camb) 74: 289
Beasley H, Boltralik J J, Baldwin H A 1975 Arch Ophthalmol 93: 184
Beattie K M, Ferguson S J, Burnie K L et al 1976 Tranfusion 16: 174
Benzi G, Arrigoni E, Sanguietti L 1970 Archs Int Pharmacodyn Thér 185: 329
Best W R 1967 J Amer Med Ass 201: 181
Bloom G P, Grillo H C 1970 J Surg Res 10: 1
Britz M L, Wilkinson R G 1978 Antimicrob Ag Chemother 14: 105
Brock T D 1964 In: Experimental chemotherapy vol 3 p 119 ed Schnitzer R J, Hawking F. Academic Press, New York
Bryan L E 1978 Antimicrob Ag Chemother 14: 154
Cambieri F, Gambini A, Lodola E 1970 Chemotherapy 15: 356
Carpenter G 1975 Lancet 2: 326
Carrizosa J, Kobasa W D, Kaye D 1975 J Lab Clin Med 85: 307
Carter H E, Gottlieb D, Anderson H W 1948, Science 107: 113
Caulfield J B, Burke J F 1971 Arch Path 92: 119
Chan T K, Chesterman C N, McFadzean A J S, Todd D 1971 J Lab Clin Med 77: 177
Chiou W L 1971 J Pharm Sci 60: 1406
Christensen L K, Skovsted L 1969 Lancet 2: 1397
Cohen H J, Huang A T-F 1973 Arch Intern Med 132: 440
Cole F S, Daum R S, Teller L et al 1979 Antimicrob Ag Chemother 15: 415
Corbett M D, Chipko B R 1978 Antimicrob Ag Chemother 13: 193
Cutler R A, Stenger R J, Suter C M 1952 J Amer Chem Soc 74: 5475
Donati R M 1971 Arch Surg 102: 132
Dunne M, Herxheimer A, Newman M, Ridley H 1973 Lancet 2: 781
Ehrlich J, Bartz Q R, Smith R M, Joslyn D A, Burkholder P R 1947 Science 106: 417
Faber O K, Mouridsen H T, Skovsted L 1975 Brit J Clin Pharmacol 2: 281
Furman K I, Koornhof H J, Kilroe-Smith T A et al 1976 Antimicrob Ag Chemother 9: 557
Glazko A J, Kinkel A W, Alegnani W C, Holmes E L 1968 Clin Pharmacol Ther 9: 472
Hansch C, Nakamoto K, Gorin M et al 1973 J Med Chem 16: 917
Harley R D, Huang N N, Macri C H, Green W R 1970 Trans Amer Acad Ophthalmol Otol 74: 1011
Hill D L, Struck R F 1973 Biochem Pharmacol 22: 127
Hughes D W O'G 1973 Med J Aust 2: 1142
Ingram J M, Hassan H M 1975 Canad J Microbiol 21: 1185
Koup J R, Lau A H, Brodsky B, Slaughter R L 1979a Antimicrob Ag Chemother 15: 651
Koup J R, Lau A H, Brodsky B, Slaughter R L 1979b Anitmicrob Ag Chemother 15: 658
Laxdal T, Hallgrimsson J 1974 Arch Dis Child 49: 235
Letters 1970 New Engl J Med 282: 343, 813, 1047
Levine P H, Regelson W, Holland J F 1970 Clin Pharmacol Ther 11: 194
Lietman P S, di Sant' Agnese P A, Wong V 1964 J Amer Med Ass 189: 924
Lindberg A A, son Nilsson L H, Bucht H, Kallings L O 1966 Brit Med J 2: 724
Lipsky J J, Anderson N D, Lietman P S 1976 Cell Immunol 23: 278
McGowan J E Jr, Terry P M, Nahmias A J 1976 Antimicrob Ag Chemother 9: 137
Mehta S, Kalsi H K, Jayaraman S, Mathur V S 1975 Amer J Clin Nutr 28: 977
Michel J, Jacobs J, Sacks T 1977 Chemotherapy 23: 32
Modan B, Segal S, Shani M, Sheba C 1975 Amer J Med Sci 270: 441
Morizono T, Johnstone B M 1975 Med J Aust 2: 634
Morley A, Trainor K, Remes J 1976 Brit J Haemat 32: 525
Orgel H A, Hamburger R N 1971 Immunology 20: 233
Rahal J J Jr, Simberkoff M S 1979 Antimicrob Ag Chemother 16: 13
Ratzan R J, Moore M A S, Yunis A A 1974 Blood 43: 363
Reeve E C R, Suttie D R 1968 Genet Res 11: 97
Schwarz M A, Firkin B G 1976 Med J Aust 1: 686
Shaw W V 1971 Ann NY Acad Sci 182: 234
Shaw W V, Brodsky R F 1968 J Bact 95: 28
Shaw W V, Bouanchaud D H, Goldstein F W 1978 Antimicrob Ag Chemother 13: 326
Skinnider L F, Ghadially F N 1976 Arch Path Lab Med 100: 601

Snyder M J, Perroni J, Gonzalez O et al 1976 Lancet 2: 1155
Symposium 1974 Postgrad Med J 50: Suppl 5
Turk D C 1977 J Med Microbiol 10: 127
Uchiyama N, Greene G R, Kitts D B, Thrupp L D 1980 J Pediat 97: 421
Wallerstein R O, Condit P K, Kasper C K et al 1969 J Amer Med Ass 208: 2045
Woodward T E, Smadel J E 1964 Ann Intern Med 60 144
Yunis A A 1974 Postgrad Med J 50 (Suppl 5) 149
Yogev R, Williams T 1979 Antimicrob Ag Chemother 16: 7
Zaidenzaig Y, Shaw W V 1976 FEBS Lett 62: 266

Chloramphenicol. Pharmaceutical preparations and dosage

Name	*Dosage*	*Preparations*	*Common international proprietary names*
Chloramphenicol	*Adult* 50 mg/kg body weight, daily in divided doses every six hours. For infections such as septicaemia and meningitis, doses of up to 100 mg/kg a day may be given. *Children* 50 mg/kg body weight, daily in divided doses every six hours. *Premature babies and Infants* 25 mg/kg a day in divided doses every six hours.	Ophthalmic preparations Injection as Sodium Succinate salt. Suspension as Palmitate. Capsules	Chloromycetin, Kemicetine (UK) Amphicol, Opthoclor (USA) Aquamycetin, Chloramsaar (Ger) Sintomicétine, Tifomycine (Fr)

7

Tetracyclines

In 1948, when aureomycin, the first of the tetracyclines, was discovered, the only other antibiotics in general use were penicillin and streptomycin. Each of these had a limited range of activity, and each had to be given by injection. Aureomycin differed from them in having a wide range of activity, including most organisms susceptible to either and some to neither of them, and a second advantage, shared with chloramphenicol, which was discovered at about the same time, of being administrable by the mouth.

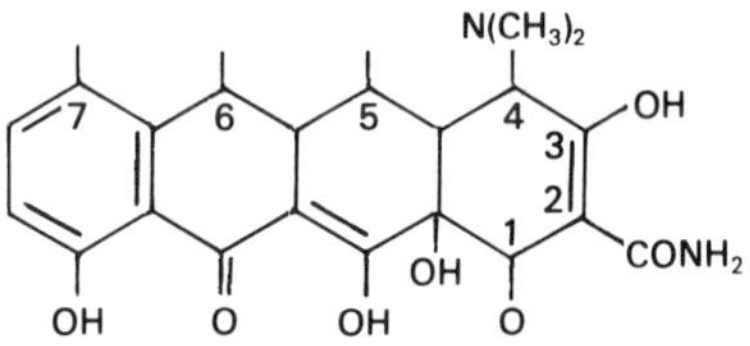

	5	6	7
Tetracycline		CH_3OH	
Chlortetracycline		CH_3OH	Cl
Oxytetracycline	OH	CH_3OH	
Demeclocycline		OH	Cl
Methacycline	OH	CH_2	
Doxycycline	OH	CH_3	
Minocycline			$N(CH_3)_2$
Clomocycline		CH_3OH	Cl

Fig. 7.1 Structure of tetracyclines

The tetracyclines are a family of closely related antibiotics, to which additions are still being made after over 20 years. The first, aureomycin, was so called from the golden yellow colour of the colony of *Streptomyces aureofaciens*, the organism forming it. Two years later (1950) 'Terramycin' derived from *Streptomyces rimosus*, was introduced, and within a further two years their structure was ascertained, which differs only in the presence of a Cl atom in one and an OH group in the other. The names chlortetracycline and oxytetracycline were then proposed for them, and in 1953 tetracycline was introduced, which has neither of these attachments: this can be obtained either by catalytic dehalogenation of chlortetracycline or directly from another *Streptomyces*. To these three compounds have since been added, in 1957, demeclocycline (formerly called demethylchlortetracycline) and, during the 1960s, methacycline, doxycycline, minocycline, clomocycline, lymecycline and rolitetracycline.

The three earlier tetracyclines are all yellow crystalline substances, amphoteric in nature and of low solubility (about 0.05 per cent): their hydrochlorides and sodium salts are much more soluble (that of tetracycline about 10 per cent) and are chiefly used in therapeutics. Their solutions are acid, and those of tetracycline and oxytetracycline are reasonably stable, but that of chlortetracycline is the most unstable of any major antibiotic, particularly in neutral and still more in alkaline solution: in nutrient broth with pH of 7.4 it loses the greater part of its activity during overnight incubation.

Antimicrobial activity

The term 'broad spectrum', denoting a wide range of activity, was coined in connection with this group of antibiotics, and in fact their spectrum is the broadest known (Table 7.1). Susceptible species include not only those, mainly Gram-positive, which are also sensitive to penicillin, but many Gram-negative species which are not, and in addition mycoplasmas, rickettsias and Chlamydia (page 428). Like penicillin the tetracyclines are active against *T. pallidum* and other treponemata: unlike it, they also have some action on the tubercle bacillus. The only large group of fully resistant pathogenic organisms are the fungi. The possible indications for administering tetracyclines, to be considered later, are therefore very numerous.

The MIC of seven tetracyclines for 421 strains of 21 varieties of bacteria is recorded in an extensive study by Steigbigel et al (1968). Table 7.1 compares the activity of three widely used compounds against a variety of bacteria.

For most organisms, individual differences in activity between the different tetracyclines are relatively small and probably insignificant in practice. An important exception is the superior activity of minocycline against staphylococci. Of the 56 strains of *Staph. aureus* they tested, 30 per cent were resistant to all the agents except minocycline, which inhibited two thirds of them at a concentration of 0.8 μg/ml and the others in a concentration of 3.1–12.5 μg/ml. This superior activity of minocycline against some strains of staphylococci resistant to other tetracyclines, which is to a lesser extent shared by doxycyline, has been confirmed by many other authors. Minuth et al (1974) found methicillin-sensitive strains of *Staph. aureus* sensitive to minocycline and doxycycline, while most of a group of 13 methicillin-resistant strains were inhibited by minocycline but not by tetracycline or doxycyline. Candanoza & Ellner (1975), in a comparative study of 200 strains of penicillin-resistant *Staph. aureus*, found that 13 per cent of them were resistant to tetracycline but sensitive to minocycline. Differences in activity between the compounds are less notable against other Gram-positive cocci, although Steigbigel et al (1968) note that minocycline is generally the most active except against enterococci. Only one fifth of the 36 strains they tested were sensitive to less than about 25 μg/ml of any of the compounds tested, with no major differences between them.

Activity against *E. coli*, Klebsiella and Enterobacter varies greatly from strain to strain but again, minocycline is in general the most active compound. None of the tetracyclines has significant activity against *Proteus mirabilis* nor against *Ps. aeruginosa* or Providencia. *H. influenzae* is inhibited by tetracyclines in the range 0.8–12.5 μg/ml, with doxycycline as most active against strains found in sinusitis.

Table 7.1 Activity of tetracyclines against Gram-positive and Gram-negative bacteria

	Minimum inhibitory concentration (μg/ml)					
	Tetracycline		Doxycycline		Minocycline	
	Range	Median	Range	Median	Range	Median
Gram-positive bacteria						
Staph. pyogenes	1.6 ->100	3.19	0.39 ->100	1.6	0.39 - 12.5	0.78
Strep. pyogenes (Group A)	0.19 - 50	0.78	50.09 - 25	0.39	0.09 - 25	0.39
Strep. pneumonice (Dip. pneumoniae)	0.2 - 100	0.8	0.1 - 12	0.2	0.1 - 25	0.2
Strep. viridans spp.	3.9 - 100	3.1	0.09 - 50	0.39	0.09 - 50	0.39
Strep. faecalis (Enterococcus, Group D)	6.3 ->100	>100	1.6 ->100	50	1.6 ->100	100
Gram-negative bacteria						
Escherichia coli	3.1 - 500	12.5	1.6 - 500	12.5	3.1 - 500	6.3
Enterobacter	6.3 - 50	25	12.5 - 25	25	6.3 - 12.5	12.5
Klebsiella	6.3 - 500	50	6.3 - 300	50	3.1 - 500	25
Serratia	200	200	50	50	25	25
Proteus mirabilis	50 ->100	>100	50 ->100	>100	50 ->100	>100
Neisseria gonorrhoeae	0.39 - 6.3	0.78	0.09 - 3.1	0.39	0.19 - 3.1	0.39
Neisseria meningitidis	0.3 - 3.1	0.8	0.8 - 6	1.6	0.8 - 1.6	1.6
Hemophilus influenzae	0.8 - 3.1	1.6	0.8 - 3.14	1.6	0.8 - 3.1	1.6
Shigella	1.6 ->500	100	1.6 - 500	100	1.6 - 500	100
Pseudomonas aeruginosa	50 - 300	200	25 - 300	100	100 - 200	
Mycoplasma and Chlamydia						
M. pneumoniae	1.6 - 3.1	1.6	1.6	1.6	1.6	1.6
T. mycoplasma	0.2 - 0.8	0.4	0.05 - 0.2	0.1		
Chlamydia	0.5 - 4.0	2.0	0.5 - 4.0		0.5 - 4.0	

(Reproduced by kind permission from Neu H J 1978 Bull New York Acad Med 54: 141)

Wood (1975) found that tetracycline-resistant strains of *H. influenzae* were inhibited by 2 μg/ml of minocycline. *Neisseria meningitidis* and *N. gonorrhoeae* are both sensitive; 20 of 25 gonococcal strains were inhibited by minocycline at 0.4 μg/ml.

Minocycline has been compared with doxycycline and tetracycline in its activity against 622 clinical isolates of a variety of anaerobic bacteria (Chow et al, 1975), and found to be significantly more active than the other two compounds when activity was expressed in terms of achievable serum concentrations. Minocycline was particularly active against a variety of anaerobic cocci, and against *B. melaninogenicus*.

Waterworth (1974) noted an inhibitory effect of minocycline against *Candida albicans* but, in a comparative study, showed no difference between the effect of tetracycline and minocycline on the vaginal yeast flora (Oriel & Waterworth 1975).

Other organisms apparently more sensitive to minocycline than to other tetracyclines include *Acinetobacter calcoaceticus var. anitratus (Herellea vaginocola)* (Montgomerie et al, 1976), and *Nocardia asteroides* (Finland, 1974).

Acquired resistance

The acquisition of resistance to tetracyclines is a slow process, and is not often observed during the treatment of an individual patient. Nevertheless resistant strains of various coliform bacilli and of staphylococci have gradually become fairly common; indeed, tetracycline resistance came to be regarded as the hall-mark of a virulent and troublesome staphylococcus. Resistance in haemolytic streptococci, was first observed as long ago as 1952 and its frequency over a number of years in London has been well documented. The proportion of resistant strains rose from 0.7 per cent in 1958 to 41 per cent in 1965 (Dadswell, 1967), remained at this high level for several years and has since decreased somewhat to 27 per cent in early 1971 (Rees, 1971). A survey covering 21 British laboratories in 1975 showed 36 per cent of 1515 group A streptococci were tetracycline-resistant, although there were wide geographical variations. Resistance to tetracyclines also emerged early in pneumococci, and the same survey (Report, 1977) documented this in 13 per cent of 1528 pneumococcal isolates, again with wide variation between regions. A survey in 1977 showed a lower incidence, 6.8 per cent of 866 strains (Howard et al, 1978). Resistance has also been observed in *H. influenzae* (Hansman, 1975).

Examples of resistance *in vitro* and of failure to prevent gas gangrene by the use of prophylactic tetracycline have been reported, and Schwartzman et al (1977) found about half of 57 strains of *Cl. perfringens* showed some degree of resistance to tetracycline.

Mode of action

Antibiotics are classified as bactericidal and bacteristatic, and the tetracyclines decidedly belong in the second category. There may be no such thing as pure bacteristasis, and there is some evidence that high concentrations of tetracyclines cause a steeper fall in the viable count than low ones, but the process is very gradual, with numerous survivors after as long as 24 hours. It is now known that tetracyclines belong to the group of antibiotics acting by interference with protein synthesis, in the case of the tetracyclines at the 30 S ribosome level, and the mechanism is discussed further in Chapter 12. Resistance may be due to decreased permeability to the antibiotic. Bacterial resistance to the tetracyclines is reviewed by Chopra & Howe (1978).

PHARMACOKINETICS

Tetracyclines are usually administered by mouth, but a number of preparations are available for intramuscular and/or intravenous use. The hydrochlorides of the original tetracyclines are much more soluble than the parent compounds and parenteral preparations of tetracycline and oxytetracycline are marketed. Lymecycline and rolitetracycline can be given by intramuscular or intravenous injection, and minocycline by intravenous injection.

Absorption

Absorption from the alimentary tract is relatively good for all compounds except chlortetracycline. Both because defective absorption militates against effective treatment and because the principal side effects are due to retention of the antibiotic in the bowel, much attention has been devoted to this problem. Two factors appear to be involved. One is simply solubility: the hydrochlorides are reasonably soluble in water, giving a highly acid solution, but in a neutral or alkaline medium they tend to be precipitated, or (as when liberated in the intestine) not to dissolve. Secondly, tetracyclines combine with divalent metals, of which calcium is likely to be present in the largest amount. The chelated compounds are not absorbed and pass out in the faeces.

Phosphate is now commonly included in the capsule to enhance absorption either as an addition or in combination with the antibiotic as a tetracycline phosphate complex, but some of the dose remains unabsorbed. Neuvonen et al (1970) showed that the concurrent administration of 200 mg of ferrous sulphate significantly reduced the peak serum concentrations of several tetracyclines.

The problems of absorption of the earlier compounds have been mitigated to a variable extent in the later tetracyclines. Lymecycline, formed by a reaction between tetracycline, formaldehyde and L-lysine, is said to be especially well absorbed by mouth but Whitby & Black (1964) obtained conflicting results in a comparison with tetracycline. Improved absorption is also claimed for demeclocycline, clomocycline and methacycline, but is best established in the case of doxycycline and minocycline, for which the proportion of administered dose absorbed is more than 90 per cent.

The blood level curve is a plateau, having a slow rise and a still slower fall. Factors contributing to this persistence are (1) continued absorption, (2) biliary excretion and reabsorption, (3) protein binding, the extent of which has been determined as 47, 20 and 24 per cent for chlor- and oxytetracycline and tetracycline respectively (Kunin et al, 1959). Demeclocycline, doxycycline and minocycline are all highly protein bound, to the extent of 80–90 per cent. Blood levels achieved after normal oral dosage are of the order of 2–4 μg/ml, with a small cumulative increase with time. Most of the compounds must be given four times daily to maintain therapeutic concentrations in the blood, but the plateau curves of demeclocycline, minocycline and doxycycline enable the two first named agents to be administered twice daily, and doxycycline to be given once daily. The serum half-life of tetracycline is about ten hours, compared with 11–17 hours for minocycline and 15–22 hours for doxycycline.

Distribution

Tetracyclines behave much like penicillin in their diffusion into serous cavities, the foetal circulation and glandular secretions. They enter the cerebro-spinal fluid somewhat more freely, concentrations of tetracycline found there being about 10–25 per cent of those in the blood. A unique feature of their behaviour is deposition in bone in areas where bone is being laid down: here they remain detectable for long periods. Similar deposition in teeth is referred to in the next section.

Tetracyclines are freely excreted into the bile; the concentrations attained are 5–20 times those in the blood, doxycyline attaining especially high levels. Tetracyclines are also found in substantial concentrations in the eye. Doxycycline appears to achieve adequate penetration into the prostate, with mean tissue/serum ratio of 0.7 after oral administration (Oosterlinck et al, 1976).

Several authors have studied the penetration of different tetracyclines into bronchial secretion. Campbell (1970) showed a good correlation between sputum and serum levels in patients receiving 1.0 g of tetracycline daily. The mean sputum level, about 20 per cent of that in serum, was high enough to inhibit all (tetracycline sensitive) pneumococci and most strains of *H. influenzae*. MacCulloch et al (1974), in a study of six patients with bronchiectasis, showed that minocycline achieved much higher levels in sputum than oxytetracycline or doxcycline. Ruhen & Tandon (1976) also found tetracycline and minocycline superior to doxycycline in their capacity to achieve satisfactory antibacterial levels in sputum.

Excretion

The main excretory route is the kidney, but tetracyclines are also eliminated to a greater or lesser extent in the faeces. Faecal excretion occurs even after parenteral administration as a result of passage of the drug into the bile. The proportion of administered dose found in the urine is, for most tetracyclines, in the range of 20–60 per cent, but is less in the case of chlortetracycline, minocycline and doxycycline. Since glomerular filtration is a main determinant of renal excretion of the tetracyclines, these drugs are retained in renal failure. The notable exception is doxycycline which does not so accumulate. The effects of tetracyclines in renal failure are discussed later in this chapter.

Side effects

At the time when the first edition of this book was in preparation, alimentary tract superinfections were almost the only side-effects recognized from the use of these drugs. After years of worldwide use, a number of new unwanted effects began to be described. There is little foundation for the claim that tetracyclines are teratogenic, but some other side-effects are now well documented and, although uncommon, are potentially important.

Gastro-intestinal disturbances

The incidence of these symptoms is dose-dependent, and they are much more common when daily doses of 2 g or more are given than when the dose is limited to 1 g daily. Nausea and vomiting are presumably due to a direct irritant effect of the drug on the gastric mucosa. Possibly diarrhoea can also be so caused, but this and other effects are more often the result of superinfection, i.e. the replacement of the suppressed normal flora by antibiotic-resistant organisms. It is here that the broad spectrum effect operates to the patient's disadvantage: most of the flora of the mouth, and even of the more complex flora of the lower bowel, including lactobacilli and clostridia as well as streptococci and the normal coliforms, are sensitive, and their suppression leaves a vacuum liable to be filled by less well-disposed inhabitants. The three main varieties of superinfection are by *Candida albicans*, by Proteus and Pseudomonas species resistant to tetracyclines, and by resistant staphylococci. Any of these may become clinically significant and the dangerous condition of staphylococcal enterocolitis has been especially well described. Staphylococcal enterocolitis has now become less common with the diminished threat from hospital staphylococci in many centres, and the growing tendency to avoid antibiotic regimens which seriously alter the bowel flora.

Although these serious consequences of superinfection are well documented, the relationship between the common minor gastro-intestinal symptoms and the undoubted changes in bowel flora is much less certain. For example, in a double-blind trial of two treatments of bronchitis, although the incidence of *Candida albicans* in the stools was significantly higher in the patients receiving tetracycline alone (37.1 per cent) than in those receiving tetracycline with nystatin (9.1 per cent), the incidence of gastro-intestinal symptoms was identical in the two groups (British Tuberculosis Association, 1968).

Staining of teeth

Tetracyclines are deposited in teeth during the early stages of calcification, just as they are in calcifying bone. This may occur *in utero* if the mother is treated after the fifth month, when calcification of the deciduous teeth begins, or be produced by treatment of the child after birth. For the effect to be visible as yellow staining a certain total dose must be exceeded: the relationship between dosage and effect was well studied by Wallman & Hilton (1962). Different tetracyclines produce different degrees and shades of pigmentation (Owen, 1963) and varying degrees of hypoplasia may accompany it. The main objection to this change is cosmetic, and this applies particularly to the second dentition. The permanent incisors begin to be formed six months after birth, the canines and premolars after two years, and the molars after three to four years (Witkop & Wolf, 1963). Tetracycline treatment is therefore to be avoided in early childhood up to the age of seven years except for imperative indications or unless a short course will suffice. Doxycycline, which binds less with calcium than other tetracyclines, is said to cause dental changes less frequently (Forti and Benincori, 1969) and should perhaps be preferred if a tetracycline must be given to a child.

The effects of tetracyclines on mineralized tissues are fully reviewed by Skinner & Nalbandian (1975).

Renal damage

The risks of tetracyclines in renal failure were described early and were fully analyzed by Shils (1963) who pointed out that clinical and biochemical deterioration may occur in patients with impaired renal function, that the changes are proportional to the degree of renal failure and to the dose and duration of tetracycline administration, and that the maximal effects are often reached some days after the course of tetracycline has finished. Despite these early reports, tetracyclines have often been used in patients with impaired renal function, leading sometimes to irreversible and even fatal deterioration in the degree of renal failure (Phillips et al 1974, Boston Collaborative Drug Survey, 1972). An exception may be made in the case of doxycycline. Several authors (Stenbaek et al 1973) have found that the half-life of this drug is unchanged in renal failure, that a progressive rise in plasma levels is not found and that blood urea and creatinine levels do not rise in patients receiving doxycycline. The reason for this difference from other tetracyclines has now been clarified. Alestig (1973) confirmed earlier studies suggesting that passive diffusion into the intestinal lumen accounts for the excretion of doxycycline in renal failure. The process has been elucidated by Whelton (1978) who shows how upper intestinal absorption is followed by excretion into the small and large bowel and cationic chelation in the alkaline lumen, thus providing a non-renal 'alternate' pathway for elimination of doxycycline in patients with renal failure. Whelton also showed that the rate of removal of doxycycline by haemodialysis is insignificant. (See also Mahon et al, 1976).

The effects of minocycline on renal function are in dispute. Welling et al (1975) showed little change in the kinetics of the drug and no evidence of renal toxicity in patients with mild renal failure, and McHenry et al (1972) also found no delay in excretion in renal failure. Another report, however (George et al, 1973), noted aggravation of renal failure even when a reduced dose was administered. Minocycline may well be harmless in mild renal failure, but should probably be avoided in renal disease. It is not removed to a significant extent by peritoneal dialysis or by haemodialysis and apparently does not accumulate in the blood in hepatic disease (Allen, 1976). Acute interstitial nephritis induced by minocycline (Walker et al, 1979) and nephrogenic diabetes insipidus from demeclocycline have been recorded (Castell & Sparks, 1965).

Liver damage

It has been known since the work of Lepper et al (1951) that tetracyclines given in excessive doses parenterally as well as orally can damage the liver. Since then a number of deaths have been reported in pregnant women given tetracycline in large intravenous doses, usually for the treatment of pyelonephritis (Schulz et al, 1963; Whalley et al, 1964; Kunelis et al, 1965). The main lesion found at autopsy was diffuse fatty degeneration of the liver.

A total daily dose of tetracycline by the intravenous route of 1 g is adequate for most purposes, and should rarely be exceeded.

Benign intracranial hypertension

A number of infants treated with tetracycline have developed bulging of the anterior fontanelle (Fields, 1961). A similar syndrome has been described in older children (Maroon & Mealy, 1971) and even in adults, with headache, photophobia and papilloedema. The signs and symptoms clear when administration of the drug is stopped, but several patients developed the same illness when tetracycline was given again. The mechanism is quite unknown.

Vertigo

Neurological symptoms including giddiness, vertigo, ataxia, and headache have been noted with variable frequency in patients receiving minocycline (Munford et al, 1974; Williams et al, 1974). The symptoms subside quickly when the drug is discountined.

Gump et al (1977), in a double blind trial, found no difference between dose schedules of 100 mg b.d. or 75 mg b.d. in causing side effects; although the serum concentrations were lower with the smaller dose, only nausea was less common with the reduced dose.

Provocation of systemic lupus

Tetracyclines are among the many drugs said to provoke exacerbation in lupus erythematosus (Domz et al, 1959) but this must be very uncommon.

Differences between tetracyclines

These have been largely discussed in the relevant sections of this chapter, but the main points may be conveniently summarized.

Of the earlier compounds chlortetracycline is notable for its poor stability in solution, while lymecycline and rolitetracycline are highly soluble and therefore suitable for parenteral use. Good absorption in the gastro-intestinal tract has been sought, especially because such a property may allow reduced dosage and a lower incidence of alimentary side effects from effects on the lower bowel. Although superior absorption is claimed for lymecycline, clomocycline and methacycline, this property is best established for doxycycline and minocycline. The infrequent dose schedules possible for demeclocycline, minocycline and especially doxycycline are notable. Tetracyclines are generally well distributed in most tissues, but antibacterial tissue concentrations have been especially studied for minocycline and doxycycline (Symposium, 1976).

As to antibacterial range, the activity of minocycline against staphylococci is the most individual feature but is of largely academic interest since tetracyclines are not the antibiotic of choice in staphylococcal infections. Adverse effects of tetracyclines are generally similar from compound to compound, but three particular aspects are notable. Doxycycline is free from adverse effects in renal failure, minocycline is particular in its vestibular side effects, and demeclocycline is the most liable to cause photosensitivity.

Cetocycline

This is a compound structually related to tetracycline which has been recently examined by Proctor et al (1978). They found it more active than tetracycline against many Gram-negative bacteria, but rather less active against staphylococci. It is inactive against Pseudomonas.

Clinical applications

Thanks to their exceptionally broad spectrum, tetracyclines are appropriate for a greater variety of infections than any other antibiotic. This fact encourages their choice, particularly by the general practitioner, when a bacteriological diagnosis is unavailable.

Much of their prescription in this country is for infections of the respiratory tract. It used to be said that all organisms capable of causing pneumonia were susceptible, but as resistant strains of pneumococci have become more prevalent this ceases to be true of the most important of them. It holds good for most Gram-negative infections, for psittacosis and infections with *Rickettsia burneti* and *Mycoplasma pneumoniae*. Resistance in haemolytic streptococci is now common, and the prescription of tetracyclines for acute throat infections is therefore inadvisable. Much the largest consumption is in the treatment of chronic bronchitis, for which the tetracyclines, the ampicillin group and, more recently, co-trimoxazole are the most commonly prescribed antimicrobial drugs.

It is disturbing that the use of tetracyclines in infections of childhood has not notably declined despite the clear evidence (page 175) of their ill effects on teeth. In the year ending June 1973, the F.D.A. certified a 5 per cent increase over previous years in tetracycline produced in liquid preparations for paediatric use (Amer. Acad. Pediatrics, 1975), and Stewart (1973), by examining the deposits in first molar teeth extracted from 505 children, showed that tetracycline usage had increased by 12 per cent over five years.

Minocycline has received extensive study in the chemoprophylaxis of meningococcal disease where sulphonamide resistance is prevalent (Sivonen et al, 1978, and p. 326).

Tetracyclines are now established as a moderately effective treatment for acne vulgaris (Pochi, 1976) used in a dose of 250–500 mg daily, and as somewhat more effective in rosacea (Sneddon, 1966). Cunliffe et al (1973), examining the action of tetracycline in acne vulgaris, demonstrated complex changes in the surface lipids of the skin, notably a decrease in fatty acids and reciprocal increase in trigylycerides probably caused by inhibition of extracellular bacterial lipase. Marples & Kligman (1971) showed that all tetracyclines except doxycycline reduced the population density of *Corynebacterium (Propionobacterium) acnes* in the skin, whereas penicillins had no effect on the numbers of this commensal. (See also p. 308.)

Other indications for the use of tetracyclines are diverse but uncommon. They are used for susceptible urinary infections, prostatitis and in brucellosis, although cotrimoxazole is now a competitor in this disease. Tetracyclines also offer an alternative to penicillin in the treatment of actinomycosis, anthrax and syphilis. Other possible or definite uses are in granuloma venereum, lymphogranuloma inguinale, leptospirosis, relapsing fever, trachoma, tularaemia and typhus. Doxycycline given for 15 days was found as effective as chloramphenicol in epidemic typhus (Huys et al, 1973) while Perine et al (1974) reported complete success in curing 26 patients with louse-borne relapsing fever and ten others with epidemic typhus by the use of one single oral dose of 100 mg of doxycycline. Single dose therapy has also been used for tick-borne relapsing fever and for gonorrhoea (page 426). In cholera, tetracyclines reduce the requirement for intravenous fluids by about half, and have also been successfully used for prophylaxis of the disease in infected families (McCormack et al, 1968). Another and surprising use, arising from the spread of drug-resistant malaria in the Far East, is as an adjunct in the eradicative treatment of *P. falciparum* infection (Rieckmann et al, 1971; Clyde et al, 1971). Claims for the value of tetracycline in the treatment of toxoplasmosis have been made, but disputed (Grossman & Remington, 1977).

Tetracyclines were formerly regarded as indicated in mixed infections, notably in patients with peritonitis but acquired resistance in several species has diminished their value. Prophylactic administration to surgical patients should be avoided if possible. A general contra-indication to the use of tetracyclines is any condition in which a bactericidal effect is essential: thus they have no place in the treatment of infective endocarditis, except that caused by *Coxiella burneti*.

Doxycycline has been used in the treatment of human infertility, on the hypothesis that genital mycoplasmas might sometimes be responsible. Both *M. hominis* and 'T' strain mycoplasmas (now called ureaplasmas) were eradicated but no change in the rate of conception was achieved (Harrison et al, 1975).

Pharmaceutical preparations and dosages are on page 181.

References

Alestig K 1973 Scand J Infect Dis 5: 193
Allen J C 1976 Ann Intern Med 85: 482
Amer Acad Pediatrics 1975 Pediatrics 55: 142
Boston Collaborative Drug Surveillance Program 1972. J Amer Med Ass 220: 377
British Tuberculosis Association 1968. Brit Med J 4: 411
Campbell M J 1970 J Clin Path 23: 427
Candanoza C, Ellner P D 1975 Antimicrob Agents Chemother 7: 227
Castell D O, Sparks H A 1965 J Amer Med Ass 193: 237
Chopra I, Howe T G B 1978 Microbiol Rev 42: 707
Chow A W, Patten V, Guze L B 1975 Antimicrob Agents Chemother 7: 46
Clyde D F, Miller R M, Dupont H L, Hornick R B 1971 J Trop Med Hyg 74: 238
Cunliffe W J Forster R A, Greenwood N D et al 1973 Brit Med J 4: 332
Dadswell J V 1967 J Clin Path 20: 641
Domz C A, McNamara D H, Holzapfel H F 1959 Ann Intern Med 50: 1217
Fields J P 1961 J Pediat 58: 74
Finland M 1974 Clin Pharmac Therap 15: 3
Forti G, Benincori C 1969 Lancet 1: 782
George C R P, Guiness M D G, Lark D J, Evans R A 1973 Med J Aust 1: 640
Grossman P L, Remington J S 1977 Brit Med J 1: 1664
Gump D W, Ashikaga T, Fink T J, Radin A M 1977 Antimicrob Agents Chemother 12: 642
Hansman D 1975 Lancet 2: 893
Harrison R F, de Louvois J, Blades M, Hurley R 1975 Lancet 1: 605
Howard A J, Hince C J, Williams J D 1978 Brit Med J 1: 1657
Huys J, Freyens P, Kayihigi J, van den Bergh G 1973 Trans Roy Soc Trop Med Hyg 67: 718
Kunelis C T, Peters J L, Edmondson H A 1965 Amer J Med 38: 359
Kunin C M, Dornbush A C, Finland M 1959 J Clin Invest 38: 1950
Lepper M H, Wolfe C K, Zimmerman H J et al 1951 Arch Intern Med 88: 271
MacCulloch D, Richardson R A, Allwood G K 1974 N Z Med J 80: 300
McCormack W M, Chowdhury A M, Jahangir N, Fariduddin Ahmed A B, Mosley W H 1968 Bull WHO 38: 787
McHenry M C, Gavan T L, Vidt D G, Jameson S, Wagner J G 1972 Clin Pharmacol Ther 13: 146
Mahon W A, Johnson G E, Endrenyi L, Kelly M F, Fenton S S A 1976 Scand J Infect Dis Suppl 9: 24
Maroon J C, Mealy J 1971 J Amer Med Ass 216: 1479
Marples R R, Kligman A M 1971 Arch Derm 103: 148
Minuth J N, Holmes T M, Musher D M 1974 Antimicrob Agents Chemother 6: 411
Montgomerie J Z, Pickett M J, Yoshimori R N, Chow A W, Guze L B 1976 Antimicrob Agents Chemother 10: 102
Munford R S, de Vasconcelos Z J S Phillips C J et al 1974 J Infect Dis 129: 644
Neu H J 1978 Bull N Y Acad Med, 54: 141
Neuvonen P J, Gothoni G, Hackman R, af Björksten K 1970 Brit Med J 4: 532
Oosterlinck W, Wallijn E, Wijndaele J J 1976 Scand J Infect Dis Suppl 9: 85
Oriel J D, Waterworth P M 1975 J Clin Path 28: 403
Owen L N 1963 Arch Oral Biol 8: 715
Perine P L, Awoke S, Krause D W, McDade J E 1974 Lancet 2: 742
Phillips M E, Eastwood J B, Curtis J R, Gower P E, de Wardener H E 1974 Brit Med J 2: 149
Pochi P E 1976 New Engl J Med 294: 43
Proctor R, Craig W, Kunin C 1978 Antimicrob Agents Chemother 13: 598
Rees T A 1971 Lancet 1: 938
Report of an *ad hoc* Study Group on antibiotic resistance 1977. Brit Med J 1: 131
Rieckmann K H, Powell R D, McNamara J V et al 1971 Amer J Trop Med Hyg 20: 811
Ruhen R W, Tandon M K 1976 Med J Aust 1: 151
Schulz J C, Adamson J S, Workman W W, Norman T D 1963 New Engl J Med 269: 999
Schwartzman J D, Reller L B, Wang W-L L 1977 Antimicrob Ag Chemother 11: 695
Shils M E 1963 Ann Int Med 58: 389
Sivonen A, Renkonen O-V, Weckström P et al 1978 J Infect Dis 137: 238
Skinner H C W, Nalbandian J 1975 Yale J Biol Med 48: 377
Sneddon I B 1966 Brit J Dermatol 78: 649
Steigbigel N H, Reed C W, Finland M 1968 Amer J Med Sci 255: 179
Stenbaek O, Myrhe E, Berdal B P 1973 Scand J Infect Dis 5: 199

Stewart D J 1973 Brit Med J 3: 320
Symposium 1976 Scand J Infect Dis Suppl 9
Wallman I S, Hilton H B 1962 Lancet 1: 827
Walker R G, Thomson N M, Dowling J P, Ogg C S 1979 Brit Med J 1: 524
Waterworth P M 1974 J Clin Path 27: 269
Welling P G, Shaw W R, Uman S J, Tse F L S, Craig W A 1975 Antimicrob Agents Chemother 8: 532
Whalley P J, Adams R H, Combes B 1964 J Amer Med Ass 189: 357
Whelton A 1978 Bull N Y Acad Med 54: 223
Whitby J L, Black H J 1964 Brit Med J 2: 1491
Williams D N, Laughlin L W, Lee Y-H 1974 Lancet 2: 744
Witkop C J, Wolf R O 1963 J Amer Med Ass 185: 1008
Wood M J, Farrell W, Kattan S, Williams J D 1975 J Antimicrob Chemother 1: 323

Tetracyclines. Pharmaceutical preparations and dosage

Name	*Dosage*	*Preparations*	*Common international proprietary names*	
Tetracycline	*Adults* The usual dose is 250 mg four times a day, and may be doubled for severe infections. i.v. infusion: 500 mg every 12 hours and not more than 2 g a day. i.m.: 200–300 mg daily in divided doses.	Capsules 250 mg Tablets 250 mg Syrup 125 mg in 5 ml i.m. injection i.v. injection	Achromycin, Tetracyn Lexacycline, Ro-cycline, SK-Tetracycline Tétracyne, Miriamycine Tetracitro S, Tetralution	(UK)
Chlortetracycline	As for Tetracycline	Capsules 250 mg Topical preparations Ophthalmic ointment Injection (USNF)	Aureomycin Auréomycine	(UK) (Fr)
Oxytetracycline	*Adults* 1–2 g daily in divided doses.	Tablets 250 mg Syrup 125 mg in 5 ml Topical preparations Injection (USNF)	Terramycin, Imperacin Oxlopar UriTet, Oxy-Kesso-Tetra	(UK) (USA)
Demeclocycline	*Adults* 600 mg daily in divided doses.	Capsules 150 mg Syrup 75 mg in 5 ml Tablets 300 mg Aqueous drop 60 mg in 1 ml	Ledermycin Declomycin Ledermycine, Mexocine	(UK) (USA) (Fr)
Rolitetracycline	i.m. injection: 150–300 mg every 12 hours. i.v. infusion: 350–700 mg every 12 hours.	Injection	Tetrex Reverin Transcycline Not available in the UK	(USA) (Ger) (Fr)
Lymecycline	Equivalent of 150 mg Tetracycline base every six hours.	Capsules 204 mg (equiv. to 150 mg of Tetracycline base)	Tetralysal	(UK)

Name	*Dosage*	*Preparations*	*Common international proprietary names*	
Methacycline	*Adults* 600 mg to 1.2 g daily in divided doses.	Capsules 150 mg Syrup 75 mg in 5 ml	Rondomycin Megamycine	(UK) (Fr)
Clomocycline	*Adults* 170 mg four times a day.	Capsules 170 mg Syrup 85 mg in 5 ml	Megaclor	(UK)
Doxycycline	*Adults* initially 200 mg, then 100 mg daily. *Children* 4 mg/kg body weight daily. (If they weigh less than 50 kg.)	Capsules 100 mg Syrup 50 mg in 5 ml	Vibramycin Doxy II, Doxychel Vibramycine Vibrveineuse	(UK) (USA) (Fr)
Minocycline	*Adult* Oral: 200 mg initially, then 100 mg every 12 hours.	Tablets 100 mg	Minocin Klinomycin Vectrin Mynocine	(UK) (Ger) (USA) (Fr)

8

Macrolides and lincosamides

The macrolides form a large group of closely similar antibiotics, the more widely used of which were discovered in 1952–4. They all consist of a macrocyclic lactone ring—to which they owe their generic name—to which sugars are attached.

ERYTHROMYCIN

This antibiotic was obtained in 1952 in the Lilly Research Laboratories, Indianapolis, from a strain of *Streptomyces erythreus* derived from soil from the Philippines. Its structure is shown in Fig. 8.1. There are three erythromycins, of which B and C possess lesser activity. Erythromycin is a weak base, soluble only to the extent of about 0.1 per cent in water, but readily so in ethanol and other organic solvents. Neutral solutions are stable for many weeks at 5 °C, but at room temperature there is some loss after a few days; at a pH below 5 loss of activity is rapid.

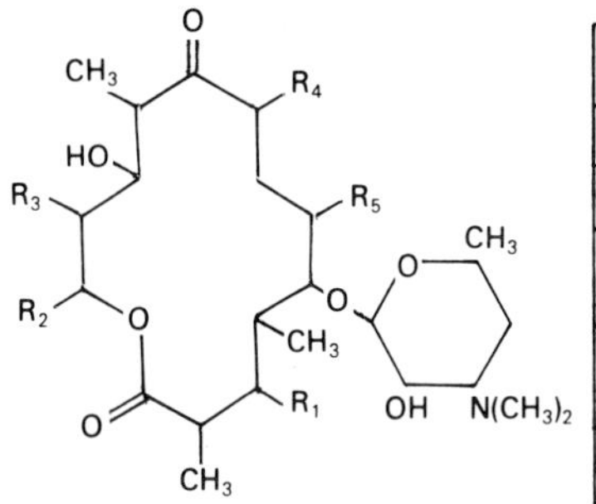

	Erythromycin A	Oleandomycin
R_1	L-cladinose	L-oleandrose
R_2	$CH_2\ CH_3$	CH_3
R_3	$<\substack{CH_3\\OH}$	CH_3
R_4	CH_3	$<\substack{CH_2\\O}$
R_5	$<\substack{CH_3\\OH}$	CH_3

Fig. 8.1 Structure of macrolides

Antibacterial activity
The sensitivity of pathogenic bacteria to erythromycin is shown in Table 8.1. Inoculum size or presence of serum has only a small effect on the MIC but pH is an important factor, activity increasing with increase in pH up to 8.5.

Noteworthy features of the spectrum are uniformly high activity against pneumococci and haemolytic streptococci of group A and rather less activity against *Staph. aureus*. The more vulnerable Gram-negative genera *Neisseria* and *Haemophilus* are also sensitive, and the hardier enterobacteria generally resistant although

Table 8.1 Sensitivity of bacteria to erythromycin

	μg/ml		μg/ml
S. aureus	0.01–2	*N. gonorrhoeae*	0.03–0.5
S. pyogenes	0.03–0.25	*N. meningitidis*	0.25–2
S. pneumoniae	0.01–0.25	*H. influenzae*	0.5–8
S. viridans	0.03–4	*B. pertussis*	0.06–0.25
S. faecalis	0.5–4	*Brucella* spp.	0.25–32
C. diphtheriae	0.25–4	*E. coli*	8–R
C. perfringens	0.25–2	*Klebsiella* spp.	R
C. tetani	0.25–0.5	*Proteus* spp.	R
M. fortuitum	R	*Salmonella* spp.	64–R
M. kansasii	0.5–2	*Shigella* spp.	8–R
M. scrofulaceum	0.5–16	*P. aeruginosa*	R
M. tuberculosis	R		

some strains of Escherichia are inhibited (and killed) by as little as 8 μg/ml. *Myoplasma pneumoniae* is sensitive to 0.004–0.016 μg erythromycin per ml (Niitu et al, 1970). Erythromycin is active against a wide variety of anaerobic bacteria. Differential sensitivity to erythromycin and lincomycin separates *Mycoplasma hominis*, which is sensitive to lincomycin and resistant to erythromycin, from T-strains (Csonka & Corse, 1970) which are sensitive to erythromycin and resistant to lincomycin. Erythromycin also exerts anti-rickettsial (*R. prowazeki*) activity in the embryonated egg, and an action inferior to that of chlortetracycline on the *Chlamydia* of lymphogranuloma venereum. Erythromycin is active against *Plasmodium berghei* and potentiates the action of chloroquine against resistant but not against sensitive strains (Warhurst et al, 1976).

Although the action of erythromycin is predominantly bacteristatic in low concentrations, somewhat higher ones are distinctly if slowly bactericidal, there being few survivors after 24 hours' exposure.

Acquired resistance

Strains of *Staph. aureus*, enterococcus and *Str. pneumoniae* develop 500-fold increases in resistance after 3–12 subcultures in the presence of the antibiotic, and strains of *Str. pyogenes* and *Str. viridans* 20-fold increases in resistance after 20 subcultures. The resistance is only moderately stable and resistant variants often consist of a mixed population, the individual cells of which have a wide variation in sensitivity to erythromycin. Resistant mutants of *Staph. aureus* produced *in vitro* frequently give rise to small colonies with relatively little pigment production and produce little or no coagulase. Similar changes may also be seen when erythromycin resistance occurs *in vivo*.

Increased resistance is not often observed to develop during successful short-term treatment, but during more prolonged treatment of infections more difficult to eradicate, such as endocarditis, it is common. Where such resistant staphylococci emerge, they may spread rapidly in a hospital where the use of erythromycin is extensive.

Resistant strains of pneumococci and of haemolytic streptococci have been reported for more than ten years and a marked increase in the prevalence of β-haemolytic streptococci of groups A, B, C and D resistant to erythromycin and lincomycin which evidently arose from epidemiologically unrelated foci was observed in northern Canada by Dixon & Lipinsky (1974). Resistance in *Mycoplasma pneumoniae* to macrolides and lincomycin (but not to the depsipeptides studied) has been observed in infected patients treated with erythromycin or in strains passaged in the presence of erythromycin (Niitu et al, 1970).

Cross-resistance

Staphylococci passaged in the presence of one of the macrolides often develop resistance not only to the agent to which they were exposed but to all the macrolides tested. The degree of resistance to the agents varies considerably from strain to strain and resistant Gram-positive cocci have generally exhibited a spectrum of unstable shared resistances with extreme strains resistant to only one agent. Several kinds of resistance are involved including what Dixon & Lipinsky (1974) call 'zonal resistance'. Some forms of resistance are due to mutations and some to the presence of plasmids which can be multiple as in the strains of *S. faecalis* studied by Clewell et al (1974).

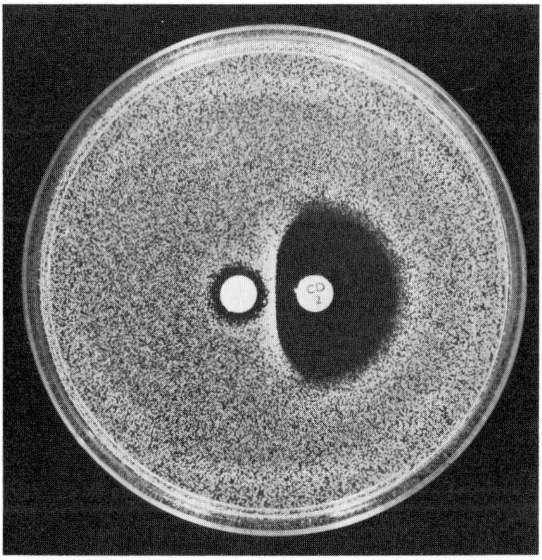

Fig. 8.2 Culture of *Staph. aureus* showing dissociated resistance to erythromycin. Discs contain: (left) erythromycin 10 μg; (right) clindamycin 2 μg. Although the organism appears sensitive to clindamycin (because resistance is induced only by erythromycin) treatment with this drug usually produces full resistance

Dissociated resistance

There also occurs in some strains of staphylococci and streptococci a most intriguing form of cross-resistance described by Garrod (1957) as *dissociated resistance.*

These strains consist of cells the majority of which are sensitive to erythromycin, but growth on a medium containing the antibiotic produces a uniformly and highly resistant population. A unique feature of the behaviour of such organisms is that in the presence of erythromycin they are also resistant to other macrolides and to lincomycin and group B depsipeptides (page 204) although in its absence they are fully sensitive (Fig. 8.2) Erythromycin is the specific inducer of this resistance which is due to the production by the bacterial cell of a second type of ribosome with reduced affinity for erythromycin, which is due not to an altered ribosomal protein as in the case, for example, of streptomycin resistance (page 120) but to methylation of adenine in the ribosomal RNA which plays an important part in the ribosomal binding of erythromycin (Saltzman & Aperion, 1976). Within 40 minutes of exposure (about one generation) more than 90 per cent of the population becomes resistant. Reversion to sensitivity is complete after 90 minutes of growth in the absence of erythromycin. Malke et al (1976) obtained evidence that this type of inducible resistance in a wild strain of *Streptococcus pyogenes* was plasmid borne. Sparling & Blackman (1973) were able to induce mutation to erythromycin dependence in *Escherichia coli* which could also be satisfied by other macrolides, lincomycin or chloramphenicol—all agents which act on the 50S sub-unit of the ribosome.

PHARMACOKINETICS

Absorption

The acid lability of erythromycin base necessitates administration in a form giving protection from gastric acid. Delayed and incomplete absorption is obtained from enteric-coated tablets and there is a good deal of individual variation, adequate levels not being attained at all in a few subjects. Alternatives are to give capsules of erythromycin stearate (which is resistant to gastric acid, and broken down in the intestine liberating the base) or the propionyl ester of erythromycin in the form of its lauryl sulphate (erythromycin estolate), which possesses the two advantages of tastelessness and resistance to gastric acid. New 500 mg preparations of the stearate are claimed to produce average peak plasma levels of 2 μg/ml which are relatively little affected, beyond being delayed, by the presence of food. The estolate is absorbed as the propionyl ester which is microbiologically inactive and must be hydrolysed in the body to the active base. Initial rapid hydrolysis affects relatively little of the drug and is followed by a period of slow breakdown during which the ratio of active to inactive compound remains fairly constant (Stephens et al, 1969). As with other compounds which depend on *in vivo* liberation of active compound from inactive precursors (see page 210) there has been some disagreement over the true concentrations of circulating active agent in patients treated with the estolate since in the course of microbiological assay further active drug could be liberated from ester in the serum by hydrolysis during the period of incubation. The serum levels obtained after single doses of various preparations are given in Table 8.2. Other salts of erythromycin sometimes administered are the propionate and the succinate.

It has been claimed that identical doses of erythromycin produce lower serum levels in women than in men. In pregnant women admitted for therapeutic abortion Philipson et al (1973) found that the estolate given in doses equivalent to 500 mg of the base produced peak serum levels of 0.29–7.2 μg per ml two hours after the dose. Levels were still detectable after 24 hours. The peak levels after the last of multiple doses were 2.45–7 μg per ml. Mean urinary concentrations were 21.6 μg per ml after one dose and 85.4 μg per ml after multiple doses. The proportion of patients who exhibited low peak levels of the drug was greater than that previously reported in non-pregnant women.

Ginsburg & Eichenwald (1976) review the properties of erythromycin, its available preparations and its uses in paediatric practice. They found that doses of 10 mg per kg produced mean peak serum concentrations of 1.78 μg per ml in infants weighing 1.5–2 kg and 1.21 μg per ml in those weighing 2–2.5 kg.

Parenteral injection
The gluceptate (glucoheptonate) and lactobionate of erythromycin are suitable for intravenous injection and are useful for attaining an immediate effect and higher blood levels (Table 8.2). Intramuscular injection is also possible but causes pain, and the dose should not exceed 100 mg.

Table 8.2 Erythromycin serum levels in man

Preparation	Dose mg	Route	Peak Hr	Peak μg/ml	Half-life hr
	250		3–4	0.25–0.5	
Base	500	oral	2–4	0.9–1.4	2–4
	1000		4	1.3–1.5	
Stearate					
fasting	250		2	1.3	
	500	oral	2–4	0.4–1.8	
after food	500		2–4	0.1–0.4	2–4
Propionate					
fasting	500		2–4	0.4–1.9	3–5
after food	500	oral	4	0.3–0.5	3–4
Estolate					
fasting	250		2–4	0.36–3.0	
	500	oral	1–2	1.4–5.0	2–4
after food	250			1.1–2.9	
	500		2–4	1.8–5.2	
Lactobionate	500	i.v.	0	11.5–30.0	1–2
Gluceptate	250	i.v.	0	3.5–10.7	

Bell S M 1971 Med J Aust 2: 1280
Davis D S, Romansky M J 1955 Antibiot Ann 1954–5, p 286
Griffith R S 1955 Antibiot Ann 1954–5, p 269
Griffith R S, Black H R 1962 Antibiot Chemother 12: 398
Griffith R S, Black H R 1964 Amer J Med Sci 247: 69
Hirsch H A, Finland M 1959 Amer J Med Sci 237: 693
Lake B, Bell S M 1969 Med J Aust 1: 449
Lopez-Belio M, Takimura Y 1955 Antibiot Ann 1954–5, p 295
Reichelderfer T E et al 1960 Antibiot Ann 1959–60, p 899

Distribution
By ultra filtration of serum containing therapeutically attainable concentrations Gordon et al (1973) found the protein binding of erythromycin base to be 73 per cent and that of the propionate to be 93 per cent. Erythromycin is distributed throughout the body water and tends to be retained longer in the liver and spleen than in the blood. Only very low levels are attained in the cerebro-spinal fluid even in the presence of meningeal inflammation and are not raised to therapeutic levels by

parenteral administration. Levels of 0.1 μg/ml aqueous humour have been found when the corresponding serum level was 0.36 μg/ml but there is no penetration into the vitreous. Bass et al (1971) gave 12.5 mg/kg of two erythromycin preparations 6-hourly to children with otitis media and measured the concentrations of drug in the serum and middle ear exudate two hours after the fourth dose. In those given the succinate the concentrations in serum and exudate were 0.45–2.6 and 0.24–1.02 μg/ml respectively; in those given the estolate: 3.9–12.3 and 1.7–>8 μg per ml.

Erythromycin appears to be concentrated by fetal liver and fetal tissue levels are considerably higher after multiple doses. Following such multiple doses the mean erythromycin concentration when the mean peak maternal serum level was 4.94 (0.66–8) μg per ml were: fetal blood 0.06 (0–0.12), amniotic fluid 0.36 (0.32–0.39) μg per ml. Levels in excess of 0.3 μg per ml were found in most other fetal tissues in some patients but the levels were variable and unmeasurable in some (Philipson et al, 1976).

Excretion

Erythromycin is excreted both in the urine and in the bile but only a fraction of the dose can be accounted for in this way. Urinary concentrations on 1 g a day of propionyl erythromycin have been reported to be 13–46 μg per ml and on similar doses of erythromycin base 11–24 μg per ml. Lake & Bell (1969) found peak concentrations of 7.4–15.2 μg per ml 3–4 hours after 250 mg of the estolate. Studies in the dog suggest that what little is excreted in the glomerular filtrate is partially re-absorbed by the tubules.

Fairly high concentrations are found in the bile in man: 10 μg per ml in subjects receiving the propionyl ester, and 64 μg per ml in those receiving the base, the bile-serum concentration ratio being about 4 for the propionyl ester, and 30 for the base. It is possible that the smaller excretion of the propionyl ester into the bile accounts in part for its better maintained serum levels. Even so, only about 1.5 per cent of the dose of the base (0.2 per cent of the ester) appears in the bile in the first eight hours. Much of the rest is presumably demethylated or otherwise degraded.

Toxicity and side effects

Erythromycin is one of the most innocuous agents in current use except that the estolate like the similar ester of oleandomycin (page 190) may give rise to signs of liver damage. These consist of upper abdominal pain, fever, hepatic enlargement, a raised serum bilirubin, with or without actual jaundice, pale stools and dark urine and eosinophilia. The condition, which is rare and usually seen 10–20 days after the initiation of treatment, may mimic viral hepatitis, cholecystitis, pancreatitis or cardiac infarction.

There have been no deaths and on stopping the drug recovery has been complete. Once patients have recovered, recurrence of symptoms can be produced by giving the estolate but not by giving the base or stearate. Studies conducted by Tolman et al (1974) on a volunteer with proven erythromycin estolate toxicity established that the essential molecular feature for toxicity was the propionyl-ester linkage. The lauryl sulphate appeared to play no part since, contrary to the findings of others using cell culture systems, it was not hepatotoxic when given alone. The relative frequency of the reaction and its rapidity of onset (within hours) after second courses of the drug, peripheral eosinophilia and other evidence of sensitivity, and the histological appearances suggest that the reaction results from a mixture of intrahepatic cholestatis, liver cell necrosis and hypersensitivity. Clarke et al (1975) demonstrate direct interaction between erythromycin and bile salts and discuss ways in which this could be responsible for cholestatic jaundice. Zimmerman et al (1974) showed that erythromycin estolate is 100 times more toxic to isolated liver cells than are the propionate or the base and postulate that primary damage to liver cells is responsible for triggering a hypersensitivity response.

Abnormal liver function tests are not uncommon in patients receiving the estolate but as increased SGOT is often the only abnormality this must be interpreted with caution since some metabolite of the estolate interferes with the measurement commonly used (Sabath et al, 1968). About 10 per cent of women in the second half of pregnancy who were infected with genital mycoplasmas and were treated by McCormack et al (1977) for six weeks with erythromycin estolate developed elevated levels of SGOT which returned to normal after cessation of treatment. Serum bilirubin was unchanged but in the patients tested, γ-glutamyl transpeptidase activity was also abnormal.

Gastro-intestinal disturbances have been found in 5–6 per cent of those patients treated with the propionate and 2 per cent of those treated with the estolate. Nausea and vomiting are said to be more common with the propionate and diarrhoea with the estolate. Allergic effects occur in about 0.5 per cent of patients.

Collectors' items amongst untoward reactions to erythromycin include transient deafness following high dosage and collapse after overdosage in the child.

CLINICAL APPLICATIONS

Since erythromycin was acclaimed as a new barrier to the onslaught of the staphylococcus our resources have multiplied remarkably and one of the newer agents will almost always be preferred for a resistant staphylococcal infection. This still leaves a large field of usefulness in pneumococcal, streptococcal and mycoplasmol infection in which there is ample evidence of its efficacy, and in clostridial infections where erythromycin is a natural second choice in patients sensitive to penicillin—as it has been for syphilis in pregnancy. The wisdom of that choice must now be doubted with the description by Fenton & Light (1976) of the fifth case of failure to eradicate fetal syphilis with erythromycin. They recommend that very convincing evidence of penicillin-hypersensitivity be obtained before alternative therapy is contemplated.

Erythromycin appears to be as effective as penicillin in the treatment of diphtheria and McCloskey et al (1974) amongst others continue to regard it as the drug of choice in the treatment of carriers. Because of the common cross-resistance between them, erythromycin and lincomycin should not be used together or sequentially (page 185). Bass et al (1971) point out that while the levels found in middle-ear exudate are more than sufficient to inhibit *Strep. pyogenes* and the pneumococcus they are unlikely to be inhibitory to many strains of *H. influenzae* which is a common cause of otitis media in the young child. Erythromycin has been used fairly often in combination both in an attempt to stem the emergence of resistant staphylococci and to secure synergy as in some cases of bacterial endocarditis (page 293). Steigbigel et al (1975) found that penicillin in combination with aminoglycosides or with erythromycin was significantly more effective in reducing mortality from an experimental penicillin-sensitive staphylococcal infection in mice than were the drugs alone.

Condon & Nichols (1975) report the satisfactory use of a combination of neomycin with erythromycin (included for its efficacy against anaerobic bowel flora) in pre-operative bowel preparation.

Intriguingly, erythromycin has found its most recent place in the treatment of two 'new' diseases due to Gram-negative rods: infection with campylobacter and Legionnella for both of which it has been commended as the drug of choice (page 340 and 357).

Some authors including Janicki et al (1975) have found that despite the higher serum levels claimed for erythromycin estolate, the clinical response is no better than that to the stearate or succinate and in Australia the Drug Evaluation Committee (Report, 1973) recommended that the estolate should not continue to be generally available except in the lower dosage paediatric combination which is used in children under the age of 6 years—a view that did not commend itself to everyone. Certainly the estolate should not be used if the patient is known to have been treated with it before. It should not be given for more than 10 days. Above all, those using the drug should be alert to the significance of any indication of hepatic derangement.

JOSAMYCIN

Josamycin was isolated in Japan in 1964 from the fermentation products of *Streptomyces narvonensis* var. *josamyceticus* (Osono et al, 1967). Its spectrum of activity is similar to that of erythromycin, susceptible organisms being inhibited by 2 μg per ml or less. It exhibits useful activity against anaerobic bacteria but less than that of clindamycin particularly against *Fusobacteria* spp. (Reese et al, 1976). Its pharmacokinetic behaviour closely resembles that of erythromycin but on repeated dosing josamycin achieved higher concentrations and was better tolerated than comparable doses of erythromycin stearate (Strausbaugh et al, 1976). Wenzel et al (1976) found josamycin to be as effective as erythromycin in the treatment of mycoplasma pneumonia.

OLEANDOMYCIN

This antibiotic was isolated in 1954 in the laboratories of Charles Pfizer & Co. from a strain of *Streptomyces antibioticus*. Its *in vitro* activity is less than that of erythromycin but greater than that of spiramycin: the factor by which that of erythromycin exceeds it was found to be two to four for *Staph. aureus* and about 10 for *Str. pyogenes*. Like erythromycin it is incompletely absorbed, and an ester, triacetyloleandomycin, gives improved blood levels (and more favourable and more consistent serum and tonsillar levels than those produced by erythromycin base—Georgiew et al, 1978), but this, like erythromycin estolate, can cause liver damage.

Oleandomycin has been extensively used as a 1:2 mixture with tetracycline (Sigmamycin) a combination for which synergic properties were claimed, but this has not been confirmed either *in vitro* or in assays of the anti-bacterial activity of the serum of subjects to whom tetracycline was given alone and in combination with oleandomycin, erythromycin or spiramycin. There is a good deal of French and a great deal of Russian literature on oleandomycin which we have not attempted to review. As far as clinical utility and safety are concerned, those who admire the drug take much the same view of it as we have taken of erythromycin.

ROSARAMICIN

This macrolide antibiotic was isolated in the laboratories of Schering Corporation from the fermentation products of *Micromonospora rosaria* (Wagman et al, 1972). Its activity is at least equal to that of erythromycin against aerobic Gram-positive organisms, against peptostreptococci and against non-spore forming Gram-positive anaerobic bacteria. Its activity is greater than that of erythromycin against Gram-negative anaerobic bacilli, peptococci and clostridia and against *N. gonorrhoeae* including β-lactamase-producing strains (Biddle and Thornsberry, 1979).

SPIRAMYCIN

Spiramycin (Rovamycin) was obtained in 1954 in the Rhone-Poulenc Research Laboratories from a strain of *Streptomyces ambofaciens* derived from a sample of soil collected near Paris (Pinnert-Sindico et al, 1955). This organism forms three closely related antibiotics, of which spiramycin A is used therapeutically.

Spiramycin has a substantially lower *in vitro* activity than erythromycin: 16–32-fold against *Staph. aureus*, 8–16-fold against *Str. pyogenes*, and 4–8-fold against *Str. pneumoniae*.

If spiramycin had no other property tending to compensate for its lesser antibacterial activity, the clinical results claimed for it would be difficult to understand. It seems that this property may be exceptional persistence in the tissues. Macfarlane et al (1968) who successfully used the drug for the prevention of post-prostatectomy staphylococcal sepsis, found levels 12 hours after a dose of 1 g in man of 0.25 μg/ml in serum, 5.3 μg/ml in bone, 6.9 μg/ml in pus, and 4 hours after the dose, 10.6 μg/ml in saliva. As with erythromycin, high levels were found in the prostate (27 μg/ml) after repeated dosage. It is evident from comparative studies of different macrolides that at a time when the spiramycin content of the blood has fallen to a low level, high concentrations persist in the organs, whereas the organ content of erythromycin, oleandomycin or carbomycin declines much more rapidly. Spiramycin has been used in the treatment of ocular toxoplasmosis, but is inferior to pyrimethamine (Nolan & Rosen, 1968). It inhibits the growth of some experimental tumours, but the claim that it might be useful in the treatment of skin cancer has not been substantiated.

LINCOSAMIDES

Lincomycin, the parent compound of this group, was isolated in the laboratories of the Upjohn Company from the fermentation products of a previously undescribed soil streptomycete, *Streptomyces lincolnensis* var. *lincolnensis* (Mason et al, 1963).

A number of derivatives have been prepared, the majority of which are less active than the parent compound, but clindamycin (7-chloro-7-deoxy-lincomycin) synthesized by Magerlein et al (1967) is substantially more active and being now available in satisfactory solid and liquid oral forms and as a parenteral preparation should replace the parent compound for therapeutic use.

Celesticetin, a naturally occurring member of the group, has only about a quarter of the activity of lincomycin *in vitro* and about 5 per cent *in vivo*.

The lincosamides are based on a novel structure unlike that of any other antibiotic (Fig. 8.3) Lincomycin is supplied as the hydrochloride which is very soluble in water, soluble in methanol and ethanol, but relatively insoluble in less polar solvents. The free base is soluble in water and most organic solvents except hydrocarbons. The dry crystalline hydrochloride is very stable.

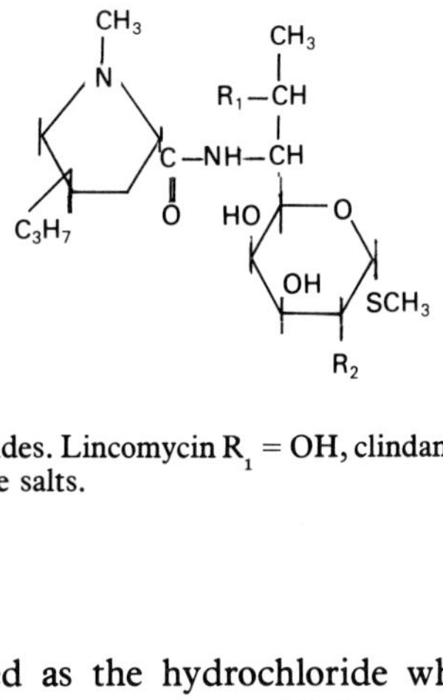

Fig. 8.3 Structures of lincosamides. Lincomycin R_1 = OH, clindamycin R_1 = Cl. R_2 (OH in the parent compounds) is substituted in the salts.

Clindamycin is supplied as the hydrochloride which is soluble in water and methanol. It has a very bitter taste, detectable in concentrations as low as 8 μg/ml water. This is absent from the ester, clindamycin palmitate, which is used in liquid preparations. Clindamycin hydrochloride is poorly soluble at neutral pH and too irritating for parenteral use so clindamycin phosphate, which is microbiologically inactive but rapidly hydrolysed to free clindamycin, is used for this purpose.

Antibacterial activity

The lincosamides closely resemble the macrolides, despite their very different chemical structure in antibacterial activity (Table 8.3) against Gram-positive organisms, notably staphylococci, haemolytic streptococci and pneumococci. There are also some interesting differences.

The enterobacteria are resistant to both lincosamides and the macrolides, but Haemophilus and Neisseria, which are sensitive to erythromycin, are resistant to lincomycin. The behaviour of Neisseria is particularly interesting since despite their Gram-negative staining they generally respond to antibacterial agents like Gram-positive organisms. Karchmer et al (1975) found that streptococci of

Table 8.3 Sensitivity of bacteria to lincosamides

	Minimum inhibitory concentrations (μg/ml)	
	Lincomycin	Clindamycin
S. aureus	0.5–2	0.1–1
S. pyogenes	0.05–1	0.01–0.25
S. pneumoniae	0.1–1	0.05
S. viridans	0.1–1	0.05
S. faecalis	2–64	0.05–64
B. anthracis	0.25–8	
Clostridium spp.	0.5–32	
A. israeli	0.1–0.5	
N. gonorrhoeae	8–64	0.5–4
N. meningitidis	>32	
H. influenzae	4–16	0.5–16
Enterobacteria	R	R
B. fragilis	2–4	0.02–0.1
Veillonella spp.	<0.1–0.5	

numerous groups and non-groupable streptococci were inhibited by 0.02–0.69 μg lincomycin/ml and <0.01–0.09 μg clindamycin/ml. Amongst group D strains, *Streptococcus faecalis* and *Streptococcus faecium* were resistant while *Streptococcus bovis* and *Streptococcus durans* were as sensitive as other streptococci.

A particular feature of the agents is their activity against anaerobic bacteria, notably the cocci and Gram-negative rods. Clostridia are more resistant than other anaerobes. *Clostridium perfringens* is generally (but not always) sensitive, but amongst the more resistant species are *C. sporogenes* and *C. tertium* which are commonly implicated in gas gangrene and anaerobic cellulitis (Wilkins & Thiel, 1973).

Halogen substituted and other analogues are as active against *Plasmodium burgei* as chloroquine even when the strains are resistant to other antimalarial agents (Lewis, 1974).

Utilizing the relative inactivity against Neisseria, Odegaard et al (1975) found improved isolation rates of gonococci on a selective medium in which lincomycin was substituted for vancomycin. Because of their antibacterial range, these agents have frequently been given to patients with grave but undiagnosed infection in combination with an agent active against aerobic Gram-negative rods, that most commonly used being gentamicin. There has been a good deal of disagreement about the nature and extent of interaction between the components of this combination but most authors have found that clindamycin inhibits the action of gentamicin or amikacin against enterobacteria and also against *S. mutans* (Snyder et al, 1975). *Mycoplasma hominis* is sensitive to lincomycin (0.4–1.6 μg/ml) and resistant to erythromycin (100 μg/ml); T-strain mycoplasma are sensitive to erythromycin (0.6–1.2 μg/ml) and resistant to lincomycin (20–80 μg/ml) according to Weström and Mardh (1971).

Acquired Resistance

There is complete cross-resistance between clindamycin and lincomycin. Resistance is relatively easily produced by passage in the presence of the drug *in vitro*. This is particularly true of erythromycin-resistant strains and the lincosamides are one of the two groups (the other being the depsipeptides) that share in the peculiar form of cross-resistance usually induced by erythromycin (page 185). Amongst *S. aureus*, with the exception of some rare strains, only erythromycin will act as the inducer but lincosamides and other macrolides are effective inducers for *S. pyogenes*. At least four independent strains of two groups, A and D, have been shown to possess inducible or constitutive cross-resistance which was plasmid-borne. The very similar molecular weights of these plasmids suggest that they had a common origin (Malke et al, 1976).

There have been wide geographical variations in the frequency with which resistant staphylococci have been found. In several series, 15–20 per cent of recently isolated, previously unexposed *Staph. aureus* have been resistant yet Phillips et al (1970) were impressed with the infrequency with which lincomycin-resistant staphylococci had been encountered in their hospital over a 4-year period. There have been reports from various parts of the world of lincomycin-resistant haemolytic streptococci and pneumococci and these strains are commonly also resistant to erythromycin. Resistance of the oral viridans streptococci to both erythromycin and lincomycin was seen by Sprunt et al (1970) to emerge in patients treated with either drug for as little as three days. They point out that patients receiving long-term penicillin for prophylaxis of rheumatic fever who require cover for dental extraction may be given erythromycin or lincomycin. Care should be taken to ensure that the patient has not received either agent in the preceding three weeks.

Table 8.4 Serum levels of lincosamides in man

Agent	Route	Dose mg	Peak Hour	Peak μg per ml	Half-life hr
Lincomycin hydrochloride	Oral	500 250, 6 hourly 500, 6 hourly	4	2–7	4–6
	i.m.	200 600	1–2	3.5–4.2 8.0–18.0	4–6
	i.v.	300	0	8.0–22.0	3.5–5
Clindamycin hydrochloride	Oral	300		3.6	2–3
Clindamycin palmitate		300	1	1.4–4.2	
Clindamycin phosphate	i.m.	300	4	3.8	1.5–4
	i.v.	300 600	0	4.3–6.6 7.9–8.7	

Based on de Haan, R M et al 1973 J Clin Pharm 13: 190
Ma P et al 1964 Antimicrob Ag Chemother 1963 p 183
Reinarz J A, McIntosh D A 1966 Antimicrob Ag Chemother 1965 p 232
Vavra J J et al 1964 Antimicrob Ag Chemother 1963 p 176

The appearance of the inducible form of resistance in streptococci causing respiratory infections and relapse of endocarditis due to the emergence of *Staph.*

aureus resistant to lincomycin and erythromycin have several times been reported in patients treated with lincosamides.

PHARMACOKINETICS

Absorption

Lincomycin is readily absorbed when given by mouth. The drug is also promptly and completely absorbed from intramuscular sites. The serum levels obtained by various authors following administration by different routes are given in Table 8.4. Several authors have commented that constant, near maximum levels can be maintained on 4–6 hourly schedules. Much the same results have been obtained in children. Food significantly delays and decreases absorption of the oral dose, the mean peak serum level from a dose given immediately after a meal being only about half the fasting levels. Capsules of clindamycin contain clindamycin hydrochloride, the syrup clindamycin palmitate and the injectable form clindamycin phosphate (page 192). The behaviour of the compounds is far from identical. Clindamycin palmitate is inactive *in vitro* but rapidly hydrolyzed in the gut before absorption occurs. The ester has not been detected in human serum after a 600 mg dose. In contrast, clindamycin phosphate is relatively slowly hydrolyzed after injection. Metzler et al (1973) found a substantial amount of unhydrolyzed clindamycin phosphate (1–2 μg per ml) at 30–60 minutes which had virtually disappeared by four hours. This probably accounts for the flat curve of the compound in plasma as compared with the other oral compound. The bioavailability in relation to dose was linear but not proportional, that is to say the plasma concentration was not doubled when the dose was doubled. It was not possible to estimate completely equivalent doses since the different behaviour of the compounds resulted in different values depending on which measure—for example average peak or area under the curve—was used. The serum concentrations produced by the different preparations are shown in Table 8.4. Clindamycin, which is 94 per cent protein bound while lincomycin is only 72 per cent, is said to be 50 times more lipid soluble than is lincomycin (Picardi et al, 1975). Unlike the finding for erythromycin (page 186) Philipson et al (1976) found fairly uniform serum levels of clindamycin in pregnant women following a single oral dose of 450 mg of clindamycin hydrochloride (3.4–9 μg per ml) which was similar to that found in non-pregnant women.

Distribution

Lincomycin is widely distributed in the body, its distribution space approximating to the total body size. It does not appear to be concentrated in any particular organ. After hydrolysis in the serum, clindamycin phosphate is rapidly distributed but in at least four different forms: the phosphate itself, clindamycin base and the demethyl and sulphoxide derivatives. Demethyl clindamycin is more, but the sulphoxide less, active than the base.

Levels in CSF are low: lincomycin up to 1.2 μg/ml and clindamycin, following a single dose of the phosphate, 0.14–0.46 μg/ml. In primates with serum concentrations in excess of 5 μg/ml Picardi et al (1975) found that clindamycin could be consistently detected in the CSF where the levels were 10–25 per cent of those of the serum. Levels in the brain were erratic and low or absent. Trauma did not increase the brain levels despite the marked increase of cerebral blood flow that occurs in those circumstances. Miyazaki (1973) recommended an intrathecal dose of 1–2 mg as being safe and efficacious in producing CSF levels in excess of 6 μg per ml.

Levels of 1.5–6.9 μg lincomycin/ml of cord serum or amniotic fluid have been found after the mother had received 600 mg intramuscularly and 0.5–2.4 μg/ml human milk after the second of two 0.5 g doses. In patients undergoing Caesarean section and receiving clindamycin (and gentamicin) as prophylaxis, Weinstein et al (1976) found peak concentrations in the cord blood after a 600 mg intravenous dose of clindamycin of about 3 μg per ml (46 per cent of the maternal level).

Particular attention has been paid to the penetration of lincosamides into dense tissues, especially bone. In patients undergoing total hip replacement and given 600 mg lincomycin intramuscularly 6 hr preoperatively, and then per-operatively by intravenous infusion over 30 min, Parsons et al (1977) found the mean and range of concentrations (μg/g or ml) to be: capsule 9.4 (<0.2–32.6), synovial fluid 5.4 (2.8–8.1); bone: cancellous 7.2 (<0.2–53.8), cortical 5.4 (0.2–8.1). In patients undergoing hip operations who received three 8-hourly injections of clindamycin phosphate, the last immediately before operation, Schurman et al (1975) found the mean and range of concentrations (μg/g) to be: cancellous bone 3.77 (0.77–6.75) and cortical bone 3.87 (1.15–9.59). Nielson et al (1976), who found the percentage of the serum concentration to be 100 in bone marrow, 50–75 in spongy and 0–15 in compact bone, make the points that allowance must be made for differential penetration into marrow, cancellous and compact bone and that levels found in normal bone are not reliably predictive for diseased bone.

Boyle et al (1971) gave 75 mg lincomycin (in 0.25 ml) subconjunctivally to 27 patients without inflammatory ocular disease who were about to undergo elective surgery (usually for cataract extraction). Peak concentrations of 30–135 μg/ml were found in the aqueous 1–2 hr after injection in all but one case. Activity was still detectable 12 hr later. Serum levels of the order of 2–3 μg/ml appeared within ten minutes of subconjunctival injection and persisted for 12 hr. Marked chemosis and subconjunctival haemorrhage frequently developed but there was little or no pain.

Excretion

Most workers have found the urinary levels of lincomycin to be low except after intravenous injection. Only 3.5 per cent of the dose has been detected in the urine over 24 hr after an oral dose, but up to 60 per cent after intravenous administration. Urinary clindamycin levels following oral administration are considerably higher after multiple (84–800 μg/ml) than after single doses (47–260 μg/ml). Less than 10 per cent of clindamycin phosphate is excreted unchanged in the urine. Bioactivity persists in the urine for up to 4 days, suggesting a slow release of the drug from tissues or fluids. In patients with severe renal disease, serum levels were 3–4 times normal and high levels persisted for over 24 hours but this has been said to result from the loss of normally important renal binding sites. Lincomycin appears to be virtually non-dialysable since its half-life in dialysed and undialysed azotaemic patients is approximately the same. Eastwood & Gower (1974) concluded that orally administered clindamycin is excreted normally in patients with renal insufficiency although urinary recovery of the drug, already low in normal subjects, can fall below one per cent in severe renal failure (Peddie et al, 1975). Investigators are agreed that the drug is not removed by haemodialysis. In uraemic patients given a 30 minute intravenous infusion of 300 mg of the more diversely handled phosphate (page 195) the average level immediately after the end of the infusion (12.8 μg per ml) was considerably higher than that observed in normal subjects (5.4 μg per ml); elimination was also greatly prolonged, possibly as a result of changes in the disposition or degradation of the drug (Joshi & Stein, 1974).

Levels of 0.9–6.8 μg lincomycin per g have been found in faeces after 1.5 g orally and 1.6–9.6 μg per g after 4 g orally. In patients with liver disease, the plasma half-life is approximately doubled. The liver also plays a significant part in the elimination of the clindamycin phosphate which may be more slowly converted to the base in patients with hepatic impairment. After 600 mg infused intravenously over 2 hours, the bile at 1 hour contained 67 μg per ml. Most of the activity was due to the demethyl metabolite. Avant et al (1975) compared the pharmacokinetics of clindamycin phosphate in patients with proven hepatic cirrhosis with those of age matched controls and showed significant impairment of clindamycin elimination. The plasma half-life of the drug in the patients was increased by about an hour over the normal value and this correlated positively with the total serum bilirubin and SGOT but not with other liver function tests. The volume of distribution and serum protein binding of the drug (79 per cent) was similar in the patients and in the normal subjects. In the patients with cirrhosis studied by Hinthorn et al (1976) clindamycin excretion was significantly delayed as compared with normal controls but the half-life still fell within the normal range.

Brown et al (1976) gave 600 mg intravenously to patients undergoing biliary tract surgery and found that in those with patent common ducts the concentrations were 2½–3 times those of the serum in gall bladder bile, common duct bile, gall bladder wall and liver. Where the common duct was obstructed, the drug could not be detected in bile and the level was lower in gall bladder wall, but the concentration in liver was slightly higher than in those without obstruction. The means and ranges of levels found (μg/ml) were: serum 19.2 (11–30), gall bladder bile 33.9 (8–100), common duct bile 41.7 (14–168), and (μg/g) gall bladder wall 12 (5–44), liver 33.9 (8–70)—in the presence of obstruction 41.5 (27–100).

Toxicity

Most authors have reported no side effects apart from diarrhoea which has commonly affected about 10 per cent of patients—more in some series—but some have developed severe, even fatal, diarrhoea, which is often bloody, and abdominal pain. This complication has followed both oral and parenteral administration of lincosamides. It has been said that no condition except epidemic cholera and the very rare non-β islet cell tumour of the pancreas produces the profound shock and dehydration associated with this disorder. The mortality is high despite vigorous treatment. Since the first report in 1970 (Editorial, 1974) this complication of lincosamide therapy has assembled a huge world literature. Nearly all the facts about it, not least its frequency and cause, are disputed, but it seems to be agreed that it is more common in older patients. It is not related to the duration or dosage of treatment, usually begins within a few days of the institution of therapy, but may develop after treatment has stopped. It usually persists for a week or two but may continue for months.

Viteri et al (1974) describe a spectrum of responses from bloodless watery diarrhoea without fever or leucocytosis through minimal proctoscopic and radiological changes to severe abdominal pain, marked leucocytosis and proctoscopic and x-ray evidence of severe mucosal ulceration with pseudomembrane and pseudopolyp formation which account for the name 'pseudomembranous' enterocolitis. The disease does not ordinarily recur but the experience of Goodacre et al (1977) indicates that it may do so.

Gorbach & Bartlett (1977) trace the history of pseudomembranous enterocolitis from the first recorded case in 1893 and compare the diseases seen after gastrointestinal surgery, the devastating necrotizing enterocolitis of the newborn (with its complication of gas invasion of the gut wall, perforation and septicaemia) and the disease that follows exhibition of antibiotics. Since, in contrast to the patients with the postoperative form of the disease, the small bowel is seldom implicated, pseudomembranous colitis is a more appropriate term for the antibiotic-induced variety of the disease than pseudomembranous enterocolitis.

In three comparisons of the incidence of complications in matched patients treated with clindamycin or ampicillin, Gurwith et al (Symposium, 1977) found diarrhoea in 11, 18 and 30 per cent of patients treated with clindamycin and 5, 8 and 17 per cent of patients treated with ampicillin and pseudomembranous colitis in 1, 2 and 2 per cent of patients treated with clindamycin and 0, 0.3 and 0.7 per cent of patients treated with ampicillin. In keeping with the apparent age relationships, the experience of Randolph & Morris (1977) suggests that this grave disorder may be less common in children.

The mechanism of the condition is disputed. It is natural to assume that disturbance of the gut flora plays a significant role and this is supported by evidence that the lethal enterocolitis produced by single doses of lincomycin or clindamycin in the hamster can be prevented by oral or parenteral vancomycin. Differential susceptibility of clostridia to lincosamides (page 193) has assumed special significance with accumulating evidence (Katz et al, 1978) that pseudomembranous colitis is due to a toxin (Larson and Price, 1977) elaborated by *Clostridium difficile* (Burdon et al, 1978). The organism studied by Bartlett et al (1977) in hamsters was resistant to clindamycin and sensitive to the protective vancomycin. In hamsters, the toxic effect of lincosamides on the gall bladder, appears to be due to a direct effect of the drug and not to its antibiotic action (Scott, 1976).

In some patients receiving large amounts of the drug by rapid intravenous injection, the blood pressure has fallen precipitately with nausea, vomiting, arrhythmias and, in a patient inadvertently given 12 g, cardiac arrest. These cardiac effects are traced by Daubeck et al (1974) to a structural similarity of the drug to quinidine. They can be avoided by giving the drug in a larger volume by slow intravenous infusion: Vacek et al (1970) suggest that the rate of infusion should not exceed 50 mg/kg per hour.

It was established fairly early in the history of the drug that lincomycin can depress neuromuscular transmission but the effect is much weaker than that of neomycin. Rubbo et al (1977) show that both lincomycin and clindamycin block neuromuscular transmission by a post-synaptic action but through a different effect. The experimental studies of Samuelson et al (1975) confirm previous findings that the block is transient and that there is no cumulative effect. Pretreatment with lincomycin failed to potentiate the action of curare but there was greater depression of neuromuscular function when the order was reversed. Hence, patients receiving lincomycin after anaesthesia should be observed carefully for respiratory depression.

Nephrotoxicity due to clindamycin has not been reported but the experience of Butkus et al (1976) suggests that the drug might potentiate the toxicity of gentamicin possibly by displacing gentamicin from its albumen binding site.

There has been disagreement about effects on the liver. Intramuscular or intravenous clindamycin phosphate can cause elevation of SGOT, SGPT and serum alkaline phosphatase but there has not generally been accompanying hyperbilirubinaemia and the relationship of these changes to any hepatotoxicity is unclear. Elmore et al (1974) report marked hepatic enzyme abnormalities in a young man, successfully treated for staphylococcal endocarditis with large doses of systemic clindamycin after a number of other antibiotic regimens had failed, in whom liver biopsy showed unequivocal evidence of injury which had substantially resolved 15 days later.

In a seven year follow up of the progeny of about 100 mothers in each of three groups treated in the trimesters of pregnancy, Mickal & Panzer (1975) detected no evidence of developmental, physical, intellectual or emotional abnormalities.

Clinical use

Lincosamides have been used for the treatment of streptococcal pharyngitis, and for Gram-positive coccal otitis, pneumonia and pyoderma with very satisfactory results in both adults and children. Clindamycin is effective in the treatment of acne (page 309) and has been described as the drug of choice (Dantzig, 1976). There is considerable concern on the part of other dermatologists about the propriety of using an agent with a potentially dangerous side effect for such a common condition (Poulos & Tedesco, 1976). The situation sounds highly reminiscent of that we have recounted for chloramphenicol (page 165): those who have seen a life-threatening complication in patients treated for a disagreeable but benign condition have no use for the drug while those who have not continue to recommend it. Lincosamides have been satisfactorily used in serious infections including diphtheria and staphylococcal septicaemia.

Because of their penetration into bone, they have been particularly commended for the treatment of both acute and chronic osteomyelitis (Geddes et al, 1977).

Their antibacterial range, low toxicity, and clinical efficacy make lincosamides a suitable substitute for penicillin in Gram-positive coccal infections where penicillin is contraindicated—circumstances in which erythromycin might otherwise be used.

Clindamycin is very effective for the prophylaxis and treatment of anaerobic infections (Symposium, 1977) and is indicated where *B. fragilis* is suspected, as in intra-abdominal sepsis and infections on the female genito-urinary tract. It is not recommended for the treatment of infections of the central nervous system nor for infections with peptococci. The drug should be supplemented with penicillin G where there are anaerobes likely to be resistant to clindamycin and with aminoglycosides where the infection is likely to include aerobic Gram-negative rods. It should be noted that Clostridia and enterococci can be resistant to both and can cause septicaemia in patients receiving the combination (Fass et al, 1977).

The relatively ready emergence of resistance and the possibility of severe colitis strongly suggests that lincosamides should not be widely used for conditions for which there are a number of satisfactory alternatives.

Several studies have suggested that despite their activity, antibacterial range and undoubted therapeutic efficacy, lincosamides are not obviously clinically superior to other agents in conditions where their properties seem particularly appropriate.

Gibbs & Weinstein (1976) found that 600 mg of clindamycin and 180 mg of gentamicin given immediately before, and again eight hours after, Caesarean section produced a decrease in the aerobic and anaerobic cocci and bacteroides in the reduced number of patients who developed endometrial sepsis but an increase in the *Escherichia coli* and enterococci. The regimen was no more effective in reducing morbidity than was ampicillin plus kanamycin. Aspiration pneumonia and lung abscess commonly involve anaerobic organisms and this has been taken to be an indication for the use of clindamycin. However, Bartlett & Gorbach (1975) were unable to show that clindamycin was therapeutically superior, even in patients infected with *B. fragilis*, to benzylpenicillin, which they still regard as the agent of choice in this condition.

References

Avant G R, Schenker S, Alford R H 1975 Amer J Dig Dis 20: 223
Bartlett J G, Gorbach S L 1975 J Amer Med Ass 234: 935
Bartlett J G, Onderdonk A B, Cisneros R L 1977 Gastroenterology 73: 772
Bass J W, Steele R W, Wiebe R A, Dierdorff E P 1971 Pediatrics 48: 417
Biddle J W, Thornsberry C 1979 Antimicrob Ag Chemother 15: 243
Boyle G L, Lichtig M L, Leopold I H 1971 Amer J Ophthalmol 71: 1303
Brown R B, Martyak S N, Barza M, Curtis L, Weinstein L 1976 Ann Intern Med 84: 168
Burdon D W, Brown J W, George R H et al 1978 New Engl J Med 299: 48
Butkus D E, de Torrente A, Terman D S 1976 Nephron 17: 307
Clarke A E, Maritz V M, Denborough M A 1975 Aust NZ J Med 5: 25
Clewell D B, Yagi Y, Dunny G M, Schultz S K 1974 J Bact 117: 283
Condon R E, Nichols R L 1975 Surg Clin N Amer 55: 1331
Csonka G, Corse J 1970 Brit J Vener Dis 46: 203
Dantzig P I 1976 Arch Dermat 112: 53
Daubeck J L, Daughety M J, Petty C 1974 Anaesthes Analges 53: 563
Dixon J M S, Lipinski A E 1974 J Infect Dis 130: 351
Eastwood J B, Gower P E 1974 Postgrad Med J 50: 710
Editorial 1974 Brit Med J 4: 65
Elmore M, Rissing J P, Rink L, Brooks G F 1974 Amer J Med 57: 627
Fass R J, Ruiz D E Gardner W G, Rotilie C A 1977 Arch Intern Med 137: 28
Fenton L J, Light I J 1976 Obstet Gynecol 47: 492
Garrod L P 1957 Brit Med J 2: 57
Geddes A M, Dwyer N St J, Ball A P, Amos R S 1977 J Antimicrob Chemother 3: 501
Georgiew S, Gröger H, Flood M C 1978 J Antimicrob Chemother 4: 472
Gibbs R S, Weinstein A J 1976 Amer J Obstet Gynec 126: 226
Ginsburg C M, Eichenwald H F 1976 J Pediat 89: 872
Goodacre R L, Hamilton J D, Mullens J E, Qizilbash A 1977 Gastroenterology 72: 149
Gorbach S L, Bartlett J G 1977 J Infect Dis 135: S89
Gordon R C, Regamey C, Kirby W M M 1973 J Pharm Sci 62: 1074
Hinthorn D R, Baker L H, Romig D A et al 1976 Antimicrob Ag Chemother 9: 498
Janicki R S, Garnham J C, Worland M C, Grundy W F, Thomas J R 1975 Clin Pediat 14: 1098
Joshi A M, Stein R M 1974 J Clin Pharmacol 14: 140
Karchmer A W, Moellering R C Jr, Watson B K 1975 Antimicrob Ag Chemother 7: 164
Katz L, Lamont J T, Trier J S et al 1978 Gastroenterology 74: 246
Lake B, Bell S M 1969 Med J Aust 1: 449
Larson H E, Price A B 1977 Lancet 2: 1312

Lewis C 1974 Fed Proc 33: 2303
MacFarlane J A, Mitchell A A B, Walsh J M, Robertson J J 1968 Lancet 1: 1
McCloskey R V, Green M J, Eller J, Smilack J 1974 Ann Intern Med 81: 788
McCormack W M, George H, Donner A et al 1977 Antimicrob Ag Chemother 12: 630
Magerlein B J, Birkenmeyer R D, Kagan F 1967 Antimicrob Agents Chemother 1966, p 727
Malke H, Jacob H E, Störl K 1976 Molec Gen Genet 144: 333
Mason D J, Dietz A, Deboer C 1963 Antimicrob Agents Chemother 1962 p 554
Metzler C M, de Haan R, Schellenberg D, Vandenbosch W D 1973 J Pharm Sci 62: 591
Mickal A, Panzer J D 1975 Amer J Obstet Gynec 121: 1071
Miyazaki Y 1973 Arzneim Forsch 23: 940
Nielsen M L, Hansen I, Nielsen J B 1976 Acta Orthop Scand 47: 267
Niitu Y, Hasegawa S, Suetake T, et al 1970 J Pediat 76: 438
Nolan J, Rosen E S 1968 Brit J Ophthal 52: 396
Odegaard K, Solberg O, Lind J, Myhre G, Nyland B 1975 Acta Path Microbiol Scand (B) 83: 301
Osono T, Oka Y, Watanabe S et al 1967 J Antibiot(Tokyo) 20: 174
Parsons R L, Beavis J P, Hossack G A, Paddock G M 1977 Brit J Clin Pharmacol 4: 433
Peddie B A, Dann E, Bailey R R 1975 Aust NZ J Med 5: 198
Philipson A, Sabath L D, Charles D 1973 New Engl J Med 288: 1219
Philipson A, Sabath L D, Charles D 1976 Clin Pharmacol Therap 19: 68
Phillips I, Fernandes R, Warren C 1970 Brit Med J 2: 89
Picardi J L, Lewis H P, Tan J S, Phair J P 1975 J Neurosurg 43: 717
Pinnert-Sindico S, Ninet L, Preud'homme J, Cosar C 1955 Antibiot Ann 1954–5, p 724
Poulos E T, Tedesco F J 1976 Arch Dermat 112: 974
Randolph M F, Morris K E 1977 Clin Pediat 16: 722
Reese R E, Betts R F, Goedde L W, Douglas R G Jr 1976 Antimicrob Ag Chemother 10: 253
Report 1973 Med J Aust 2: 192
Rubbo J T, Gergis S D, Sokoll M D 1977 Anaesthes Analges 56: 329
Sabath L D, Gerstein D A, Finland M 1968 New Engl J Med 279: 1137
Saltzman L, Aperion D 1976 Molec Gen Genet 143: 301
Samuelson R J, Giesecke A H, Kallus F T, Stanley V F 1975 Anaesthes Analges 54: 103
Schurman D J, Johnson B L, Finerman G, Amstutz H C 1975 Clin Orthop 111: 142
Scott A J 1976 Gastroenterology 71: 814
Snyder R J, Wilkowske C J, Washington J A II 1975 Antimicrob Ag Chemother 7: 333
Sparling P F, Blackman E 1973 J Bact 116: 74
Sprunt K, Leidy G, Redman W 1970 Pediatrics 46: 84
Steigbigel R T, Greenman R L, Remington J S 1975 J Infect Dis 131: 245
Stephens V C, Pugh C T, Davis N E, et at L 1969 J Antibiot 22: 551
Strausbaugh L J, Bolton W K, Dilworth J A et al 1976 Antimicrob Ag Chemother 10: 450
Symposium 1977 J Infect Dis 135: S25–88
Tolman K G, Sannella J J, Freston J W 1974 Ann Intern Med 81: 58
Vacek V, Tesarova-Magrova J, Stafova J 1970 Arzneim Forsch 20: 99
Viteri A L, Howard P H, Dyck W P 1974 Gastroenterology 66: 1137
Wagman G H, Waitz T A, Marquez J, et al 1972 J Antibiot Tokyo 25: 641
Warhurst D C, Robinson B L, Peters W 1976 Ann Trop Med Parasitol 70: 253
Weinstein A J, Gibbs R S, Gallagher M 1976 Amer J Obstet Gynec 124: 688
Wenzel R P, Hendley J O, Dodd W K, Gwaltney J M Jr 1976 Antimicrob Ag Chemother 10: 899
Weström L, Mardh P-A 1971 Acta Obstet Gynaec Scand 50: 25
Wilkins T D, Thiel 1973 Antimicrob Ag Chemother 3: 136
Zimmerman H J, Kendler J, Libber S, Lukacs L 1974 Biochem Pharmacol 23: 2187

Pharmaceutical preparations and dosages are on page 202.

Macrolides and lincosamides. Pharmaceutical preparations and dosage

Name	*Dosage*	*Preparations*	*Common international proprietary names*	
Erythromycin	*Adult* Oral: 1–2 g daily in divided doses every 6, 8, or 12 hours. i.m.: 5–8 mg/kg daily in 3–6 divided doses. i.v.: 300 mg every six hours or 600 mg every eight hours. The i.v. or i.m. dose can be increased in very severe infections. *Children* Oral: 30–50 mg/kg daily in divided doses. i.m.: (for children over 15 kg) 50 mg at 4–6 hourly intervals. i.v.: 30–50 mg/kg daily in divided doses.	Erythromycin: tablets. Erythromycin estolate: suspension, capsules. Erythromycin ethylsuccinate: syrup, i.m. injection. Erythromycin stearate: syrup, tablets. Erythromycin lactobionate: i.v. injection.	Erythrocin, Erythromid, Ilosone, Ilotycin, Erythroped. Abboticine Bristamycin, Pfizer E, SK-Erythromycin Erycinum	(UK) (Fr) (USA) (Ger)
Spiramycin	*Adult* Oral: 2–4 g daily in 2–3 divided doses. *Children* Oral: 50–100 mg/kg body weight daily in 2–3 divided doses.	Tablets	Selectomycin No longer available in U.K.	(Ger)
Lincomycin	*Adult* Oral: 500 mg every 6–8 hours depending on the severity of the infection. i.m.: 600 mg every 12–24 hours. i.v.: 600 mg every 8–12 hours as an infusion. *Children* Oral: 30–60 mg/kg body weight daily in divided doses every 6–8 hours. i.m.: 10 mg/kg body weight every 12–24 hours depending on the severity of the infection. i.v.: 10–20 mg/kg a day in divided doses every 8–12 hours as an infusion.	Capsules Syrup Injection	Lincocin, Mycivin Albiotic, Cillimycin	(UK) (Ger)
Clindamycin	*Adult* Oral: 150–450 mg every 6 hours, depending on the severity of the infection. i.m., i.v.: 600–2700 mg a day depending on the severity of the infection. This dose is given in 2, 3 or 4 divided doses. No more than 600 mg should be given as a single i.m. dose, and 1200 mg i.v. as a single infusion. A maximum daily dose of 4.8 g may be given in life-threatening situations. *Children* Oral: 3–6 mg/kg body weight every 6 hours. i.v., i.m.: 15–40 mg/kg daily in 3–4 divided doses depending on the severity of the infection. The daily dose should not exceed a maximum of 300 mg.	Capsules Syrup Injection	Dalacin C Cleocin Sobelin	(UK) (USA) (Ger)

9

Peptides

The peptide antibiotics form a large group (Storm et al, 1977) of which very few have found any therapeutic application. They are composed of peptide-linked amino acids which commonly include both D- and L-forms and some unusual compounds. Characteristic non-amino acid moieties, like the long chain fatty acids of the polymyxins (page 206), also occur. Ring formation is common. The whole group has fascinated biochemists because of the way in which molecular changes allow the compounds to interact with the cell membrane (Veatch & Stryer, 1977) and because of the light this interaction throws on the process of ion transport (Haavik, 1976).

Antibiotic peptides are commonly produced in families of closely related compounds which sometimes differ only in one amino acid residue. The separation of these close relatives may be so difficult that there is doubt about the homogeneity of some of the compounds and hence doubt about the number of members of the family. There are also strong resemblances between some of the members of different families. This kind of inter-relationship is illustrated in Fig. 9.1, which shows that the tyrocidines not only closely resemble one another but that half the tyrocidine molecule is made up of the amino acid sequence of gramicidin S.

There is a connection between antibacterial range and the number of basic groups in the molecule. Bacitracin and gramicidin are most active against Gram-positive organisms and each has two basic groups. The compounds of greatest therapeutic importance, colistin and polymyxin B, are more active against Gram-negative organisms and have 5 and 6 basic groups respectively.

It is of interest that almost all peptide antibiotics have been isolated from the genus *Bacillus*, and that few other antibiotics have emerged from this genus. Those that have found a place in clinicial medicine are gramicidin, bacitracin, isolated in the United States in 1945, and the polymyxins, discovered independently in Britain and America in 1947.

BACITRACIN

Bacitracin was the outcome of a study of the bacterial flora of contaminated civilian wounds in the Presbyterian Hospital, Columbia University (Johnson et al, 1945). It was observed that following direct plating of material from the injured tissue, bacteria sometimes appeared on blood agar plates that were not subsequently recovered from broth cultures made at the same time from the same material. This occurred most frequently when the broth cultures contained a large number of aerobic Gram-positive sporing bacilli. The cell-free filtrate of one such bacillus was found to have strong antibiotic activity. Further extraction and purification led to the isolation of a group of closely related peptide antibiotics, designated bacitracin A, B and C after Tracy, the patient from whom the bacillus was originally isolated.

Anti-bacterial activity

Bacitracin is highly active against many species of Gram-positive bacteria and the pathogenic *Neisseriae*. Although strains of *Staph. aureus* are usually sensitive, they are rather less so than most other Gram-positive bacteria. Haemolytic streptococci of Lancefield's Group A are so much more sensitive than streptococci of other groups that bacitracin sensitivity is used as a screening test for the identification of Group A streptococci, although it has been claimed that co-agglutination is as quick and provides definitive grouping (Stoner, 1978).

Toxicity and clinical use

The bacitracins are not absorbed by the oral route. All are nephrotoxic when given parenterally, and depression of renal function may persist for weeks.

With the steady accumulation of less toxic antibiotics it has been recommended that it be removed from human use (Report, 1969). It is still included in some preparations for local application (page 306); absorption may occur from application to ulcerated areas and resulting anaphylaxis has been described (Roupe & Strannegård, 1969).

DEPSIPEPTIDES

This large group of natural cyclic peptides is of great general biological interest. They occur, like their relatives, in families of compounds some of which are antibiotics, some powerful poisons and others devoid of biological effect. They were given the name *peptolides*—which expresses well their kinship (Fig. 9.2) with the peptides on the one hand and the macrolides on the other—but the name was withdrawn when it was found that *depsipeptides* had priority. Many antibiotic members of the group have been isolated and characterized but few have been pursued with any vigour into the therapeutic field. They are particularly active against streptococci and staphylococci, but include *H. influenzae* and the pathogenic *Neisseria* in their spectrum. Vazquez (1975) reviews the whole group of which the better studied are ostreogrycin, virginiamycin, streptogramin, mikamycin and pristinamycin. With the exception of viridogrisein, which is intrinsically the most active member of the group, they each consist of two components, which act synergically. The combined action of the two components of virginiamycin was found by Varon et al (1976) to be a thousand times greater than that of either component alone.

The group A components of the differently named agents are very closely related if not identical and it is the Group B components that share in the plasmid-borne variety of resistance to macrolides and lincomycins (Malke et al, 1976) which is induced by erythromycin (page 185). Some have been used in the treatment of staphylococcal septicaemia with 'spectacular' results. Two have been developed commercially: virginiamycin (Staphylomycine, *R.I.T.*, Belgium) which has been fairly extensively studied (Van Dijck, 1969) and is used as an animal feed additive and

Tyrocidine	R_1	R_2
A	L-Phe	D-Phe
B	L-Try	D-Phe
C	L-Try	D-Try

GRAMICIDIN S

[L-Val — L-Orn — L-Leu — D-Phe — L-Pro
L-Pro — D-Phe — L-Leu — L-Orn — L-Val]

TYROCIDINES

[L-Val — L-Orn — L-Leu — D-Phe — L-Pro
L-Tyr — L-Glu-NH_2 — L-Asp-NH_2 — R_1-R_2]

Fig. 9.1 Structure of gramicidin S and tyrocidines (Ruttenberg et al, 1965)

pristinamycin (Pyostacine, *Rhone Poulenc*) which has been used a good deal in France almost exclusively for the treatment of infections by staphylococci, most strains of which are inhibited by less than 1 μg/ml. Administration is oral, 2–3 g being given daily in divided doses.

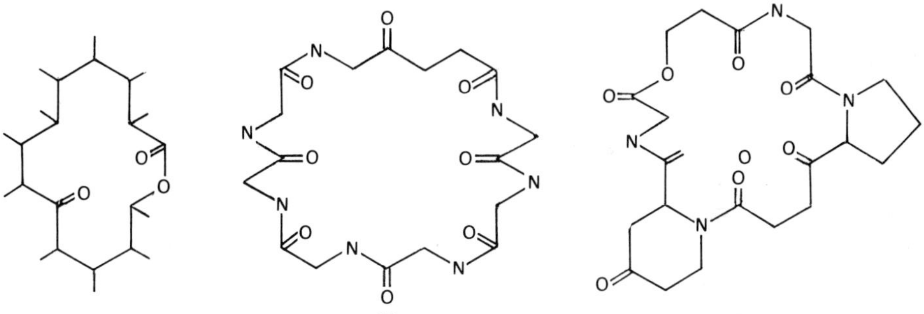

I II III

Fig. 9.2 Skeleton structures of a typical macrolide (I) peptide (II) and depsipeptide (III) to show the general similarity of their large cyclic molecules, closed in the case of the macrolide through oxygen (O), in the case of the peptide through nitrogens (N) and in the case of the depsipeptide through both

GRAMICIDIN

This was the first in the field and came from the pioneer work of Dubos (1939) which preceded the extraction and purification of penicillin. It is produced by an aerobic sporing bacillus, *B. brevis*, originally isolated from soil. Crude extracts of cultures of this bacillus yielded an alcohol-soluble bactericidal substance, tyrothricin, from which two antibiotics, gramicidin and tyrocidine, were separated (Dubos & Hotchkiss, 1941). There are at least four gramicidins in the substance isolated by Dubos and a further compound designated gramicidin S (Soviet), the structure of which is indicated in Fig. 9.1, was obtained from a strain of *B. brevis* by Gause & Brazhnikova (1944).

Antibacterial activity

Gramicidin is active against most species of aerobic and anaerobic Gram-positive bacteria, including mycobacteria. Gram-negative bacilli are completely insensitive probably due to the presence of surface phospholipids which inhibit the action of gramicidin.

Tyrothricin, which contains only 15 to 20 per cent gramicidin, is about as active against pneumococcal infection in mice as gramicidin itself, although the other component of tyrothricin, tyrocidine, is inactive *in vivo*. It has been suggested therefore, that there is a synergic action between tyrocidine and gramicidin, a situation reminiscent of the more recently discovered depsipeptides.

Toxicity and use

By intravenous injection gramicidin is highly toxic to erythrocytes, liver and kidney and therapeutically is of historical interest only. It has no special properties to justify its inclusion in mixtures for local application (page 306).

POLYMYXINS

The polymyxins are a group of basic peptide antibiotics derived from a spore-bearing soil bacillus and with a selective action against Gram-negative bacilli. They were first isolated in 1947 independently in one laboratory in Britain (Ainsworth et al, 1947) and two in the United States (Stansly et al, 1947; Benedict & Langlykke, 1947). The British investigators called the antibiotic 'aerosporin' since they identified the bacillus as *B. aerosporus*. The American investigators identified the bacillus as *B. polymyxa* and called the antibiotic polymyxin. Comparative studies in the two laboratories proved the identity of the two bacilli and the name polymyxin was accepted (Symposium, 1949).

Chemical properties

Five polymyxins, A, B, C, D and E were originally isolated and characterized and others have since been added. Polymyxin A is the antibiotic originally named aerosporin and polymyxin D is the polymyxin isolated by Stansly et al in 1947. Interestingly, neither has come into therapeutic use for which the less toxic polymyxin B and colistin (Koyama et al, 1950)—shown to be identical with polymyxin E by Suzuki et al (1964)—have been commercially developed. Polymyxins are composed of amino acids linked in the form of a ring with a tail adorned at its end by a characteristic fatty acid. The close relationship of the two components of polymyxin B, B1 and B2, and one of the two components of colistin (colistin A, which is identical with polymyxin E1) is shown in Fig. 9.3. Both polymyxin B and colistin are supplied as the sulphate. Both were available as sulpho-methyl derivatives, but the polymyxin preparation has been withdrawn.

The sulphates are highly soluble in water and methanol; solutions are fairly stable and withstand heating to 60°C for one hour. If solutions are sterilized by filtration, there is some loss in either Seitz or sintered glass filters.

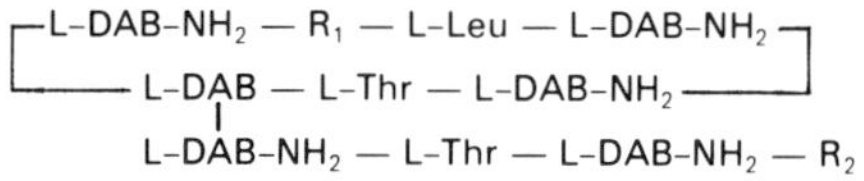

$$
\begin{array}{c}
\text{┌── L–DAB–NH}_2 \text{ — R}_1 \text{ — L–Leu — L–DAB–NH}_2 \text{ ┐} \\
\text{└──── L–DAB — L–Thr — L–DAB–NH}_2 \text{────┘} \\
\text{L–DAB–NH}_2 \text{ — L–Thr — L–DAB–NH}_2 \text{ — R}_2
\end{array}
$$

	R₁	R₂
Polymyxin B₁	D-Phe	6-methyl-octanoyl
Polymyxin B₂	D-Phe	6-methyl-heptanoyl
Polymyxin E₁ Colistin A	D-Leu	6-methyl-octanoyl

Fig. 9.3 Structure of polymyxins
Leu = leucine; Thr = threonine; Phe = phenylalanine; DAB = di-amino-butyric acid.

Suzuki T et al 1963 J Biochem (Japan) 54: 173, 412, 555
Suzuki T et al 1964 J Biochem (Japan) 56: 335
Wilkinson S, Lowe L A 1964 Nature (Lond) 204: 993

Sulphomethyl polymyxins

By treatment with formalin and sodium bisulphite, some or all of the 5 amino-groups of the polymyxins can be replaced by sulpho-methyl groups. The sulphomethyl derivative of polymyxin B is also known as sulphomyxin and that of colistin as colistimethate. The substituted compounds differ considerably in their properties from the parent antibiotics. They are relatively painless on injection, less toxic, less active antibacterially (Table 9.1), and more rapidly excreted by the kidney.

There has been some argument about the basis of these differences. The situation is complicated by the fact that the derivatives consist of undefined mixtures of the mono-, di-, tri-, tetra- and penta-substituted compounds—all of which might theoretically have different properties—and by the fact that the more substituted compounds readily dissociate in solution. The experimental toxicity of the colistin sulphomethate commercially available in America (ColyMycin) is so different from that available in this country (Colomycin) that the two compounds probably differ considerably in their degree of sulphomethylation.

Solutions of the compounds increase progressively in antibacterial activity on incubation until activity approaching that of the parent polymyxin is obtained. It has been argued from this and other evidence that the sulphomethyl derivatives are relatively non-toxic, inactive compounds which owe their effect to the liberation of the parent polymyxin but other evidence suggests that the less substituted compounds must possess intrinsic antibacterial activity.

The liberation of more active compounds on incubation considerably complicates the determination of minimum inhibitory concentrations, since the results are compounded of the activities of substances liberated during incubation of the cultures. Direct comparisons of the antibacterial activity of colistin and polymyxin sulphates with their sulphomethyl derivatives have generally shown the sulphates to be 4–8 times more active.

Against dense cultures of *Escherichia coli* Greenwood (1975) found that polymyxin and colistin sulphates had similar activity. The concentration of polymyxin sulphomethate required to produce lysis was four times that of polymyxin sulphate while colistin sulphomethate produced delayed lysis consistent with the liberation of the parent compound. Adaptation to the agent allowing regrowth during the overnight period easily occurred—most readily to colistin sulphomethate and least readily to polymyxin B sulphate.

Davis (1975) found polymyxins to be more active than the aminoglycosides he tested against *Pseudomonas aeruginosa* in a mouse protection test while colistimethate had little effect. Similarly, in a model simulating conditions of bacterial growth in the urinary bladder, Greenwood & O'Grady (1977) found that polymyxins were effective (although they exerted less effect than in static cultures) whereas the sulphomethyl derivatives had very little effect.

Anti-bacterial activity

All the polymyxins have a similar anti-bacterial spectrum. Although there are slight quantitative differences in their activity *in vitro* there is effectively complete cross-resistance between them. Nearly all species of Gram-negative bacilli including Pseudomonas, but excluding Proteus, are highly sensitive to polymyxin and on a weight for weight basis are usually more sensitive to polymyxin than to almost any other antibiotic (Table 9.1).

Table 9.1 Sensitivity of bacteria to polymyxins

	Colistin sulphate	Sulphomethyl colistin	Polymyxin B sulphate
S. aureus	64–R	R	64–R
S. pyogenes	32	32	16–R
S. viridans	32–R	32–R	32–R
S. faecalis	R	R	R
H. influenzae	0.5–1		0.03
E. coli	0.01–32	0.05–R	0.02
K. pneumoniae	0.01–1	0.01–4	0.03–0.5
E. aerogenes	0.03–32	0.5–R	0.03–16
Proteus spp.	R	R	R
Salmonella spp.	0.01–1	0.03–0.5	0.01–1
Shigella spp.	0.01–1	0.1–0.25	0.01–1
P. aeruginosa	0.03–4	2–32	0.03–4

Based on
Graber C O et al 1960 Antibiot Ann. 1959–60, p 77
Ross S et al 1960 Ibid, p 89
Schwartz B S et al 1960 Ibid, p 41
Wright W W, Welch H 1960 Ibid, p 61
Courtieu A L et al 1961 Ann Inst Pasteur Suppl 4: 14
Postic B, Finland M 1961 Amer J Med Sci 242: 551
Fekety F R et al 1962 Ann Intern Med 57: 214
Taylor G, Allison H 1962 Brit Med J 2: 161

With the exception of some atypical strains (Goodwin et al, 1971), all species of *Proteus* are resistant, evidently because of a peculiarity of cell-wall structure which renders it impermeable to the drug (Sud & Feingold, 1970). It is possibly through modification of such a cell-wall component that Proteus growing in the presence of sulphonamide becomes susceptible to polymyxin and that this is the mechanism of the well-known synergy between the two agents which can be extended to triple synergy against some strains by the addition of trimethoprim (page 28). Resistance of *Vibrio el tor* to polymyxin distinguishes it from the classical vibrio (Gugnani & Pal, 1974).

The pathogenic Gram-negative cocci, *N. gonorrhoeae* and *N. meningitidis*, and nearly all species of Gram-positive bacteria and fungi are also resistant. *Candida tropicalis* is exceptional in this regard in that its sensitivity to 30–75 μg colistin/ml can be used as a screening test for its identification, and utilized therapeutically in eradicating it from the urine (Nichols, 1970). *Coccidioides immitis* is even more sensitive, being inhibited by concentrations of 5–10 μg polymyxin B per ml. Collins & Pappagianis (1976), who had previously shown polymyxin to enhance the action of amphotericin B, successfully used polymyxin B to control experimental coccidioidomycosis of mice.

Because of its wide activity against Gram-negative organisms, polymyxin has been used in a number of selective media (see for example Orth & Anderson, 1970) and in combination with nalidixic acid, for the selective isolation of Group B streptococci in Todd Hewitt broth (Fenton and Harper, 1979). Because of its effect in disrupting the cell membrane (page 260) it has been commended as a gentle means of releasing from the bacterial cell enzymes (Page & Tsang, 1976) and the heat-labile enterotoxin elaborated by some strains of *Escherichia coli* (Evans et al, 1976).

Interactions

Complex interactions occur with serum because polymyxins act synergically with the natural bactericidal systems, but are adversely affected by the calcium and magnesium present in serum. For example, Traub & Kleber (1975) found that strains of *Serratia marcesens* resistant to the bactericidal action of fresh human serum alone were killed by the addition of therapeutically attainable concentrations of polymyxin B, while of the antibiotics tested against 13 species of Pseudomonas, D'Amato et al (1975) found polymyxin B to be the most affected by the presence of calcium and magnesium ions in the medium.

Polymyxin (like aminoglycosides) is inhibited by polyanethol sulphonate (liquoid), presumably through a charge effect, and this has been used as the basis of an assay of unaffected antibiotics, such as penicillins, in the presence of polymyxin (Edberg et al, 1976).

Polymyxins bind specifically to the lipid A region of lipopolysaccharide—the biologically active portion of the molecule—and this interaction is probably responsible for its depressant effect on phage attachment (Koike & Iida, 1971) and for its effect on the biological responses to lipopolysaccharide (Corrigan et al, 1974; Jacobs & Morrison, 1977) including the development of endotoxin shock (From et al, 1979).

Acquired resistance

Polymyxin has been remarkably free from the problem of emergence of resistance in initially susceptible species that has plagued so many other antibiotics, and that despite the fact that adaptation to growth in high concentrations of the drug is readily achieved in a variety of enterobacteria (Greenwood, 1975; Shimizu et al, 1977)—a further indication that ease of laboratory acquired resistance is not a reliable guide to epidemiological significance.

PHARMACOKINETICS

Polymyxins are not absorbed from the alimentary tract or from the uninflamed bladder into which they are sometimes instilled to control infection (Chamberlain & Needham, 1976). After parenteral administration of the sulphates blood levels are usually low. Somewhat higher levels are obtained in children, and by repeated administration, peak levels around 1.5 μg/ml are obtained about an hour after a dose of 60 mg.

Substantially higher plasma levels are obtained from intramuscular injections of sulphomethyl polymyxins but (as in the determination of inhibitory concentrations, page 207) because the drug concentration has to be measured microbiologically there is an opportunity during incubation for the liberation of active agent which was not present in the serum at the time of collection of the samples. Levels reported by various authors are given in Table 9.2. Froman et al (1970) give rather lower values for all the parameters: peak plasma levels of 5–6 μg/ml at 1–2 hr with a half-life of 2.75–3 hr after an intramuscular dose of 150 mg. Ten minutes after a similar intravenous dose, the level was 18 μg/ml falling after 4 hr to 2 μg/ml. Cox & Harrison (1971) treated some patients with urinary infection with an intravenous priming dose of 1.5–2.5 mg/kg followed by continuous infusion of 4.8–6 mg/hr for 20–36 hr (after which they continued with intramuscular therapy). During the period of infusion they found steady-state levels around 5–10 μg/ml.

Table 9.2 Serum levels of sulpho-methyl colistin in man

Dose i.m.	Patients	Peak Hr	Peak μg per ml	Half-life hr
2 mg/kg		2–3	6–15	6–12
4 mg/kg	Adult	3–5	17–25	6–10
5 mg/kg		4	25	5
2.5 mg/kg	Children	1	5	2–3

Forni P V, Guidetti E 1956 Minerva Med 2: Suppl 77: 823
Ross S et al 1960 Antibiot Ann 1959–60, p 89
Wright W W, Welch H 1960 Antibiot Ann 1959–60, p 61
Colley E W, Frankel H L 1963 Brit Med J 2: 790

Polymyxins bind to both bacterial (page 260) and mammalian cell membranes. Because of this binding, the agents persist in the liver, kidneys, brain, heart, muscle and lungs (at least of the rabbit) for as long as 72 hours (Kunin & Bugg, 1971). On repeated dosage the drugs accumulate in the tissues although they disappear from the serum. Such behaviour greatly complicates the general pharmacokinetics of the agents and may of course have special importance in relation to both toxicity and therapy of infection in the organs in which they accumulate. Binding is through the amino groups of the molecules and consequently only free colistin and not the sulpho-methyl derivatives, in which the amino groups are occluded, is bound.

Following a dose of 150 mg colistin sulphomethate intravenously, none could be detected in the amniotic fluid three hours later. Very low plasma levels (about 0.45

μg/ml) were found in both mothers and infants born 6–20 hours later. A dose of 30–40 mg injected into the amniotic fluid of patients not in labour was still present 18 hours later (MacAulay & Charles, 1967).

Excretion

Polymyxin sulphates are excreted mainly by the kidneys but after a considerable lag. With a daily dose of 3 mg/kg, only about 0.1 per cent of the dose is recovered in the first 12 hours, but concentrations varying from 40 to 400 μg/ml can be found from 24 hours onwards.

The sulphomethyl derivatives are much more rapidly excreted and this accounts for their shorter half-lives. Froman et al (1970) found that 67 per cent of an intramuscular dose and 75 per cent of an intravenous dose were excreted within 24 hours. Urinary levels around 100 to 200 μg/ml were found at 2 hr and 15–45 μg/ml at 8 hr. A rather wider range of the same order (73–315 μg/ml) was found by Cox & Harrison (1971) on their continuous intravenous regimen. Serum levels are not augmented by probenecid and extra-renal mechanisms probably take part in excretion. There is disagreement about the effect of peritoneal dialysis on the plasma half-life, but it is in any case insufficient for the management of overdosage for which Brown et al (1970) successfully resorted to exchange transfusion. Described differences in the effect of haemodialysis may well depend on the membrane used (Curtis & Eastwood, 1968). There does not seem to be excessive retention of sulphomethyl colistin in the newborn.

Toxicity

Like other members of the family, but to a lesser degree, polymyxin B and colistin are nephrotoxic and neurotoxic. Possible hazards of their use must, therefore, be considered, but when appropriately given their therapeutic efficiency outweighs their nephrotoxicity.

Pain (and tissue injury) can occur at the site of injection of the sulphates but the sulphomethyl derivatives are less aggressive. Neurological symptoms such as paraesthesiae with typical numbness and tingling around the mouth, dizziness and weakness are relatively common and neuromuscular blockade, sometimes severe enough to impede respiration, occurs. In a review of 317 courses of treatment, Koch-Weser et al (1970) found evidence of renal damage in 20.2 per cent, with acute tubular necrosis in 1.9 per cent. Neurotoxicity was encountered in 7.3 per cent with respiratory insufficiency in 2.1 per cent. Reactions appeared early in the course of treatment, often within the first four days. Most patients had received no more than conventional doses but toxic manifestations occurred more frequently in heavier patients. Apparently dosage on a direct weight basis results in such patients receiving toxic amounts of the drug. It is suggested that a dosage regimen based on the square root of the weight might ensure adequate treatment for the lighter patient and avoid overdosage in the heavier. The appearance of any evidence of deterioration of renal function or of neuromuscular blockade calls for immediate cessation of treatment. All the toxic manifestations appear to be reversible but complete recovery may be slow.

Nephrotoxicity

In the mouse, the sulphates and sulphomethyl derivatives differ considerably in their toxicity but the more toxic the compound, the more effective it is therapeutically: polymyxin B is more toxic to white mice than colistin; the sulphomethyl derivatives are considerably less toxic but for a given antibacterial effect, an equally toxic dose of each of the compounds has to be given.

In the dog, Vinnicombe & Stamey (1969) found that an intravenous dose of 5 mg/kg polymyxin B sulphate, which produced average serum and urine levels of 30 and 60 μg/ml depressed the GFR and renal plasma flow by about 60 per cent. The same dose of sulphomethyl polymyxin B produced average serum and urine levels of 14.5 and 165 μg/ml and depressed renal function by 20–25 per cent. In contrast, 40 mg/kg of sulphomethyl colistin, which produced much higher serum and urine levels of 57 and 1020 μg/ml, had no depressant effect on renal function. When sulphomethyl polymyxin B was given in a dose (25 mg/kg) which produced about the same urine levels (999 μg/ml) but higher serum levels (143 μg/ml), both the GFR and renal plasma flow were reduced by more than 80 per cent.

In human volunteers studied by Caldwell et al (1969) creatinine clearance was depressed less by colistin sulphomethate than by sulphomyxin. In all subjects renal function returned to normal in 5–8 days. An effect on the renal tubules may have been responsible for the association described in leukaemic patients by Rodriguez et al (1970) between polymyxin B therapy and low levels of sodium, potassium, chloride and calcium—sometimes with tetany.

Neurotoxicity

In addition to the common paraesthesiae, several cases of apnoea have been reported following polymyxin therapy, some with other pareses. This effect has not been described in patients with normal renal function and presumably results from the high plasma levels which may develop (100 μg/ml in one patient). It is possible that the cationic polymyxins, which owe their antibacterial effect to interaction with the lipid-rich anionic bacterial cell membrane, exert a similar effect on the lipid-rich synaptic membranes so interfering with conduction. McQuillen & Engbaek (1975) showed that the presynaptic effect of colistin differed from that of neomycin and several workers, for example White (1977), have studied the details of the electrochemical effect of peptide antibiotics at the synaptic membrane.

It is plainly unwise to give polymyxins to patients who are likely to receive muscle relaxants or anaesthetics, or to those suffering from hypoxia or impaired neuromuscular activity. A single dose of 150 mg colistin sulphomethate produced complete flaccid paralysis with respiratory arrest in an elderly man suffering from myasthenia gravis (Decker & Fincham, 1971) who subsequently recovered fully.

Histamine liberation

Polymyxins liberate histamine and serotonin and their intraperitoneal injection depletes the mast cells and in some way alters the peritoneal membrane so that absorption of the drug (and others) is facilitated (Reite & Hausken, 1970). Morrison et al (1975) showed that polymyxin B covalently bound to sepharose beads caused mast cells to degranulate thereby demonstrating that the effect was at the membrane rather than following penetration of the cell. Marschke & Sarauw (1971) observed two patients who developed acute respiratory distress on inhaling polymyxin B but concluded that this was due not to neuromuscular blockade but to airways obstruction possibly related to histamine liberation. Hypersensitivity to polymyxin has been rarely reported and the immunological basis of this response is discussed by Lakin et al (1975).

Clinical applications

Before the advent of gentamicin (page 142) and carbenicillin (page 82), polymyxins were unchallenged as the drug of choice for the treatment of infections due to *Ps. aeruginosa* and also in infections with some other resistant coliform bacilli.

Where systemic polymyxin therapy is indicated, relative painlessness on intramuscular injection and lower toxicity have caused colistin sulphomethate to be generally used. For oral and local application, the more active polymyxin sulphates should be used. Oral polymyxins have been used for the treatment of gastrointestinal infection and in combination with other agents for the suppression of bowel flora in leukaemic patients and preoperatively (page 288). The use of oral colistin sulphate by Hirschhorn et al (1975) in an attempt to reduce the prevalence of diarrhoea in undernourished children increased the frequency of both diarrhoea and isolation of enteropathogenic *E. coli*.

Prophylactic use of polymyxin aerosols by Klick et al (1975) administered to patients in an intensive therapy unit in doses of 2.5 mg/kg per day divided into six doses reduced respiratory colonization and pneumonia due to *Pseudomonas aeruginosa* but did not affect overall mortality.

Since the development of resistance to polymyxin has not been a problem, and the antibiotic does not appear to damage healing wounds, it can be used as a spray, powder or cream, for the treatment of any superficial infection with *Ps. aeruginosa* such as superficial wounds, ulcers or otitis externa. A cream containing 1 mg per g polymyxin has had considerable success in preventing burns becoming colonized by *Ps. aeruginosa*.

Pharmaceutical preparations and dosages are on page 216.

References

Ainsworth G C, Brown A M, Brownlee G 1947 Nature (Lond) 160: 263
Benedict R G, Langlykke A F 1947 J Bact 54: 24
Brown J M, Dorman D C, Roy L P 1970 Med J Aust 2: 923
Caldwell A D S, Martin A J, Trigger D J 1969 Brit J Pharmacol 37: 283
Chamberlain G, Needham P 1976 J Urol 116: 172
Coleman D J, McGhie D, Tebbutt G M 1977 J Clin Path 30: 421
Collins M S, Pappagianis D 1976 Antimicrob Ag Chemother 10: 318
Corrigan J J Jr, Sieber O F Jr, Ratajczak H, Bennett B B 1974 J Infect Dis 130: 384
Cox C E, Harrison L H 1971 Antimicrob Agents Chemother 1970, p 269
Curtis J R, Eastwood J B 1968 Brit Med J 1: 484
D'Amato R F, Thornsberry C, Baker C N, Kirven L A 1975 Antimicrob Ag Chemother 7: 596
Davis S D 1975 Antimicrob Ag Chemother 8: 50
Decker D A, Fincham R W 1971 Arch Neurol 25: 141
Dubos R J 1939 J Exper Med 70: 1
Dubos R J, Hotchkiss R D 1941 J Exper Med 73: 629
Edberg S C, Bottenbley C J, Gam K 1976 Antimicrob Ag Chemother 9: 414
Evans D J, Evans D G, Richardson S H, Gorbach S L 1976 J Infect Dis 133: S97
Fenton L J, Harper M H 1979 J Clin Microbiol 9: 167
From A H L, Fong J S C, Good R A 1979 Infect Immun 23: 660
Froman J, Gross L, Curatola S 1970 J Urol 103: 210
Gause G F, Brazhnikova M G 1944 Nature (Lond) 154: 703
Goodwin C S, Kliger B N, Drewett S E 1971 Brit J Exper Path 52: 138
Greenwood D 1975 J Gen Microbiol 91: 110
Greenwood D, O'Grady F 1977 J Med Microbiol 10: 255
Gugnani H C, Pal S C 1974 J Med Microbiol 7: 535
Haavik H I 1976 Acta Path Microbiol Scand 84(B): 117
Hirschhorn N, Woodward W E, Evans L K et al 1975 Amer J Trop Med Hyg 24: 320
Jacobs D M, Morrison D C 1977 J Immunol 118: 21
Johnson B A, Anker H, Meleney F L 1945 Science 102: 376
Klick J M, du Moulin G C, Heldley-White J et al 1975 J Clin Invest 55: 514
Koch-Weser J, Sidel V W, Federman E B, et al 1970 Ann Intern Med 72: 857
Koike M, Iida K 1971 J Bact 108: 1402
Koyama Y, Kurosasa A, Tsuchiya A, Takakuta K 1950 J Antibiot (Tokyo) 3: 457
Kunin C M, Bugg A 1971 J Infect Dis 124: 394
Lakin J D, Strong D M, Sell K W 1975 Ann Intern Med 83: 204
MacAulay M A, Charles D 1967 Clin Pharmacol Ther 8: 578
Malke H, Jacob H E, Störl K 1976 Molec Gen Genet 144: 333
Marschke G, Sarauw A 1971 Ann Intern Med 74: 296
McQuillen M P, Engbaek L 1975 Arch Neurol 32: 235
Morrison D C, Roser J F, Cochrane C G, Henson P M 1975 J Immunol 114: 966
Nichols M W N 1970 J Med Microbiol 3: 529
Orth D S, Anderson A W 1970 Appl Microbiol 20: 508
Page L V, Tsang J C 1976 Microbios 15: 153
Reite O B, Hausken O 1970 Europ J Pharmacol 10: 101
Report 1969 Joint Committee on the Use of Antibiotics in Animal Husbandry and Veterinary Medicine. Her Majesty's Stationery Office, London
Rodriguez V, Green S, Bodey G P 1970 Clin Pharmacol Ther 11: 106
Roupe G, Strannegård Ö 1969 Arch Derm 100: 450
Ruttenberg M A, King T P, Craig L C 1965 Biochemistry 4: 11
Shimizu S, Iyobe S, Mitsuhashi S 1977 Antimicrob Ag Chemother 12: 1
Stansly P G, Shepherd R G, White H J 1947 Bull Johns Hopk Hosp 81: 43
Stoner R A 1978 J Clin Microbiol 7: 463
Storm D R, Rosenthal K S, Swanson P E 1977 Ann Rev Biochem 46: 723
Sud I J, Feingold D S 1970 J Bact 104: 289
Suzuki T, Hayashi K, Fujkawa K, Tsukamoto K 1964 J Biochem 56: 335
Symposium 1949 Ann NY Acad Sci 51: 875, 879, 891, 897, 909, 952
Traub W H, Kleber I 1975 Chemotherapy 21: 189
Van Dijck P J 1969 Chemotherapy 14: 322
Varon M, Cocito C, Siejffers J 1976 Antimicrob Ag Chemother 9: 179

Vazquez D 1975 Antibiotics III, Mechanism of action of antimicrobial and antitumour agents. In: Corcoran J W, Hahn F E (eds) Springer-Verlag, p. 459
Veatch W, Stryer L 1977 J Molec Biol 113: 89
Vinnicombe J, Stamey T A 1969 Invest Urol 6: 505
White T D 1977 J Neurochem 29: 193

Peptides. Pharmaceutical preparations and dosage

Name	*Dosage*	*Preparations*	*Common international proprietary names*	
Bacitracin	Topical application only	In combination with other antibiotics in topical preparations. Aural and ophthalmic preparations.	Baciguent	(USA)
Gramicidin	As above	In combination with Neomycin in topical applications.		
Pristinamycin	*Adult* 2-3 g daily in 2 or 3 divided doses *Children* 50-100 mg/kg body weight daily in divided doses.		Pyostacine	(Fr)
Polymyxin B Sulphate	*Adult* Intrathecal injection: A maximum of 100 000 i.u. twice a day (for meningitis). i.v. 2000-4000 i.u./kg body weight hourly for five doses. i.v. Infusion 25 000 i.u./kg body weight in 24 hours, either as a single infusion or divided into 2 infusions, each given 12 hourly. The total daily dose should not exceed 2 000 000 i.u. and should be reduced if renal function is impaired. Oral: 1 000 000 i.u. every 4 hours. *Children* Intrathecal injection: 20 000-40 000 i.u. twice daily i.v: 10 000-20 000 i.u./kg body weight daily, in divided doses every 4 hours, with a maximum of 200 000 i.u. daily Oral: 40 000 i.u./kg body weight three times a day.	Injection	Aerosporin	(UK)
Colistin sulphate Polymyxin E sulphate	*Adult* Oral: 1 500 000-3 000 000 u every 8 hours *Children* Oral: (up to 15 kg) 250 000-500 000 u every 8 hours (15-30 kg) 750 000-1 500 000 u every 8 hours	Tablets Syrup Sterile powder	Colomycin Colimycine Coly-Mycin S	(UK) (Fr) (USA)
Colistin sulphomethate Sodium Colistimethate Sodium (USP)	*Adult* i.m., i.v: 6 000 000 units daily in 3 divided doses *Children* i.m., i.v: (up to 60 kg body weight) 50 000 units/kg body weight in 3 divided doses.	Injection	Colomycin Colimycine Coly-Mycin M	(UK) (Fr) (USA)

10

Various anti-bacterial antibiotics

Here follow accounts of antibiotics not classifiable among the main groups described in other chapters. Those of some of the less important are necessarily brief, but some mention of them may be more helpful than none at all. Only those are included which have been used in human therapeutics; we do not, for example, include tylosin, a macrolide, or nisin, a peptide, for which the only uses have been non-medical. Other exceptions are antibiotics used exclusively in tuberculosis, which are referred to in Chapter 23.

CYCLOSERINE

Cycloserine is a product of *Streptomyces orchidaceus* and other organisms, and has also been synthesized. Chemically it is D-4-amino-3-isoxazolidone, with a molecular weight of only 102, and thus almost the simplest known substance possessing antibiotic activity. A fairly wide range of bacteria, both Gram-negative and Gram-positive, including *Myco. tuberculosis*, are sensitive to it. Early studies of *in vitro* activity produced discouraging results, but these were carried out before it was recognized that the action of cycloserine is specifically antagonized by D-alanine, a fact which provides the clue to its mode of action (page 257). Tests in a medium free from this amino acid produce more realistic results.

Cycloserine is well absorbed after oral administration, attaining high and well sustained concentrations in the blood and being excreted unchanged in the urine. Cycloserine may induce confusional states, depression, acute psychotic reactions, hyperreflexia, tremors and dysarthria. Convulsions are said to occur in about 5 per cent of patients when the plasma concentration exceeds 20 μg per ml but the relationship to dose is not particularly close. No permanent damage appears to be caused. Sustained release preparations may be helpful in mitigating side effects; this and other aspects of the pharmacokinetics of this drug were discussed at an International Symposium (1970).

As a result of attempts to trace the neurotoxic effects to vitamin deficiency it was found that convulsions could be abolished by simultaneous administration of pyridoxine. Nair et al (1976) found evidence in tuberculous patients of deranged tryptophane metabolism, presumably due to pyridoxal phosphate deficiency, but could not show that cycloserine is a pyridoxine antagonist. Cycloserine inhibits mammalian transaminases and Yasumitsu et al (1976) attribute this and the convulsant effects of the drug to a metabolite, amino-oxyalanine. They conclude that any improved derivative of cycloserine should be resistant to hydrolysis. One attempt to improve on cycloserine led to the development of terizidone, a Schiff's base incorporating two molecules of cycloserine (Bianchi et al, 1965) which produces higher plasma concentrations than does an equivalent dose of cycloserine (Zítková & Tousek, 1974).

Its principal use is as a second-line drug for the treatment of tuberculosis. Horsfall (1972) discusses the use of the drug in combination with other second line antituberculous agents, mainly ethionamide and pyrazinamide, in the treatment of drug-resistant tuberculosis. It requires mention here because it also has advocates as a remedy for urinary tract infection, notably Murdoch and his colleagues who have continued to use the drug over the course of twenty years for both short- and long-term treatment without encountering significant problems of bacterial resistance or toxicity (Murdoch, 1979). At ages greater than 45 or if renal function is impaired the dose must be reduced. All authors advise blood assays to ensure that the concentration attained shall not exceed 20–25 μg per ml.

References

Bianchi S, Felder E, Tiepolo U 1965 Farmaco 20: 366.
Horsfall P A L 1972 Tubercle 53: 166
International Symposium 1970 Scand J Resp Dis Suppl 71: 13
Murdoch J McC 1979 In: Proudfoot A T (ed) Prospects for prevention. Royal College of Physicians, Edinburgh, p. 47
Nair S, Maguire W, Baron H, Imbruce R 1976 J Clin Pharmacol 16: 439
Yasumitsu T, Takao T, Kakimoto Y 1976 Biochem Pharmacol 25: 253
Zítková L, Tousek J 1974 Chemotherapy 20: 18

FOSFOMYCIN

This small molecule is unrelated to any other antibiotic. Originally called phosphonomycin, it is produced by several species of streptomyces: *Streptomyces fradii*, *Streptomyces irridochromogenes* and *Streptomyces wedmonensis*, and was jointly described by workers in the laboratories of Merck Sharp and Dohme and the Compagnia Espanola de la Penecilina y Antibioticos (Hendlin et al, 1969). The compound was shortly after synthesized by a process appropriate for commercial production (Glamkowski et al, 1970). The calcium salt, which is relatively insoluble, is used in the oral preparation and the very soluble sodium salt in the parenteral form of the drug. Its properties and therapeutic utility have recently been comprehensively reviewed (Symposium, 1977).

Fosfomycin is moderately active against a wide range of pathogens (Table 10.1) but as it depends for its action on active transport into the bacterial cells by the α-glycerophosphate and glucose-phosphate systems, its transport and hence its antibacterial activity *in vitro* are inhibited by the presence of glucose and phosphate in the medium. Addition of glucose-6-phosphate to the medium enhances the activity of the drug and the degree to which this is successful no doubt accounts in part for the wide range of sensitivities reported. Phosphate ions are present at a lower level in blood and mammalian tissues than in culture media and the drug is effective on oral administration.

Bacterial populations contain variants which are highly resistant to the drug but these have not proved to be a problem *in vivo* and there did not appear to have been any significant increase in the prevalence of resistance in the two years after the drug was released for use in Spain. There is no cross-resistance with any other therapeutic antibiotic and the agent is active against many resistant strains including those with plasmid-borne resistance. Olay et al (1978) claim that a useful degree of interaction with various antibiotics can be demonstrated both *in vitro* and *in vivo.*

About 30–40 per cent of the drug is absorbed orally, producing peak plasma levels about 4 hr after 2 g doses of around 7 μg per ml. Absorption is not affected by food. Peak blood levels occur about 1 hour after intramuscular injection and are 3–5 times higher than those produced by the oral route, average values being 17 and 28 μg per ml after 0.5 and 1 g doses. There is some accumulation after repeated doses given 6-hourly. Intravenously a similar dose gives a peak level of around 100 μg per ml. Constant intravenous infusion of 500 mg per hour produces a steady state blood level of about 60 μg per ml. The serum half-life is 1.5–2 hours.

Fosfomycin is not bound to plasma protein and the large volume of distribution (20–22 litres) indicates free diffusion into interstitial fluid and tissues. Relatively high concentrations have been found in fetal blood (17.6 μg per ml) and amniotic fluid (45.3 μg per ml). In patients with acute meningitis Drobnic et al (1977) found CSF levels of 10.9 μg per ml when the serum level was 65.2 μg/ml.

The drug is excreted almost entirely unchanged by glomerular filtration to produce urinary levels in excess of 1000 μg per ml after a parenteral dose or 300–500 μg per ml after an oral dose.

Adverse reactions have been observed in about 10–17 per cent of patients, mostly slight gastrointestinal disorders, although there has been some rise in the SGOT and SGPT levels. The drug has been successfully used in Spain for a wide variety of conditions including respiratory, urinary, gastrointestinal, generalized and genito-urinary infections (Symposium, 1977).

Table 10.1 Sensitivity of bacteria to fosfomycin

	MIC μg/ml*
S. aureus	2–32
S. pneumoniae	8–64
B. anthracis	64
E. coli	1–16
Klebsiella spp.	8–64
Enterobacter spp.	1–R
P. mirabilis	0.5–R
Proteus spp.	2–R
Salmonella spp.	1–8
Shigella spp.	1–8
V. cholerae	64–R
S. marcescens	4–128
P. aeruginosa	4–R
B. fragilis	R
Sphaerophorus spp.	4–64

*Medium supplemented with glucose-6-phosphate

References
Drobnic L, Quiles M, Rodriguez A 1977 Chemotherapy 23: (Suppl 1) 180
Glamkowski E J, Gal G, Purick R, Davidson A J, Sletzinger M 1970 J Org Chem 35: 3510
Hendlin D, Stapley E O, Jackson M et al 1969 Science (Wash) 166: 122
Olay T, Rodriguez A, Oliver L E, et al 1978 J Antimicrob Chemother 4: 569
Symposium 1977 Chemotherapy 23: Suppl 1

FUSIDANES

Several antibiotics with a basic steroid structure have been isolated from natural sources and collectively described as 'fusidanes' (Carey et al, 1975). Three have received a fair amount of study: cephalosporin P_1, helvolic acid and fusidic acid (Fig. 10.1). They have in common a narrow antibacterial range, synergic activity with penicillin and some other agents, and ready emergence of resistant mutants on passage *in vitro*. Their principal interest lies in their activity against penicillinase-producing staphylococci. Fusidic acid is about 10 times as active as the others and is the only one commercially available.

Table 10.2 Sensitivity of bacteria to sodium fusidate

	MIC µg/ml
S. aureus	0.03–0.1
S. pyogenes	4–16
S. pneumoniae	2–16
S. viridans	1–8
S. faecalis	1–4
C. diphtheriae	0.004–0.008
Bacillus spp.	0.06–2
Clostridium spp.	0.01–0.5
N. gonorrhoeae	0.03–1
N. meningitidis	0.06–0.25
M. tuberculosis	0.5–2
K. pneumoniae	4–R
Enterobacteria	R
N. asteroides	0.5–4

Based on Godtfredsen W et al 1962 Lancet 1: 928; Barber M, Waterworth P M 1962 Lancet 1: 931; Black W A, McNellis D A 1971 J Med Microbiol 4: 293

FUSIDIC ACID

Fusidic acid is a colourless crystalline compound sparingly soluble in water, isolated from a strain of *Fusidium coccineum* and supplied as the sodium salt which is readily soluble in water (Godtfredsen et al, 1962).

Anti-bacterial activity

Sodium fusidate is active against species of Gram-positive bacteria and the Gram-negative cocci. Nearly all strains of *Staph. aureus* are outstandingly sensitive regardless of their sensitivity to other antibiotics. It is bactericidal for many strains in concentrations close to the MIC (although a proportion of the cells, increasing with inoculum size, always remains) and has been shown by stereoscan electron microscopy to exert a

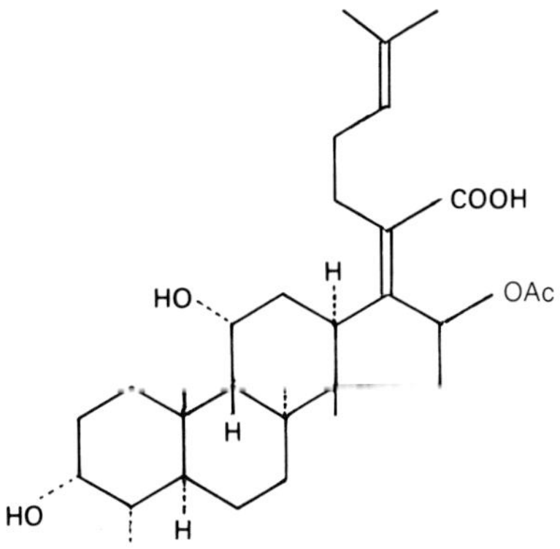

FUSIDIC ACID[1]

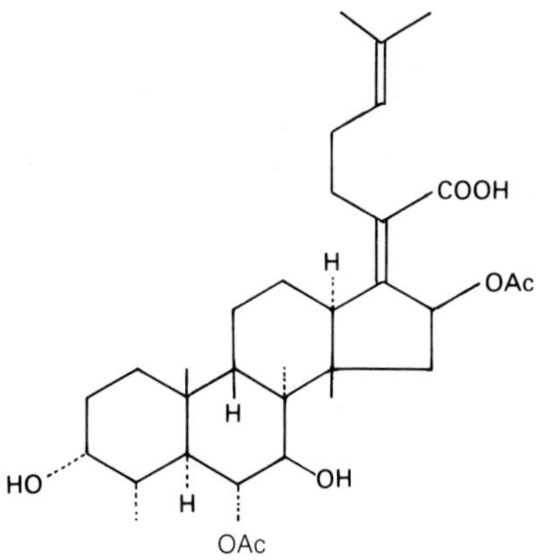

CEPHALOSPORIN P_1[2]

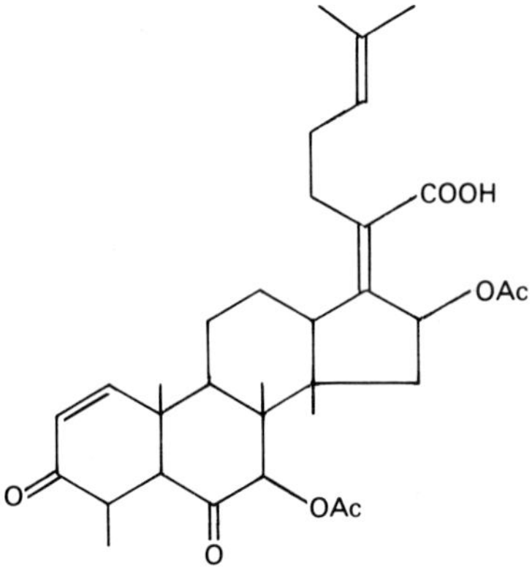

HELVOLIC ACID[3]

Fig. 10.1 Structure of steroid antibiotics.
[1]Gotfredsen, W O et al 1965 Tetrahedron 25: 3505
[2]Halsall T G et al 1966 Chem Comm 1966 p 685
[3]Okuda S et al 1964 Chem Pharm Bull (Japan) 12: 121

marked destructive effect on staphylococci. *Nocardia asteroides* and some *C. diphtheriae* and many strains of *Clostridia* are also highly sensitive. Strains of *Myco. tuberculosis* have been shown to be partially inhibited by from 0.5 to 5.0 μg per ml. Streptococci and pneumococci are relatively resistant and coliform bacilli and fungi are highly resistant (Table 10.2). In 50 per cent serum the MIC may increase 50–100-fold and the drug is slightly more effective at pH 6–7 than at pH 8.

Acquired resistance

A large inoculum of most strains of *Staph. aureus* contains a small number of resistant mutants and this appears to be responsible for the effect of inoculum size on the efficacy of sodium fusidate. As would be expected from this, sodium fusidate resistant strains of *Staph. aureus* emerge rapidly *in vitro* and sometimes during clinical therapy. The growth rate, coagulase, haemolysin and penicillinase production of these mutants appear to be unimpaired. There is a cross-resistance between fusidate and cephalosporin P_1.

Pattison & Mansell (1973) were prompted to review the hospital prevalence of staphylococci resistant to sodium fusidate after observing relapse of staphylococcal septicaemia associated with the development of resistance in a patient receiving cloxacillin and sodium fusidate. The prevalence proved to be 1.4 per cent, half the strains being associated with sepsis and less than half isolated from patients who had received the drug.

The gene specifying resistance may be located on the chromosome or on a plasmid. In a survey of staphylococci from different sources 70 per cent of the strains resistant to penicillin and to sodium fusidate carried the genes for penicillinase and sodium fusidate resistance on the same plasmid and Lacey (1975) concluded that the same plasmid had been transmitted to a number of strains. Chromosomal mutation results in a change in protein synthesis while in the plasmid-mediated form the protein synthetic activity of cell-free extracts remains sensitive. Chopra (1976) concluded from changes in the phospholipid composition of the cells that plasmid-mediated resistance is due not to degradation, as it is with several other agents (page 262), but to drug exclusion, as in the case of tetracycline, although this could not be measured directly. A number of R factors in enterobacteria have been shown to confer resistance to sodium fusidate and Datta et al (1974) speculate on the persistence of this property in organisms already resistant to the agent on which it confers no selective advantage.

Interactions with penicillins

Because resistant mutants of staphylococci readily emerge *in vitro* it has generally been recommended that this should be prevented as far as possible in patients by simultaneous administration of a penicillin which will kill any emergent resistant mutants while fusidic acid destroys the bulk of the bacterial population and thus prevents generation of sufficient penicillinase to destroy penicillin. The benefits of this peculiar form of 'synergy' in controlling the minority population is clear, but the wisdom of giving fusidic acid and penicillins together has been questioned because the effect of the two agents on the bulk of the bacterial population can commonly be shown to be antagonistic.

Contradictory findings in the literature probably arise from the fact that different strains of staphylococci respond differently to the combination. O'Grady & Greenwood (1973) describe three distinct patterns of interaction. In the commonest, exhibited by more than half their penicillinase-producing strains and almost all their penicillin-sensitive strains, there was two-way antagonism: more staphylococci survived overnight incubation in the presence of fusidic acid and a penicillin than in the presence of either agent alone. In the second kind of interaction, least survivors were recovered after incubation with a penicillin alone, more from the mixture and most from fusidic acid. In this case there was one-way antagonism of penicillin by fusidic acid. The remaining strains showed 'indifference' in that the effect of the more bactericidal agent (which against some strains was fusidic acid) prevailed. In the *in vitro* situation, antagonism of one or other form is evidently the commonest form of interaction between the two agents but it is important to note that even where the effect of penicillin against the bulk of the bacterial population was antagonized, it always prevented the emergence of fusidic acid-resistant mutants. (See p. 224.)

PHARMACOKINETICS

Absorption

Sodium fusidate is well absorbed after oral administration in the adult and in children absorption is more rapid. Milk appears to delay absorption, peak concentrations not being reached for 4–8 hours. In a comparison of the disposition of sodium fusidate in six volunteers after oral and rapid or slow intravenous infusion Wise et al (1977) found considerable intersubject variation in the concentrations obtained after 500 mg doses given orally and by infusion but little difference when 100 mg was given by rapid intravenous injection (the larger dose not being given because of the possibility of venospasm or thrombosis). The mean peak concentrations obtained were 31 μg per ml from the oral capsules, 23 μg per ml from the suspension and 43 μg per ml from the infusion. The areas under the serum concentration curves showed that only about 70 per cent of the suspension was assimilated as compared with the capsule. Calculations based on the areas under the intravenous infusion curve indicated that the drug was virtually completely absorbed from the capsule and they support the practice of giving the drug orally except when this route is unavailable. Because of slow elimination, considerable accumulation of the drug occurs on repeated administration of doses above 250 mg: 500 mg t.d.s. for four days produced plasma concentrations of 11–41 μg per ml after 24 hours and 30–144 μg per ml after 96 hours. On doses of 3 g/day (40 mg/kg) plasma levels can reach 200 μg/ml. Güttler & Tybring (1971) found that the relative concentrations in plasma and pus (20.8 and 17.2 μg/ml) corresponded with the ratio of their protein contents. The extravascular albumen pool is as large as that of the plasma and together with protein in oedema fluid and exudate constitutes an important depot of the drug. About 95 per cent is reversibly bound to plasma protein.

Distribution

Sodium fusidate is well distributed in the tissues and most organs of the body, but does not reach the cerebro-spinal fluid. Inhibitory levels are obtained in muscle, kidney, lungs and pleural exudate.

Bone concentrations in samples taken at operation from patients with chronic osteomyelitis treated for at least five days were 1.7–14.9 μg per g in patients receiving 1.5 g of the drug per day and 3.4–14.8 μg per g in patients receiving 3 g per day (Hierholzer et al, 1974).

Levels in excess of 7 μg per ml have been demonstrated in aspirated synovial fluid from patients with osteo- or rheumatoid arthritis treated with 0.75 or 1.5 g sodium fusidate daily after 3–7 days' treatment (Deodhar et al, 1972). The drug has been detected in brain, milk and placenta which it crosses to reach the fetus. In patients treated with 1.5 g per day, levels of 0.08–0.84 μg/ml were found in the aqueous humour after one day and 1.2–1.28 μg/ml after three days' treatment (Williamson et al, 1970). Others have found levels up to 2.0 μg/ml and in contrast to other agents (page 385), levels in the vitreous 2–3 times as high. Wise et al (1977) conclude from their analysis that in the post-distribution phase about half of the drug is in the peripheral compartment in keeping with the known ability of sodium fusidate to penetrate into tissues including bone.

Excretion

Sodium fusidate is excreted and concentrated in the bile as a number of metabolites, much in the form of glucuronides and very little unchanged. Having shown that glycine and taurine conjugates of sodium fusidate exhibit many features of conjugated bile salts, Carey et al (1975) found that derivatives actively secreted into the bile of primates significantly influenced biliary secretion of bile salts, phospholipid and cholesterol.

About two per cent of the administered dose can be recovered in active form in the faeces. Little or no active antibiotic is excreted in the urine: less than 1 per cent, producing concentrations of only 0.8 μg per ml after four days' treatment. Combined with the fact that very little of the drug is dialysed (no doubt because such a high proportion is bound to protein) this means that in anuric patients on haemodialysis dosage does not need to be modified (Hobby et al, 1970).

Side effects

When given by mouth sodium fusidate appears to be well tolerated and apart from mild gastro-intestinal disturbance and occasional rashes no untoward symptoms have been reported. Too rapid infusion (see dosage) of the parenteral form of the drug may lead to venospasm or thrombosis but Liddy (1973) gave 20 mg per kg per day to new-born infants with severe staphylococcal sepsis, giving the infusion over 4-hour periods separated by 4-hour periods of drug-free infusion for 4–5 days with no evidence of local or systemic side effects.

Clinical application

Sodium fusidate is a particularly interesting agent in that it precisely fits the demand frequently made for agents of very narrow antibacterial spectrum, well absorbed by mouth and remarkably free from untoward effects yet it is relatively little used: certainly it is not the automatic choice of most prescribers for staphylococcal sepsis. Cost may well have been a major factor since there is no doubt that the drug has been successfully used for the treatment of a variety of severe staphylococcal infections often after other potent antistaphylococcal agents have failed. Particular benefit has been claimed for fusidate treatment of bone and joint infections in both the acute and intractable chronic forms of the disease (page 318).

Several authors have reported outstanding success with combinations of fucidin and penicillins despite the fact that the mixture may show antagonism *in vitro* (page 222). Two findings in the study by O'Grady & Greenwood (1973) indicate that in the therapeutic situation the prevention by penicillin of the emergence of sodium fusidate-resistant mutants is likely to outweigh any antagonistic effect. Even where two-way antagonism was most marked, the combination still exerted a substantial bactericidal effect. Moreover the great difference between the half-lives of fusidic acid and penicillins means that (apart from the first dose) penicillin will be given when substantial concentrations of fusidic acid are already present. In these circumstances antagonism did not occur.

Nevertheless, the possibility of antagonism should be borne in mind when treating severe infections such as endocarditis. An imperfect response from this cause can only convincingly be demonstrated by improvement on withdrawal of one or other agent.

One other pharmacokinetic factor is likely to operate against significant interaction of the two agents *in vitro*. As discussed in the case of combined therapy with trimethoprim and sulphonamide, pairs of agents can only behave in the body as they do *in vitro* if they resemble one another closely in their absorption and distribution characteristics. Fusidic acid is apparently widely distributed in the body while, in the absence of active inflammation, penicillins commonly are not. It may therefore be argued that a second agent used with fusidic acid should follow its distribution more closely than do the penicillins. Erythromycin or lincomycin may be considered for this role. Both have been used with sodium fusidate in the treatment of osteomyelitis (page 317) and Jackson & Saunders (1973) successfully treated four of seven patients with prosthetic valve endocarditis due to diphtheroids with a mixture of sodium fusidate and erythromycin, this mixture being chosen on the grounds that sodium fusidate was bactericidal to the organism in therapeutically attainable concentrations and that synergy was obtained with erythromycin which would also be likely to be effective against any L-forms.

Local therapy has been successfully used for a number of skin infections including erythrasma (page 311) and it has been suggested that it may be of value in the treatment of psoriasis (Kurwa & Abdel-Aziz, 1973).

References

Carey M C, Montet J-C, Small D M 1975 Biochemistry 14: 4896
Chopra I 1976 J Gen Microbiol 96: 229
Datta N, Hedges R W, Becker D, Davies J 1974 J Gen Microbiol 83: 191
Deodhar S D, Russell F, Dick W C, Nuki G, Buchannan W W 1972 Scand J Rheumatol 1: 33
Godtfredsen W, Roholt K, Tybring L 1962 Lancet 1: 928
Güttler F, Tybring L 1971 Brit J Pharmacol 43: 151
Hierholzer G, Rehn J, Knothe H, Masterson J 1974 J Bone Joint Surg 56B: 721
Hobby J A E, Beeley L, Whitby J L 1970 J Clin Path 23: 484
Jackson G, Saunders K 1973 Brit Heart J 35: 931
Kurwa A, Abdel-Aziz A-H M 1973 Brit J Clin Pract 27: 92
Lacey R W 1975 Bact Rev 39: 1
Liddy N 1973 Lancet 1: 621
O'Grady F, Greenwood D 1973 J Med Microbiol 6: 441
Pattison J R, Mansell P E 1973 J Med Microbiol 6: 235
Williamson J, Russell F, Doig W M, Paterson R W W 1970 Brit J Ophthal 54: 126
Wise R, Pippard M, Mitchard M 1977 Brit J Pharmacol 4: 615

NOVOBIOCIN

Cathomycin, isolated from a new species of streptomycete which was given the name *Streptomyces spheroides* (Wallick et al, 1956) and streptonivicin isolated from *Streptomyces niveus* (Smith et al, 1956) were shown to be identical and given the generic name novobiocin. Novobiocin and the coumermycins derived from *Streptomyces rishiriensis spinicoumarensis* (Kawaguchi et al, 1965), are related to the coumerol group of anticoagulants.

Chemical properties

Novobiocin is a dibasic acid usually supplied as the calcium or monosodium salt. The calcium salt is soluble at 3 mg/ml water and 125 mg/ml alcohol. The monosodium salt is much more readily soluble: 200 mg/ml water, 140 mg/ml ethyl alcohol and 350 mg/ml methyl alcohol. With both salts a 2.5 per cent solution has a pH of 7.0 to 8.5. Both salts are moderately stable if kept dry, stored in the cold and protected from light.

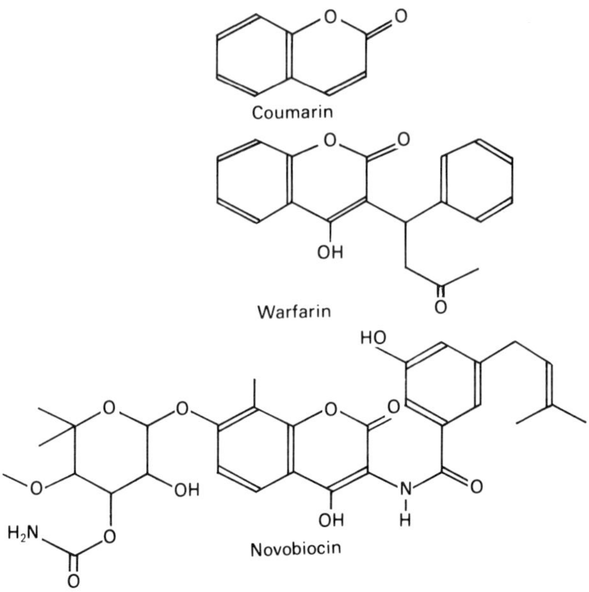

Fig. 10.2 Structures of coumarins and coumarin antibiotics

Antibacterial activity

Novobiocin has a rather unusual antibacterial spectrum (Table 10.3). It is outstandingly active against *Staph. aureus*; other highly sensitive species are *Str. pneumoniae, C. diphtheriae, H. influenzae, N. gonorrhoeae* and *N. meningitidis*.

Novobiocin sensitivity (to a disc containing 5 μg) serves to make very simply the taxonomic distinction between staphylococci, which are almost universally sensitive, and micrococci, which are almost universally resistant. According to Wren et al (1977) all strains of peptococci tested showed no zone of inhibition around a disc containing 5 μg of novobiocin while all strains of peptostreptococci showed a zone of at least 15 mm.

Some strains of Pasteurella, Citrobacter and Proteus, particularly *Proteus vulgaris*, are sensitive to moderate concentrations but other enterobacteria are resistant. This selective activity has been utilized for the suppression of Citrobacter and Proteus in a medium selective for Salmonella (Hoben et al, 1973) although in some media the agent is inhibitory to *Salmonella typhi* (Shanson, 1975).

Novobiocin is primarily a bacteristatic drug, but with highly sensitive species a concentration two to ten times that required for bacteristasis has a slow killing effect. The MIC is eight or more times greater at pH 8.0 than at pH 5.4, and markedly increased by the presence of 10 per cent or more serum or by increase in the magnesium or nutrient content of the medium.

The fact that novobiocin acts on DNA replication (page 260) induced McHugh & Swartz (1977) to examine its capacity to eliminate plasmids from a variety of hosts which it did at growth inhibitory concentrations in 8 out of 14 cases involving 4 bacterial species.

Table 10.3 Sensitivity of bacteria to novobiocin

	MIC μg/ml		MIC μg/ml
Staph. aureus	0.1–2	*H. influenzae*	0.2–0.8
Str. pyogenes	0.5–4	*N. meningitidis*	0.5–4
Str. pneumoniae	0.2–2	*N. gonorrhoeae*	4
Str. faecalis	1 –16	*Pasteurella*	2–16
C. diphtheriae	0.4	*Proteus vulgaris*	2–50
Cl. welchii	1.0	*Proteus mirabilis*	8 100
B. anthracis	1.0	*Proteus morgani*	16–>100
Ery. insidiosa	>64	*Proteus rettgeri* }	
L. monocytogenes	2.0	*Escherichia, Klebsiella,* }	>100
Actino. israeli	2.0	*Salmonella, Shigella* }	
Myco. tuberculosis	R	*Pseudomonas* }	

Jones W F, Nichols R L, Finland M 1956 J Lab Clin Med 47: 783
Frost B M et al 1956 Antibiot Ann 1955–56 p 918
Schneierson S S, Amsterdam D 1957 Antibiot Chemother 7: 251

Many species of bacteria initially sensitive to novobiocin readily develop resistance to it *in vitro* and a considerable increase in the resistance of the infecting staphylococcus during treatment has been recorded by several investigators. There is no cross resistance with other common antibiotics.

Interaction

It has several times been claimed that novobiocin and tetracycline act synergically and this mixture continues to be available in some countries although it has been removed from the U.S. market. Table 27.5 on page 484 shows that against the strain of *Staph. aureus* tested, so far from any synergy being demonstrable, the effect of this combination was not even additive, the inhibitory concentration of each remaining the same regardless of the presence of a sub-inhibitory concentration of the other. Low magnesium concentration in the test medium may allow tetracycline to enhance the effect of novobiocin by chelating antagonistic magnesium ions (Garrett & Won, 1973). Bactericidal synergy has been claimed against *Pseudomonas pseudomallei* (Calabi, 1973).

On the basis of reports that novobiocin enhances the activity of idoxuridine against herpes simplex and vaccinia viruses *in vitro*, House et al (1973) used this combination, they believed to some effect, in a new-born infant suffering from infection with cytomegalovirus.

Absorption, distribution and excretion

Novobiocin is well absorbed from the alimentary tract, producing peak plasma levels of 10.9 and 18.8 μg/ml 1–4 hr after doses of 250 and 500 mg. The plasma half-life is 1.7–4 hours. After repeated doses serum levels of 50 to over 100 μg/ml may be reached. About 90 per cent of the drug is reversibly bound to serum albumen. Brand & Toribara (1975) have shown that the binding sites are multiple and differ between human and bovine albumen—a further warning against the use of non-human albumen for the purpose of preparing serum standards for microbiological assay.

Concentrations rather lower than those in the blood are found in serous effusions, but cerebrospinal fluid contains little or none. The amount found in the urine does not usually exceed three per cent of the dose and in single specimens of urine the concentration may be considerably lower than that in the blood.

Novobiocin is excreted mainly in the bile, in which the concentration is high. Biliary recirculation plays an important part in maintaining the high blood levels but much of the antibiotic eventually escapes by this route and high concentrations are found in the faeces.

Toxicity and side effects

Maculopapular, morbilliform or urticarial skin eruptions with or without fever are common, often developing about the ninth day. The rashes disappear on stopping the drug but may promptly re-appear if the drug is re-administered together with a prompt and profound fall in circulating basophils indicative of sensitization. Novobiocin may displace other substances from protein binding sites and can lower the plasma-bound iodine by displacing thyroxine.

Eosinophilia and moderate transient leucopenia are occasionally seen. Thrombocytopenia, which may be severe, and haemolytic anaemia have also been reported.

Novobiocin gives rise to a yellow pigment metabolite in the serum, which may give an indirect positive van den Bergh reaction, but in addition the drug exerts a profound effect on hepatic excretory function by interfering with uptake of various compounds by hepatic cells, inhibiting glucuronyl transferase—the enzyme concerned with glucuronide conjugation—and suppressing excretion of conjugates into the bile (Duvaldestin et al, 1976). Particularly severe effects may occur in the new-born where glucuronide formation is imperfectly developed. Novobiocin exerts a different depressant effect on the biliary excretion of different compounds and on the excretion of the same conjugate when this is produced endogenously or infused. This has been taken to indicate that the drug exerts its effect at several different sites (Smith & Fujimoto, 1974).

Clinical application

Novobiocin is an interesting and active compound but its once useful place as an anti-staphylococcal agent has been overtaken by numerous other agents. This, combined with its high-grade competition for albumin binding sites, its unequivocal depressant effect on hepatic function and its capacity to produce skin reactions with a frequency which many physicians regard as unacceptably high, makes it hard for the drug to look good in any risk/benefit analysis. Its activity against certain strains of *Proteus* has led to its prescription for urinary tract infection—a use for which there is no possible justification.

References

Brand J G, Toribara T Y 1975 Arch Biochem Biophys 174: 541
Calabi O 1973 J Med Microbiol 6: 293
Duvaldestin P, Mahu J-L, Preaux A-M, Berthelot P 1976 Biochem Pharmacol 25: 2587
Garrett E R, Won C M 1973 Antimicrob Ag Chemother 4: 626
Hoben D A, Ashton D H, Peterson A C 1973 Appl Microbiol 26: 126
House R F, Person D A, Smith T F, Harris L E 1973 Lancet 1: 39

Kawaguchi H, Tsukiura H, Okanishi M et al 1965 J Antibiot (Tokyo) Ser A 18: 1
McHugh G L, Swartz M N 1977 Antimicrob Ag Chemother 12: 423
Shanson D C 1975 J Med Microbiol 8: 357
Smith C G, Dietz A, Sokoloski W T, Savage G M 1956 Antibiot Chemother 6: 135
Smith D S, Fujimoto J M 1974 J Pharm Exp Therap 188: 504
Wallick H, Harris D A, Reagan M A, Ruger M, Woodruff H B 1956 Antibiot Ann 1955–6 p 909
Wren M W D, Eldon C P, Dakin G H 1977 J Clin Path 30: 620

RIFAMYCINS

The rifamycins are a family of antibiotics produced by *Streptomyces mediterranei* and studied in the laboratories of Lepetit, Milan. Rifamycin B is the most active, and its molecule has been modified with advantage in various ways. Large numbers of rifamycins have now been synthesized. They are structurally related to the streptovaricins, tolypomycins and geldanamycin, all of which possess an aromatic ring system spanned by an aliphatic bridge called the 'ansa ring' to which the whole group owes the name 'ansamycins' (Wehrli & Staehelin, 1971). The early history of the group is reviewed by Riva & Silvestri (1972). The compounds so far developed for therapeutic use have been based on rifamycin B and rifamycin SV.

Rifamide

Rifamycin diethylamide was released for therapeutic use in man under the name 'rifamide' but subsequently withdrawn . Extremely low concentrations (0.01 to 0.1 μg per ml) inhibit the growth of staphylococci, streptococci (other than *S. faecalis*) and *Myco. tuberculosis*; Gram-negative species require 10–100 μg per ml or more. There are small numbers of much more resistant cells in populations of staphylococci. The action is bactericidal, and there is no cross-resistance with other common antibiotics.

Rifamide is little absorbed from the alimentary tract. Intramuscular injection of 500 mg produces a therapeutic blood level for up to eight hours, but protein binding is extensive: with a blood level of 5 μg per ml only 14 per cent is said to be free. Elimination is mainly via the bile, in which a concentration as high as 2.8 mg per ml has been observed. Some re-circulation occurs, but much is excreted in the faeces and little in the urine. The compound may not be missed now that it is no longer commercially available except possibly for its action in the biliary tract which appears to have been promising.

Rifampicin

This derivative of rifamycin SV (Fig. 10.3), represents perhaps the greatest advance over the original properties of an antibiotic which has yet been achieved by synthetic modification. It is one of 500 derivatives prepared by Ciba of Basel and Lepetit of Milan in collaboration (Kradolfer, 1968). It has the same spectrum as other rifamycins but much higher activity, the MIC for highly sensitive species (Table 10.4) being almost incredibly low (e.g. for *Staphylococcus aureus* 0.002 μg/ml). Other bacteria are correspondingly more sensitive to rifampicin than to earlier rifamycin derivatives; 0.5 μg/ml is actively bactericidal for *Myco. tuberculosis* and 20 μg/ml for *E. coli*. According to Mandell & Vest (1972) rifampicin has a much superior bactericidal effect to that of any other antibiotic tested on intra-leucocytic staphylococci. *Mycobacterium tuberculosis*, *Mycobacterium kansasii* and *Mycobacterium marinum* are susceptible to rifampicin, the majority of strains being inhibited by <0.01 μg per ml of the drug. *Mycobacterium fortuitum* is uniformly resistant (Woodley et al, 1972), as are most organisms of the *M. avium–intracellulare* group (Wolinsky, 1979).

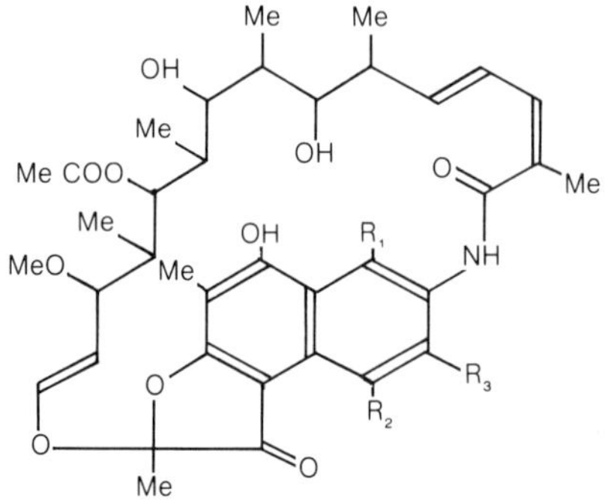

	R_1	R_2	R_3
Rifamycin B	OH	$OCH_2 \cdot COOH$	H
S	O	O	H
SV	OH	OH	H
Rifampicin	OH	OH	–CH=N–N N–Me

Fig. 10.3 Structure of rifamycins

Rifampicin was the most active of the antibiotics tested by Blackman et al (1977) against *Chlamydia trachomatis*, 0.25 μg per ml suppressing inclusion formation by all the strains tested; 50 per cent end points were achieved at 0.03 or less μg per ml.

Considerable interest has been generated by the activity of some rifamycins and streptovaricins against a number of viruses including RNA tumour viruses (through a specific inhibitory effect on reverse transcriptase—Horoszewicz et al, 1977) but this activity is insufficient for therapeutic purposes and is, in a number of cases, as with bacteria, complicated by the emergence of resistant mutants.

It is most important to recognize that large bacterial populations may contain resistant mutants. Hence the MIC as determined in a fluid medium with a generous inoculum may be enormously higher than that in the plate dilution method with a light one.

The mutation rate to resistance in *S. aureus*, *S. pyogenes*, *S. pneumoniae*, *E. coli* and *P. mirabilis* is about 10^{-7}. The mutation rates to resistance in *Mycobacterium kansasii* and *Mycobacterium marinum* were calculated to be 4.9×10^{-10} and 1.7×10^{-9} respectively (Woodley et al, 1972). The growth rates and biochemical properties of the mutants are unchanged. Resistance is not due to enzymic destruction, is not transferable and is stable on subculture. It is due to a change in the DNA-dependent RNA polymerase, such that the normal stable complex is no longer formed with the mutant enzyme. There is no cross-resistance with antibiotics of any other groups which have been tested.

An important consequence of the high mutation rate to resistance is that, at least in treating most infections, rifampicin should never be given alone, but together with another drug to which the organism is sensitive.

Combined action

Rifampicin and ampicillin are antagonistic *in vitro* against enterococci (Iannini et al, 1976) and *E. coli*. Some workers have found antagonism with some penicillins and cephalosporins against strains of staphylococci but Tuazon et al (1978) found the combination of rifampicin with nafcillin to be synergic for 12 of 20 strains of *S. aureus* isolated from patients with endocarditis while the combination with vancomycin was synergic for 5 of the 20 strains. No antagonism was found with either combination.

Rifampicin is synergic *in vitro* with aminoglycosides against *E. coli* and with polymyxin B against multi-resistant *S. marcescens*. The rifampicin-polymyxin combination has been successfully used to treat patients infected with these organisms (Ostenson et al, 1977).

Combination with trimethoprim was first studied by Kerry et al (1975), who found the combination to be synergic, although to only a limited degree, against some organisms, including streptococci and Proteus spp., additive against many others and antagonistic against *S. aureus*. They also showed that mutation to high resistance to rifampicin was prevented by the presence of trimethoprim, thus claiming a second advantage for the combination. Farrell et al (1977) tested the combination on 61 strains of 11 Gram-negative species resistant to gentamicin, and observed synergy against 24 of them in concentrations attainable in the urine, but against only two in those attainable in the blood. Arioli et al (1977) report what they claim are encouraging results in tests of several species of enterobacteria both *in vitro* and in protection tests in mice, although the method of tabular presentation of results is somewhat obscure. A discordant note is struck by Harvey (1978), who claims to have shown that the combined action of the two drugs on *Kl. aerogenes* and *Strep. faecalis* is actually antagonistic, and suggest that a better combination with rifampicin would be with an inhibitor of protein synthesis such as tetracycline.

Rifampicin acts synergically with amphotericin B against *Candida albicans* (the combination has been successfully used in the treatment of Candida endophthalmitis —Lou et al, 1977) and against the mycelial, but not the spherule-endospore phase of *Coccidioides immitis*. Combined therapy was no more effective against murine coccidioidomycosis than was amphotericin alone (Huppert et al, 1976).

Pharmacokinetics

The second advantage of rifampicin over other rifamycin derivatives is that it is well absorbed when administered orally. Not only is a high initial concentration reached in the blood, but, owing in part to entero-hepatic re-circulation, the subsequent fall is slow, a therapeutic level being maintained for 12 hours or more according to the dose. Blood levels fall somewhat after the first week of treatment. The peak plasma levels reported in the literature vary greatly and differ to an important degree amongst the different pharmaceutical preparations. Following the administration of 600 mg of the drug as a syrup (20 mg/ml) Mannisto (1977) obtained peak levels of about 14 μg/ml from syrup compared with 4–6 μg/ml from various capsules. Hence he suggests that the dose of syrup could be reduced. Differences between tablet preparations were particularly marked. The apparent plasma half-life was about 3 hours and protein-bound fraction 65–80 per cent—less than the 90 per cent reported by Boman & Ringberger (1974) who found the bound proportion to be unaffected by the presence of

INH, PAS, streptomycin or ethambutol. The pKa is 2.9. Administration of 600 mg of an intravenous form of the drug at present under trial over 3 hours was well tolerated and gave plasma levels and half-lives similar to those obtained when the same dose was administered orally (Nitti et al, 1977) though the urinary recovery was less (Acocella et al, 1977).

The main excretory route is biliary, although concentrations in the bile are lower than those of rifamide, and biliary obstruction raises blood levels. The quantity normally excreted by the liver appears to be fixed, and any excess is dealt with by the kidney; thus the larger the dose the greater the proportion of it excreted in the urine. Renal insufficiency is said not to affect this. Haemodialysis does not reduce blood levels. The rest of the drug is metabolised mostly to the desacetyl form, the bulk of which is rapidly excreted in the bile (50 per cent by the fourth hour) and is not reabsorbed.

The drug has a particular capacity to penetrate into cells and abscess cavities and an interesting fact with regard to distribution is that concentrations of 5–10 μg/ml are demonstrable in sputum. An admirable account of the early studies, including clinical, is given in a review with 847 references by Binda et al (1971).

Side effects

Various rashes and gastro-intestinal disturbances may occur. Some patients, particularly those who take the drug irregularly, develop an influenza-like syndrome. This and effects of the drug on hepatic and renal function and on immune responses are discussed on page 396. Hepatic dysfunction, manifested first by raised transaminase levels and then by a raised serum bilirubin, is not uncommon and not necessarily an indication for stopping treatment (Lal et al, 1972).

Clinical Uses

Much the most important use of rifampicin is for the treatment of tuberculosis, which is discussed from both experimental and clinical standpoints in Chapter 23 where its use in leprosy is also considered.

Because of its outstanding importance in the treatment of tuberculosis, the view has been taken that it should be reserved solely for this purpose because of the danger that widespread use could lead to the emergence of resistant organisms in patients with unsuspected tuberculosis. This danger has been exaggerated, but there is no clear reason for preferring rifampicin to other agents in the wide variety of pulmonary, skin and soft tissue, bone and other, even including intestinal, infections that have been treated.

It has been proposed that the combination of rifampicin with trimethroprim (page 28) could be safely used for wider indications but a fixed ratio might well be unsatisfactory. The degree of synergy achieved is never great, and the effect on most species is inconstant, so securely based treatment would require tests of the action of the combination, which are time-consuming. Most of the bacteria shown to be susceptible occur chiefly in such infections as those of the urinary tract, which are rarely life-endangering and often susceptible to treatment with any of several more ordinary drugs. It is arguable that so valuable—and costly—a drug as rifampicin should not be used for such conditions, but reserved for individual cases of more serious infection in which its use is specially indicated.

Although rifampicin has relatively low activity against enterobacteria the high concentrations achieved in the bile make it an appropriate agent to consider for the treatment of biliary tract infection (page 345). The treatment of trachoma is considered later in the book.

It may exceptionally be indicated in staphylococcal infection. One of us found rifampicin and erythromycin to be the most bactericidal of many antibiotic combinations for a strain of *Staph. aureus* from an infection of a patent interventricular septum in a child aged three (Peard et al, 1970). The fact that both drugs could be given orally was welcome at this age, and the infection was rapidly eliminated. The synergic effect of this combination on *Staph. aureus* was subsequently demonstrated by Banič and Stropnik (1971). Rifampicin in combination has been commended for the treatment of *S. epidermidis* infection of prosthetic valves and CSF shunts by Archer et al (1978) and for the treatment of endocarditis due to *S. aureus* or *S. epidermidis* by Massanari & Donta (1978), but any combination proposed for clinical use should be tested on the causative organism.

A practical use to which the drug has been put is the treatment of meningococcus carriers. This is immediately very effective, but in each of four papers on this subject published within one year in the United States (e.g. Eickhoff, 1971; Weidmer et al, 1971) it is acknowledged that the meningococcus may rapidly become highly resistant and this is confirmed by the experience of Sivonen et al (1978). Not only would this change soon deprive the treatment of efficacy, but the possible effect of mass administration on other bacterial species is a strong objection.

References

Acocella G, Bonollo L, Mainardi M, Margaroli P, Tenconi L T 1977 Arzneim Forsch 27: 1221
Archer G L, Tenenbaum M J, Haywood H B III 1978 J Amer Med Assoc 240: 751
Arioli V, Berti M, Carniti G, Rossi E 1977 J Antimicrob Chemother 3: 87
Banič S, Stropnik Z 1971 Zbl Bakt I Orig 216: 418
Binda G, Domenichini E, Gottardi A et al 1971 Arzneim Forsch 21: 1907
Blackman H J, Yoneda C, Dawson C R, Schachter J 1977 Antimicrob Ag Chemother 12: 673
Boman G, Ringberger V-A 1974 Europ J Clin Pharmacol 7: 369
Eickhoff T C 1971 J Infect Dis 123: 414
Farrell W, Wilks M, Drasar F A 1977 J Antimicrob Chemother 3: 459
Harvey R J 1978 J Antimicrob Chemother 4: 315
Horoszewicz J S, Leong S S, Carter W A 1977 Antimicrob Ag Chemother 12: 4
Huppert M, Pappagianis D, Sun S H, et al 1976 Antimicrob Ag Chemother 9: 406
Iannini P B, Ehret J, Eickhoff T C 1976 Antimicrob Ag Chemother 9: 448
Kerry D W, Hamilton-Miller J M T, Brumfitt W 1975 J Antimicrob Chemother 1: 417
Kradolfer F 1968 Schweiz Med Wschr 98: 622
Lal S, Singhal S N, Burley D M, Crossley G, 1972 Brit Med J 1: 148
Lou P, Kazdan, J, Bannatyne R M, Cheung R 1977 Amer J Ophthlamol 83: 12
Mandell G L, Vest T K 1972 J Infect Dis 125: 486
Mannisto P 1977 Clin Pharmacol Therap 21: 370
Massanari R M, Donta S T 1978 Chest 73: 371
Nitti V, Virgilio R, Patricolo M R, Iuliano A 1977 Chemotherapy 23: 1
Ostenson R C, Fields B T, Nolan C M 1977 Antimicrob Ag Chemother 12: 655
Peard M C, Fleck D G, Garrod L P, Waterworth P M 1970 Brit Med J 4: 410
Riva S, Silvestri L G 1972 Ann Rev Microbiol 26: 199
Sivonen A, Renkonen O-V, Weckström P, et al 1978 J Infect Dis 137: 238
Tuazon C U, Lin M Y C, Sheagren J N 1978 Antimicrob Ag Chemother 13: 759
Wehrli W, Staehelin M 1971 Bact Rev 35: 290
Weidmer C E, Dunkel T B, Pettyjohn F S, Smith C D, Leibovitz A 1971 J Infect Dis 124: 172
Wolinsky E 1979 Amer Rev Resp Dis 119: 107
Woodley C L, Kilburn J O, David H L, Silcox V A 1972 Antimicrob Ag Chemother 2: 245

VANCOMYCIN

Vancomycin, isolated in 1956 in the laboratories of Eli Lilly from strains of *Streptomyces orientalis*, is now a well recognized antibiotic with very limited if important uses. Despite a presumably limited demand the manufacturers have kept it on the market, whereas a very similar antibiotic, *ristocetin* ('Spontin', Abbott) was withdrawn some years ago.

Antibacterial activity

The spectrum of vancomycin includes only Gram-positive organisms, and only its activity against staphylococci and streptococci and to a lesser extent clostridia is of clinical interest (Table 10.4).

Pharmacokinetics

For practical purposes, vancomycin is not absorbed from the normal alimentary tract. Bryan and White (1978) gave 2 g of the drug orally for 16 days to five functionally anephric patients without inflammatory bowel disease and found just detectable levels in two of them. Intramuscular injections cause pain and necrosis and administration

Table 10.4 Sensitivity of bacteria to vancomycin

	MIC µg/ml
Staph. aureus	0.2–2
Str. pyogenes	0.1–1
Str. pneumoniae	0.5–1
Str. faecalis	0.5–4
Bacillus spp.	0.2–4
Corynebacterium	0.5–1
Cl. perfringens	0.25–1
Clostridium spp.	0.1–4

Based on McCormick, M H et al, Antibiot Ann 1955–6, p. 606;
Griffith R S, Peck F B Jr Antibiot Ann 1955–6, p.619;
Kirby W M M, Divebliss C L Antibiot Ann 1956–7, p. 107;
Geraci J E et al Antibiot Ann 1956–7, p.90

has therefore to be intravenous. The levels 2 hr after doses of 0.5, 1 and 2 g have been reported to be 10, 25 and 50 µg/ml respectively.

When doses were repeated at 6- or 12-hour intervals there was slight accumulation. Therapeutic levels could be maintained by a regimen of 0.5 g six-hourly, 1.0 g 12-hourly, or 2.0 g once a day. A regimen of 1.0 g 12-hourly appeared to be the most satisfactory from the standpoint of ease of administration and effective blood levels.

In patients with impaired renal function much higher blood levels are obtained, and one such patient had a serum concentration of 5 µg/ml nine days after vancomycin had been discontinued. Organ distribution shows no noteworthy features, except that little of the antibiotic is found in either cerebrospinal fluid or bile. Some authors (Hawley & Gump, 1973) have reported that it reaches the cerebrospinal fluid in acute meningitis, but recommend additional 20 mg intrathecal injections if 2 g daily intravenously does not sterilize the fluid in 48 hours. A very high proportion (about 90 per cent) of a dose of vancomycin administered intravenously is excreted in the urine.

Toxic effects

Thrombophlebitis and febrile reactions are common, a rash may occur, and neutropenia, sometimes severe but reversible, occurs, but the most serious risk is that of producing deafness. As usual with ototoxicity, the excessively high blood levels responsible are liable to be attained in patients with impaired renal function, and this unfortunately sometimes exists in patients requiring this treatment. Dosage should be controlled by blood assays: the aim should be to limit the peak level to 50 μg/ml, although according to some authors otoxicity results only if it exceeds 80 μg/ml. The vancomycin level in the blood is little affected by renal dialysis.

Clinical applications

These are well reviewed by Cook & Farrar (1978). The chief indication for vancomycin is the treatment of endocarditis caused by staphylococci or streptococci resistant to penicillin or when the use of penicillin is precluded. Hook & Johnson (1978) in an account of 15 cases treated in the New York Hospital, state infection by a resistant organism as the indication in six, severe reactions to penicillin, including anaphylaxis, in seven, and failure of response to penicillin in one. These infections were caused by several different organisms, and eight involved valve prostheses, in view of which the recovery of all but two patients with prosthetic valve infections who relapsed, was a remarkable achievement. Valves had to be replaced in three others. Vancomycin was given usually in a dose of 2 g daily and usually for from 4 to 6 weeks. Another antibiotic was given in addition and for a full course to seven patients. The reasons for this are not clear, but combinations have been studied by other workers mainly with the object of securing an enhanced bactericidal effect on enterococci, which are more resistant to the bactericidal action of vancomycin than other species. Combined treatment has apparently not been found necessary in other infections, and whether it would enable a shorter course to succeed has not been studied. Mandell et al (1970) found that vancomycin + streptomycin had often a synergic action on enterococci, and Harwick, et al (1973), while confirming this, found that of vancomycin + gentamicin to be superior. Vancomycin and aminoglycosides are both ototoxic, but there need apparently be no reluctance to use them together for fear of synergy in this property as well; no such effect has been reported.

Of the different infections for which vancomycin has been found effective, those due to *Staph. aureus* were the first to be well studied, and included simple septicaemia and severe soft tissue infections as well as endocarditis. Later experience has confirmed these findings, and even methicillin-resistant strains are invariably susceptible. Treatment for endocarditis has been with doses of 500 mg at 6-hour intervals for 4 to 6 weeks, although shorter courses have sometimes been successful. A peculiar form of this infection is that involving shunt sites. As already mentioned, effective concentrations of vancomycin persist in the blood for long periods in advanced renal failure, and Eykyn et al (1970) controlled this infection with doses of 1 g at weekly intervals. *Staph. epidermidis* is a common cause of infection of prosthetic valves; there were four such cases in the series of Hook & Johnson (1978). This organism, although liable to be resistant to almost any other antibiotic, is invariably sensitive to vancomycin. This statement also applies to diphtheroids, responsible for four other infections in this series, and recently reported by others as causing this and other serious infections. *Strep. viridans* is also a fully sensitive organism, and vancomycin is required for endocarditis due to it only when penicillin has unaccountably failed or had to be stopped because of serious intolerance. *Strep. faecalis*, although sensitive by ordinary test, is resistant to the bactericidal action of vancomycin, and combined treatment with an aminoglycoside is indicated. Efficacy in single cases has been reported, but not in any series, perhaps because aminoglycoside combination with penicillin has been so successful.

For the prophylaxis of bacterial endocarditis when teeth are extracted during a course of treatment for this disease itself, when much of the salivary streptococcal population will be resistant to the antibiotic(s) being administered, a single 1 g dose of vancomycin was first suggested by Garrod & Waterworth (1962). It has rightly been objected that this is impracticable in a dentist's surgery, but the recommendation is nonetheless in the latest pronouncement on this subject by the American Heart Associaton (A.H.A. Report, 1977). This subject is further discussed on page 301.

Another use reported on very favourably is oral administration for acute staphyloccal enterocolitis, usually resulting from treatment with other antibiotics. Uniform success has been obtained by giving 0.5 g in 30 ml water or fruit juice at 4–6 hrs intervals. The same treatment has been found effective in pseudomembranous colitis, a condition now attributed to the toxin of *Cl. difficile*, a species reported to be sensitive to vancomycin (page 198).

Tedesco et al (1978) report on the treatment of nine established cases in five widely scattered centres in the United States, and Keighley et al (1978) on a study in Birmingham in which 44 patients with post-operative diarrhoea were first randomly allocated to treatment with vancomycin or placebo; 16 among these were later found to have the specific toxin in their stools as well as *Cl. difficile* itself, nine being in the treated and seven the placebo group. The dose of vancomycin given in this study was 125 mg at 6-hour intervals, and was shown to be adequate; that used by Tedesco et al was 500 mg at the same interval, yielding a faecal content of 3 mg/g. In both studies the treatment was almost uniformly successful in relieving symptoms, promoting resolution of the lesions, and eliminating the organism and its toxin from the bowel.

References

A.H.A. Report 1977 Circulation 56: 139A
Bryan C S, White W L 1978 Antimicrob Ag Chemother 14: 634
Cook F V, Farrar W E Jr 1978 Ann Intern Med 88: 813
Eykyn S, Phillips I, Evans J 1970 Brit Med J 3: 80
Garrod L P, Waterworth P M 1962 Brit Heart J 24: 39
Harwick H J, Kalmanson G M, Guze L B 1973 Antimicrob Agents Chemother 4: 383
Hawley H B, Gump D W 1973 Amer J Dis Child 126: 261
Hook E W, Johnson W D Jr 1978 Amer J Med 65: 411
Keighley M R B, Burdon D W, Arabi Y et al 1978 Brit Med J 2: 1667
Mandell G L, Lindsey E, Hook E W 1970 Amer J Med Sci 259: 346
Tedesco F, Markham R, Gurwith M, Christie D, Bartlett J G 1978 Lancet 2: 226

Various antibacterial antibiotics. Pharmaceutical preparations and dosage

Name	*Dosage*	*Preparations*	*Common international proprietary names*	
Cycloserine	*Adult* Oral: 250–750 mg daily in divided doses, with a maximum daily dose of 1g	Tablets 250 mg Capsules 125, 250 mg	Cycloserine Roche, Cycloserine Lilly Oxamycin, Seromycin	(UK) (USA)
Sodium fusidate	*Adult* Oral: 500 mg three times a day. i.v. 500 mg every 6–8 hours. *Children* Oral: 20–30 mg/kg body weight daily in three divided doses. i.v.: 20 mg/kg body weight daily in three divided doses.	Capsules 250 mg Tablets (enteric coated) 250 mg Suspension in 5 ml equivalent 175 mg i.v. Infusion equivalent 500 mg (contains tetracycline) Topical Preparations	Fucidin Fucidine	(UK) (Fr) (Ger)(USA)
Novobiocin	Available in UK only with tetracycline.	Capsules	Albamycin T Cathomycine Inamycin	(UK) (Fr) (Ger)
Rifampicin	See Chapter 23.			
Vancomycin	*Adults* Oral: 125–500 mg every 6 hours. i.v. infusion: 500 mg every six hours or 1 g every 12 hours. *Children* i.v. infusion: 45 mg/kg body weight daily in divided doses.	Injection 500 mg Oral solution	Vanococin	(UK)

11

Anti-fungal antibiotics

Most of the major antibiotics are produced by fungi, and it is thus not surprising that others should be resistant to them. So resistant are they that quantities of penicillin and streptomycin, enough to inhibit any bacterial growth can be added to culture media used for the isolation of pathogenic fungi: this is a useful proceeding in dealing with, for instance, material from secondarily infected lesions of histoplasmosis. All other mycoses, systemic or surface, are susceptible only to certain highly specialized antibiotics or other drugs, which in general have no anti-bacterial action. These have different specificities among the fungi themselves, very different pharmacokinetic properties, and hence quite separate indications. They include both antibiotics and synthetic compounds.

Some of the more serious systemic mycoses, such as cryptococcosis, coccidioidomycosis and histoplasmosis, are rare or non-existent in this country. Even in the United States, in areas of which they are endemic, the arduous treatment which may be necessary, calling for advanced laboratory facilities, is concentrated for the most part in special centres. For obvious reasons this is no place for a full account of such work, and only outlines will be given.

POLYENE ANTIBIOTICS

The polyenes are a large group of antibiotics—over 60 have been described although few have come into clinical use—all formed by *Streptomyces* spp. and sharing a common structure. They are characterized by a large macrolide ring, closed as in the case of macrolides by the formation of an internal ester or lactone, which contains a series of conjugated double bonds the number of which gives the different groups of agents their names; tetraenes (four double bonds), pentaenes (five double bonds) and so on. Another highly characteristic feature of the molecule is the large number of hydroxy groups, usually on alternate carbon atoms, which are arranged on the opposite side of the molecule to the hydrophobic double bonds, an arrangement which confers an amphapathic property which is probably important in the interaction of the compounds with biological membranes.

The polyenes are now known to have a common mode of action, which is combination with the cell membrane causing increased permeability and ultimately fatal leakage of cell constituents. Moreover it is known that the elements in the membrane with which they combine are sterols. This is illustrated by the fact that resistant organisms do not contain sterols and susceptible do, including not only fungi but algae, protozoa, flatworms and mammalian cells (Kobayashi & Medoff, 1977). Moreover the addition of sterols to the medium protects susceptible cells from the action of polyenes. This effect on mammalian cells is believed to be the main basis of the toxicity of these antibiotics for man.

NYSTATIN

Originally named fungicidin, this antibiotic was the product of a soil survey by members of the staff of the New York State Department of Health (Hazen & Brown, 1951), and this is the derivation of its present name. It is formed by *Streptomyces noursei*, the original strain of which came from dairy farm soil in Virginia, and has a tetraene structure. This was the first of the polyenes to be discovered, and was well established in clinical use before any others were described. (Fig. 11.1).

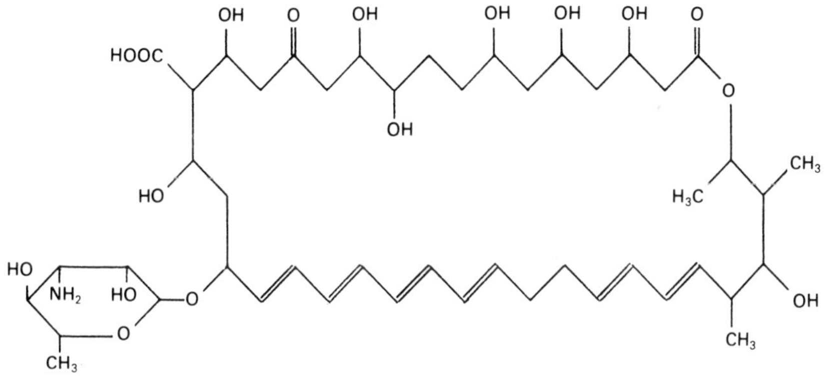

Fig. 11.1 Nystatin

The very low solubility of nystatin has compelled investigators to work with suspensions prepared in various ways. Its discoverers used them not only to demonstrate *in vitro* activity, which is highest against yeast-like fungi, but therapeutically in animals by subcutaneous injection. In their experiments and those of Campbell et al (1954, 1955) some effect was observed in infection by *Histoplasma capsulatum, Cryptococcus neoformans* and *Coccidioides immitis*. Drouhet (1955) not only had similar success from parenteral treatment of *Candida albicans* infection in rabbits, but good results from *oral* administration in 25 patients, some of whom had systemic infection. In human infections the primary and most extensive lesions are usually in the alimentary tract, where they are directly accessible, and it seems possible that when the organism is destroyed in these, the task of its elimination from inaccessible sites may become easier. How much of a systemic effect can be obtained with nystatin is now of less practical interest since the effect is certainly inferior to that obtainable with the more recently discovered amphotericin and perhaps with other drugs.

The local action of nystatin in controlling candidiasis involving any part of the alimentary tract from the mouth to the anus is now so generally familiar as to call for no further discussion. The only aspect of it on which there can be two opinions is whether or when it should be given together with tetracyclines as a preventive, since this class of broad spectrum antibiotic, with its suppressive action on the normal flora, is a common cause of intestinal candidiasis. This question is discussed later (page 242). Nystatin is available in suitable form for the local treatment of *Candida* infections elsewhere (skin, vagina, etc.).

Full purification of nystatin is impracticable, and it is usually prescribed in units, an average dose for candidiasis of the alimentary tract being 500 000 units adminstered three times a day: 3500 units is the activity of 1 mg of the pure substance.

AMPHOTERICIN B

This is the more useful of two antibiotics formed by a strain of *Streptomyces nodosus* found in soil from Templadora on the Orinoco river (Fig. 11.2). It is a heptaene, and like other polyenes almost insoluble in water; early studies were carried out with suspensions. It is active against all the important pathogenic fungi, both yeast-like and filamentous, most species being inhibited by concentrations of <0.5 μg/ml.

In early studies amphotericin B was shown to be effective in various mycotic infections in mice, including some caused by filamentous (e.g. *Aspergillus fumigatus, Rhizopus oryzae*) as well as yeast-like fungi. The intravenous route was chiefly used, but there is some evidence of an effect from much larger doses given orally. That there could be such an effect is shown by the human pharmacological studies of Louria (1958), who gave oral doses of 1.6–5.6 g daily and found amounts up to 0.3 μg/ml in the blood: on the other hand, an intravenous dose of about 1 mg/kg gave blood levels of 0.5 to 3.5 μg/ml and these were found still to be 0.5 to 1.5 μg/ml 20 hours later, indicating very slow elimination. Later studies of intravenous administration have verified these findings, particularly the very slow elimination, such that a dose at 2-day intervals is now generally agreed to maintain an adequate effect. Only about 3 per cent of the dose is excreted in the urine; both distribution and fate of the greater part of it are still uncertain. Haemodialysis is without effect, but dosage need not be reduced on account of renal impairment.

For some years past the antibiotic has been 'solubilized' for intravenous injection with sodium desoxycholate. Much more recently salts of the methyl ester, which are apparently freely water-soluble, have been proposed as an alternative (Hoeprich, 1978) and given with some success to a few patients. In this form a larger dose can be given, and higher levels are attained in the body, but the half-life is shorter. Although these findings were first reported in 1976 they appear not to have been followed up, and we are indebted to Dr P. D. Hoeprich (personal communication, May 1979) for important information bearing on this. He and his colleagues have continued to use the methyl ester, and have treated 50 patients, but have had difficulties with its toxicity. It is not nephrotoxic, but ototoxicity has been seen after intravenous administration, whereas in its ordinary form amphotericin B is ototoxic only when given intrathecally. Secondly, nervous and mental disturbances have been produced (tremor, exaggerated reflexes, confusion and disorientation), and although it seems that these may be due to an antimycotically active impurity and not to the methyl ester itself, clinical trial has been suspended for the present.

The conduct of a course of treatment and the results to be expected have been well described by Cartwright (1975) and by Drouhet (1978). Amphotericin B is now the accepted treatment for any systemic mycosis endangering life, including histoplasmosis, coccidioidomycosis, North American blastomycosis and cryptococcal meningitis. For this condition additional small (e.g. 0.5 mg) intrathecal doses are

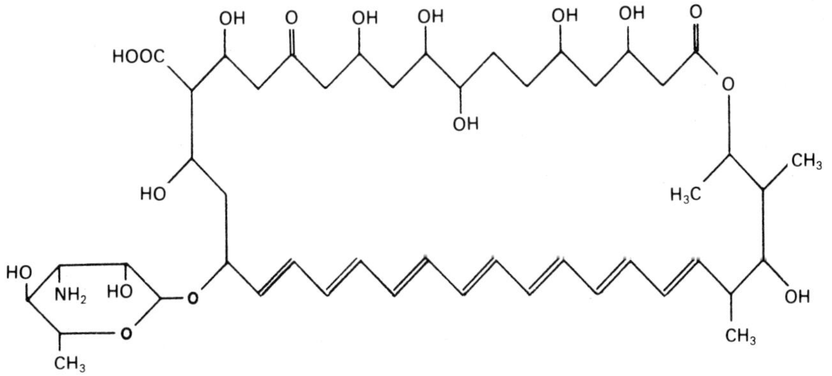

Fig. 11.2 Amphotericin B

advisable. Other possible indications are severer forms of aspergillosis and of candidiasis; there are even recorded instances of cure of *C. albicans* endocarditis, a condition which formerly was invariably fatal. An initial intravenous dose of 1 mg is progressively increased, steeply if toleration is good, until a dose of 1 mg/kg is reached, which is then repeated on alternate days and continued if possible until 3 g have been given. Various toxic effects are common, including fever and nausea and vomiting (which are usually mitigated by also giving aspirin and an antihistamine), local thrombophlebitis resulting from the injection, anaemia, hypokalaemia and a rise in blood urea. The latter is usually said to be 'reversible', but Sanford et al (1962) who performed renal biopsies on three successfully treated cases of coccidioidomycosis, found proliferative changes in glomeruli, degenerative tubular changes and interstitial deposits of calcium, indicative of some degree of permanent damage.

A conference at the National Institutes of Health, Bethesda (Utz et al, 1964) on the toxic effects of amphotericin B includes two contributions in which effects on the kidney are fully described, in both patients and experimental animals. It is emphasized that some effect is invariable if a certain total dose is exceeded. A rise in blood urea and decreased clearance of creatinine may occur without albuminuria. In this paper and another from the same source (Tynes et al, 1963) hydrocortisone is commended for reducing the frequency of immediate reactions such as fever and vomiting: its effect on actual tissue changes was not examined.

This is the only antibiotic used in the treatment of microbic infections of which so small a total dose can have such effects. It is therefore clear that this treatment should not be undertaken except in certainly diagnosed cases, and when, as in coccidioidomycosis, the severity of the infection is variable, only in the more severe and disseminated form.

The efficacy of this treatment is unquestioned but the course is difficult to administer, arduous for the patient, and not without risk. A promising development, discussed later (page 243), is combined treatment with flucytosine, which may enable the effective dose of amphotericin B to be reduced.

OTHER POLYENES

Of many other antibiotics in this group only a few have reached the stage of clinical trial, and, despite some contrary claims, none has proved useful except as a local application. The following have attracted most interest.

Candicidin, a heptaene, formed by *Streptomyces griseus*, is said to be more active than nystatin against Candida spp; good results are claimed in vaginal candidiasis by no less an authority than S. A. Waksman himself (Waksman et al, 1965).

Hamycin, a heptaene from *Streptomyces pimprina* recovered from local soil in the Research Laboratories of Hindustan Antibiotics, was also claimed to be more active than nystatin against Candida. It attracted widespread interest because in further studies in India a systemic effect in experimental infections was claimed from oral administration. It was nearly ten years before work done elsewhere showed that although absorbed to some extent after large oral doses it is both nephrotoxic and relatively ineffective. We understand that it is no longer being produced.

Pimaricin (*Natamycin*), a tetraene, so-called because *Streptomyces natalensis* forming it was derived from soil near Pietermaritzburg (Struyk et al, 1958), has been successfully used in vaginal candidiasis and has some effect also on trichomoniasis (Korteweg et al, 1963). Bronchopulmonary aspergillosis and candidiasis were treated successfully in 7 out of 10 cases by inhalation (Edwards & La Touche, 1964). Fungal keratitis responded very well in 8 cases to the application of a 5 per cent suspension (Newmark et al, 1971).

Trichomycin, a heptaene, so-called because of its activity against *Trichomonas vaginalis*, a product of *Streptomyces hachijoensis*, was discovered in Japan (Hosoya et al, 1952). This property, together with the usual susceptibility of Candida to a polyene, enables this antibiotic to be used successfully for the treatment of both common forms of vaginitis. Efficacy in vaginal candidiasis has been confirmed (Smith et al, 1963) although only an 80 per cent cure rate is claimed, and some of the patients were also given trichomycin orally, whether in expectation of some systemic effect or merely to prevent re-infection from the bowel is not clear.

Prophylactic use of polyenes

Several preparations are on the market in which a polyene, usually nystatin, is mixed with a tetracycline, with the object of preventing overgrowth of *Candida* in the alimentary tract. The merits of this combination require to be considered, and particularly the pros and cons of its regular use, as suggested by some manufacturers. This question was discussed at length in the previous edition, and the arguments now need only be summarized.

There are three objections to this practice. The first is that it usually fails to achieve any useful object. With a single exception no study has revealed any difference in the frequency of side effects. In fact the common assumption that the ordinary side effects result from the proliferation of *Candida* is baseless. More extensive proliferation and actual tissue invasion can occur in debilitated patients, and in them only does the treatment appear to be indicated.

The second objection is one which applies to the indiscriminate and unnecessary use of any antibiotic: that it may lead eventually to increased microbic resistance. This has not yet been seen in clinical isolates of *Candida albicans*, but it has in other Candida (Woods et al, 1974). The margin between the present effective concentrations of amphotericin B and the maximum achievable blood levels is dangerously narrow, and even a small increase in the former might be disastrous.

A different objection applies to preparations, the first of which was intended only for administration to children, which contain tetracycline and amphotericin B. Amphotericin B is the most toxic antibiotic in therapeutic use and the studies of Louria (1958) and observations in mice show that it is absorbed when administered orally. The organ most likely to suffer damage is the kidney, and such damage is likely to be undetected, since proteinuria has been described in only a few patients, and is not characteristic.

OTHER ANTI-MYCOTIC DRUGS

FLUCYTOSINE (5-FLUOROCYTOSINE)

This substance, an anti-metabolite of the pyrimidine base cytosine, acts exclusively on certain yeast-like fungi and not at all on filamentous fungi or any bacteria. According to Shadomy (1969) it inhibits *Cryptococcus neoformans* in concentrations of 0.46–3.9 μg/ml and kills it at 3.9–15.6 μg/ml. *Candida albicans* is about equally sensitive. Since the drug can be given orally in doses of 100 mg/kg daily, and then attains concentrations in the blood and cerebro-spinal fluid of 10–30 and 8–20 μg/ml respectively, an effect in these two infections is to be expected, and this has been confirmed clinically. *Histoplasma capsulatum* and *Blastomyces dermatitidis* are resistant.

Although it was at first supposed that this drug acts as an anti-metabolite, since its inhibitory action is prevented *in vitro* by the presence of cytosine, it now appears that its main effect is of a different nature. It is believed to be converted in the body to 5-fluorouracil. Using this compound labelled with ^{14}C and studying its action on many strains of *Candida albicans* with different degrees of resistance to flucytosine, Polak and Scholer (1975) showed that the extent of uptake correlated well with degree of sensitivity. It is believed that 5-fluorouracil is incorporated in DNA, in consequence of which abnormal proteins are formed.

The drug has been extensively used in treating *C. albicans* infections at various sites and to a smaller extent those due to *C. neoformans*, and an extensive literature has grown up which cannot be reviewed here. Treatment is sometimes successful, but sometimes fails owing to microbial resistance to the drug. Some degree of this may exist initially, or a usually higher degree may develop, even within a short time, in response to treatment, precluding its success. (Fig. 11.3). The hypothesis of its mode of action proposed by Polak & Scholer (1975) is consistent with several mechanisms which could explain resistance. Although some cases of severe *Candida* infection have responded, including septicaemia (but not endocarditis) it may be unwise to rely on flucytosine alone in infections seriously endangering life. Some patients tolerate large doses well, but in others bone marrow depression (leucopenia, etc.), hepatic dysfunction or diarrhoea may be produced.

Combined treatment

Combined treatment is a well recognized resource for overcoming defects in a therapeutic agent, including toxicity, since combination with another agent may reduce the necessary dose. Treatment with amphotericin B and flucytosine rests on a sound theoretical basis, namely that the former, by increasing permeability enables a higher concentration of the latter to be attained in the cell. It is well ascertained that the permeabilizing and lethal effects of amphotericin B are distinct, and exerted respectively by low and higher concentrations. The low one is inadequate for independent therapeutic effect, but might enable another drug to exert this. Experimental verification has been achieved in a series of therapeutic studies in mice, reviewed by Kobayashi & Medoff (1977), who are themselves responsible for most of this work. These involved several different fungal infections, and consistently showed a synergic effect from amphotericin and flucytosine, and in some experiments amphotericin and rifampicin, the latter alone having little or no action. Proof was also obtained that during combined treatment the uptake of flucytosine by the cells was increased.

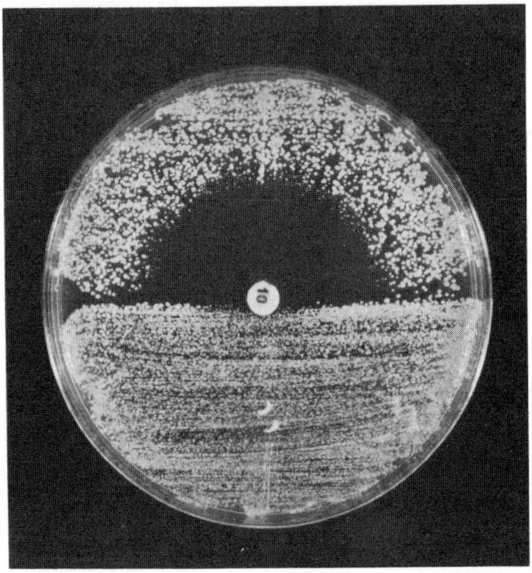

Fig. 11.3 Strain of *C. albicans* isolated from the blood of a patient with endocarditis before (top) and after (lower) treatment with flucytosine. Disc contains 1 μg flucytosine

It is not surprising in view of the arduous and complex nature of such treatment with all its necessary controls that its clinical exploitation has not been extensive. Utz et al (1975) treated disseminated cryptococcosis with 20 mg amphotericin and 150 mg/kg flucytosine daily for 6 weeks; of 15 culturally verified cases there were three early deaths, four died later of other causes and eight survived. More recent experience published from the National Institutes of Health, Bethesda (Bennett et al, 1979) of the treatment of cryptococcal meningitis with this combination has had encouraging results. Of 27 patients treated with amphotericin alone for 10 weeks, 11 were improved or cured compared with 16 of 24 treated with a combination of a somewhat lower dose of amphotericin together with flucytosine for 6 weeks. Dosage of amphotericin used alone was 0.4 mg/kg daily for 42 days changing to 0.8 mg/kg on alternate days for 28 days. In the combined treatment, the doses were amphotericin 0.3 mg/kg daily and flucytosine 150 mg/kg daily in 6-hourly doses. CSF cultures became negative more quickly with the combination although few patients received any intrathecal treatment. Flucytosine toxicity from the large dose given for a long time has been a problem: neutropenia, thrombocytopenia and diarrhoea were associated with blood levels of more than 100 mg/ml. It is advisable to monitor blood levels and renal function and to adjust the dose accordingly.

CLOTRIMAZOLE

This compound, one of a long series of tritylimidazole derivatives prepared in the Bayer laboratories, is fully described by Plempel et al (1969). It inhibits all the principal fungi causing systemic infections in concentrations of the order of 1 μg/ml. It is well absorbed from the alimentary tract. Efficacy has been demonstrated in mice in *Candida, Histoplasma* and *Aspergillus* infections. Shadomy (1971) obtained less favourable results than these in experimental infections, and observed that pre-treatment worsened them; this paradoxical effect is confirmed by Waitz et al (1971), who found that after pre-treatment for 5 days the blood levels during subsequent post-inoculation treatment were much reduced. It seems therefore that habituation to the drug enables the body to dispose of it more rapidly.

Some favourable results from systemic treatment have been reported in candidiasis and aspergillosis (the latter disputed) but an additional drawback to falling blood levels has been recognized in toxicity. Nausea and vomiting have been troublesome, and even mental disturbances have been reported (Cartwright 1975). Evidently for these reasons systemic use has declined, and at a Conference (1974) attention was concentrated mainly on local application, a 1 per cent cream being advocated for dermatomycoses and 100 mg tablets for vaginal candidiasis.

MICONAZOLE

This substance was developed by Janssen Pharmaceutica of Belgium. Like clotrimazole it has a wide anti-fungal spectrum, and considerable activity also against Gram-positive bacteria. Morphological and other studies have shown that its action is on the cell wall, increasing permeability and causing leakage of cell constituents. It has similar efficacy to that of clotrimazole in the treatment of superficial mycoses, but differs from it in being administrable parenterally (no suitable form of clotrimazole for this purpose has been devised). It can also be given orally. Again unlike clotrimazole, it is free from serious toxicity. A further advantage over some other treatments is that fungal resistance to it does not develop.

There is an extensive literature on its topical use, which cannot be reviewed here, and convincing evidence of systemic efficacy, although not yet enough to compare this with the performance of other drugs; indeed it may be several years before its place can be finally assessed.

Antimycotic activity. We are aware of no fully comprehensive and exact study (the most comprehensive reported hitherto employed 10-fold differences) but there is scattered information in more detail about several important species. Most strains of *Candida albicans* are inhibited by <1 μg/ml, and the sensitivity of *Cryptococcus neoformans* seems to be similar. *Blastomyces brasiliensis* and *Histoplasma capsulatum* are reported to be more sensitive than this and *Aspergillus* spp. less so. Most dermatophytes are also sensitive.

Pharmacokinetics. Intravenous infusion of 500 mg gives an initial blood level of about 7 μg/ml, falling at first rapidly and then progressively more slowly. Protein binding is 95 per cent. Levels are lower after oral doses, one of 1000 mg reaching a peak of only 1 μg/ml, with a similar subsequent gradual fall (Boelaert et al, 1976). In order to sustain adequate levels three daily doses are advised. The drug is excreted unchanged only into the intestine; much of the dose is converted in the liver to inactive metabolites, and only these appear in the urine.

Clinical application. The most extensive source of information hitherto is the report of a Symposium (1977). Administration was either oral, usually at the rate of 1 g three times a day, or by intravenous infusion, somewhat smaller doses being given. Success is claimed in various forms of deep-seated candidiasis, in coccidioidomycosis, the susceptibility of which in experimental infections is convincingly demonstrated by Levine et al (1975), cryptococcosis, South American blastomycosis and (rather less convincingly) in aspergillosis. The account by Deresinski et al (1977) of the treatment of fungal meningitis (ten *C. immitis* and two *C. neoformans*) includes a study of the cerebrospinal fluid concentrations attained after not only intravenous but intrathecal injections; doses of 20 mg by this route were well tolerated. All investigators are agreed that miconazole causes few side effects, none being serious; pruritus has been the chief complaint, sometimes accompanied by a rash, and phlebitis has been troublesome, but can be avoided by passing the cannula into the superior vena cava. Other useful reports are those by Sung et al (1977) and Stevens (1977). No attempt is made here to analyse any of these results in detail, because none prove superior benefit conclusively. The patients treated were heterogeneous, some being previous amphotericin failures and others not, with variations also in the severity both of the infection itself and of underlying disease, these factors sometimes rendering the prognosis almost hopeless. Findings are often qualified by the proviso that more prolonged treatment might have been more successful, and such arduous courses call for facilities available in few institutions.

ECONAZOLE

This drug is closely related in structure to miconazole, and differs very little from it in other properties, although it seems to have been rather differently used. Its properties and therapeutic achievements are revealed by Heel et al (1978). Its range of antimycotic activity is almost identical to that of miconazole. The nitrate is used for local application and the base for systemic administration. Almost all published information so far concerns topical use, mainly for vaginal candidiasis or for infections by dermatophytes, including those of the skin, hair and nails. Satisfactory results are claimed, but few studies have been comparative. Although support for systemic use is afforded by the result of animal studies, confirming both safety and efficacy, very few patients have yet been so treated.

Two remaining anti-fungal drugs to be described are antibiotics other than polyenes. For one of these, saramycetin, the reader is referred to the previous edition; little more has been heard of it, and we understand that it is now unobtainable. The second is now a well established remedy for one class of mycoses only.

GRISEOFULVIN

This antibiotic was discovered as a product of *Penicillium griseofulvum* by Oxford, Raistrick and Simonart (1939). It was re-discovered some years later as the product of a *Penicillium* in soil at Wareham Heath, Dorset, in which conifers grew poorly because of its action on mycorrhizal fungi: from its effect on these organisms it was called 'curling factor'. Its identity with a sample of griseofulvin supplied by Raistrick was verified by Grove & McGowan (1947). Its anti-fungal action was then further examined and exploited in the field of plant pathology. Clinical use was at first considered inadvisable because of the observation of an anti-mitotic effect, but this was produced by large doses given intravenously in animals and there is not now believed to be any risk of such an effect from the doses employed clinically.

The highest activity of griseofulvin is against dermatophytes: yeast-like fungi are less susceptible, although O'Grady and his colleagues (1963), by giving large doses to mice, obtained a reduction in the size of *Candida* lesions in the mouse thigh, possibly by some indirect mechanism. Total inhibition of the growth of dermatophytes *in vitro* may require concentrations exceeding those obtainable at the site of infection, but much lower concentrations retard growth, and Jesenská & Danilla (1971) suggest determination of sensitivity by comparing colony diameters on solid media containing 0.1 to 3 μg/ml with those on drug-free medium. A curative effect was first demonstrated in experimental *Microsporum canis* infection in guinea-pigs by Gentles (1958) who was also responsible (Gentles et al, 1959) for showing that the antibiotic is actually in the hair of treated animals, some of it being only extractable with methanol. The fact that griseofulvin when administered orally is actually incorporated in keratin as it is formed explains its unique activity in fungus infections of the hair and nails.

The results in *Microsporum audouini* and other infections of the scalp hair are uniformly good. A good account of results in onychomycosis is given by Davies et al (1967). Treatment was continued for up to two years, 0.5 g being given three times a day for one month and thereafter twice daily. Finger nail infections responded better than those of the toes, and *Trychophyton rubrum* infections better than *T. mentagrophytes*, the former being the more sensitive organism. (See also Chapter 16).

The antibiotic is better absorbed when in finely divided form, and its absorption is also said to be promoted by fat in the diet (Crounse, 1961). Blood levels are much reduced by administration of phenobarbitone. Other systems of dosage have been proposed for short courses. Atkinson et al (1962) contest the suggestion made by others that scalp ringworm can be cured by a single massive dose, and showed that divided doses give higher blood levels than a single daily dose. Grin & Nadaždin (1965) observed effects by microscopy of hairs plucked at intervals, and confirmed that a single large dose is ineffective, but achieved economy by initial large doses (50 mg per kg daily) for five days followed by only 6.25 mg per kg daily for the remainder of a 28-day course.

Even long courses of treatment are usually well tolerated. Rashes, headache and gastric discomfort are uncommon and rarely severe. The disturbance of porphyrin metabolism and liver damage produced by large doses in mice (De Matteis & Rimington, 1963) appear to have little or no counterpart in patients given conventional doses.

Pharmaceutical preparations and dosages are on page 249.

References

Atkinson R M, Bedford C, Child K J, Tomich E G 1962 Antibiot Chemother 12: 225
Bennett J E, Dismukes W E, Duma D J et al 1979 New Engl J Med 301: 126
Boelaert J, Daneels R, Van Landuyt H, Symoens J 1976. In: Williams J D, Geddes A M (ed), Chemotherapy, Plenum Press, New York, London, Vol 6 p165
Campbell C C, Hodges E P, Hill G B 1954 Antibiot Ann 1953–54 p 210
Campbell C C, O'Dell E T, Hill G B 1955 Antibiot Ann 1954–55 p 858
Cartwright R Y 1975 J Antimicrob Chemother 1: 141
Conference 1974 Clotrimazole. Proceedings of a Conference held May 17–18 1973 Postgrad Med J 50: Suppl 1
Crounse R G 1961 J Invest Dermatol 37: 529
Davies R R, Everall J D, Hamilton E 1967 Brit Med J 3: 464
De Matteis F, Rimington C 1963 Brit J Dermatol 75: 91
Deresinski S C, Lilly R B, Levine H B et al 1977 Arch Intern Med 137: 1180
Drouhet E 1955 Ann Inst Pasteur 88: 298
Drouhet E 1978 Antibiotic Chemother 25: 253
Edwards G, La Touche C J P 1964 Lancet 1: 1349
Gentles J C 1958 Nature Lond 182: 476
Gentles J C, Barnes M J, Fantes K H 1959 Nature Lond 183: 256
Grin E I, Nadaždin M 1965 Bull Wld Hlth Org 33: 183
Grove J F, McGowan J C 1947 Nature Lond 160: 574
Hazen Elizabeth L, Brown Rachel 1951 Proc Soc Exp Biol NY 76: 93
Heel R C, Brogden R N, Speight T M, Avery G S 1978 Drugs 16: 177
Hoeprich P D 1978 Scand J Infect Dis Suppl 16: 74
Hosoya S, Komatsu N, Soeda M, Sonoda Y 1952 Jap J Exp Med 22: 505
Jesenská Z, Danilla T 1971 Zbl Bakt I Orig 217: 104
Kobayashi G S, Medoff G 1977 Ann Rev Microbiol 31: 291
Korteweg G C, Szabo K L H, Rutten A M G, Hoogerheide J C 1963 Antibiot Chemother 11: 261
Levine H B, Stevens D A, Cobb J M, Gebhardt A E 1975 J Infect Dis 132: 407
Louria D B 1958 Antibiot Med 5: 295
Newmark E, Kaufman H E, Polack F M, Ellison A C 1971 Sth Med J 64: 935
O'Grady F, Thompson R E M, Cotton R E 1963 Brit J Exp Path 44: 334
Oxford A E, Raistrick H, Simonart P 1939 Biochem J 33: 240
Plempel M, Bartmann K, Buchel K H, Regel E 1969 Dtsch Med Wschr 94: 1356
Polak A, Scholer H J 1975 Chemotherapy 21: 113
Sanford W G, Rasch J R, Stonehill R B 1962 Ann Intern Med 56: 553
Shadomy S 1969 Appl Microbiol 17: 871
Shadomy S 1971 Antimicrob Agents Chemother 1970 p 169
Smith A G, Taubert H D, Martin C W 1963 Amer J Obstet Gynec 87: 455
Stevens D A 1977 Amer Rev Respirat Dis 116: 801
Struyk A P, Hoette I, Drost G et al 1958 Antibiot Ann 1957–8, p 878
Sung J P, Grendahl J G, Levine H B 1977 West J Med 126: 5
Symposium 1977 New Possibilities in the Treatment of Systemic Mycoses. Reports on the Experimental and Clinical Evaluation of Miconazole Proc Roy Soc Med 70: Suppl 1
Tynes B S, Utz J P, Bennett J E, Alling D W 1963 Amer Rev Resp Dis 87: 264
Utz J P, Bennett J E, Brandriss M W, Butler W T, Hill G J 1964 Ann Intern Med 61: 334
Utz J P, Garriques I L, Sande M A et al 1975 J Infect Dis 132: 368
Waitz J A, Moss E L, Weinstein M J 1971 Appl Microbiol 22: 891
Waksman S A, Lechevalier H A, Schaffner C P 1965 Bull Wld Hlth Org 33: 219
Woods R A, Bard M, Jackson I E, Drutz D J 1974 J Infect Dis 129: 53

Anti-fungal agents. Pharmaceutical preparations and dosage

Name	*Dosage*	*Preparations*	*Common international proprietary names*	
Nystatin	*Adult* Oral: 500 000–1 000 000 U every six hours (for intestinal candidiasis) *Intravaginal* 200 000 U daily *Children* Oral: 100 000 U every six hours	Tablets Suspension Topical and Vaginal preparations	Nystan Moronal Mycostatin, Nilistat Mycostatine	(UK) (Ger) (USA) (Fr)
Amphotericin	*Adults* i.v. infusion, see text. Oral: Lozenges 10–20 mg every 6 hours Tablets 100–200 mg every 6 hours *Children* Reduced dosage according to weight	Lozenges Tablets Suspension Topical and Vaginal preparations Intravenous Injection	Fungizone, Fungilin Ampho-Moronal	(UK) (Ger)
Candicidin	*Intravaginal:* 3–5 mg inserted twice a day for 14 days	Pessaries Ointment	Candeptin Vanobid	(UK) (USA)
Natamycin (Pimaricin)	*Adults* By inhalation: 2.5 mg three times a day for four weeks and 2.5 mg twice a day thereafter, until sputum cultures are negative. *Children* By inhalation: as for adults Also topical and vaginal application	Suspension Pessaries	Pimafucin	(UK)
Clotrimazole	Topical application as a 1% preparation. Vaginal tablets containing 100 mg	Cream Pessaries Powder Atomiser spray	Canesten Lotrimin	(UK) (USA)
Miconazole	*Adult* Oral: 250 mg four times a day after meals i.v. Infusion: 600 mg three times a day Topical and vaginal application	Tablets Oral Gel Intravenous solution Local application	Daktarin, Gyno-daktarin, Monistat	(UK)

Name	*Dosage*	*Preparations*	*Common international proprietary names*	
Econazole	Topical and vaginal application	Cream Pessaries	Ecostatin	(UK)
Flucytosine	*Adult* Oral: 100–200 mg/kg daily in four divided doses, depending on the sensitivity of the infecting organism. i.v. infusion: 100–200 mg/kg daily in divided doses. The dose should be reduced if renal function is impaired *Children* Oral: 100–200 mg/kg daily as for adults. i.v. infusion, as above	Tablets Infusion	Alcobon Ancobon Ancotil	(UK) (USA) (Fr)
Griseofulvin	*Adult* Oral: 500 mg–1 g daily, but not less than 10 mg/kg body weight. To be taken after food *Children* oral: 10 mg/kg body weight daily	Tablets Suspension	Fulcin, Grisovin Fulvicin -U/F, Grifulvin V Griséfuline Likuden M	(UK) (USA) (Fr) (Ger)

12

Modes of action

An antibacterial agent suitable for human therapy must possess a remarkable array of attributes, but above all it must exhibit a high degree of selective toxicity—that is to say its detrimental effect on the infecting organism must greatly exceed any detrimental effect on the patient. Extreme degrees of selective toxicity depend on possession by bacteria of processes or structures (for example bacterial cell wall) which are not represented in man. Unacceptably low degrees of selective toxicity result from the fact that many essential processes (for example, protein synthesis) are common to widely separate species in which they differ only in detail. These processes have now been the subject of intensive biochemical investigations for many years and a great deal of what is said about metabolic processes in general derives from studies of bacteria, notably *E. coli* and from the use of antibiotics as tools in the elucidation of their details. Many of these studies have been conducted in cell-free systems, often with substitution of modified or synthetic components in order to simplify, isolate or identify precisely certain steps in complex and often interwoven chains of reactions. For cells to metabolize, grow and divide a very high degree of interaction and control must be exerted over these processes so that the overall progress is orderly and balanced. It is disorder and uncontrolled progress of the unaffected processes that follow interference with a particular reaction by an antibiotic rather than the loss of the specific reaction itself that is generally responsible for the grave effects that antibiotics can exert on microbes. If fragments of such a balanced system are removed, as they must be, in order to study and dissect them, it is not surprising that their behaviour is not always immediately interpretable in terms of the activities of the agent against the whole bacterial cell, nor can the results of different workers using different approaches always be reconciled.

We are not competent to adjudicate on the enormous amount of work which is still in progress and we feel that the needs of most of our readers will be met by a general overview of the kinds of ways in which antibacterial agents work. Many excellent reviews on the topic have appeared in the last few years and those who would wish to know more should consult Gale et al (1972), Franklin & Snow (1975), Corcoran & Hahn (1975). Antibacterial agents may be conveniently divided into four groups which exert their effects on (1) nucleic acids (2) protein synthesis (3) the cell wall (4) the cell membrane.

Nucleic acids

Replication of the nucleic acids of the bacterial cell is prevented directly by nalidixic acid and rifamycins and remotely by sulphonamides and certain diaminopyrimidines.

It was early postulated that sulphonamides compete with the structurally similar para-aminobenzoic acid for the same enzyme. The majority of bacteria have an essential requirement for para-aminobenzoate which they use in the first step towards the synthesis of folate. Sulphonamides inhibit the enzyme which catalyses this step—tetrahydropteroate synthetase—and exposed organisms develop the signs of folate deficiency.

Preformed folate possessed by the organism continues to function and it is only when this has been diluted by division amongst the organism's progeny that the growth stops. It has been argued that the successful, albeit slow, arrest of bacterial growth cannot be the result of simple competition for enzyme sites between structural analogues because the natural substrate would simply accumulate until its concentration was sufficient to dispel the competitor. Either, therefore, the inhibitor must have a much higher affinity for the enzyme than has the natural substrate—an unlikely state of affairs since the enzyme has evolved to handle the natural substrate—or it must act in some other way.

It often appears that successful antibacterial agents act in several ways and sulphonamide not only has a greater affinity than has para-aminobenzoate for tetrahydropteroate synthetase, but it may also act at an earlier stage (and we shall see shortly also at a later stage) by acting on the control mechanisms, which are always vital to the balancing of the growth process, to switch off the supply of natural substrate.

Tetrahydrofolate

From the precursors with which sulphonamides interfere, bacteria construct tetrahydrofolate which plays a crucial part in the synthesis of the purines and some amino-acids. Amongst the purines thymidilate is particularly important because it is produced through the catalytic agency of thymidilate synthetase from tetrahydrofolate which is thereby consumed.

In other syntheses tetrahydrofolate is converted to dihydrofolate and must be regenerated—a process which is brought about through the agency of the enzyme dihydrofolate reductase. Inhibition of this enzyme is a general property of 2 : 4 diaminopyrimidines which exhibit remarkable selectivity in that modification of the molecule can greatly increase the activity against the enzyme of one species while decreasing it against another (Hitchings, 1969).

Amongst therapeutically important examples of this class of agent, pyrimethamine inhibits mammalian and bacterial enzymes approximately equally but only in a concentration about 2000 times that needed to produce comparable inhibition of the plasmodial enzyme. In contrast, trimethoprim is extremely active against the bacterial enzyme, much less active against the plasmodial enzyme, and very feebly active against the mammalian enzyme which requires for comparable inhibition about 50 000 times the concentration which inhibits the bacterial enzyme, and 2000 times that which inhibits the plasmodial enzyme. Although its anti-plasmodial effect is plainly much less than its anti-bacterial effect, it is nevertheless sufficient to produce a useful degree of anti-malarial activity.

Loss by mutation of the ability to produce thymidilate synthetase renders the organism incapable of utilizing tetrahydrofolate for the synthesis of thymidilate and makes the organism resistant to trimethoprim but dependent on an exogenous supply of thymine. Such thymine-dependent trimethoprim-resistant mutants have occasionally been encountered in clinical practice (page 29).

Differential affinity for the enzymes of different species is clearly of great importance in determining the selective toxicity of trimethoprim, but there is an additional important difference in the way in which animals and parasites obtain their folate requirements. Bacteria and protozoa synthesize folate from para-aminobenzoate, while man and animals utilize preformed folic or folinic acid (leucovorin) from the diet. These two processes appear to be mutually exclusive: parasites which synthesize folic acid cannot absorb it preformed, and man and animals which absorb it preformed cannot synthesize it.

This difference has two important consequences. Firstly, any depressant effect of diaminopyrimidines on human folate metabolism may be overcome by feeding tetrahydrofolate supplements which the parasite cannot utilize. Secondly, since sulphonamides inhibit the incorporation by parasites of para-aminobenzoate into dihydrofolate, sulphonamides and trimethoprim act sequentially in the same metabolic pathway. As a result, their combined action is strongly synergic. There is about a 10-fold increase in activity when the agents are given together. Figure 12.1 shows the difference between parasite and human folic acid metabolism diagrammatically, and indicates the point at which sulphonamides and such folic acid antagonists as pyrimethamine and trimethoprim work.

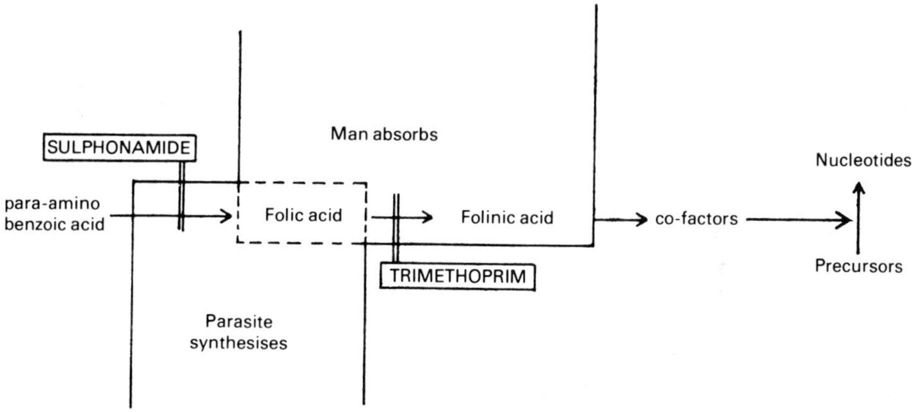

Fig 12.1 Sequential interruption of folate synthesis in parasites by sulphonamide and trimethoprim (based on Hitchings G H 1961 Trans NY Acad Sci 23: 700).

The claim that action at sequential points in the same pathway is responsible for the striking synergy that can commonly be demonstrated between trimethoprim and sulphonamides has—like the explanation that sulphonamides themselves act by competitive inhibition—been viewed by some with scepticism. Poe (1976) offers the explanation that sulphonamides are certainly potent inhibitors of dihydropteroate synthetase but also significant inhibitors of dihydrofolate reductase. Those diaminopyrimidines that permit simultaneous binding of sulphonamide by dihydrofolate reductase produce synergy while those that prevent sulphonamide binding do not.

DNA

The effect of sulphonamides and diaminopyrimidines is ultimately to deprive the cell of nucleic acid; the effect of nalidixic acid is to prevent its replication. Nalidixic acid specifically inhibits bacterial DNA synthesis both *in vitro* and *in vivo* yet it does not bind to DNA, it does not interfere with the biosynthesis of purines or pyrimidines and does not inhibit any of the enzymes known to be concerned in DNA synthesis. It has no effect on RNA synthesis or on the production of DNA initiator protein and its bactericidal effect is probably due to this induced imbalance since if RNA and protein synthesis are constrained the bactericidal action of the drug is abolished. Termination of a round of DNA synthesis is the signal for completion of cross septation and separation of daughter cells and its inhibition causes these cells to form into long filaments.

Construction of the very long DNA molecules appears to proceed in stages of which the first is formation of short elements which are then joined into longer strands. These strands are then linked to form a complete molecule and Crumplin and Smith (1975) present evidence that it is this linkage which is inhibited by nalidixic acid. It also affects the cell membrane and synchronous premature resumption of chromosome replication occurs on removal of the drug. By its effect on chromosomal replication nalidixic acid interrupts conjugation between enterobacteria if the male organism is sensitive but not if it is resistant (Hane, 1971).

RNA

Rifamycins specifically inhibit the bacterial enzyme—RNA polymerase—concerned with replication of RNA. This effect is brought about by binding of one molecule of the antibiotic to one molecule of the enzyme (Lill et al, 1970). The corresponding mammalian enzyme is unaffected by the antibiotic and this undoubtedly accounts for its selective toxicity. On the other hand it exerts a certain degree of antiviral activity and is of particular interest in its activity against the RNA dependent DNA polymerase of oncogenic viruses. Inhibition of RNA synthesis is usually bacteristatic since it results in a relatively balanced decline in other functions. In the presence of an RNA inhibitor the supply of m-RNA—which is rapidly turned over in bacteria—soon fails with cessation of protein synthesis and deprivation of initiator protein brings DNA synthesis to a halt.

Protein

For bacterial growth to proceed all the biochemical events of the cell must be repeated cyclically: some over the long term from one division to the next, some over very short periods when a particular event has to recur many times in the course of construction of new material as, for example, in the linking together of the large number of amino-acids which make up a single molecule of protein. As each component makes its contribution to the cycle it is altered and must be regenerated before the cycle can begin again. Interruption of the cycle locks the process at that point and growth halts. Because of the continuation of unaffected processes the overall integration of cell metabolism is disrupted and the long-term effect of this may be so severe that the cell dies. On the DNA template the cell assembles three kinds of RNA: transfer-RNA (t-RNA), ribosomal-RNA (r-RNA) and messenger-RNA (m-RNA). Ribosomal-RNA is utilized, with protein, in the construction of ribosomes, lying free in the cytoplasm or attached to the cytoplasmic membrane, on which protein is synthesised. Messenger-RNA takes from DNA to the ribosomes the code which fixes the order in which amino acids are assembled into protein.

In the metabolic pool, uncommitted ribosomes exist as separate 30S and 50S components (the figures indicate the speed at which the components sediment in the ultracentrifuge). Close to the end of a thread of m-RNA a specific initiation complex brings together the 30S and 50S components to form a functional ribosome on which there are two attachment sites for amino-acids. From the metabolic pool, amino-acids are transported to the ribosome, each kind of amino-acid being carried by its own specific t-RNA. The region of the messenger thread which is attached to the ribosome is 'recognized' by the appropriate t-RNA which attaches to it and to the ribosome in such a way that the carried amino-acid is brought into contact with the first of the two ribosome sites. The energy required to effect this process of attachment is provided by ATP together with other factors, all of which have to be regenerated once the appropriate amino-acid has been attached to the 'receptor' site of the ribosome and the carrier t-RNA released to collect another amino-acid. Once the amino-acid has been attached, the ribosome is moved to the next 'codon' of the messenger which stipulates the amino-acid next to be added.

With this movement, called 'translocation', the amino-acid is transferred to the second or 'donor' site of the ribosome. The delivery and attachment process is now repeated so that the second specified amino-acid is brought on to the vacated receptor site. When both amino-acids are in position, the first is detached from the donor site and coupled to the newly attached amino-acid to form a dipeptide in a process called 'transfer'. The processes of translocation and transfer consume energy which is again supplied by cycling factors which must be regularly regenerated in each cycle.

In the meantime, a second ribosome is assembled from its two components at the first site on the messenger and the specified first amino-acid attached as before. In the second translocation move the dipeptide attached to the first ribosome is transferred to the donor site and in due course transferred to the third amino-acid specified by the messenger.

This process continues until a 'polysome' is assembled which consists of the messenger completely threaded with ribosomes the first of which, having traversed the whole length of the messenger, carries a completed protein. In its final move, the ribosome releases the completed protein, dissociates into its two components and returns to the pool through the agency of a termination complex.

Sites of antibiotic action

The key step of initiation of polysome construction in which the first ribosome is attached to the messenger is halted by streptomycin and this is now thought to be the main mode in which it prevents protein synthesis. There is rapid initial uptake of the drug resulting in some efflux of ions from the cell followed by binding to 30S ribosomes at 1 molecule per ribosome. There is also evidence that binding to the attached RNA is also implicated. It appears that interference with almost every aspect of protein synthesis follows. The attachment renders the initiation complex unusually unstable, there is binding to t-RNA and translation is inhibited, there is inhibition of release factor function and, finally, there is the extremely intriguing malfunction called 'miscoding'. In this the presence of streptomycin causes the messenger code to be misread and the wrong amino acid to be incorporated into the growing peptide chain.

The degree of infidelity introduced into protein replication by this process is very small. Major deletions of amino-acid sequences do not occur and it appears that the lesion involves misplacement of a single amino-acid. This very discrete lesion is sufficient for the continuation of the peptide sequence to fail, or for protein to be manufactured which is unable to fulfil its enzymic or structural function. The effect of streptomycin on cell growth is relatively slow and it is probable that considerable accumulation of faulty protein occurs before cell function ceases. Streptomycin produces a number of later effects on the cell, such as permeability changes and impairment of respiration, which might result from imperfections in the protein molecules concerned in those functions or might be independent effects of the drug. Either way it is probable that it is these effects, rather than the protein derangement itself, which are directly responsible for cell death. The action of other aminoglycosides has been much less extensively studied but appears to follow generally similar lines. Miscoding appears to be a function of true aminocyclitol aminoglycosides since it is shown by neither kasugamycin nor spectinomycin (page 117).

Tetracycline interrupts the cycle by which amino-acid is carried and attached to the ribosome. It has been generally held that transfer of the growing peptide chain to the newly attached amino-acid which is to be next added is interrupted by chloramphenicol (Teraoka, 1970). However, Pongs & Messer (1976), who have identified the specific ribosomal proteins concerned with chloramphenicol binding, still regard the mechanism of action of the drug as being ill understood. Several agents appear to exert their major effect on the translocation step. Erythromycin acts after activation of the amino-acid and its attachment to the t-RNA and appears to influence both transfer and translocation. It binds to the 50S sub-unit of the ribosomes of susceptible bacteria at a site which, at least in some organisms, also binds other macrolides, lincosamides and chloramphenicol—an association which is no doubt related to the cross-resistances sometimes seen amongst them. Translocation is mediated by an elongation factor which forms a labile complex with the ribosome and GDT. This complex is frozen by fusidate, preventing the regeneration of the components and thus the next round of translocation. As protein synthesis declines DNA synthesis levels off but RNA synthesis continues. Some of this is t-RNA, some accumulates as incomplete ribosome-like particles ('chloramphenicol particles') but most is m-RNA. When protein synthesis is released from the action of chloramphenicol the excess RNA is degraded and normal growth is resumed. Interestingly enough, the similarity of the translocation lesion produced by these three agents is reflected in the similarity of the characteristic morphological injury which they exert on staphylococci as seen in the stereoscan electron microscope.

The translocation step may be peculiarly accessible to modification since all three agents, erythromycin, lincomycin and sodium fusidate, which affect it are particularly liable to give rise to resistant mutants. It is not known why interruption of protein synthesis at the point of attack adopted by tetracycline and chloramphenicol halts bacterial growth while the effect of the agents which interfere with translocation is frequently lethal.

The process of protein synthesis is essentially the same in all cells and the differential toxicity of antibacterial agents for different species (both in terms of selective toxicity and antimicrobial spectrum) depends either on differences in the ribosomes or on impermeability of the cell to the agent. The resistance of enterobacteria to lincomycin, erythromycin or fusidic acid (all of which will interfere with protein synthesis by the isolated ribosomes of *E. coli*—the biochemists' favourite tool—is due to failure of the agent to penetrate the cell. By using radioactively labelled antibiotics it is possible to show that the greater sensitivity of Gram-positive organisms to macrolides is due to the fact that they are not only permeable to the agents (which the resistant Gram-negative organisms are not) but actually concentrate the agent within the cell.

Cell wall

The outstanding difference between bacteria and mammalian cells is the tough, thick cell wall external to the cell membrane which fixes the shape of bacterial cells and gives to them their extraordinary resistance to osmotic damage. This remarkable structure is absent from mammalian cells and any agent which interfered solely with its construction would be entirely without effect on a mammalian host. Several groups of antibacterial agents exert their effects through interference with cell wall synthesis, and setting aside the special problem of hypersensitivity, the most important of them, the penicillins and cephalosporins, are amongst the most innocuous of therapeutic agents.

The walls of Gram-positive organisms consist largely of a characteristic wall component called mucopeptide, while those of Gram-negative bacteria, which are much thicker, consist of a sandwich of mucopeptide and lipoprotein. The steps by which mucopeptide is synthesized differ in detail between bacterial species but the sequence of events follows a similar general pattern.

The process begins with the conversion of natural L-alanine into the D-form and the linking of two D-alanine molecules together. Both these events are inhibited by cycloserine which is a close structural analogue of alanine. Other amino-acids are linked to the di-alanine to create a short peptide which is united with a sugar characteristic of bacterial cell wall, acetylmuramic acid. This is coupled to a molecule of acetylglucosamine and this complex constitutes the brick from which the wall is constructed. The hod which carries the brick across the cell membrane to the site of cell wall construction is a phospholipid which is released once the brick is in place and returns to carry more bricks (Fig. 12.2) until alternating acetylmuramic acid-acetylglucosamine molecules are united into long glycan strands with their trailing peptides. Layer upon layer of these strands are set down upon one another until the proper thickness of the wall is achieved. In the final step—the one which gives the wall its shape-retaining rigidity—the short peptides of one layer are fixed to the short peptides of the next (Fig. 12.2).

Since there is no analagous structure in mammalian cells the attraction of the cell wall as a prime target for antibacterial action is obvious and the possibility that structural analogues of cell wall components would prove to be potent inhibitors of cell wall synthesis has attracted a good deal of attention. The fluorination of alanine by Kollonitsch et al (1973) produced a potent bacterial inhibitor and Roche have investigated an interesting group of phosphonated oligopeptides which are potent inhibitors of cell wall synthesis (Allen et al, 1978). Cycloserine can be seen as a naturally occurring D-alanine analogue and is particularly interesting in that it exerts its inhibitory effect on cell wall synthesis by sequential blockade of both reactions concerned with the production of the alanine dimer: conversion of the natural L-form of the amino-acid to the D-form and ligation of the two molecules (Fig. 12.2).

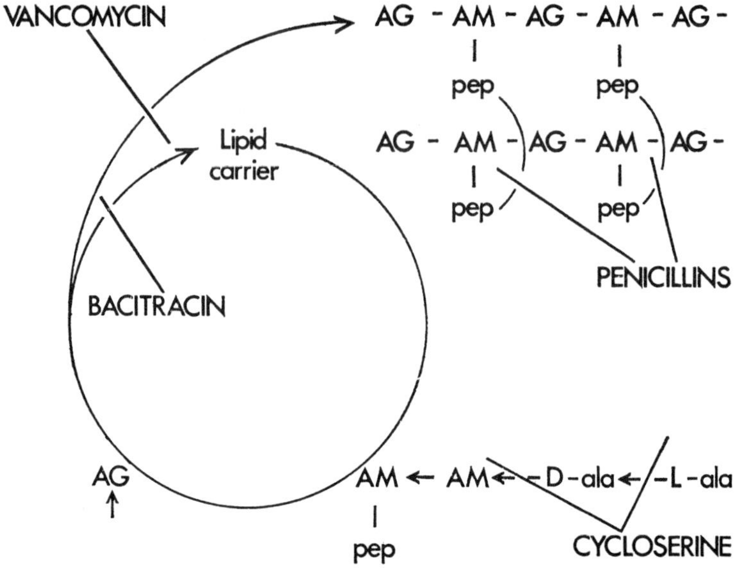

Fig. 12.2 The cell-wall consists of layers of 'glycan' strands composed of units in which N-acetylglucosamine (AG)—made from alanine (ala)—is linked to N-acetylmuramic acid (AM) with a peptide tail (pep). The units are transported to the site of insertion into the wall by a lipid carrier which returns to carry more units. The wall is made rigid by joining the peptide tails together. The points of interruption by antibiotics are shown.

Fosfomycin is an analogue of phosphoenolpyruvate which in bacteria functions as a link in the movement of N-acetylglucosamine. In mammals the role of phosphoenolpyruvate is different and fosfomycin does not interfere with peptide utilisation in man.

Vancomycin and bacitracin act on the operation and release of the lipid carrier and to the extent that this is a membrane-bound component resembling mammalian analogues it is perhaps not surprising that these agents should be the most toxic of the anti-cell wall agents.

Therapeutically much the most important antibiotics acting on the cell wall are the penicillins and cephalosporins. Benzylpenicillin, itself, is by far the most completely studied but the mode of action is believed to be essentially similar for all (Tipper, 1979). The effect of penicillins and cephalosporins is to prevent the formation of the final solidifying cross-links in the cell wall. Precisely how this is done is still not clear despite intense study for many years (Frere, 1977). On purification, the enzyme responsible for the peptide cross-linking—transpeptidase—is certainly inhibited by penicillin and in the presence of the drug uncrosslinked peptidoglycan is formed. There is, however, another enzyme—a carboxypeptidase—which cuts off the terminal alanine which is left hanging free when the peptide cross-link is formed. The precise significance of this tidying-up operation is obscure, but the carboxypeptidase is also very sensitive to penicillin. In some bacteria its inhibition appears to be without effect but in others the pair of enzymes provides another example of the need for processes to be in balance and both must operate for normal cell wall to form. Extraction of the membrane underlying the cell wall yields eight separate proteins which will bind penicillin. It has been possible to ascribe enzymic (usually carboxypeptidase) or structural roles to some of these, the most intriguing being to associate the manufacture of surface and septal wall with separate proteins (Spratt, 1975). This distinction is brought out very clearly by the morphological effects of β-lactam antibiotics.

The completed cell wall consists of a single giant bag-shaped molecule occupying the whole of the surface of the cell. For the cell to grow this tough envelope must be expanded in such a way that throughout the process its strength is preserved so that the cell does not succumb to osmotic damage, and when the time comes for division the shape of the original cell is reproduced in each of the progeny. Much elegant work has revealed a great deal about the structure and synthesis of the cell-wall polymer but the processes by which such remarkably controlled remodelling of the cell coat is achieved are at present unknown.

For the cell to grow, the bonds which give the wall its strength must be opened in order to allow the insertion of fresh components as the cell expands. That expansion of the surface cell wall and the construction and ultimate cleavage of the septum when the cell divides are to an important extent separate is shown by the effect of low concentrations of penicillins or cephalosporins which interfere with septum formation but do not otherwise interfere with cell wall synthesis sufficiently to prevent cell growth. In such conditions Gram-negative bacilli continue to grow but instead of separating into new cells, expand into longer and longer filaments. In higher concentrations of these agents the cell membrane is progressively deprived of external support as the wall weakens and in conditions of low osmolality the cell ruptures. It is this osmotic or other external force which is directly responsible for the death of susceptible cells exposed to penicillins or cephalosporins. In conditions of suitably high osmolality—such as may occur in body fluids—the cell membrane remains intact and continues to grow. Through the weakened wall it may expand into a spherical cell covered only by membrane—a *protoplast*—or one which retains some cell-wall elements—a *spheroplast*. Being highly deficient in wall components these cells are unaffected by the continuing presence of penicillin and may remain dormant until therapy is stopped when synthesis of cell wall can be resumed and infection re-emerges.

Such survival in the presence of penicillin has been held to account for the phenomenon of 'persisters', the small number of cells first described by Bigger (1944) which survive when sensitive staphylococci are exposed to concentrations of penicillin to which the majority of the bacterial cells succumb. Such organisms are not resistant in the ordinary sense of the term since on subculture their progeny respond to exposure to penicillin in just the same way: the majority die and a few survive.

Morphological and other evidence strongly suggests that the minority of cells that persist in the presence of penicillin are not all in cell wall deficient forms and that at least some of them are cells which happen to be at a particular stage of their metabolic cycle at the moment of exposure, and in that stage are not accessible to the effect of the agent (Elliott et al, 1979). The inhibitory effect of low concentrations of β-lactam antibiotics on septal synthesis and of higher concentrations on both septal and surface wall synthesis indicates that the two processes are separate but much the most convincing evidence comes from the action of agents which exert an almost pure effect on one or other process. Cephalexin and, generally the orally absorbed cephalosporins, induce only filamentation in Gram-negative bacteria in concentrations greatly above those achievable in any body fluid except urine. Conversely, mecillinam has little or no effect on division but produces serious weakness and deformity of the cells by interfering with the laying down of surface wall. Examination of the affinity of these agents for the penicillin binding proteins extracted from bacterial cell membranes shows that they are respectively specifically bound to proteins believed to be associated with wall synthesis at the two sites.

Cell membrane

Beneath the cell wall is the lipoprotein layer of the cell membrane which corresponds with the limiting membrane of mammalian cells. It is this layer that is to a large extent concerned with the control of ingress and egress of material from the cells. The simplest model of the membrane sees it as bundles of lipoprotein molecules held together by magnesium ions in such a way that gaps are left through which molecules of suitable size can move. Chelating agents which compete with the membrane for its essential magnesium, increase the permeability of the cell bringing about direct lysis or permitting more ready access. and hence greater antibacterial effect, of other agents.

Some antibiotics unite with the membrane and function as ionophores—compounds which provide a way for abnormal movement of ions through the membrane. This process has excited a great deal of biochemical interest and it appears that agents acting in this way may trap ions which are then transported within the enveloping agent across the membrane, or, like gramicidins, may wind into helical forms which join end to end to form channels which are sufficiently long to traverse the membrane and allow the ions to pass through them.

Therapeutically the most important agents which act on the membrane are the peptides. These consist of circular molecules (page 206) the attachment of which to the membrane modifies the ion flux and brings about lysis of the cell. Subinhibitory doses of colistin make *Escherichia* susceptible to penicillin and erythromycin presumably by facilitating their entry to the cell.

Above the cell membrane is the cell wall and beneath it the point of attachment of the chromosome. Interference with the construction of the membrane may, therefore, affect these adjacent structures. Bacitracin, which interferes with cell wall synthesis (page 258), does so at the level of the membrane and because of this differs from penicillins and cephalosporins, which affect only mucopeptide synthesis, in being active against protoplasts.

Novobiocin acts at a site on the cell membrane such that it affects both the synthesis of cell wall and the replication of the underlying attached chromosome. The resulting incoordination of growth produces peculiar morphological changes in staphylococci not so far seen with any other agent.

The study of the modes of action of antibiotics has contributed greatly to our understanding of cellular metabolism particularly to that of protein synthesis. Nevertheless much still remains to be done since agents which produce apparently similar effects on isolated enzyme or ribosomal systems commonly show marked differences in the degree or range of their activities against living bacteria. No doubt elucidation of the reasons for these differences will in due course be forthcoming and with that increased chance of synthesizing agents which possess precisely those properties which appear most desirable.

References

Allen J G, Atherton F R, Hall M J et al 1978 Nature 272: 56
Bigger J H 1944 Lancet 2: 497
Corcoran J W, Hahn F E (eds) 1975 Antibiotics Series Vol III: Mechanism of action of antimicrobial and antitumour agents, Springer-Verlag, New York
Crumplin G C, Smith J T 1975 Antimicrob Ag Chemother 8: 251
Franklin T J, Snow G A (1975) Biochemistry of Antimicrobial Action, 2nd edn. Halsted Press, New York
Frere J-M 1977 Biochem Pharmacol 26: 2203
Gale E F, Cundliffe E, Reynolds P E, Richmond M H, Waring M J 1972 The molecular basis of antibiotic action. Wiley, London
Hane M W 1971 J Bact 105: 46
Hitchings G H 1969 Postgrad Med J 45: Suppl Nov, 7
Kollonitsch J, Barash L, Kahan F M, Kropp H 1973 Nature 243: 346
Lill H, Lill W, Sippel A, Hartmann G 1970. In: RNA Polymerase and Transcription. Ed L Silvestri, Amsterdam, North-Holland, p 55
Poe M 1976 Science 194: 533
Pongs O, Messer W. 1976 J Molec Biol 101: 171
Spratt B G 1975 Proc Nat Acad Sci USA 72: 2999
Teraoka H 1970 Biochem Biophys Acta 213: 535
Tipper D J 1979 Rev Infect Dis 1: 39

13

Drug resistance

The adaptability of bacteria in the presence of poisonous agents has been well-known since the early days of bacteriology and a paper on this subject appeared in the first volume of the *Annales de l'Institut Pasteur*, published in 1887, under the patronage of the master himself (Kossiakoff, 1887). Ehrlich, in his pioneer work on chemotherapy at the beginning of this century, appreciated the significance of this and attempted to cure syphilis with a single massive dose. As it affects antibiotics, this problem is of exceptional magnitude, since the degree of abnormal resistance which may appear is often enormously greater than that capable of being acquired to any other type of drug.

Abnormal resistance to antibiotics and other drugs as seen in the clinical sphere may arise by selection or by adaptation.

Selection

Here no change is induced in the bacteria by exposure to the drug which eliminates the sensitive majority of the bacterial population and allows overgrowth of a minority of resistant cells. Cross infection and the maintenance by widespread use of the drug of a selection pressure in favour of the ordinarily disadvantaged resistant cells play crucial roles in the emergence of such resistant strains. The rapidity and extent of the change vary widely among different antibiotics. An organism may become highly resistant to streptomycin overnight ('single step' mutation), or within a few days to erythromycin or novobiocin, but to most other antibiotics the development of resistance is a more gradual process. In some cases the number of steps involved may be so great, and the increase in resistance with each step so slight, that the development of resistance may appear to be an almost continuous process. To some antibiotics, no substantial degree of resistance has developed: these include the peptides and vancomycin.

Drug degradation

Over comparatively recent years it has emerged that most clinically important resistance is due not to modifications in the cell biochemistry such as those already described, but to protection of the unmodified economy of the cells from attack by antibiotic degradation. In this way the cell incurs none of the potential penalties of having to alter processes that have presumably evolved to serve its needs optimally and the growth, behaviour and virulence of the cells, apart from their ability to degrade the drug, appear entirely normal. The first and best known example of this form of resistance was provided by penicillin-resistant *Staphylococcus aureus*. The normal virulence of this organism, which became the major scourge of hospitals in the 1950s, contrasts sharply with the behaviour of staphylococci 'trained' to resistance to penicillin which are poor shadows of the wild sensitive strains.

It has since emerged that enzymes capable of destroying penicillins and the related cephalosporins can be synthesized by a large variety of species. These enzymes, collectively called β-lactamases, are classified according to their ability to utilize certain penicillins and cephalosporins as substrate (page 105) and their synthesis is the major cause of resistance to these agents in both Gram-positive and Gram-negative bacteria.

Reliance on drug destruction for resistance is, of course, not without its hazards since the organism remains intrinsically vulnerable to the drug and absolutely dependent on high and rapid activity of the enzyme. *B. anthracis*, for example, is so susceptible to penicillin that production of modest amounts of β-lactamase will not protect it from the drug's action. In addition, there is the possibility of finding or synthesizing related antibiotics that retain antibacterial activity but are insusceptible to enzyme degradation. This possibility has been pursued with great success in the production of the β-lactamase resistant penicillins (page 73) and cephalosporins (page 104).

Alternatively, there are compounds which have little antibacterial activity but bind strongly to the enzymes, thus allowing agents to which the organism remains intrinsically sensitive to exert its normal effect. So far this principle has not been exploited therapeutically to a useful degree, but the discovery of such compounds as clavulanic acid, a naturally occurring potent inhibitor of a broad range of β-lactamases, raises the possibility that the concomitant use of such agents will restore the original sensitivity of β-lactamase producing organisms.

Resistance to other antibiotics can also depend on drug inactivation. That in staphylococci to chloramphenicol is due to an enzyme which acetylates the antibiotic (page 157) and enzymes which inactive aminoglycosides (page 137) are responsible for the great bulk of clinically important resistance to this group of drugs. These enzymes, like the β-lactamases, show a range of substrate specificities for different aminoglycosides by which they are classified (page 138). Even in the case of streptomycin, where mutation leading to drug-resistant modification of the ribosome is a relatively common event, the majority of organisms encountered in practice owe their resistance not to this mechanism but to the synthesis of a streptomycin-degrading enzyme. The possibility that appropriate chemical modification could produce derivatives resistant to bacterial degradation has been responsible for much activity in the semi-synthetic aminoglycoside field.

Cross-resistance

Depending on the substrate specificity of the enzymes they synthesize, bacteria can be resistant to several aminoglycosides and other 'cross-resistances' are seen in organisms trained to grow in different aminoglycosides. 'Cross-resistance' is also seen between other agents where the resistance mechanism is shared. Thus bacteria which have developed resistance to one sulphonamide will show a corresponding increase in resistance to all sulphonamides. Similarly there is almost complete cross-resistance between the different tetracycline antibiotics although minocycline is an exception (page 170). The macrolides are in a special category. Thus strains of staphylococci which have developed resistance by passage in one of the macrolides *in vitro* usually show a similar increase in resistance to all other members of the group. On the other hand, erythromycin-resistant staphylococci isolated from clinical infections are fequently sensitive to spiramycin and oleandomycin and exhibit a special form of inducible resistance (page 185).

Adaptation

It has been fashionable to attribute all drug resistance in a previously sensitive culture to mutation, and many ingenious methods have been devised to prove that this is so: among these perhaps the most convincing is the use of replica plating by Lederberg & Lederberg (1952) to prove the presence of resistant bacterial cells before exposure to an antibiotic. It should nevertheless be recognized that Hinshelwood and his colleagues (Dean & Hinshelwood, 1964) have long been publishing studies providing evidence that increased bacterial resistance to various noxious agents, including some antibiotics, can arise by a process of adaptation. Such adaptive resistance, developed in response to exposure to the drug, has been generally regarded as a laboratory artefact partly because the steps by which resistance changes are generally small and partly because organisms 'trained' to high degrees of resistance by serial passage in progressively increasing concentrations of the drug are often defective by comparison with their sensitive parents in that properties such as growth rate, colony size, pigment production and virulence are reduced.

It is now plain that adaptive resistance is important in at least two respects. In the first place antibiotics can often be shown to exert an inhibitory effect on bacteria in concentrations well below the conventional MIC—the concentration called by Lorian (1975) the minimum antibacterial concentration (MAC). The difference between the MAC and the concentration that inhibits growth of the organism overnight (MIC) is due to adaptive resistance. The potential clinical importance of this is that the concentration which suppresses growth for 8 hours (the normal interdose interval) may be therapeutically more relevant than the higher concentration that suppresses growth overnight. The clearest therapeutic importance of adaptive resistance comes with the aminoglycosides, notably gentamicin, where the therapeutic ratio is small and a relatively minor increase in resistance to the drug threatens effective and safe therapy. Such increase has been seen principally in staphylococci exposed to topical aminoglycosides but also in enterobacteria recovered from the urine of treated patients. A special and notable feature of such resistance is that it affects not only the inducing agent, in this case gentamicin, but other aminoglycosides and the degree of resistance to new agents such as amikacin may be greater than that to gentamicin itself.

Biochemistry of resistance

Resistance arises either from a change in the target within the cells such that the effect of the antibiotic is nullified, or by exclusion of the antibiotic from the still sensitive target, either by decreased permeability of the cell to the drug or by enzymic destruction of the drug before it can reach the sensitive target. Antibiotics act on various functions of the cells including protein and nucleic acid synthesis and specific enzyme systems (Chapter 12). Many of these processes are central to the cell's economy and cannot be drastically altered in order to render them insusceptible to antibiotic attack without also rendering the cells inoperative. It is presumably for this reason that resistance to tetracycline due to a change in that part of the protein synthetic mechanism affected by the drug has not been encountered. Further details of the changes associated with resistance to specific agents are given in the relevant chapters but good examples of the kind of changes that occur are provided by streptomycin, rifampicin and trimethoprim.

Classical single step mutation to high level resistance, such as that seen when strains of *Escherichia coli* initially sensitive to 1 μg streptomycin per ml require 10 mg per ml to inhibit their growth, results from a change in the chromosome at the streptomycin locus which codes for a ribosomal protein to which streptomycin attaches, such that the ribosome no longer binds the drug and is consequently not affected by it. Rifampicin acts on RNA synthesis and in resistant mutants there is a modified RNA polymerase. In trimethoprim-resistant organisms the target enzyme of the drug, dihydrofolate reductase, is modified and no longer binds the drug. An analagous state exists in sulphonamide-resistant strains where the target enzyme is synthesized in both the modified, and hence resistant, and the native sensitive form but the sensitive enzyme is inactivated.

Drug exclusion

The best example of resistance due to drug exclusion is provided by tetracycline, but it is probable that an element of relative impermeability plays a part in resistance to other agents even where the major mechanism of resistance is different.

Genetics of resistance

Exposure of *E. coli* to streptomycin in appropriate conditions will allow the outgrowth of highly resistant cells which have undergone a spontaneous change of genetic information such that they synthesize a new ribosomal protein which no longer binds the drug. That genetic change occurs in the bacterial chromosome but in many cases the new genetic information is produced in the cell not by mutation of chromosomal genes but by acquisition of the new genetic information in the form of extra-chromosomal plasmids.

These can confer all sorts of properties on the recipient cell, including the ability to synthesize toxins, but they are of special importance in relation to antibiotic resistance. They are acquired in the case of Gram-positive cocci through the transfer of genetic information from one cell to another by bacteriophage (transduction) and in the case of Gram-negative rods by physical contact between cells—which need not be of the same species—during conjugation. These processes and their molecular biology have been the subject of intense activity for some years now and have generated an enormous and complex literature. We propose to review the subject very briefly; those interested to know more might begin with Falkow (1975) and Bukhari et al (1977).

Transduction

The transmission of capacity to produce penicillinase by a phage (transduction) to a penicillin-sensitive staphylococcus was first demonstrated by Ritz & Baldwin (1958). Since then the same mechanism has been shown capable of transmitting resistance to streptomycin, tetracycline, chloramphenicol and macrolides (page 186). Co-transduction of resistances to two antibiotics can occur, as does that of the two properties of penicillinase formation and mercury resistance, which appear therefore to be genetically linked. There are strong reasons for believing that the elements transduced are usually plasmids although in appropriate circumstances chromosomal material can also be transduced.

Transduction has also been achieved *in vivo* as in the convincing experiments of Novick & Morse (1967). They inoculated mice intravenously with cultures of two strains of staphylococcus, a lysogenic strain possesing erythromycin resistance and another resistant to streptomycin, and recovered from the kidneys organisms resistant to both antibiotics in numbers much greater when the mice were also treated with both. Linked penicillin-erythromycin resistance was also transduced *in vivo*.

It is not certainly known whether, and if so to what extent, transduction is responsible for antibiotic resistance in clinical isolates of staphylococci, but the probability is very high that it plays a major part. Lacey (1971) achieved transference of resistance to neomycin in *Staph. aureus* to a sensitive strain not only in mixed culture but on the skin surface of volunteers, and adduces reasons for attributing this to transduction.

Drug resistance can also be transduced in various enterobacteria. Owing to the limited host range of phages, such transduction is for the most part intra-species, but the mechanism of transfer now to be described can operate between organisms of many different genera.

Conjugation

'Infectious' resistance of this type was first observed in Japan in 1959 (Watanabe, 1963) and reported in Europe first by Datta (1962) in England and by Lebek (1963) in Germany. The earlier studies showed that in a mixed culture of Shigella or Salmonella possessing multiple resistance (e.g. to sulphonamide, tetracycline, chloramphenicol and streptomycin) and a sensitive *E. coli*, this resistance may be transferred to a minority of cells of the latter organism, usually en bloc but sometimes in part. This organism can then retransfer resistance so that it spreads rapidly through the pathogenic population. Clear clinical evidence of such transfer within the human bowel was obtained. It is now known that transfer can occur between organisms of all genera of the enterobacteria and the transfer of resistance to *Serratia marcescens*, *Vibrio cholerae* and *Pasteurella pestis* among others has also been observed. The plasmids determining such resistance can only be transferred to another cell when a second element is present, the 'resistance transfer factor' (R factor) (Anderson, 1965).

A finding of outstanding importance has been the relative ease with which segments of DNA which have the same terminations can be substituted for one another. This process, utilising restriction endonucleases, has enabled plasmids to acquire and exchange information with one another and with bacterial chromosomes to the point at which they have assembled a remarkable assortment of genetic information, frequently freely transmissible to other cells, even those of other species, not the least of which is resistance to several unrelated antibiotics. This situation is quite different from that described as 'cross-resistance' where the shared mechanism confers resistance to related agents. In the case of the plasmid, distinct pieces of information have been collected together like beads on a string which confers a package of resistances which have different underlying mechanisms. The importance of this—in addition to the obvious therapeutic problem of multiple antibiotic resistance—is that exposure to any of the agents to which the strain is resistant will serve to select it from the normally sensitive population.

Plasmids have been classified according to a number of features and this makes it possible to trace their passage from one organism or species to another. Generally speaking the information conferred is the ability to synthesize antibiotic-degrading enzymes but in the case of tetracycline it is the information required to establish the permeability block that is the basis of resistance to that group of agents. Characterization of plasmids and of the antibiotic-degrading enzymes for which they code makes it possible to compare those found in different organisms. Thus, an organism acquiring plasmid-borne resistance to ampicillin can be shown to produce a β-lactamase and the same enzyme specified by the same plasmid can be demonstrated in different species. The β-lactamase responsible for the relatively recently observed ampicillin resistance in *H. influenzae* (Sykes et al, 1975) and probably also that acquired by penicillinase-producing gonococci is the familiar TEM enzyme of the enterobacteria. Transmissible chloramphenicol resistance is due to the formation of chloramphenicol acetyltransferase and the enzyme responsible for resistance in staphylococci is again indistinguishable from that obtained from a resistant *E. coli* carrying an R plasmid. Transmissible resistance to aminoglycosides also results from acquisition of the genetic information required to synthesize aminoglycoside degrading enzymes.

It is indeed fortunate that in the absence of further exposure to any of the drugs involved this form of resistance is often spontaneously lost within weeks or months of its acquisition. In view of the ease with which transfer can be obtained, the speed with which it spreads through the bacterial population and the promiscuity with which conjugation occurs between different bacterial species, it can well be imagined that but for this, resistance to commonly used drugs would by now be almost universal. Exposure to acridine dyes and some other agents will 'cure' bacteria of carried plasmids but no way of utilizing this approach to the problem of plasmid-borne resistance for therapeutic purposes has yet been found.

The epidemiological importance of the capacity to transfer multiple antibiotic resistance between bacterial species can hardly be overemphasized and it has emerged that plasmids in one way or another have played a dominant role in the production of resistant strains. Spread of these strains, however, requires antibiotic exposure to select them from the sensitive majority and hygienic conditions that encourage the transfer to fresh susceptible subjects. It is the changing interplay between these different factors that makes the epidemiology of antibiotic resistance so complex and any but the most general predictions so uncertain.

Epidemiology of antibiotic resistance

Staphylococcus aureus

Rare strains of *Staph. aureus* isolated before the introduction of penicillin formed penicillinase. The increasing prevalence of such strains in the hospital environment after penicillin had come into general use was first described (see previous editions) by our late co-author, Mary Barber: the frequency of their occurrence was 14, 38 and 59 per cent in the successive years 1946–48. During the next few years similar reports followed from hospitals all over the world and by about 1950 the majority of staphylococcal infections in most general hospitals were penicillin-resistant. Resistance has since become increasingly common in strains from the general population.

Resistance subsequently appeared in certain staphylococci to all the major antibiotics. Streptomycin and tetracyclines were first affected: triple resistance to these two and to penicillin has been common in epidemic strains, and resistance to tetracycline came to be regarded as the hallmark of a dangerous strain. Chloramphenicol resistance also appeared early, but diminished in frequency when consumption diminished following recognition of marrow toxicity. Similar resistance to erythromycin has been observed to spread rapidly in hospitals where the agent was much used, and to decline (less rapidly) when it was withdrawn—clear examples of the role of antibiotic usage in maintaining the prevalence of such strains.

It is not to be supposed that any staphylococcus can acquire these characters. Multiple resistance is largely confined to a few notorious types in phage groups I and III which are also those commonly responsible for epidemics of staphylococcal sepsis. Multiple resistance is also linked with mercury resistance and with high penicillinase production. The selective effect of the therapeutic use of other antibiotics as well as penicillin has in fact been to bring into prominence what must have been an originally very small minority of staphylococci of a few phage types.

Experience up to the time of the introduction of the first of the penicillin-resistant penicillins had led to the expectation that the staphylococcus would continue to exhibit its capacity to become resistant to each new agent in turn. These expectations appeared to be fulfilled as the prevalence of methicillin-resistant staphylococci rose in the U.K. from less than 0.1 per cent in 1960 to 4–5 per cent in 1969 and in Denmark reached a record 40 per cent. In fact, in many places methicillin-resistant staphylococci have never been a serious problem and even where they were common their prevalence has declined. It may be that the peculiar nature of methicillin resistance and the need for special properties in staphylococci to exploit it has protected us so far. Some experiences with streptococci and Neisseria, however, caution us that the prevalence of resistance can remain low for years before increasing to high levels over relatively short periods.

Streptococci

Strains of both *Str. pyogenes* and *Str. pneumoniae* resistant to sulphonamides were beginning to interfere with the efficacy of treatment and to cause grave apprehension for the future when penicillin came to the rescue. *Str. pyogenes* appears incapable of developing resistance to penicillin, and resistance in pneumococci was first reported from the Antipodes, but has since been occasionally encountered elsewhere and resistance to tetracycline and to macrolides (page 184) now occurs in both.

The prevalence of resistance to tetracycline remained very low in both haemolytic streptococci and pneumococci, despite the widespread use of the agent until the early 1960s when within five years it rose to 44 per cent in strains recovered from patients attending ENT clinics. Notwithstanding what has been said about the disadvantage suffered by resistant as compared with the fully sensitive parent strains, as in the case of staphylococci and enterobacteria, the prevalence of resistant strains, once established, has been slow to decline. A survey covering much of the U.K. in 1975 showed that in some parts of the country the prevalence of tetracycline resistance in haemolytic streptococci was still as high as 50 per cent (Report, 1977).

The capacity of the haemolytic streptococcus and the pneumococcus to become resistant is not in doubt, therefore, and the contrast between their behaviour and the rapidity and ease of development of resistance in the staphylococcus is all the more remarkable. Still more remarkable is the contrast in behaviour between the two pathogenic Neisseria.

Neisseria

Sulphonamide resistance appeared promptly in *N. gonorrhoeae* and was eventually followed after many years by the development of a degree of resistance to penicillin that was unimpressive by laboratory standards but sufficient to compromise treatment (page 422). After a delay of many more years these difficulties have been greatly compounded by the acquisition by rare strains of *N. gonorrhoeae* of the plasmid coding for the TEM β-lactamase of enterobacteria.

In contrast to the prompt appearance of sulphonamide resistance in *N. gonorrhoeae*, cerebrospinal fever remained for many years the only acute bacterial infection for which treatment with sulphonamides remained equal or superior to that with antibiotics. Sulphonamide resistance of a degree precluding successful treatment was first reported in 1963 in a Naval Training Depot in California. A report from the same State extended these observations to civilians and by 1968 the majority of strains isolated from a large epidemic at Fort Lamy (Chad) were sulphonamide-resistant (Lefevre et al, 1969). Resistant strains have also been found in Norway, Germany, Britain and other countries. Plainly freedom from resistance for many years is not a guarantee that it will not appear or that the prevalence of resistance, once established, will rise gradually.

All the Los Angeles strains were sensitive to penicillin and to ampicillin, with which the patients were treated. It is not to be expected that this alternative treatment will remain effective indefinitely since it was shown long ago that meningococci could be trained to a high degree of penicillin resistance, not only *in vitro* but in experimentally infected mice. With the gonococcus as an example, resistance may be expected in the meningococcus at some time in the future.

Enterobacteria

These form a group among which apparently increasing antibiotic resistance presents difficulties only exceeded by similar changes in staphylococci. No purpose would be served by reviewing the extensive and confused literature of this subject. Several processes have evidently been at work. Many authors have found that isolates in successive periods of the normally more drug-sensitive species, notably *E. coli*, show an increasing frequency of resistance although in recent years amongst urinary pathogens, there has been little change (Grüneberg, 1980). Secondly, the therapeutic use of antibiotics has favoured the survival and spread of organisms possessing a high degree of natural resistance, notably Aerobacter, Pseudomonas, and some species of Proteus. It seems impossible to determine whether organisms of this kind are more drug-resistant now than they were originally, but this seems highly probable. A good deal of multiple resistance in intestinal bacteria has been acquired by conjugation and in a number of important instances the responsible plasmids have had their origins in animal strains.

Transmissible resistance

It seems strange that not until 1966 was any serious attempt made to discover how much drug resistance in human intestinal bacteria generally is transmissible. From this time onwards a series of studies of strains from various sources has yielded remarkably consistent results. The proportion of drug-resistant strains has varied with both species and source (hospital strains being more often resistant than those from elsewhere), but a constant finding has been that transference has been achieved from over 50 per cent of cultures so tested. The organisms examined include Salmonella species, *Shigella sonnei*, *E. coli*, Klebsiella and Proteus.

Several of these studies have shown a higher frequency of transmissible resistance, which is also more often multiple, in organisms from patients under treatment with antibiotics. This emerges from a comparison by Dailey et al (1972) of the intestinal flora of infants in a well baby and a high risk nursery. The results of Datta et al (1971) and others show the capacity of different drugs for selecting resistance. In the faeces of women treated for urinary tract infections, sulphonamide or ampicillin caused moderate increases in the frequence of resistance in *E. coli* only to the drug given, but during tetracycline treatment resistance to tetracycline itself was invariable, and usually accompanied by resistance to other drugs as well.

Resistance transfer has been thought of as occurring only in the bowel, where purely physical factors impede it, although it unquestionably occurs. It is becoming recognized that it can occur, perhaps with more facility, elsewhere in the body. Roe et al (1971) have shown that it happens in burns and Witchitz & Chabbert (1972) point out that peritoneal dialysis fluid is an ideal medium; in a patient undergoing this and being treated with gentamicin, strains of four different species carrying an R factor determining resistance to this and several other drugs were recovered at different times from the dialysate. Other organisms carrying this factor were subsequently recovered from patients in this intensive care unit.

These studies have transformed our outlook on drug resistance in human enterobacteria and related organisms. Most of this is transmissible and much of it may have arisen by transference rather than by exposure to the drug itself. Although its existence severely limits the possibilities of antibacterial therapy, it is reassuring that of 95 strains of *Ps. aeruginosa* and 429 of enterobacteria from various infections in a general hospital, there were none which were not sensitive to at least one applicable antibiotic (Anderson et al, 1972).

Role of animal strains

The study of farm animals owes much to the alarming revelations of Anderson and his colleagues beginning in 1965 (Anderson, 1968). The later papers in this series deal with an epidemic of type 29 *S. typhimurium* infection in calves which lasted several years, during which the strain developed transferable resistance successively to six or more drugs. It also caused at least 500 human infections, its source being made certain not only by its phage type but by its resistance pattern, sometimes including furazolidone, a drug used only in animals. The main danger apprehended from such human infection by resistant animal pathogens was the transmission of resistance via human *E. coli* to organisms of the enteric group, notably *S. typhi*: the possible prospect of resistance in this species to both chloramphenicol and ampicillin was disastrous. Again strangely, transferable resistance to chloramphenicol in *S. typhi* remained almost unknown until an epidemic strain possessing it appeared in Mexico (Anderson & Smith, 1972).

At the same time the frequent existence of multiple infectious resistance in *E. coli* from calves and pigs, and less commonly lambs and fowls, was attributed to antibiotic feed supplementation, and a campaign to restrict this culminated in the adoption of the report of the Swann Committee (Report, 1969) which proposed that the use of medical antibiotics for this purpose be prohibited.

The extent of the contribution made by animal organisms to infectious resistance in the human intestinal flora has been the subject of much dispute. There is no question of the capacity of animal *Salmonella* to colonize the human bowel but any large scale transmission of resistance from animals to man must be via commensals such as *E. coli* which are found in meat and meat products and can be widely spread in the kitchen to other foods that are consumed uncooked (Shooter et al, 1970; Cooke et al, 1970). Unequivocal evidence of implantation from this source in the human bowel has not been obtained. The more frequent occurrence of resistant *E. coli* in country than in urban populations (Moorhouse, 1971; Linton et al, 1972) has been adduced as an argument in this connection, but it must be remembered that the farming community handle antibiotics in preparing supplemented feeds, and the effect may be a direct one on their own flora. Schön et al (1972), while confirming such findings, found an even higher frequency of resistance in workers in antibiotic production plants and in fodder plants where antibiotic supplements are mixed. It is interesting in this connection that Guinée et al (1970) found transmissible resistance in *E. coli* to be as frequent in vegetarians and in infants under six months as in either of two groups of meat eaters; indeed in one of these groups the frequency was decidedly lower.

Evidence has also been sought from deliberate implantation experiments such as those of Williams Smith (1969). Resistant strains of *E. coli* (from pigs, oxen and fowls) swallowed in large numbers by a human subject often failed to establish themselves at all, although two human strains were recoverable for periods up to 35 days later, and in the few instances in which transfer of resistance from an animal to the native human strain occurred, the resistant variant disappeared within a few days. Wiedeman et al (1970), although using a resistant human strain, obtained similar results.

This question can only be decided by a large extension of such studies as these, but they need to be so laborious that reluctance to pursue them is not surprising. An implanted strain can only be recognized serologically, and if only five colonies are examined there can be no certainty either that it is not present among others or that it was not there originally. Nevertheless the emergence of resistance in animal enterobacteria presents a hazard both to animals and to man and if it is to be controlled two other measures in addition to prohibition of the use of therapeutic antibiotics as feed additives seem called for.

The first is hygienic: the root cause of widespread animal salmonellosis is bad methods of animal husbandry, notably the wholesale trade in very young calves, conducted under conditions strongly favouring the spread of infection. Secondly, resistance in these organisms is attributable at least in part to therapeutic use; that to ampicillin which appeared in 1964 was clearly the result of attempts to control enteritis in calves with therapeutic doses. While feed supplementation has been prohibited, therapeutic use remains entirely uncontrolled, and is said often to be misdirected and ineffective. The single step of prohibiting the administration of chloramphenicol to animals would afford some reassurance, but the right of the medical profession to some say in the treatment of animals, which are an important source of human disease, although repeatedly asserted has never been acknowledged.

Control of the emergence of antibiotic-resistant strains is one of the important goals of antibiotic prescribing policies, the general aspects of which are discussed in the next chapter.

References

Anderson E S 1965 Brit Med J 2: 1289
Anderson E S 1968 Brit Med J 3: 333
Anderson E S, Smith H R 1972 Brit Med J 3: 329

Anderson F M, Datta N, Shaw E J 1972 Brit Med J 3: 82
Bukhari A I, Shapiro J A, Adhya S L 1977 In: DNA insertion elements, plasmids and episomes, Cold Spring Harbour Laboratory, New York
Cooke E M, Shooter R A, Kumar P J et al 1970 Lancet 1: 436
Dailey K M, Sturtevant A B Jr, Feary T W 1972 J Pediat 80: 198
Datta N 1962 J Hyg (Lond) 60: 301
Datta N, Faiers M C, Reeves D S et al 1971 Lancet 1: 312
Dean A R C, Hinshelwood C 1964 Nature Lond 202: 1046
Falkow S 1975 In: Infectious multiple drug resistance. Pion, London
Grüneberg R N 1980 J Clin Path 33: 853
Guinée P, Ugueto N, van Leeuwen N 1970 Appl Microbiol 20: 531
Kossiakoff M G 1887 Ann Inst Pasteur 1: 465
Lacey R W 1971 J Med Microbiol 4: 73
Lebek K 1963 Zbl Bakt I Abt Orig 188: 494
Lederberg J, Lederberg E M 1952 J Bact 63: 399
Lefevre M, Sirol J, Vandekerkove M, Faucon R 1969 Bull Wld Hlth Org 40: 331
Linton K B, Lee P A, Richmond M H et al 1972 J Hyg Lond 70: 99
Lorian V 1975 Antimicrob Ag Chemother 7: 864
Moorhouse E 1971 Ann NY Acad Sci 182: 65
Novick R S, Morse S I 1967 J Exp Med 125: 45
Report 1977 Brit Med J 1: 131
Report 1969 Joint Committee on the Use of Antibiotics in Animal Husbandry & Veterinary Medicine, Her Majesty's Stationery Office, London
Ritz H L, Baldwin J N 1958 Bact Proc p 40
Roe E, Jones R J, Lowbury E J L 1971 Lancet 1: 149
Schön E, Wagner V, Wagnerova W et al 1972 Rev Czech Med 18: 1
Shooter R A, Cooke E M, Rousseau S A, Breaden A L 1970 Lancet 2: 226
Sykes R B, Matthew M, O'Callaghan C H 1975 J Med Microbiol 8: 437
Watanabe T 1963 Bact Rev 27: 87
Wiedemann B, Knothe H, Doll E 1970 Zbl Bakt I Orig 213: 183
Williams Smith H 1969 Lancet 1: 1174
Witchitz J L, Chabbert Y A 1972 Ann Inst Pasteur 122: 367

Part II

14

General principles of treatment

Not one of the drugs with which this book is concerned can be administered without some risk of ill effects. Many of them are costly, and many will preserve their value only if they are used with discrimination. For these and other reasons it is unjustifiable to prescribe a powerful antibacterial drug for most trivial infections. It is impossible to be fully dogmatic on this point, because admittedly some specially predisposing factor may convert a minor into a major infection unless steps are taken to prevent this. Such situations are exceptional, and it must regretfully be admitted that much prescribing for minor conditions goes on unnecessarily. If figures of consumption in relation to population were available, it would doubtless be found that some countries sin more gravely in this way than others.

Prescribing habits are revealed in a brilliant and tragic light in reports of fatalities from the administration of antibiotics. An astonishing proportion of deaths from penicillin shock have followed an injection given for what seems an inadequate indication, including even a common cold, toothache and a sprained toe. Likewise, some deaths from marrow aplasia have been caused by chloramphenicol administered for minor catarrhal conditions: in some instances this has even been self-administration from a left-over bottle kept in the bathroom. These are extreme examples, but they can be supported by thousands of others in which more harm than good has been done, and by untold millions in which the drug has merely been wasted because the condition treated is by nature insusceptible to it.

Clinical diagnosis

Successful chemotherapy must be rational, and rational treatment demands a diagnosis. This may only be provisional, and it may later be proved wrong, but the treatment chosen should be based on some explicit assumption as to the nature of the disease process. This may or may not carry with it an implication that the cause is a particular micro-organism.

Bacteriological diagnosis

This is in a sense more important, because treatment, to be successful, must be aimed at the micro-organism and not at the disease as such. There are fortunately many diseases which have only one microbic cause: if a clinical diagnosis of erysipelas, scarlet fever, typhoid fever, typhus or anthrax can be made, the microbic diagnosis is implicit in the clinical, and furthermore all the organisms concerned here are regularly susceptible to certain antibiotics. On the other hand pneumonia, meningitis, urinary tract infections and wound infections can be caused by any of a number of different bacteria, and the most astute clinician may sometimes be wrong if he has to guess with which of these he is dealing.

It is here that any writer on this subject is faced with his greatest difficulty. Given a patient in a hospital with a good laboratory service, a bacteriological diagnosis should soon be forthcoming. Where laboratory facilities are distant or even non-existent, how is treatment to be directed? It must be insisted that in the more serious of these infections of multiple causation, certainly in meningitis, suspected septicaemia or severe pneumonia, a bacteriological diagnosis must at all costs be made, but for the patient whose life is not in danger, it may often be necessary to dispense with laboratory aid. The choice of treatment may then be based on past experience in similar situations or on bacteriological guesswork. Some attempt will be made in this book to point to probabilities in the commoner of these situations.

Sensitivity tests

A simple bacteriological diagnosis is not always enough. If the organism is a staphylococcus or one of the tougher coliform bacilli, there is no guarantee that it will be sensitive to the drug of obvious choice or indeed to any of those which would naturally be preferred for their usual efficacy, ease of administration and freedom from toxicity. Here again it may be a counsel of perfection to advise that an appropriate range of sensitivity tests be carried out, but there can be no certainty of effect unless this is done. Fortunately not all pathogenic bacteria are so unpredictable, and it is helpful to the clinician to know which should regularly be susceptible and which he should mistrust.

Choice of drug

This depends in the first place on the causative organism being sensitive to the drug chosen. A comprehensive statement of normal sensitivities is given in Table 14.1.

There are few diagnoses which point unequivocally to a single drug for treatment. There is usually a choice, and it may be of either of two kinds.

Some infections, such as those caused by pneumococci and haemolytic streptococci, respond to a variety of drugs, including sulphonamides (usually), penicillin, and several other antibiotics. Because of the certainty and rapidity of its action, its harmlessness (except in sensitized patients), and incidentally its cheapness, penicillin is to be preferred for these infections. A suitable alternative in a sensitized patient would be erythromycin, a cephalosporin or cotrimoxazole (sulphamethoxazole + trimethoprim).

The second kind of choice is between a relatively harmless but less efficacious drug and one which is more potent but also more potentially toxic. This choice must take into account the severity of the condition, since naturally in a desperate situation risks not otherwise justifiable may rightly be taken, and the likelihood that toxic effects will be produced. A vital factor in this is renal function: to the extent that this is already impaired, so do the chances increase of further renal damage by nephrotoxic drugs and of damage to the eighth nerve by those which are ototoxic. Adequate laboratory control of treatment, referred to in Chapter 27, can be a valuable safeguard against these effects.

Dosage and route of administration

The object of systemic treatment is to attain a drug concentration in the blood and tissues which is calculated to exert the effect desired, and to maintain this, either continuously or with only short intermissions, until the infection has been overcome. To devise effective treatment it is necessary to know (1) the minimum concentration of the drug necessary to inhibit or kill the infecting organism; (2) the concentration attained in the blood after a given single dose (which should exceed (1) by several-fold for most of the time between one dose and the next), and (3) the rate of elimination of the drug, on which the frequency of dosage must depend. This question therefore involves two other large subjects, the sensitivity of different microbic species, and the pharmacological behaviour of the drugs concerned, both of which are dealt with elsewhere in this book.

When there is a choice between the oral and parenteral routes of administration (as there is, for instance, for sulphonamides, penicillin and tetracyclines) the latter may be preferred in severely ill patients for the greater certainty of its effect, since the whole dose must be absorbed, whereas the whole of an oral dose never is; or to initiate treatment, since its effect is immediate. If the oral route only is used, a 'loading' dose larger than those which follow may be advantageous, particularly with drugs which are more slowly and incompletely absorbed.

Necessary accompanying treatment

There are many kinds of condition in which chemotherapy cannot be expected to do the whole job of getting the patient well. It is most successful in acute uncomplicated infections, and least in those predisposed to by some structural abnormality. An obstructive lesion of the urinary tract or the bronchial dilatation and mucosal changes of bronchiectasis will cause the infection to recur unless they can be dealt with surgically. Chemotherapy does not obviate the necessity for draining an abscess or removing sequestra or calculi. General causes of diminished resistance to infection—nutritional, metabolic or due to disorders of blood formation—also require attention.

A minor example of accessory treatment which is often neglected is the control of urinary pH at the optimum for the drug administered in urinary tract infections. This is fully discussed in Chapter 21.

Laboratory control of the effects of treatment

Whether treatment is succeeding is best judged by clinical criteria, but it is also useful to know whether the infecting organism has been eliminated: this is particularly helpful in deciding how long treatment should continue. Repeated cultures are therefore sometimes indicated if facilities for them are available. They are more decidedly called for when treatment is *not* succeeding, because one cause of failure is the replacement of the original sensitive organism by a resistant one requiring a different drug.

A more difficult service perhaps not within the competence of every laboratory is the assay of antibiotics in body fluids. This may be desirable to verify either that the concentration attained is adequate, or that it is not excessive. In the blood the level may prove inadequate if absorption from the alimentary tract is poor, or if long intervals between injections are adopted: in the cerebro-spinal fluid in meningitis treated without intrathecal injections it is reassuring to know that enough antibiotic is

Table 14.1 Sensitivity of important pathogenic bacteria to the principal antibiotics. Usual minimum inhibitory concentration (μg/ml)

	Benzyl penicillin	Cloxacillin/ Flucloxacillin	Ampicillin Amoxycillin	Carbenicillin	Cephaloridine	Cefuroxime	Cefoxitin	Erythromycin	Clindamycin	Fusidate	Tetracycline	Chloramphenicol	Streptomycin	Amikacin	Gentamicin	Polymyxin
Staph. aureus a.	0.03	0.12	0.06	0.5	0.12	1	4	0.12	0.1-1	0.06	0.12	4	2	2	0.06	32
Staph. aureus b.	R	0.25	R	R	5	1	4	0.12	0.1-1	0.06	0.12	4	2	2	0.06	32
Str. pyogenes	0.01	0.06	0.03	0.25	0.01	0.03	0.5	0.03	0.03	8	0.25	2	32	R	8	R
Str. faecalis	2	32	1	64	16	R	R	0.5	4-16	4	0.5	2	32	R	4	R
Str. pneumoniae	0.01	0.25	0.06	0.5	0.03	0.03	1	0.03	0.03	8	0.25	2	64	R	16	R
Cl. welchii	0.12	1	0.25	0.25	0.5	2	2	2	0.03-1	0.25	0.25	4	R	R	R	R
B. anthracis	0.01	0.25	0.06	0.25	0.12			0.25	0.1	0.5	0.12	4	1		0.06	R
Ery. insidiosa	0.03	0.25	0.12	0.5	0.25	1-8		0.06		0.12	0.12	8	16		R	R
L. monocytogenes	0.25	4	0.5	2	1	R		0.25		16	0.25	8	2		0.12	R
A. israeli	0.06	0.25	0.06		0.01			0.12		0.5	2	2	16			R
Myco. tuberculosis	R	R	R	R	10	R		R		64	10	30	1	2.5	5	R
N. gonorrhoeae	0.01	0.5	0.04	0.01	0.2-8	0.06	0.25	0.06	4	0.5	1	1	4	32	2	R
N. meningitidis	0.03	0.5	0.06	0.06	0.1-1	0.06	0.25	0.5		0.12	1	1	1		2	R
H. influenzae	0.5-2	16	0.25	1	8	0.5	4	1-8	2-8	8	1	0.5	4	2	0.5	0.5

Bord. pertussis	1	16	0.5	0.25	16	4		0.06		0.25	2	2	4		1	0.5
Esch. coli	32	R	8	4	4	4		R	R	R	1	2-8	2	4	0.5	0.25
Klebsiella	R	R	16	16	4	4	4	R	R	R	2-4	2-16	2	2	0.28	0.25
Enterobacter	R	R	R	R	R	8	R	R	R	R	2-8	2-16	2	2	0.28	0.25
Pr. mirabilis a.	32	R	2	1	4	1	4	R	R	R	32	8	8	4	0.5	R
Pr. mirabilis b.	R	R	R	R	4	1	4	R	R	R	32	8	8	4	0.5	R
Indole + Proteus	R	R	R	1-8	R	2-R	8	R	R	R	4-R	4-16	1-4	2	0.5	R
Serratia spp.	R	R	8-R	4-R	R	8-R	16	R	R	R	16-R	8	4	4	0.5	R
Providencia	R	R	16-R	4-R	32-R	2-R	8	R	R	R	2-R	4-R	8		2-128	R
Salmonella spp.	4-16	R	1-8	2-8	2	4	4	64-R	R	R	1	2	2	4	0.25	0.25
Shigella spp.	16	R	8	2-8	2	4	4	8-R	R	R	1-2	8	4	4	0.25	0.25
Ps. aeruginosa	R	R	R	16-128	R	R	R	R	R	R	32-R	R	16	4	1	0.5
Br. abortus	2-8	R	1-4	4-16		64		32	R	4-16	1	2	2		0.25	8-16
Past. septica	0.5	1-8	0.5	2	1			1		1-8	0.5	0.5	2		1-4	0.5
Bact. fragilis	8-R	32	16	8-32	8-64	4-32		1-4	0.0-1	1-R	0.5-2	8	R	R	R	>16
Blood level†	0.5*	2.5*	2.5*	5*	5	5	5	1.5	5	20	2.5	5	10	10	2.5	2

†These figures are necessarily arbitrary, but they are intended to represent a concentration which is exceeded in the blood after the usual ordinary full dose for at least half the interdose interval. It is assumed that administration is at short intervals as in the treatment of an acute infection.

*Much higher levels can be attained if necessary by giving larger doses.

diffusing into the infected area. It is no less important to know that the blood level of a potentially toxic drug is not excessive: this possibility should be borne in mind when streptomycin, gentamicin, kanamycin or vancomycin has to be given to a patient with impaired renal function.

Treatment with drug combinations

There are five alleged indications for prescribing two antibacterial drugs together:

1. As a temporary expedient during the investigation of an obscure illness.
2. To prevent the development of bacterial resistance.
3. To achieve a synergic effect.
4. Mixed infections.
5. To permit reduction in dose of a potentially toxic drug.

Of these indications for combined treatment, their initial use in serious infections when the precise bacteriological diagnosis is doubtful is often justifiable provided that specimens have been taken. The importance of combined treatment in delaying the emergence of bacterial resistance has been amply verified in tuberculosis, and is particularly relevant to chronic infections. This function of antibiotic combinations also applies, however, to some more acute infections, for example, those caused by *Pseudomonas aeruginosa*. Antibacterial synergy is discussed in the following pages. Although its operation is more readily shown *in vitro* than in the patient, bactericidal synergy is clearly related to success in treatment of several difficult infections, notably certain forms of bacterial endocarditis and septicaemia in the immune-suppressed.

No general rule can be established about the treatment of mixed infections or that of different infections (i.e. at different sites) in the same patient. This purpose may sometimes be served best by a drug combination, sometimes by a broad-spectrum antibiotic. The last indication to permit reduction in dosage of a potentially toxic drug, although proposed by Ehrlich, is now rarely necessary; the combination of amphotericin and flucytosine in severe fungal infections provides a good example.

Types of combined effect

The attainment of a synergic effect, when this is possible, may be the most important indication of all. When two anti-bacterial drugs act together *in vitro* they may show indifference, when their combined action is no greater than that of the more active alone. They may be antagonistic, when the activity of one is reduced by the presence of the other, or they may be synergic, when their combined effect is significantly greater than that of either acting alone: small increases of activity are usually considered to be an additive effect rather than synergy.

These effects may apply to the bacteristatic action of the drugs, for example, the synergy seen between trimethoprim and sulphonamides, and the antagonism between nalidixic acid and nitrofurantoin or between erythromycin and clindamycin against staphylococci and streptococci resistant to the former. These effects are readily demonstrated by ordinary bacteristatic tests described on page 484 and illustrated in Table 27.5 and Fig. 27.12.

In contrast the effect of such drug combinations on their bactericidal action is of a different nature and requires special tests: it is also of much greater clinical significance. In bacteristatic synergy a significantly smaller amount of the two drugs acting together will produce the effect of a greater amount of either acting alone (Table 27.5). This is not the case with bactericidal action. Bactericidal synergy is only seen between two drugs which individually are incompletely bactericidal, though acting together they may completely kill the inoculum. An inhibitory concentration of one drug will be required but complete killing may be produced by the addition of a sub-inhibitory concentration of the second. Special tests are required to demonstrate this effect (see page 485), such combinations showing indifference or slight additive effect in bacteristatic tests. Two drugs which individually are fully bactericidal will show indifference or possibly slight additive effect when acting together.

It has been suggested that combined bactericidal action can be predicted, depending on whether the component drugs are bactericidal (penicillins, cephalosporins, aminoglycosides) or bacteristatic (tetracyclines, chloramphenicol, erythromycin) as follows:

Bacteristatic + bacteristatic is simply additive.
Bactericidal + bacteristatic may be antagonistic.
Bactericidal + bactericidal may be synergic.

It cannot be pretended that this law proposed so many years ago is universally valid. Manten & Meyerman-Wisse (1962) sought to elaborate it by sub-dividing both classes of antibiotic. Among the bactericidal penicillin and vancomycin are antagonized by bacteristatic, but polymyxin, streptomycin, neomycin and bacitracin are said not to be, because their action is exerted on non-multiplying bacteria. We dispute the truth of this as regards the aminoglycosides. Among bacteristatic antibiotics, tetracycline and chloramphenicol antagonize bactericidal, but others, including cycloserine (and sulphonamides) do not because their action is exerted too slowly. In fact no law based on such classification will apply to all combinations. Derivatives of rifamycin behave exceptionally; they are bactericidal but act synergically with tetracycline, and the best bactericidal combination for a staphylococcus in a patient referred to on page 293 was found to be rifampicin + erythromycin. Other exceptions depend on some peculiarity in the action of one of the pair. Michel et al (1975) found a combination of chloramphenicol and cephaloridine to be strongly synergic against some strains of otherwise highly resistant Gram-negative bacilli (Enterobacter etc.), their interpretation being that chloramphenicol, by inhibiting β lactamase formation, enables cephaloridine to exert its bactericidal effect on strains owing their resistance to this enzyme.

Commercial combinations

The claims made for most commercial combinations are exaggerated, and the use of these preparations is in general to be discouraged. Many consist of penicillin and streptomycin, and although this has an important use just described, no one is likely to use such a commercial combination for treating endocarditis, since the proportions of the two constituents are wrong for this purpose; that of penicillin needs to be higher. These products are mainly used for purposes which often do not require such a combination at all, whether the 'blind' treatment of infection of unknown nature, or as cover for surgical operations, including those for which no such precaution should be necessary. Many patients have quite unnecessarily suffered eighth nerve damage from streptomycin or dihydrostreptomycin in such combinations administered in this way: such damage is most likely to occur in those with unrecognized impairment of renal function, who fail to excrete the antibiotic at the normal rate.

Most other commercial combinations contain bacteristatic antibiotics, and there is no evidence in the extensive studies of Finland and his colleagues (reviewed by Garrod, 1965) that any of these exert an effect superior to that of the more active of their constituents. In a separate category are mixtures of tetracyclines with anti-fungal antibiotics, the merits of which are discussed on page 242.

Prophylactic administration

This is a subject on which much has now been written, and no attempt will be made to review the literature, but only to define some principles and to propose what we hope will be considered a rational plan. Some accepted forms of prophylaxis are dealt with elsewhere in this book, including that of rheumatic fever (page 351) and of bacterial endocarditis (page 298) and pre-operative bowel preparation (page 342).

Antibiotics have often been given in clinical situations which involve a special risk of autogenous infection, especially of the lungs. These include inhalation anaesthesia in elderly and 'chesty' patients, and particularly for operations on the upper abdomen which limit the depth of subsequent respiration. In the medical field, supposed indications have been virus infections such as measles, and various comatose and paralytic states. We are aware of no evidence that any of these proceedings is beneficial; indeed, studies have usually shown a higher infection rate in treated than in control patients. The principle involved here is that treatment does nothing to remove the predisposing cause; if this is strongly operative infection will always follow, and all that the antibiotic does is to select a resistant pathogen. In place of, say, a pneumococcus, infection due to which, if it does occur, is amenable to treatment, the more likely cause is a Klebsiella or some other Gram-negative organism relatively resistant to any treatment.

In the surgical field prophylaxis aimed at the wound itself is a different matter. An imperative indication for it is a serious risk of gas gangrene, as in extensive trauma with gross soiling of the wound, or thigh amputation for obliterative arterial disease, when *Cl. welchii* may be derived from the peri-anal skin and the disease itself for which the operation is undertaken ensures the reduced tissue oxygen tension to enable its spores to germinate. There is also general agreement that antibiotic cover is advisable for open heart surgery. At the other extreme are commonplace clean operations involving no risk of sepsis, for which most surgeons, in this country at least, consider antibiotic cover quite superfluous, yet serious harm has commonly been caused by such treatment (see preceding section).

Between these two extremes lies debatable ground. Various particular operations have been thought to require cover, usually because highly susceptible tissues are exposed, or because bacterial contamination cannot be prevented, or because the consequences of any infection can be particularly disastrous. We would only suggest that, the decision having been made, it should further be decided exactly what the antibiotic is intended to do. If the aim is to destroy bacteria accidentally implanted in the wound during operation, what purpose is served by starting treatment 24 hours beforehand? Yet this is very common practice. A logical aim would be to maintain an adequate concentration of a bactericidal antibiotic throughout the operation and for a few hours after it. That such simple treatment can be effective is supported by the findings of many recent studies of peri-operative prophylaxis in abdominal surgery, which are reviewed in Ch. 18. The same principles can be applied to other forms of surgery which carry a high infection risk, or in which infection, although rare, is especially dangerous. Much controversy has, for example, centred on prevention of infection after total hip replacement and Pollard et al (1979) showed that a three-dose cephaloridine scheme gave the same results as did a course of flucloxacillin which continued for 14 days; two infections were recorded with each regimen in a total of 310 operations. The fortunately low infection rate following such operations makes assessment of prophylactic regimens difficult.

So short a course as this may not provide for all situations, but it may well be adequate for many, and those in the habit of continuing antibiotic prophylaxis for days—or even, in connection with heart surgery, for weeks—might perhaps with advantage ask themselves what exactly the later stages of such a course are supposed to be achieving. If some fresh autogenous infection is feared it is likely, owing to the selective effect of such treatment on the normal flora of the body, to be due to a highly resistant organism. After open heart surgery the sites of insertion of intravenous cannulae are a special possible source of infection, and prophylaxis should be continued until after these have been removed.

ANTIBIOTIC CONTROL POLICIES

The spread of resistant strains, the incidence of unwanted effects from antimicrobial drugs and their high cost have all led to the study of prescribing policies for hospitals, hospital groups or even on a national scale. The principles of antibiotic policy are easily stated. Avoidance of antibiotics in patients who do not have bacterial infections, notably their use for prophylactic purposes or in patients with respiratory viral infections; optimum choice of agents and regimens for patients who do have bacterial infections, critical examination of the need to apply antibiotics topically or to use by any route agents known to be prone to the emergence of resistance and limitation of the opportunities for resistant organisms to spread. Offences against the first two of these requirements on a world-wide scale are massive since in many countries antibiotics are freely available to the public and studies even in some of the world's premier medical institutions (recently reviewed by Jones et al 1977) have indicated considerable room for improvement.

However, while there has been much railing against 'antibiotic misuse' there has been relatively little specification of the precise nature of this abuse and fewer still plans to bring the abuse under control. There are essentially two options open to us: direction and education. Direction as to which antibiotics may be prescribed inside or outside hospital has been adopted on a national scale, for example in Czechoslovakia, and removal of antibiotic combinations from the market in the United States could be seen as a move in this direction. Many hospitals have adopted by internal agreement restriction on the prescribing of certain agents thought to be too valuable for the treatment of severe infection, or too expensive, to be squandered in the widespread treatment of assorted conditions for which ample well tried agents are available. In an endeavour of this kind undertaken at one London hospital at the instigation of our late co-author, Mary Barber, agreed prescribing policies for the treatment of staphylococcal infection undoubtedly affected the pattern of emergence of staphylococcal resistance, but in this and a few similar studies conducted elsewhere it was acknowledged that other measures taken at the same time—notably those to contain the possible spread of any resistant strains—played a significant part in the fall of their prevalence (Rosendal et al, 1977).

There is abundant evidence that the lavish use of antibiotics favours the spread of resistant species. A remarkable illustration of this is reported by Price & Sleigh (1970) from a neuro-surgical intensive care unit in which *Klebsiella aerogenes* infection was endemic and had caused numerous chest and urinary infections and eight deaths from meningitis. The occurrence of these infections was abruptly halted by stopping all antibiotic treatment, both therapeutic and prophylactic; the antibiotic largely used for the prophylaxis of both chest and wound infections had been ampicillin. Restricted use was resumed four months later. A comparable achievement was the elimination of a highly carbenicillin-resistant strain of *Ps. aeruginosa* from a burns unit by stopping the use of this antibiotic (Lowbury et al, 1972). This resistance was multiple and determined by an R factor, and other species carrying this also disappeared when the use of other antibiotics was restricted.

Educational programmes have enjoyed mixed success. In a hospital where the prescriber was required to justify his choice of antibiotic to an infectious diseases consultant, the consumption of expensive and potentially toxic agents appeared to be substantially reduced (McGowan & Finland, 1974). On the other hand Jones et al (1977) found that a survey of antibiotic usage in hospital followed by presentation to the staff of the data drawing attention to the prescribing errors revealed had little noticeable effect. In particular, prophylaxis continued to be the most common form of abuse. Shapiro et al (1979) recently found that 10 per cent of the patients in 20 short stay hospitals received prophylactic chemotherapy, and that this accounted for 30 per cent of the antibiotics used, with cephalosporins in first place. Contrary to the principles stated on page 278, and justified by many clinical studies, these drugs were mostly continued throughout the patient's hospital stay.

Nevertheless, pressure for retrospective antibiotic 'audits' and usage surveillance will no doubt increase in the expectation that these will lead to more rational (and more restrictive) prescribing policies. The justification for such policies is that the policy makers know better than the prescribers what is good for the patient. Where this concerns individual agents (for example restriction of the availability in hospital of a new antibiotic or in domiciliary practice of an agent indicated predominantly for conditions for which the patient needs to be in hospital) the issues are contentious but fairly simple. Where it concerns individual patients, the issues are much more complicated as illustrated in Figure 14.1. Perhaps reluctance on the part of those at the bedside to accept the views of those elsewhere at the time the prescription was written will be overcome by bowing to the ultimate of modern arbiters, the computer. Yu et al (1979) asked their computer, prescribers of various degrees of seniority and experts in infectious diseases the most appropriate treatment for seven complicated cases of meningitis. The computer came top.

Methods of promoting education in antimicrobial drug use and of administering agreed antibiotic policies are discussed in reviews by Phillips (1979) and Buckwold & Ronald (1979).

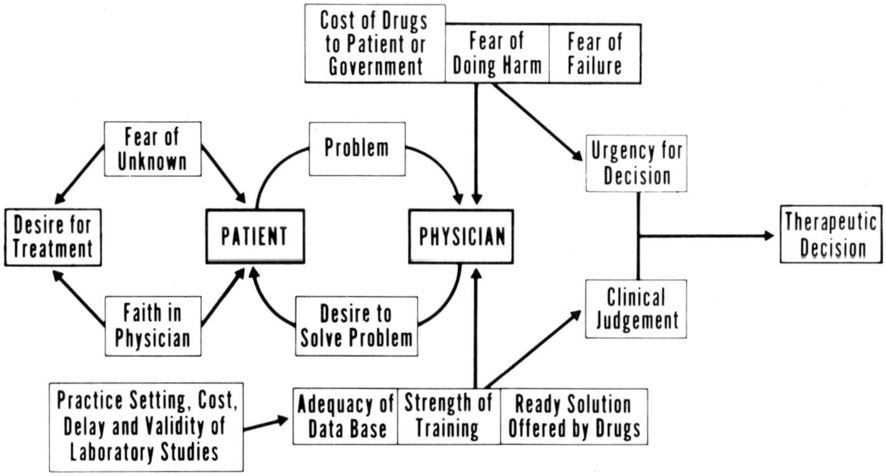

Fig. 14.1 Interactive network of pressures affecting the use of antimicrobial drugs, designed by and reproduced with kind permission of Dr Calvin Kunin

References

Buckwold F J, Ronald A R 1979 J Antimicrob Chemother 5: 129
Garrod L P 1965 S Afr Med J 39: 607
Jones S R, Pannell J, Barks J et al 1977 Amer J Med Sci 273: 79
Lowbury E J L, Babb J R, Roe E 1972 Lancet 2: 941
Manten A, Meyerman-Wisse M J 1962 Antonie van Leeuwenhoek J Microbiol & Serol 28: 321
McGowan J E Jr, Finland M 1974 J Infect Dis 130: 165
Michel J, Bornstein H, Luboshitzky R, Sacks T 1975 Antimicrob Agents Chemother 7: 845
Phillips I 1979 In: Reeves D, Geddes A (eds) Recent Advances in Infection. Churchill Livingstone, Edinburgh p 151
Pollard J P, Hughes S P F, Scott J E, Evans M J, Benson M K D 1979 Brit Med J 1: 707
Price D J E, Sleigh J D 1970 Lancet 2: 1213
Rosendal K, Jessen O, Bentzon W, Bülow P 1977 Acta Path Microbiol Scand 85(B): 143
Shapiro M, Townsend T R, Rosner B, Kass E H 1979 New Engl J Med 301: 351
Yu V L, Fagan L M, Wraith S M et al 1979 J Amer Med Ass 242: 1279

15

Septicaemia and endocarditis

Profound changes in the aetiology of septicaemia have taken place during the antibiotic era. Of those which develop in previously well patients, meningococcal septicaemia is still a life-threatening infection (see Chapter 17) but serious infection from group A streptococci (*Str. pyogenes*) is now rarely encountered, and clostridial septicaemia is now almost unknown in many communities. By contrast, septicaemia arising in patients with various forms of impaired defence against bacterial infection has assumed great importance, especially for patients in hospital. During the 1960s staphylococcal infection presented the chief threat, but, although still common, this cause of septicaemia in hospital is now outnumbered by others, notably a large increase in infections caused by Gram-negative bacilli. The resurgence of interest in anaerobic bacteriology has led, also, to increased recognition and reporting of anaerobic infection.

Three factors interact in causing these changes in the pattern of hospital-based septicaemia. A large number of patients possess lowered resistance to infection by reason of age, underlying disease or drug treatment. Breaches in local defence mechanisms are now commonly inflicted on patients in the course of treatment, for example, intravenous or urinary catheters, endotracheal intubation, tracheostomy, and patients may be admitted with injury or disease causing damage to skin or mucous membranes. Finally, hospital environments have promoted the selection of a dangerous flora, so that nosocomial infection is often a serious danger to patients especially in high-technology areas such as in intensive care units, neuro-surgical units or special care nurseries. Moreover, these infections are often caused by antibiotic-resistant organisms as a result of the selective pressures imposed by the use of these drugs. The problem of nosocomial infection and antibiotic use has been reviewed by Jackson (1979).

Because the causes of septicaemia are so diverse, the clinical syndrome is rarely an accurate guide to the microbial cause and the antibiotic susceptibility of many species causing septicaemia varies greatly, accurate and early bacteriological diagnosis is most important. The sensitivity of any isolate should be determined to individual appropriate antibiotics and if necessary, to combinations of drugs. In the following sections, provisional suggestions are made for each common causal organism in septicaemia, some of which can only be tentative, since optimal treatment must often be based on laboratory studies of the individual strain, and a scheme of management is proposed for initiating treatment before bacteriological diagnosis is made, or in circumstances in which laboratory facilities are not available.

ANTIBIOTIC MANAGEMENT OF SEPTICAEMIAS OF KNOWN CAUSE

Streptococcus pyogenes

Benzyl penicillin by intravenous or intramuscular injection in a dose of 1 mega unit (600 mg) four to six-hourly. Group B streptococcal infections have their main impact on the neonate (Chapter 20) but are occasionally encountered in adults. Bayer et al (1976) record 24 examples, mostly of pyelonephritis, endometritis or pneumonia, in patients with diabetes or other chronic disease. The strains were all susceptible to penicillin but the MIC for group B strains is appreciably higher than those of group A and it is possible that, as in the neonate, these infections would best be treated by a combination of penicillin with an aminoglycoside. Group B strains are, like other streptococci, resistant to aminoglycosides given alone, and most of the strains in Bayer's series were tetracycline-resistant.

Staphylococcus aureus

Penicillin resistance should be assumed even in patients acquiring staphylococcal septicaemia in the community and treatment begun with cloxacillin in Britain. In other countries other, equally suitable isoxazolyl penicillins are available rather than cloxacillin (see Chapter 3) in a dose of 1 g four-hourly by intravenous or intramuscular injection. If the strain proves penicillin-sensitive, benzyl penicillin can then be substituted. Some physicians begin treatment with both drugs but, if this is done, full dosage of both must be ensured. The treatment regimen is modified if endocarditis is established or even suspected, and this aspect is considered later in the chapter (page 292).

Gram-negative rods

It is in this group of infections, now so common in hospital practice, that the most difficult antibiotic decisions lie. The responsible organisms have a widely variable and changing pattern of drug susceptibility, and many of the appropriate antimicrobials have a low therapeutic ratio. In general, initial policy for septicaemias of this type is based on the use of an aminoglycoside, most commonly gentamicin but sometimes tobramycin or amikacin, depending on local patterns of drug sensitivity, but treatment can sometimes be changed, when bacteriological data becomes available, to an agent with more favourable pharmacokinetic characteristics. For example, some enterobacteria are still susceptible to ampicillin/amoxycillin, and co-trimoxazole, which also can be administered by mouth or parenterally, is active against a wide range of Gram-negative (as well as Gram-positive) organisms, and has been used successfully in Gram-negative septicaemias (Franzen & Brandberg, 1976). The range of available drugs for Gram-negative infections is large and changing rapidly. The new cephalosporin, cefotaxime (HR 756) has been shown very active *in vitro* against a large number of isolates, including those resistant to other cephalosporins and cefoxitin. It is also more active than carbenicillin against *Ps. aeruginosa* (Hamilton-Miller et al, 1978; Drasar et al, 1978).

The agents most likely to be indicated for the bacterial species causing Gram-negative septicaemias can be listed as follows:

E. coli, Proteus, Providencia. Gentamicin, other aminoglycosides, ampicillin/amoxycillin, co-trimoxazole, cephalosporins.

Klebsiella. Choice is especially difficult, aminoglycoside-cephalosporin combination may often be most suitable.

Pseudomonas. Gentamicin or tobramycin together with carbenicillin or ticarcillin. Azlocillin, mezlocillin and cefotaxime are active *in vitro* and are under clinical trial for severe Pseudomonas infection.

Serratia marcescens. This species has emerged as an important agent of nosocomial infection, affecting especially patients with lowered resistance, and also causing endocarditis, notably in intravenous drug abusers. Ball (1976) reviewing choices of treatment, noted the very variable pattern of *in vitro* susceptibility. All strains were, until recently, inhibited by gentamicin, but gentamicin-resistance has now increased greatly in frequency in some hospitals in the U.S.A. If an aminoglycoside cannot be used, other possible treatments may be applicable. Co-trimoxazole is active against some strains, and a combination of polymyxin B and rifampicin, found by Ostenson et al (1977) to be synergic *in vitro* against a large number of clinical isolates, was used by them in 12 patients with multi-resistant serratia infections, with apparent success in eight of them. Cephalosporins and cefoxitin are active against some strains, and Lin et al (1979) showed that, in a number of resistant strains, bactericidal synergy could be demonstrated between aminoglycosides and carbenicillin.

Anaerobic septicaemia

Of the anaerobes cultivated from blood, *Bacteroides fragilis* is most commonly found, but is the least fastidious and most easily grown. Sensitivity testing in this group is difficult and does not always correlate well with *in vivo* efficacy. Assessment of treatment is also especially difficult, since patients with bacteroides septicaemia are often very ill, with serious underlying bowel or pelvic disease, abscesses and other complex medical problems. Antibiotics, as with other septicaemias, form only part of the management and Chow & Guze (1974) noted that, while appropriate antibiotic treatment apparently reduced the mortality of anaerobic septicaemia, drainage of abscesses had about the same degree of benefit in patients not receiving appropriate antibiotics. The two agents most uniformly effective against *B. fragilis* are clindamycin and metronidazole, while cefoxitin is also active against most strains. In the U.S.A. clindamycin has hitherto been used most extensively since metronidazole has not been approved for use in anaerobic infection, whereas in the U.K., the justifiable fear of clindamycin-associated colitis, and the favourable pharmacokinetic characteristics of metronidazole, have led to widespread use of the latter agent. Good results have been reported from both drugs. Clindamycin has the advantage that, in the phase before diagnosis is established, Gram-positive coccal infection as well as anaerobes are being 'covered' and the incidence of unwanted effects is relatively low in many centres; Leigh et al (1977), for example, treated 219 patients with parenteral clindamycin without seeing pseudo-membranous colitis, although 13 per cent of the patients had gastro-intestinal side effects. On the other hand metronidazole achieves excellent blood and tissue levels when given by mouth, by suppository or intravenously, is active against nearly all clinically important anaerobes, has few unwanted effects and sometimes succeeds when clindamycin has failed (Sharp et al, 1977). We generally favour the choice of metronidazole for known or presumed Bacteroides infections (Tally et al, 1975). It must be remembered, however, that many other agents have variable activity against bacteroides, and may sometimes be suitable. These include carbenicillin, chloramphenicol, erythromycin and tetracyclines, although the proportion of bacteroides species susceptible to the last of these has greatly diminished in recent years.

There is much evidence, strongly supported by recent experimental studies (Bartlett, 1978), of the importance of bacterial synergy in initiating and maintaining anaerobic sepsis, and in practice patients with known or suspected bacteroides septicaemia are usually also treated simultaneously with a drug, usually an aminoglycoside, active against coliforms. Single drug treatment with cefoxitin may prove appropriate in this context (Tally et al, 1979). Severe clostridial infections are still treated with high doses of benzyl penicillin, although metronidazole has been used successfully on occasion.

Fungal septicaemia See Chapter 10 and page 295

INITIAL TREATMENT OF SEPTICAEMIA

The clinical syndrome presented by patients with septicaemia is sometimes specific enough to allow accurate initial treatment before bacteriological findings are available. A familiar example is meningococcal meningitis when the characteristic purpuric rash is present. Slightly less familiar are the equally characteristic lesions sometimes seen in gonococcal, staphylococcal and Pseudomonas septicaemia. In other patients rapid help from the laboratory may be possible, for example, by Gram-stain examination of pus from an abdominal abscess, by counterimmune electrophoresis of CSF, gas liquid chromatography of pus or other emerging methods which aid rapid microbial diagnosis.

In many patients with suspected septicaemia no such early diagnostic guidance is available, and the patient's condition demands treatment as soon as blood cultures and other appropriate specimens have been taken. Unfortunately this need for treatment before diagnosis arises commonly in those patients, neonates, the immune-suppressed and those with serious abdominal, pelvic or genito-urinary tract disease, who are especially liable to septicaemia of varied causation. The great recent emphasis on Gram-negative septicaemias is in one sense seriously misleading for the clinician, since a notable minority of the patients in whom such septicaemias are common may in fact have infection by staphylococci, streptococci or anaerobes, while mixed infections are increasingly recognized, especially the polymicrobial nature of infections involving anaerobes. The bacterial shock syndrome may be associated with any of these septicaemias and is not confined to those caused by Gram-negative aerobes.

A rational approach to initial treatment can be devised by considering first, those patients in whom the clinical and laboratory data available within an hour or two of admission give a high probability of the agent and its drug sensitivity and second, those patients in whom this initial narrowing of the diagnostic possibilities cannot be achieved. Even for the latter, however, the likely range of causal organisms can be inferred from the age of the patient, the nature of any underlying disease or immune deficiencies, and the epidemiological setting in which the illness arises. In this way it becomes unnecessary to consider, as is often done, an excessively wide group of 'septicaemia of unknown origin' for initial choice. An attempt to cover all possible causes of septicaemia leads to unnecessarily complex and dangerous treatments. For example, the recent interest in anaerobic infection often leads to the inclusion of anti-anaerobic drugs in patients in whom this type of infection would be excessively unlikely.

In Tables 15.1 and 15.2 an initial treatment policy is proposed on the foregoing principles.

Table 15.1 Initial treatment of septicaemia

When early clinical/microbiological information indicates probable cause

Presumed cause	Treatment
Meningococcus	Benzyl Penicillin
Gonococcus	Benzyl Penicillin
Pneumococcus	Benzyl Penicillin
Str. pyogenes	Benzyl Penicillin
Staph. aureus	Benzyl Penicillin + (flu) cloxacillin (but see also bact. endocarditis)
Enterobacteria	Gentamicin
Pseudomonas	Gentamicin or Tobramycin + Carbenicillin or Ticarcillin
Clostridium	Benzyl Penicillin
Bacteroides, other non-sporing anaerobes	Metronidazole

Table 15.2 Initial treatment of septicaemia

Best guess policies when early clinical/microbiological information does *not* indicate cause

Probable source and/or associated disease	Treatment
Lower gut, pelvis	Penicillin + Gentamicin + Metronidazole *or* Gentamicin + Clindamycin
Urinary tract	Ampicillin (Amoxycillin) + Gentamicin
Biliary tract	Ampicillin (Amoxycillin) + Gentamicin
Neutropenia	Gentamicin + Carbenicillin or Ticarcillin
Intravenous catheters	Cloxacillin + Gentamicin
Neonate	See Chapter 20

SEPTICAEMIA IN PATIENTS WITH IMMUNE SUPPRESSION

Infection is a common cause of illness and death in patients with a number of blood diseases in which host defences are impaired both by the disease and its treatment. Patients who receive transplants are also at prolonged risk because of their long-term immunosuppressive treatment. The onset of serious infection in these patients may be very sudden and accompanied by few or no pointers to the likely causal organism, while the range of possible pathogens, viral, bacterial and fungal, is very wide. In general the policy most commonly adopted in suspected septicaemia is to take appropriate cultures and then immediately begin treatment aimed at the common Gram-positive and Gram-negative bacterial pathogens. If this is ineffective and no causal diagnosis is made, it may be necessary to carry out more invasive procedures (for example, trans-tracheal aspiration or lung biopsy if a pulmonary source is suspected) since the risk of such procedures may be less than those of the antimicrobial agents necessary to treat all the possible causal organisms.

Most formal trials of infection control have centred around patients with acute leukaemia or with a wider range of malignant disease who develop fever during a period of neutropenia, since neutropenia is known to be the most important predisposing factor in their liability to infection. A huge number of regimens has been used, depending much on the experience of the unit involved and the local patterns of nosocomial infection, but international comparative trials have also been completed. One of the largest (EORTC International Antimicrobial Therapy Project Group, 1978) compared, in febrile neutropenic patients with cancer, three regimens, carbenicillin with cephalothin, carbenicillin with gentamicin, and cephalothin with gentamicin. The difficulties of such trials can be realized when it is noted that, although 625 episodes of suspected infection were included, infection was documented in only 396 episodes, with Gram-negative bacteraemia in 86. Of the pathogens isolated, 61 per cent were Gram-negative rods and 16 per cent were *Staph. aureus*. As with other studies, the response rate is closely related to recovery of neutrophil function during treatment. A satisfactory response was obtained in about 70 per cent of patients on any of the three regimens, with a notably higher incidence of disturbed renal function with the cephalothin and gentamicin scheme than with the other two. The group recommends a combination of carbenicillin (or ticarcillin) with an aminoglycoside for initial therapy in these patients. The importance of *Ps. aeruginosa* septicaemia in leukaemic patients in some centres, and the evidence of synergy between carbenicillin and aminoglycosides for this infection, also favour this approach, although the frequency of Pseudomonas infection varies greatly. Falk et al (1977) for example, used tobramycin and clindamycin successfully in febrile leukaemic patients without other elaborate control measures, isolating *Ps. aeurginosa* in only one of the 16 proved infections in 39 febrile episodes. Similar findings were reported by Hahn et al (1977), with two Pseudomonas infections of 17 bacteraemias. They used a combination of amikacin and cephalothin in 93 patients, two of whom showed evidence of ototoxicity and six of possible antibiotic renal damage.

Prevention of infection in immune-suppressed patients

This large and important problem cannot be treated in detail here. Controversy has centred round the importance of various types of isolation system in protecting the patient from exogenous infection and the value of reducing the endogenous microbial flora by bowel disinfection and by the application of topical agents to normally colonized skin and mucosal sites. The construction and staffing of advanced isolation systems, and the long term administration of complex antibiotic schemes are expensive procedures which may also impose further physical and psychological burdens on already ill patients; hence much effort has been put into controlled trials designed to test the value of various methods, especially in acute leukaemia. As regards the antimicrobial drug aspect, several trials have shown a reduction of infective episodes and deaths from infection in patients receiving prophylactic regimens, although the remission rate of leukaemia has not always been reduced (Editorial 1978; Rodriguez et al, 1978). The method used at Hammersmith Hospital consists of gut decontamination with a mixture of framycetin, colistin and nystatin (FRACON), with topical chlorhexidine to mucosal and skin colonization sites (Storring et al, 1977). Oral co-trimoxazole has recently been used in an attempt to make infection prophylaxis in leukaemia less difficult and less expensive. Hughes et al (1977) reduced the incidence of Pneumocystis and bacterial infections in childhood leukaemias by this means, and Enno et al (1978) significantly improved the efficacy of the FRACON regimen by the addition of oral co-trimoxazole. It remains to be seen whether the benefits of this simple method will be vitiated by an increasing incidence of bacteria resistant to the combination, or by a higher frequency of infections with organisms, for example, Pseudomonas or fungi, normally resistant to it.

Other forms of immune suppression

Although most discussion of infection control in immune suppression has been concerned with leukaemia and other malignant disease, other forms of impaired resistance must also be considered. Patients with renal failure, for example, are at increased risk of septicaemia, and infection remains an important cause of death. Shunts used in chronic haemodialysis are an important source of potentially dangerous organisms. Dobkin et al (1978) reporting on 60 episodes of septicaemia in patients receiving haemodialysis, thought that 44 of them had their origin in the vascular access site, despite the change in method towards the use of internal fistulas. Thirty-one of the septicaemias were caused by *Staph. aureus*, and 11 by Gram-negative bacilli. Contrary to previous experience, they were usually able to eradicate infection by appropriate antibiotics without removal of the shunt.

Other patients suffer from more specific forms of lowered resistance to infection. Patients with sickle cell disease or whose spleens have been removed are at special risk of overwhelming infection by pneumococci and other Gram-positive cocci, and many examples of genetic defects of the immune system are now being analysed, some of which lead to fairly specific infective risk, such as those of severe meningococcal or gonococcal infection in otherwise healthy patients with deficiencies of certain late complement components (C6, 7 and 8). This type of defect, more specific than those usually encountered in generally ill patients in hospital, may be amenable to prevention by immunization or chemoprophylaxis.

Other aspects of treatment and prevention in septicaemia

This book is concerned with antimicrobial agents in the treatment and prevention of infection, but many other aspects of management in septicaemia must also be considered. Best established and most dramatic in its beneficial effect is the drainage of abscesses, sometimes associated with duct obstruction as in the biliary and urinary tract. Another important complication of septicaemia is the bacterial shock syndrome, presenting many problems of diagnosis and management and the pathogenesis of which is still much in dispute. Rapid changes in renal function are common in septicaemia, whether or not the patient has been hypovolaemic or hypotensive, and this tendency to renal failure has an important influence on antibiotic choice and dosage (Chapter 26). Patients with prolonged septicaemia become anaemic, hypoproteinaemic and malnourished, and the underlying disease which predisposed them to serious infection will also need continued attention.

Finally, although also beyond the scope of our present discussion, the dramatic challenges presented to the clinician by septicaemic illnesses may have diverted attention from the need to prevent illnesses, as far as possible, by cross-infection control programmes, the development of rational antibiotic policies, and the use, where applicable, of specific methods of prophylaxis (see page 279).

INFECTIVE ENDOCARDITIS

The pattern of infective endocarditis has changed in many ways during the antibiotic era. Classical subacute bacterial endocarditis is less often seen. Culture-negative endocarditis remains an important problem, especially in elderly patients, while in contrast improved bacteriological technique has led to increasing reports of endocarditis caused by unusual organisms of fastidious growth requirements. Rheumatic heart disease as an underlying lesion has become less common in wealthier countries, but the importance of other lesions, some of them revealed by technical advances such as echocardiography, has become recognized. These include bicuspid aortic valve and prolapsed mitral valve, as well as the more familiar congenital defects known to predispose to endocarditis, while infection occasionally occurs in degenerative and other forms of heart disease. The largest change in pattern has, however, been brought about by the advance of cardiac surgery. While this has allowed successful treatment in many patients with endocarditis who would otherwise have died of cardiac failure or uncontrolled infection, cardiac surgery, especially the insertion of prosthetic valves, is itself followed by a substantial incidence of endocarditis. Other medical procedures, notably haemodialysis, may be followed by endocarditis, while intravenous drug abusers ('main-line' addicts) suffer a definite risk of right-sided and left-sided endocarditis. These changes in pattern and in predisposing factors have made the time-honoured distinction between acute and subacute bacterial endocarditis less valuable than it was, and it is now more useful to distinguish between naturally occurring, or primary endocarditis, and extraneous, or secondary infective endocarditis, associated with such factors as prosthetic cardiac valves, haemodialysis or intravenous drug abuse (Gray, 1975; Schnurr et al, 1977).

Table 15.3 Causes of infective endocarditis

	Predisposing factor	Organisms
'Primary'	Underlying heart disease, or unknown	*Str. viridans* *Staph. aureus* *Str. faecalis* and other streptococci (see text) Rare causes, e.g. *Staph. epidermidis* Haemophilus, Acinetobacter, Anaerobes, Coxiella (see text)
'Secondary'	Cardiac surgery, prosthetic heart valves	*Staph. aureus* *Staph. epidermidis* *Str. viridans* Gram-negative bacilli Fungi
	Intravenous drug abuse	*Staph. aureus* *Staph. epidermidis* *Strep. faecalis* Gram-negative bacilli, inc. Pseudomonas and Serratia Fungi Mixed infections
	Haemodialysis	*Staph. aureus* *Str. viridans* Other streptococci Gram-negative bacilli

As regards causal organisms (Wilson & Washington, 1977) viridans streptococci still constitute by far the largest group in primary endocarditis. Group D streptococci and *Staph. aureus* cause an appreciable minority but all other causes are rare. In secondary endocarditis, causes are more diverse and vary to some extent according to the extraneous factors. These relationships are summarized in Table 15.3

ANTIBIOTIC TREATMENT

The diagnosis must be verified by blood culture and the organism should be exactly identified. In addition to standard sensitivity tests, the MBC for the isolate of penicillins and of other appropriate agents should be determined by tube dilution tests with no more than two-fold differences. If this concentration proves unduly high, a bactericidal effect cannot be assumed and further tests undertaken as discussed in Chapter 27. Culture-negative endocarditis is discussed below.

Streptococcus viridans

This is not really a species, but a heterogeneous group of streptococci having little else necessarily in common except the property of alpha-haemolysis. In addition endocarditis may be caused by streptococci, presumably derived from the mouth, which are non-haemolytic or have some other peculiar character: some, for instance, are micro-aerophilic. What follows refers also to these atypical strains.

These organisms are usually highly sensitive to penicillin, and their degree of sensitivity is an important determinant of the correct mode of treatment. Highly sensitive *Str. viridans*, with an MIC of less than 0.1 μg/ml have traditionally been treated with penicillin alone. Although success has been claimed for oral administration, most workers prefer injection treatment, at least in the initial phase, either as 6-hourly benzyl penicillin or 12-hourly procaine penicillin. In recent years a tendency to add an aminoglycoside, at least in the initial phase of treatment (see later discussion on other streptococci) has developed. One reason for this is that treatment may thus be shortened from the traditional 6 weeks. Tan et al (1971) treated small numbers of patients for 2 weeks only; two of 13 given high dose penicillin relapsed, but a small group given parenteral penicillin with streptomycin had satisfactory results, as did 27 patients given oral phenoxymethyl penicillin (600–750 mg 4-hourly) with streptomycin 0.5–1.0 g twice daily. Another reason is that an aminoglycoside improves the killing rate of penicillin for penicillin-sensitive *Str. viridans in vitro*, as it does for enterococci (see below), and the combination gives improved results in experimental *Strep. viridans* endocarditis (Durack and Petersdorf, 1973). Finally, although the results of penicillin alone are good, relapses may apparently be prevented completely by the addition of an aminoglycoside. Wolfe & Johnson (1974), at New York Hospital, have treated over 100 patients with a scheme of 2 weeks' parenteral penicillin (average 10–12 mega units daily) with streptomycin for 2 weeks, followed by parenteral penicillin for another 2 weeks, with no relapses.

We would agree with this general pattern of treatment but would prefer, pending the results of sensitivity tests which should always guide treatment, to use gentamicin rather than streptomycin, and would normally be prepared to use an oral preparation, preferably amoxycillin, after the first 2 weeks. The reasons for these variations are discussed in the following section.

Enterococci and less sensitive Str. viridans

The treatment of endocarditis caused by viridans streptococci resistant to more than 1 μg/ml of penicillin is identical to that of enterococcal endocarditis and can be considered jointly. It should be noted, however, that *Str. bovis* although a group D streptococcus is not an enterococcus (distinguished by bile-esculin hydrolysis and growth on 6.5 per cent NaCl broth) is much more penicillin-sensitive than an enterococcus and can be treated in the same way as ordinary viridans streptococci (Hoppes & Lerner, 1974). Success claimed in several papers quoted in the previous edition of this book in treating enterococcal endocarditis with penicillin alone can best be explained by assuming that these were *Str. bovis* infections.

An effective bactericidal regimen is essential for the successful treatment of endocarditis caused by *Str. faecalis* and other relatively resistant streptococci. It is this group of infections which provides the best established example of the correlation of bactericidal synergy *in vitro* with success in therapy, since it was first shown that penicillin alone did not eradicate a population of *Str. faecalis*, whereas addition of subinhibitory doses of streptomycin to the penicillin did so, and that such a combination was effective in clinical practice. Changes in antibiotic resistance patterns and of available antibiotics have now made it necessary to reconsider the choice of both penicillin and aminoglycoside components of this form of combined therapy. Enterococci are now often streptomycin-resistant, and if this resistance is of high degree (some authors have defined this as a MIC of >2000 μg/ml) it precludes synergy with penicillin (see page 20). Ruhen & Darrell (1973) studied 100 strains at the Royal Postgraduate Medical School and found 25 of them highly resistant to streptomycin, 11 to kanamycin but none to gentamicin. They verified that a synergic combined bactericidal action was unobtainable with penicillin + streptomycin against the 25 resistant strains, but was achieved with penicillin + gentamicin against every strain. There have been other reports of similar results, and gentamicin is now generally regarded as preferable to streptomycin for this purpose, although naturally its suitability for every patient should be verified by an *in vitro* test where possible. According to Sanders (1977) netilmicin and sissomicin may also suitably be combined with penicillin against strains resistant to the earlier aminoglycosides.

The optimum concentration of benzyl penicillin for bactericidal effect on enterococci is 6 μg/ml, and dosage (including that of probenecid) can with advantage be aimed at maintaining something like this level in the blood. The corresponding concentration of ampicillin, with its rather higher activity against this organism, is somewhat lower, and either ampicillin or amoxycillin, which is much better absorbed, and acts well on these and other streptococci both alone and in combination with an aminoglycoside (Basker & Sutherland, 1977), may be preferred to parenteral penicillin if a stage in treatment is reached at which oral administration is thought to be safe.

Staph. aureus endocarditis

Penicillin, if the strain is sensitive to it, cloxacillin if not, should be the mainstay of treatment, but since a total bactericidal effect is often not achieved even by an antibiotic to which the strain is fully sensitive, full tests of bactericidal action by single antibiotics and combinations should be carried out. It may well be found that the addition of an aminoglycoside to the penicillin will convert incomplete bactericidal action to complete, and if so, this combination, which should be used as provisional initial treatment, should unhesitatingly be continued. For a methicillin-resistant strain such a combination is essential, and Bulger (1967) showed that kanamycin together with methicillin or cephalothin exerted a synergic effect against such organisms. Gentamicin would now be preferred. Penicillin-aminoglycoside synergy has also been reported by Watanakunakorn & Glotzbecker (1974) and in the treatment of the experimental infection by Sande & Courtney (1976).

Combined treatment is also absolutely required for infection by penicillin-tolerant strains, i.e. those which although sometimes normally sensitive to bacteristatic action, are killed only by unattainably high concentrations (see page 59). Such strains have been reported from several sources to be quite common in serious infections such as endocarditis. It is arguable that a full range of tests of combined bactericidal action should be carried out in every case of this infection. Other possible combinations should be considered if necessary; Peard et al (1970) achieved immediate success with rifampicin + erythromycin, and in the hands of Shafqat et al (1971) infection of a prosthetic valve responded to penicillin + co-trimoxazole. Another combination which has been commended (Jensen & Lassen, 1969) is that of a penicillin with fusidic acid, but this is less soundly based in theory since its *in vitro* effect may actually be antagonistic (page 222). It is sometimes possible, provided blood levels prove satisfactory, to implement a long course of continuation treatment with a combination of oral flucloxacillin and fusidate.

Staph. epidermidis (albus) endocarditis

This is an infection, the existence of which may be overlooked because the organism in a blood culture is taken for a contaminant. It occurs in two types of patient. It has always been recognized as an uncommon variety of endocarditis of usually unknown origin. Recently it has become an important problem in patients after cardiac surgery, and in patients with shunts for the relief of hydrocephalus. Quinn & Cox (1964) describe 16 *Staph. albus* infections, nine of the first type and seven of the second. In all the idiopathic cases the staphylococcus was sensitive to penicillin, and penicillin, usually with streptomycin, cured the eight treated. From the 'post-cardiotomy' cases, six of the seven strains were penicillin-resistant, and despite a variety of antibiotic treatments, three of these patients died. Geraci et al (1968) describe 23 patients with *Staph. epidermidis* endocarditis. Most of their strains were penicillin-sensitive, but this is now uncommon, although most are susceptible to cloxacillin. Methicillin-resistant strains may be sensitive to cephalosporins. A recent collection of isolates from patients with prosthetic valve endocarditis, showed variable resistance to methicillin, and 11 of 25 methicillin-resistant isolates were also resistant to aminoglycosides. All strains were susceptible to vancomycin and all but one to rifampicin (Archer et al, 1979).

Provisional initial treatment can be given with flucloxacillin (or cloxacillin) with gentamicin, but individual susceptibility testing is particularly important and the definitive treatment of choice may be changed to one of the following regimens: a cephalosporin, a penicillin or cephalosporin with rifampicin, vancomycin alone or in combination with a cephalosporin or other β-lactam antibiotic. Synergy has been demonstrated *in vitro* with several of these combinations.

Table 15.4 Provisional choice of treatment in bacterial endocarditis. (Laboratory control of chemotherapy is most important)

Cause	First line of treatment				Reserve treatment (penicillin allergy, etc.)
Str. viridans	1. Benzyl penicillin i.v. or i.m. + Gentamicin i.v. or i.m.	2 wks	followed by oral Amoxycillin	2 wks	1. Cephalosporin 2. Vancomycin
	OR				
	2. Oral amoxycillin + Gentamicin i.m. or i.v. first	4 wks 2 wks			
Str. faecalis Relatively resistant *Str. viridans*	1. Benzyl penicillin i.v. or i.m. + Gentamicin i.v. or i.m.	4–6 wks			1. Vancomycin 2. Vancomycin + Gentamicin
	2. Benzyl penicillin i.v. or i.m. + Gentamicin i.v. or i.m.	2 wks	followed by oral Amoxycillin + Gentamicin i.m.	2–4 wks	
Staph. aureus	1. Cloxacillin i.v. or i.m.* + Gentamicin i.v. or i.m.	4–6 wks			1. Vancomycin 2. Special combinations indicated by tests e.g. Erythromicin/ Rifampicin
	2. Cloxacillin i.v. or i.m.* + Fusidic acid	4–6 wks			
Staph. epidermidis	Sensitivity tests especially important 1. Cloxacillin i.v. or i.m.* + Gentamicin i.v. or i.m.				See text

*It may be possible to substitute flucloxacillin given by mouth after initial control has been achieved.

Alternative treatments for staphylococcal and streptococcal endocarditis

The treatment regimens outlined may be, or may become, unsuitable by reason of drug hypersensitivity or other unwanted effects. A suitable alternative can usually be achieved by careful laboratory study of the bactericidal effect of individual agents and combinations. Cephalosporins have been successful in a number of patients with endocarditis, but are not in general drugs of first choice for this group of conditions and failures have especially been noted in enterococcal and staphyloccal endocarditis (Bryant & Alford, 1977). An important alternative choice for staphylococcal (both species), and streptococcal endocarditis is vancomycin and a renewed interest in this agent (Hook & Johnson 1978; Cook et al, 1978) has defined its mode of use, showing that ototoxicity need not generally be feared if a dose of 0.5 g is given intravenously six-hourly in patients with normal renal function, renal and auditory function are monitored, and peak blood levels do not rise above about 50 μg/ml. Vancomycin is usually indicated in patients with serious penicillin-cephalosporin allergy, or whose organisms are resistant to the penicillins or whose treatment, although apparently soundly based, has failed. It is commonly used as a single drug, but a combination of vancomycin with an aminoglycoside has been proposed and used for enterococcal endocarditis in penicillin-allergic subjects, while resistant *Staph. aureus* endocarditis has been cured by vancomycin with rifampicin. A recent example is that of a patient with pneumococcal endocarditis after cardiac surgery, which proved resistant to two courses of appropriate therapy but was then cured with vancomycin (Borland & Farrar, 1979).

FUNGAL SEPTICAEMIA AND ENDOCARDITIS

Candida endocarditis usually arises after cardiac surgery, in drug addicts or occasionally in patients who have received prolonged intravenous treatment for bacterial endocarditis. Early diagnosis and treatment are both difficult and the disease carries a grave outlook. Patterns of infection in 91 cases are well described by Seelig et al (1974). The main methods used in treatment have been removal of the affected valve, and administration of the anti-fungal agents amphotericin B and flucytosine. Turnier et al (1975) described 15 patients in their unit in Los Angeles and reviewed 116 published cases. The mortality in patients treated by surgery alone or by anti-fungal drugs alone was very high, 9 of 11 and 37 of 46 patients respectively. Of the 11 treated by surgery together with pre- and post-operative antibiotics, four died.

The advent of flucytosine made it possible that an orally administered and relatively non-toxic drug could be used for eradicative treatment of candidal septicaemia and endocarditis, but the mainly fungistatic action of this drug and the rapid emergence of drug resistance soon made it evident that flucytosine alone provided inadequate treatment. Stone (1975), for example, gave it for two months to a patient who developed *C. albicans* endocarditis after aortic valve replacement. He relapsed when the drug was stopped but was then cured by a combination of amphotericin B and flucytosine.

Stiehm et al (1978) recommends using both drugs, both because the rapid action of flucytosine is available immediately compared with the slow build up of amphotericin, and because advantage might be gained by the more modest dose schedule of amphotericin which simultaneous use of flucytosine allows. Many strains of Candida, moreover, are synergistically inhibited by the drug combination. Although *in vitro* and *in vivo* evidence (Chapter 11) favours the combination, recent work on an experimental model of *C. albicans* endocarditis in the rabbit aortic valve makes it uncertain whether the flucytosine component contributes much to the fungicidal effect (Sande et al, 1977). Amphotericin alone greatly reduced the fungal population of the infected valve, from a mean of $10^{8.8}$ to $10^{3.1}$, whereas flucytosine reduced the count to $10^{7.4}$. The rate of killing was not increased by the use of both drugs together, and killing curves *in vitro* were also not increased with the combination, although fungistatic synergy could be detected in the *in vitro* system. In view of this equivocal evidence, we agree with the conclusion (Stiehm et al, 1978) that both drugs should be used. Other possible improvements in treatment have yet to be evaluated, the role of miconazole and econazole, and the possible use of the enhanced killing of Candida *in vitro* by addition of rifampicin to amphotericin.

UNUSUAL CAUSES OF ENDOCARDITIS

Haemophilus spp, *Actinobacillus*

Endocarditis caused by a number of Haemophilus species has been reported more commonly in recent years, and is reviewed by Lynn et al (1977), Chunn et al (1977), Geraci et al (1977). Most patients are young adults, many have cardiac abnormalities and embolism appears to be a common complication. The treatment usually recommended is ampicillin with gentamicin for six to eight weeks, although Geraci et al (1977) recommends ampicillin alone in a dose of 12 g daily for three weeks, for those strains (which include all isolates of *H. aphrophilus*) sensitive to this drug. If ampicillin resistance becomes common in *H. influenzae* and *H. parainfluenzae* (the latter a more common causes of endocarditis than the former), the value of chloramphenicol, which is bactericidal against this organism, or the newer cephalosporins and cefamycins will need to be evaluated.

Actinobacillus actinomycetemcomitans, superficially similar to *H. aphrophilus*, has also been cultivated successfully in recent years from several cases of endocarditis (Page & King, 1966; Macklon et al, 1975).

Gonococcal endocarditis

Although long recognized, few cases of gonococcal endocarditis have been reported in recent years. John et al (1977) report three patients with this complication, two of them fatal and the other running a subacute course. Antibiotic treatments used have included intravenous penicillin and intravenous erythromycin.

Anaerobic endocarditis

Several examples have been reported in recent years. Although optimal treatment is uncertain, one patient with *Bacteroides fragilis* endocarditis was cured by a combination of metronidazole and clindamycin without valve replacement (Galgiani et al, 1978), and another, with fusobacterial endocarditis, was successfully treated by metronidazole and ampicillin after the failure of high dose penicillin and streptomycin (Seggie, 1978).

Coliform endocarditis

Now less uncommon than formerly because of their association with prosthetic heart valves and with intravenous drug abuse, treatment of these infections of course depends on careful sensitivity testing. An aminoglycoside will usually be needed but the possible value of co-trimoxazole should be considered (Fowle & Zorab, 1970).

Endocarditis caused by *Erysipelothrix rhusiopathiae* and by *Streptobacillus moniliformis* should be responsive to penicillin; strains of *Listeria monocytogenes* vary in their antibiotic susceptibility but most are sensitive to ampicillin. Endocarditis occasionally occurs in brucellosis (page 302).

Coxiella burneti endocarditis

This occurs mainly in patients with rheumatic heart disease and occasionally in prosthetic heart valves; it is a rare but important cause of culture-negative endocarditis. The diagnosis is made by finding a high titre of complement-fixing antibody to phase 2 antigen. The disease, often accompanied by visceral involvement and thrombocytopenia, carries a bad prognosis. Treatment is based on the administration of tetracycline for a long period, at least one or two years. Of 13 patients with Q fever endocarditis studied by Wilson et al (1976), the infected valve was probably sterilized in one patient who received tetracycline alone. Turk et al (1976) as a result of a chance observation, propose the addition of lincomycin to tetracycline. Whether or not valve replacement is necessary for cure of the condition is uncertain, but the operation may often be necessary for haemodynamic reasons. Another possible advance in treatment is the proposed addition of co-trimoxazole (Freeman & Hodson, 1972).

Culture-negative endocarditis

Repeatedly negative blood culture in the face of strongly suspicious clinical features presents a difficult problem. Later blood cultures are rarely positive if the first two are negative, but most people prefer to go on taking cultures up to a total of 8 or 10 over several days when endocarditis is suspected. A number of additional laboratory methods can be employed when fastidious organisms are suspected, and in this way some of the unusual causes of endocarditis just discussed will be revealed. Antibodies to *Coxiella burneti* should be measured. Recently recognized as a cause of apparently negative blood cultures are nutritionally deficient strains of streptococci, which require cysteine or pyridoxine. They should be suspected if organisms seen in the Gram-stain of the initial thioglycollate broth culture fail to grow on subculture to unsupplemented solid medium (Editorial, 1977).

Prosthetic valve endocarditis

This problem has already been mentioned on several occasions, and the salient features of this increasingly important problem are summarized here. Although endocardial infection may follow any form of heart surgery, the greatest risk arises after the insertion of prosthetic valves. In discussing the complications of these prostheses Kloster (1975) estimates the incidence of endocarditis at 4 per cent. During the first two months after surgery, this development carries a high mortality, more than 70 per cent in most series, and is mainly caused by staphylocci including *Staph. epidermidis*, Gram-negative bacilli and fungi. After this stage, although gram-negative bacillary endocarditis may still occur, endocarditis is often caused by viridans streptococci, and the complication, although still very serious, is less often fatal (35–40 per cent mortalilty). The organism responsible for early endocarditis after these operations may sometimes be found at the time of operation in the pump oxygenator, in intravenous catheters or at wound sites. Medical treatment alone may succeed in eradicating some of these infections, but further surgery for replacement of the prosthesis is often needed. In a large series of 45 patients at the Mayo Clinic, 20 patients survived this complication, of whom 11 were cured by medical treatment alone, and the other nine by antibiotics together with surgery (Wilson et al, 1975).

Prevention of prosthetic valve endocarditis is discussed below.

Endocarditis in patients on haemodialysis

Local infections and septicaemia (page 289) are important complications of haemodialysis; a few patients may also develop endocarditis, usually with *Staph. aureus*. *Str. viridans*, enterococci and Gram-negative bacilli are sometimes responsible and Cross & Steigbigel (1976) report that two of 30 episodes were caused by Listeria. Antibiotic treatment must be based on the normal principles with dosage modifications necessary for patients on haemodialysis (Chapter 26); removal of the shunt site is often but not always necessary to achieve cure.

Laboratory control of treatment

The methods are discussed fully in Chapter 27. The principles are the accurate identification of the causal organism and its sensitivity testing, first by conventional disc methods and then tests to determine the MBC. Serum levels may need to be determined, especially when aminoglycosides are used. The value of other tests used in managing endocarditis is hard to judge. One of the most widely used is to determine the maximum dilution in which the patient's serum has a bactericidal effect on his own organism (the method is described in Chapter 27), with the aim of achieving a titre of at least eight. Carrizosa & Kaye (1977) correlated success in the treatment of experimental streptococcal endocarditis in rabbits with maximum bactericidal levels in serum maintained at about 1:8 or 1:16.

Finally tests of bactericidal synergy for proposed antibiotic combinations are used to give some guidance with difficult problems in endocarditis and septicaemia. Their theoretical basis is discussed in Chapter 14 and the methods employed in Chapter 27.

PROPHYLAXIS

Dental extraction, tonsillectomy and other operations causing bacteraemia should not be undertaken in predisposed patients, i.e. past sufferers from rheumatic fever or those with a known predisposing congenital abnormality, without antibiotic 'cover'. The object of this is to destroy bacteria which enter the circulation before they can colonize a valve, and penicillin, which kills the great majority of a susceptible bacterial population within four hours, is very suitable for the purpose. Penicillin should therefore be given at such a time that the maximum concentration in the blood after the first dose is being reached at the time of the operation: appropriate intervals are a few minutes before if 'soluble' penicillin is given, or one to two hours for procaine penicillin. A single dose containing both these forms of penicillin, such as

Fortified Procaine Penicillin Injection B.P. (300 mg procaine penicillin and 60 mg benzyl penicillin) given immediately before extraction provides both an immediate high level and a persistent effect, and should not require repetition.

For dental extraction in a patient already receiving penicillin, even in small doses for the prophylaxis of rheumatic fever, treatment needs to be more vigorous. Penicillin is excreted in saliva, and its presence leads to the suppression of sensitive strains of *Str. viridans* and their replacement by resistant ones; these may first appear after only two days' treatment, and persist in diminishing numbers for some weeks after it (Garrod & Waterworth, 1962). This change was demonstrated not only by diffusion tests, but studied quantitatively in subcultures from colonies of different morphology. Of 40 strains from 16 controls (untreated) the MIC of all but one (0.6 μg/ml) were between 0.15 and 0.01 μg/ml. There were 74 strains from 31 treated patients all but four of whom were receiving only small oral doses, in most cases for the prophylaxis of rheumatic fever. Only eight of these strains were inhibited by <1 μg/ml (lower end-point of 5 not reached); of the remaining 66 strains three had a MIC of 1 μg/ml, but the rest were all higher than this, usually 1.2–19.2 μg/ml. A culture with a normal sensitivity pattern was never seen in this series. To say that in patients having oral penicillin for the prophylaxis of rheumatic fever 'streptococci relatively resistant to penicillin are occasionally found in the oral cavity' (Report, 1977) is a travesty of the truth. They are found not occasionally but invariably, and their degree of resistance is often out of proportion to the small dose being administered. The experiments illustrated in Figure 15.1A & B have been done recently in order to confirm and emphasize these facts in the present edition.

In the same paper two case histories illustrate the dangers of: (1) starting penicillin prophylaxis too early (in this case three days) before dental extraction, (2) of performing extractions during a course of treatment for endocarditis. This is sometimes thought to be an ideal time, since the patient is already under generous antibiotic cover; in fact it is the worst possible time, since not only will oral streptococci be resistant to the antibiotic(s) administered, but the rough surface of the vegetations is almost certain to entrap some of them. The patient whose relapse closely followed extraction during treatment, was being given both penicillin and streptomycin; his original infection had been due to a fully sensitive organism, but the MIC of that causing the relapse were penicillin 8 μg/ml and streptomycin >512 μg/ml. It was in this paper that it was first suggested that cover in patients already under treatment with penicillin should be with vancomycin. This has been considered impracticable, but it is recommended for some categories of patient in the latest official pronouncement from the United States (Report, 1977). An alternative suggested by Tozer et al (1966) is 0.5 g cephaloridine either repeated or followed by a short course of erythromycin.

Recently much more has been written on this highly controversial subject. A notable advance was an experimental method of studying the subject; Durack & Petersdorf (1973) passed catheters into rabbits' hearts, securing them there, causing small vegetations to form on valves with which they were in contact. These are infected intravenously with *Str. viridans* and a single dose of antibiotic given; 24 hours later the animal is killed and the vegetations are cultivated. Sterility was achieved only by bactericidal antibiotics acting for some hours, either a large dose of procaine penicillin, penicillin or ampicillin + streptomycin, or vancomycin; no orally

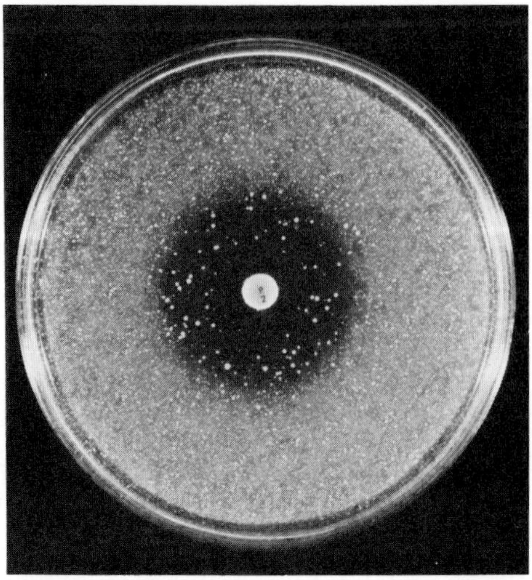

Fig. 15.1A Culture of normal saliva. The disc contains 2 units of penicillin. The streptococci are all sensitive to penicillin, the colonies within the zone of inhibition being *Neisseria*

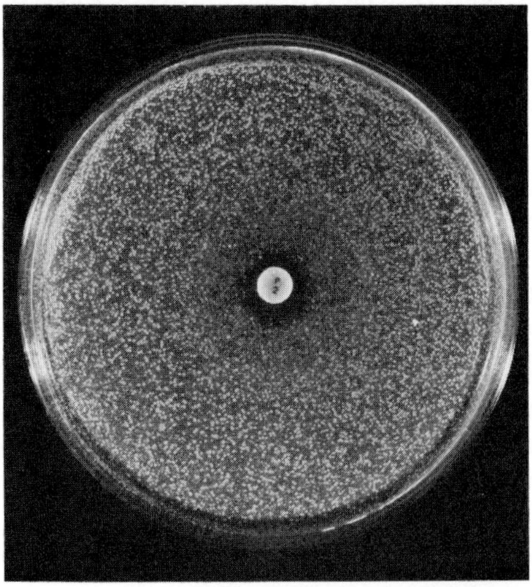

Fig. 15.1B Culture of saliva from a patient undergoing treatment with penicillin. The disc contains 2 units of penicillin. The majority of the colonies are streptococci, most of which are relatively resistant to penicillin

administered antibiotic was effective. Later Durack (1975) made an inquiry into prophylactic methods actually used by dentists, and found most of them faulty in the nature of the drug used, dosage or timing; most relied on oral administration. Durack was also one of the 11 authors of a Report (1977) already quoted, the latest pronouncement on this subject by the American Heart Association. This proposes that prophylaxis for dental extraction should be with 1.6 mega units of mixed soluble and procaine penicillin, followed by eight oral doses of 500 mg penicillin V at six-hour intervals. Patients with prosthetic valves receive 1 g streptomycin in addition to the same large dose of penicillin. Oral courses of penicillin V or erythromycin are alternatives in some circumstances. Vancomycin is proposed for those allergic to penicillin, combined if necessary with streptomycin. For those subjected to proceedings on the intestinal or urinary tract liable to cause bacteraemia, which is then likely to be due to enterococci, there is no escape from three full parenteral doses at 12-hour intervals of penicillin or ampicillin + streptomycin or gentamicin.

These are formidable proposals, and a protest against them is not surprising; it is interesting that one should come from Petersdorf, Durack's colleague in the experimental study on which these drastic recommendations are mainly based. In a paper with the subtitle 'Prudent caution or bacterial overkill?' Petersdorf (1978) criticizes their rabbit experimental model as too severe a test; although he does not so describe it, it seems an exercise in treating endocarditis rather than in preventing it. He points out that these recommendations may entail three days in hospital and an outlay of up to $1000. He suggests further that only high risk patients, such as those with prosthetic valves, need parenteral penicillin and streptomycin, and that others be given 2 g penicillin V orally followed by three further doses of 0.5 g. Penicillin-allergic patients are treated with erythromycin.

Shanson et al (1978) propose even further simplification. Groups of 40 patients undergoing extractions each received 2 g oral doses of penicillin V or of amoxycillin one hour before the operation or no treatment. Multiple blood cultures were made two minutes after extraction, penicillinase being added to one of each pair after four and 24 hours. The eventual result of these cultures showed aerobic streptococci and various anaerobes to have survived in few bloods from treated patients compared with controls even after four hours (only a single culture contained a streptococcus after 24). A separate experiment was done to compare the blood levels attained by the two antibiotics. Penicillin V, although acid-stable and thus preferable to penicillin G for oral administration, is far from being completely absorbed, less so indeed than other phenoxypenicillins; only about one-third of the dose is excreted in the urine, and according to Hellström et al (1974) much of the drug is degraded in the body to penicilloic acid. The results of Shanson et al show a striking contrast between the mean blood levels attained in 12 volunteers by amoxycillin and penicillin V after a single oral dose of 2 g. These were in μg/ml, at 2 hours after the dose respectively 24.7 and 8.4, at 6 hours 5.0 and 0.7, and at 9 hours 0.7 and <0.1. Since the activity, both static and cidal, of the two antibiotics against many strains of *Str. viridans* was indistinguishable, it is clear that amoxycillin is much the more likely of the two to sterilize the blood completely, and reliance on a single dose may well be justified. Could there be a greater contrast between this and the elaborate regimens proposed in the United States?

We suggest that amoxycillin is used in the manner suggested by Shanson for routine prophylaxis. For penicillin-allergic subjects erythromycin can be substituted, used in the manner recommended by the American Heart Association, i.e. 1.0 g by mouth 1½–2 hours before the procedure, and 500 mg 6-hourly after it for eight doses.

Antibiotic cover is also required for procedures in other parts of the body. Outstanding among these are operations on the heart itself, including mitral valvotomy and the insertion of prosthetic valves. The best method of protecting these patients seems not yet to have been defined. If the object is simply to destroy any staphylococci accidentally implanted at operation, a logical choice would be a penicillinase-resistant penicillin or cephalosporin with an aminoglycoside, and this is supported by the findings in experimental endocarditis, since single dose benzyl penicillin with streptomycin was successful in preventing *Str. sanguis* endocarditis, when penicillin alone failed (Pelletier et al, 1975). The large number of papers published on this subject do not reveal an optimal regimen, since in many of them the incidence of post-operative endocarditis was fortunately low. Cephalosporins are often administered as a single agent in this context, but Newsom (1978) proposes a loading dose of cloxacillin, benzyl penicillin and gentamicin with the premedication, followed by an intravenous infusion of these agents during the next 48 hours. Penicillin-allergic patients are given a cephalosporin or vancomycin.

It is difficult to decide how often prophylaxis is necessary for some manoeuvres below the diaphragm. Enterococcal endocarditis is said to be a disease of women of 25 and men of 60, the sources being respectively the uterus after septic abortion and the urinary tract after surgery, including the dilatation of a urethral stricture. These are genuine risks, but what are we to think of those involving the intestinal tract? It is understandable that biopsies anywhere in the large bowel should cause bacteraemia, but so according to some authors may sigmoidoscopy or even a barium enema (Editorial, 1975); nevertheless these are almost unheard-of causes of endocarditis. If there is thought to be a risk of enterococcal endocarditis, prophylaxis is best attempted by a combination of ampicillin and gentamicin, from one hour before to 48 hours after operation.

BRUCELLOSIS

Although a number of antimicrobials have an inhibitory action against Brucella species, the optimal type and duration of treatment is still uncertain, since no formal comparisons have been made between several of the possible regimens. Tetracyclines, with or without streptomycin in the first few weeks of therapy, formed the mainstay of treatment for some years. Buchanan et al (1974) reviewing a large outbreak in abattoir workers, noted a significantly lower relapse rate in patients treated with regimens including streptomycin (1/116, 0.9 per cent), compared with those receiving tetracycline alone or tetracycline with drugs other than streptomycin (4/41, 10 per cent, $P<0.001$). Treatment should be given for three weeks with the combination, followed by at least three weeks more with tetracycline alone.

The introduction of co-trimoxazole has provided an alternative form of therapy and good results in small numbers of patients were reported both in *Br. abortus* (Lal et al, 1970) and *Br. melitensis* infections (Hassan et al, 1971). Daikos et al (1973), using one or two months' treatment with co-trimoxazole in 86 patients (39 confirmed by positive blood culture), recorded a good immediate response in 78, with a relapse rate of 4 per cent. Patients with brucellosis of long duration form a difficult group, and Kontoyannis et al (1975) treated 20 such patients, who had been ill for six to 12 months, with co-trimoxazole for two months. Two relapsed and the rest were well during a two year follow-up.

It seems likely that co-trimoxazole, given for at least six or eight weeks, will become treatment of first choice for acute brucellosis. In the rare event of brucella endocarditis (Pratt et al, 1978; O'Meara et al, 1974) both *in vitro* and *in vivo* findings suggest that rifampicin should be given, together with either streptomycin and tetracycline, or with co-trimoxazole.

PLAGUE

Y. pestis is susceptible to many antimicrobials *in vitro*, and of them sulphonamides, streptomycin, tetracycline and chloramphenicol have been shown effective clinically. Earlier experience of the disease has been greatly increased by observations made during the war in Vietnam. Streptomycin alone is effective but most patients in Vietnam were treated additionally with another agent. At first a sulphonamide was used, but resistant strains of *Y. pestis* soon emerged (Reiley & Kates, 1970), and tetracycline or chloramphenicol was used. Only one death was reported by Butler (1972) in 40 patients treated with regimens of this type, the untreated disease having an overall mortality of 60–70 per cent. Butler et al (1977) suggest streptomycin in a dose of 30 mg per kg per day in two divided doses for 10 days as routine treatment, and that hypotensive patients needing i.v. therapy or those with meningitis be given chloramphenicol 25 mg per kg followed by 60 mg per kg per day in four divided doses, followed by oral chloramphenicol to complete 10 days.

Two other antimicrobial choices are also available. Some strains resistant to streptomycin but susceptible to kanamycin have been reported, and Cantey (1974) reported good results in 23 patients treated with kanamycin. Nguyen-Van-Ai et al (1973), noting that 50 strains of *Y. pestis* were all sensitive to co-trimoxazole and that this combination was effective in mice, treated 12 patients, usually giving two tablets twice daily for periods of five to 17 days depending on severity. All were cured although some had the septicaemic form of plague.

TULARAEMIA

This disease responds well to streptomycin, a course lasting about seven days eradicating the infection. Chloramphenicol or tetracyclines have a similar immediate effect, but with some tendency to relapse. The fact that streptomycin, by virtue of its bactericidal action, eliminates the organism, whereas chloramphenicol only suppresses it, has been shown by preventive administration to volunteers inoculated subcutaneously. A report by Overholt et al (1961) concerns 42 infections in laboratory staff at Fort Detrick despite previous vaccination: the infection was acquired by inhalation, and was therefore of the 'typhoidal' type with pulmonary lesions, although of very varying severity. A streptomycin-resistant strain was responsible for 75 per cent. Treatment with 2 g tetracycline daily for 10 days or more was followed by relapse in five out of 15 cases treated during the first week, but in none of 16 in whom it was begun after this time, suggesting that an adequate immune response combines to render tetracycline alone effective. On the other hand, Knothe & Helpap (1965) in patients treated with tetracycline during an epidemic in Schleswig-Holstein, obtained good results when the antibiotic was given early and less satisfactory when it was delayed. These authors' poor results with streptomycin may have been due in some patients to inadequate dosage, but it also seems possible that American and European strains of *Br. tularensis* differ in their drug susceptibility. The importance of tularaemia as a possible cause of exudative pharyngitis in patients exposed to this organism, and the efficacy of streptomycin in treatment, have been stressed by Tyson (1976).

References

Archer G L, Karchmer A W, Dismukes W E 1979 Abstracts, 11th International Congress of Chemotherapy—19th Interscience Conference on Antimicrobial Agents and Chemotherapy
Ball A P 1976 J Antimicrob Chemother 2: 317
Bartlett J C 1978 J Antimicrob Chemother 4: 392
Basker M J, Sutherland R 1977 J Antimicrob Chemother 3: 273
Bayer A S, Chow A W, Anthony B F, Guze L B 1976 Amer J Med 61: 498
Borland C D R, Farrar W E Jr 1979 J Amer Med Ass 242: 2392
Bryant R E, Alford R H 1977 J Amer Med Ass 237: 569
Buchanan T M, Faber L C, Feldman R A 1974 Medicine (Baltimore) 53: 403
Bulger R J 1967 Lancet 1: 17
Butler T 1972 Amer J Med 53: 268
Butler T, Mahmoud A A F, Warren K S 1977 J Infect Dis 136: 317
Cantey J R 1974 Arch Intern Med 133: 280
Carrizosa J, Kaye D 1977 Antimicrob Ag Chemother 12: 479
Chow A W, Guze L B 1974 Medicine 53: 93
Chunn C J, Jones S R, McCutchan J A et al 1977 Medicine 56: 99
Cook F V, Coddington C C, Wadland W C, Farrar W E 1978 Amer J Med Sci 276: 153
Cross A S, Steigbigel R T 1976 Medicine 55: 453
Daikos G K, Papapolyzos N, Marketos N 1973 J Infect Dis 128: Suppl 731
Dobkin J F, Miller M H, Steigbigel N H 1978 Ann Intern Med 88: 28
Drasar F A, Farrell W, Howard A J et al 1978 J Antimicrob Chemother 4: 445
Durack D T 1975 Brit Heart J 37: 478
Durack D T, Petersdorf R G 1973 J Clin Invest 52: 592
Editorial 1975 Brit Med J 3: 396
Editorial 1977 Culture-negative endocarditis. Lancet 2: 1164
Editorial 1978 Infection prevention in acute leukaemia. Lancet 2: 769
Enno A, Catovsky D, Darrell J et al 1978 Lancet 2: 395
EORTC International Antimicrobial Therapy Project Group 1978 J Infect Dis 137: 14
Falk R H, Gillett A P, Wise R, Melikian V 1977 J Antimicrob Chemother 3: 317
Fowle A S E, Zorab P A 1970 Brit Heart J 32: 127
Franzen C, Brandberg A 1976 Scand J Infect Dis Suppl 8: 96
Freeman R, Hodson M E 1972 Brit Med J 1: 419
Galgiani J N, Busch D F, Brass C et al 1978 Amer J Med 65: 284
Garrod L P, Waterworth P M 1962 Brit Heart J 24: 39
Geraci J E, Hanson K C, Giuliani E R 1968 Mayo Clin Proc 43: 420
Geraci J E, Wilkowske C J, Wilson W R, Washington J A 1977 Mayo Clin Proc 52: 209
Gray I R 1975 Quart J Med 44: 449
Hahn D M, Schimpff S C, Young V M et al 1977 Antimicrob Ag Chemother 12: 618
Hamilton-Miller J M T, Brumfitt W, Reynolds A V 1978 J Antimicrob Chemother 4: 437
Hassan A, Erian M M, Farid Z, Hathout S D, Sorensen K 1971 Brit Med J 3: 159
Hellstrom K, Rosen A, Swahn A 1974 Clin Pharmacol Ther 16: 826
Hook E W, Johnson W D 1978 Amer J Med 65: 411
Hoppes W L, Lerner P I 1974 Ann Intern Med 81: 588
Hughes W T, Kuhn S, Chaudhary S et al 1977 New Engl J Med 297: 1419
Jackson G G 1979 J Antimicrob Chemother 5: 1
Jensen K, Lassen H C A 1969 Quart J Med 38: 91
John J F, Nichols J T, Eisenhower E A, Farrar W E 1977 Sex Trans Dis 4: 84
Kloster F E 1975 Amer J Cardiol 35: 872
Knothe H, Helpap B 1965 Dtsch Med Wschr 90: 2361
Kontoyannis P A, Papapoulos S E, Mortoglou A A 1975 Brit Med J 2: 480
Lal S, Modawal K K, Fowle A S E, Peach B, Popham R D 1970 Brit Med J 3: 256
Leigh D A, Simmons K, Williams S 1977 J Antimicrob Chemother 3: 493
Lin M Y C, Tuazon C U, Sheagren J N 1979 J Antimicrob Chemother 5: 37
Lynn D J, Kane J G, Parker R H 1977 Medicine 56: 115
Macklon A F, Ingham H R, Selkon J B, Grimley Evans J 1975 Brit Med J 1: 609
Newsom S W B 1978 J Antimicrob Chemother 4: 389
Nguyen-Van-Ai, Nguyen-Duc-Hanh, Pham-Van-Dien, Nguyen-Van-Le 1973 Brit Med J 4: 108
O'Meara J B, Eykyn S, Jenkins B S et al 1974 Thorax 29: 377
Ostenson R L, Fields B T, Nolan C M 1977 Antimicrob Ag Chemother 12: 655
Overholt E L, Tigertt W D, Kadull P J, Ward M K 1961 Amer J Med 30: 785
Page M I, King E O 1966 New Engl J Med 275: 181

Peard M C, Fleck D G, Garrod L P, Waterworth P M 1970 Brit Med J 4: 410
Pelletier L L, Durack D T, Petersdorf R G 1975 J Clin Invest 56: 319
Petersdorf R G 1978 Amer J Med 65: 220
Pratt D S, Tenney J H, Bjork C M, Reller L B 1978 Amer J Med 64: 897
Quinn E L, Cox F 1964 Antimicrob Agents and Chemother 1963: 635
Reiley C G, Kates E D 1970 Arch Intern Med 126: 990
Report 1977 American Heart Association. Circulation 56: 139A
Rodriguez V, Bodey G P, Freireich E J et al 1978 Medicine 57: 253
Ruhen R W, Darrell J H 1973 Med J Australia 2: 114
Sande M A, Bowman C R, Calderone R A 1977 Infect Immun 17: 140
Sande M A, Courtney K B 1976 J Lab Clin Med 88: 118
Sanders C C 1977 Antimicrob Ag Chemother 12: 195
Schnurr L P, Ball A P, Geddes A M, Gray J, McGhie D 1977 Quart J Med 46: 499
Seelig M S, Speth C P, Kozinn P et al 1974 Progr Cardiovasc Dis 17: 125
Seggie J 1978 Brit Med J 1: 960
Shafqat S H, Shah S A A, Syed S A 1971 Brit Heart J 33: 974
Shanson D C, Cannon P, Wilks M 1978 J Antimicrob Chemother 4: 431
Sharp D J, Corringham R E T, Nye E B et al 1977 J Antimicrob Chemother 3: 233
Stiehm E R, Fischer T J, Young L S 1978 Ann Intern Med 89: 91
Stone D L 1975 Brit Heart J 37: 1191
Storring R A, Jameson B, McElwain T J 1977 Lancet 2: 837
Tally F P, Miao P V W, O'Keefe J P, Gorbach S L 1979 J Antimicrob Chemother 5: 101
Tally F P, Sutter V L, Finegold S M 1975 Antimicrob Ag Chemother 7: 672
Tan J S, Terhune C A Jr, Kaplan S, Hamburger M 1971 Lancet 2: 1340
Tozer R A, Boutflower S, Gillespie W A 1966 Lancet 1: 686
Turck W P G, Howitt G, Turnberg L A et al, 1976 Quart J Med 45: 193
Turnier E, Kay J H, Bernstein S et al 1975 Chest 67: 262
Tyson H K 1976 Pediatrics 58: 864
Watanakunakorn C, Glotzbecker C 1974 Antimicrob Agents Chemother 6: 802
Wilson H G, Neilson G H, Galea E G et al 1976 Circulation 53: 680
Wilson W R, Jaumin P M, Danielson G K et al 1975 Ann Intern Med 82: 751
Wilson W R, Washington J A 1977 Mayo Clin Proc 52: 254
Wolfe J C, Johnson W D 1974 Ann Intern Med 81: 178

16

Infections of skin, soft tissues and bones

SKIN INFECTIONS

Antibacterial preparations for topical application to the skin should have a wide spectrum since many superficial infections have a mixed bacterial flora. Local applications are very liable to lead to the development of drug-resistance, so that agents to which bacteria rapidly become resistant should be avoided.

The agent must be non-irritating and non-toxic to leucocytes and other phagocytic cells and granulation tissue, and antibacterial drugs liable to give rise to hypersensitivity should not be used. Antibiotics suitable for systemic administration should be avoided, so that if drug-resistance or skin hypersensitivity should occur the patient is not thereby deprived of the benefits of a valuable drug for systemic treatment should this become necessary. The skin is neither entirely impervious to topically applied antibiotics nor unaffected by systemically administered agents. Experimentally, sodium fusidate has been shown to penetrate the skin rapidly, while penicillin, tetracycline and erythromycin penetrate at lower rates and ampicillin very slowly.

Preparations

Many antibacterial agents are available in proprietary preparations as creams, ointments, powders, lotions and sprays. The attributes of wide antibacterial spectrum, little chance of emergent resistance and very limited parenteral usage are provided in various combinations of bacitracin (or its relatives), neomycin (or its relatives) and polymyxin.

Amongst those commercially available are:

Bacitracin and neomycin. Neomycin and bacitracin ointment B.N.F. contains neomycin sulphate 5 mg and bacitracin zinc 500 units per g. Numerous similar proprietary preparations are available some of which *e.g.* Cicatrin (Calmic: powder and aerosol) contain added amino acids which are said to promote wound healing. Graneodin (Squibb) is a similar preparation in which bacitracin is replaced by gramicidin; in Ecomytrin (Warner) bacitracin is replaced by amphomycin (a peptide antibiotic produced by *Streptomyces canus* principally active against Gram positive cocci). Soframycin (cream and ointment) contains framycetin 1.5 per cent and gramicidin 0.005 per cent.

Bacitracin, neomycin and polymyxin. Available as creams, *e.g.* Polybactrin (Calmic): bacitracin zinc 400 units, neomycin sulphate 3300 units and polymyxin B 5000 units per g; as powders or as sprays: Polybactrin (Calmic); Rikospray Antibiotic (Riker); Trispray (Pigot and Smith) and others. Framspray (Fisons) is a similar mixture with framycetin substituted for neomycin.

Several other combinations of neomycin with polymyxin, or bacitracin with polymyxin and many similar mixtures with added corticosteroids are also available.

It may not be widely known that antibiotics are incorporated in some cosmetics and deodorants. The presence of neomycin in such preparations may contribute to the development of sensitization and the emergence of resistant strains.

Antiseptics

There is, in addition, a very wide choice of antiseptics, singly or in combination, for local application. They include:

Cetrimide (Cetavlon, *I.C.I.*, and numerous other proprietary preparations) B.P., B.N.F.: 0.5 per cent cream.

Chlorhexidine (Hibitane, *I.C.I.*) cream B.P.C., B.N.F.: 1 per cent. Naseptin (*I.C.I.*) contains chlorhexidine hydrochloride 0.1 per cent and neomycin sulphate 0.5 per cent. It is most commonly used for application to the nose in treatment of nasal carriers of staphylococci.

Dibromo-propamidine isethionate B.P. (Brulidine *M. and B.*); Propamidine isethionate, B.P.C.: 0.15 per cent creams.

Iodophors: Povidone iodine (Betadine, *Napp*) 10 per cent ointment and paint.

Polynoxylin (Anaflex, *Geistlich*) 10 per cent cream and paste.

Quinolines: Clioquinol (Vioform, *Ciba*) 3 per cent cream. Halquinol (Quinolor, *Squibb*) 0.5 per cent ointment; Potassium hydroxyquinoline sulphate, B.P.C. (Quinoderm, *Quinoderm Ltd.*) 0.5 per cent cream.

Many preparations for local dermatological use also contain steroids, and numerous warnings have been given about the possible facilitation of superinfection, especially with fungi. While the danger is undoubtedly real and must be watched for, it appears that in the majority of cases the benefits of inflammation control outweigh any deleterious effect on infection (Davis et al, 1968). Necrosis of the skin from applications of 2 per cent cetrimide solution or powder under occlusive dressings has occasionally been described (August, 1975).

SUPERFICIAL INFECTIONS

Impetigo contagiosa

This is an infection of the superficial layers of the epidermis which occurs in two forms. The commoner is the vesicular, golden-crusted variety which is classically of streptococcal origin but is commonly superinfected with staphylococci. In Britain the majority of infections are due to staphylococci rather than streptococci (Noble et al, 1974). Less common is the bullous variety, a pure staphylococcal infection, which may occur in hospital nurseries in the severe epidemic form called impetigo (or pemphigus) neonatorum. The streptococci and staphylococci are often of unusual types peculiar to skin infections. Distinct streptococcal types are involved in respiratory and skin infections with a few unusual types able to infect both sites (Anthony et al, 1976).

It was held that mild cases respond fairly readily to removal of heavy crusting and local treatment, but most patients are now treated with oral penicillin or erythromycin. The benefits of both systemic therapy and local scrubbing have been disputed. Ruby & Nelson (1973) obtained unimpressive results from penicillin treatment which were uninfluenced by the presence or absence of staphylococci or the use of hexachlorophane skin scrubbing.

In some parts of the world, it may be felt that systemic treatment of mild crusted impetigo is necessary in order to prevent the sequelae of streptococcal infection. It is currently unsettled how important the unusual streptococcal types peculiar to skin infections are in this respect but some patients are infected with classical nephritogenic strains. In an outbreak encountered in Cairo, which was mainly of streptococcal origin, post-impetigo nephritis was encountered in 11 per cent, almost all of which was due to two of the 15 types of streptococci identified (El Tayeb et al, 1978). Derrick & Dillon (1970) confirm that while oral penicillin and erythromycin are clinically effective, systemic benzathine penicillin is superior in eradicating streptococci. Of their 708 cases of streptococcal skin infection, 91 yielded nephritogenic strains and amongst patients infected with those strains, five developed acute nephritis.

Impetigo neonatorum (*Pemphigus neonatorum*)

Bullous exfoliative disease of the new-born belongs to a group of diseases, including the scalded skin syndrome, which are associated with phage group II *Staphylococcus aureus*. Melish et al (1974) give a comprehensive account of these diseases and the role of staphylococcal epidermolytic toxin. Scalded skin syndrome may be seen in adults whose immunological status is impaired (Elias & Levy, 1976). Milder cases in the new-born may respond to local treatment as for impetigo contagiosa, but the condition occurs in a severe epidemic form, in which case early systemic treatment is essential and measures to control the outbreak are required (Albert et al, 1970). Since in this hospital-acquired disease the infecting staphylococcus is likely to be resistant to penicillin, while waiting for laboratory reports treatment should be started at once with flucloxacillin or sodium fusidate.

Sycosis barbae

Mild and early cases usually respond to local treatment as for impetigo contagiosa, but relapses are frequent. The source of infection is sometimes nasal carriage, in which case the nose should be treated as described on page 312. Quinoline derivatives, e.g. iodochlorhydroxyquinoline (Vioform) may be helpful in intractable cases. Adult pyoderma (also due to streptococci and staphylococci acting alone or in concert) usually responds to oral treatment with a penicillinase-resistant penicillin where local therapy fails.

Erysipeloid of Rosenbach (*Erythema serpens*)

This is an acute infection of the skin by *Erysipelothrix rhusiopathiae*. The organism is very widely distributed in nature and infection in man usually occurs in those who handle meat, particularly pork, or fish. The disease tends to be limited and in the absence of treatment usually clears up in three or four weeks, but may persist for longer. The condition responds rapidly to benzyl penicillin or tetracycline.

Acne vulgaris

Various aspects, including treatment, of this common and disfiguring condition are reviewed by Kaminester (1978), Leyden & Kligman (1976) and by Rasmussen (1978). There have always been those who doubted that normal follicular bacteria, principally *Propionibacterium acnes* (Izumi et al, 1970), split the triglycerides of sebum liberating free fatty acids causing the inflammation of acne (Ray & Kellum, 1971) and that suppression of the lipolytic activity of these organisms is responsible for the improvement which occurs on tetracycline. Disbelievers will be heartened by the work of Weeks et al (1977) who showed that topical application of haloperidyl phosphates which are potent inhibitors of purified bacterial lipases dramatically decreased the skin fatty acids but had no effect on the clinical severity of acne. While tetracycline has been shown to lower the fatty acid content of sebum, a placebo effect also occurs and the efficacy and mode of action of tetracycline in this condition are disputed. The extent of this disagreement is plain from a review (Report, 1975) of 12 trials of tetracycline *v.* placebo, six of which showed tetracycline to be superior and six showed no statistically significant difference. It was nevertheless concluded that tetracycline and erythromycin are safe and effective for the treatment and suppression of papules and pustules but not for the treatment of comedones.

Leyden & Kligman (1976) recommend gentle washing without friction, topical retinoic acid which 'reverses the abnormality in follicular keratinisation' and, in patients suffering from moderate to severe inflammatory lesions, tetracycline or erythromycin. They recommend 500–1000 mg per day initially with gradual withdrawal as the inflammatory lesions subside. In severe (cystic, papulo-pustular or conglobated) acne, Baer et al (1976) obtained good results from high dose tetracycline—usually 2 g per day for many weeks or months. The drug was well tolerated and improvement was usually noted after 2–3 months. Side effects were observed in half the 31 patients treated but were severe enough to require withdrawal of treatment in only three. One occult but important side effect results from the potent effect of oral tetracycline in encouraging the proliferation in the gut of resistant enterobacteria. In a group of patients receiving long term treatment with 100 mg tetracycline per day, Valtonen et al (1976) found that enterobacteria from the faeces of treated patients were almost all tetracycline-resistant and almost all carried plasmids.

Clindamycin has been used as an alternative to tetracycline in a number of trials. The clinical results of low dose oral tetracycline and clindamycin were found to be identical by Poulos & Tedesco (1976) but several of the patients treated with clindamycin developed diarrhoea and one pseudomembranous colitis. They believe that there is no justification for the use of clindamycin in acne and Basler (1976) believes that clindamycin should be restricted to nodulo-cystic acne which is not responsive to other measures.

Proper concern about possible side effects from the long term administration of oral agents has attracted several investigators to re-examine the value of topically applied antibiotics. Topical tetracycline was as effective as oral tetracycline in the hands of Blaney & Cook (1976) and this may be a safe and effective mode of application of clindamycin (Algra et al, 1977). While this may prove to be the method of the future (Leyden & Kligman, 1976; Rasmussen, 1978) when suitable preparations are available, we must reiterate the warning (page 129) that topical antibiotic applications are particularly likely to facilitate the emergence of bacterial resistance.

Cutaneous anthrax

The clinical aspects of this uncommon disease are reviewed by Christie (1973).

B. anthracis is highly sensitive to benzyl penicillin which, like streptomycin, is superior to tetracycline or chloramphenicol in the treatment of experimental infection. Unlike the generally lethal pulmonary and intestinal forms, most cases of cutaneous anthrax respond well to penicillin (4–6 mega units per day for 10–12 days) which reduces the local inflammation and systemic symptoms but does not affect the evolution of the typical local lesion and eschar. Despite treatment, some patients die of generalized disease. Excision of the lesion increases and prolongs both the local and the systemic manifestations and has no place in treatment. In describing a case of fatal cutaneous anthrax, McSwiggan et al (1974) remind us of two important features: that there may be no history of occupational exposure to alert the physician to the diagnosis and that sudden death may occur at a time when response to what would be expected to be adequate therapy is apparently satisfactory. They raise again the question whether antitoxin would be a useful adjunct to therapy in bacteraemic patients.

Fungal infections

Before starting treatment, accurate identity of the fungus should be established. Griseofulvin, the most important agent for dermatophyte infections, has no effect on Candida, *Malassezia furfur* (the causative organism of pityriasis versicolor), or other non-dermatophytes which occasionally infect the skin.

Pettit (1975) reviews the treatment of superficial fungus infections and concludes from the plethora of local treatments that there is not much to choose between them. Whitfield's ointment has been recommended for its keratolytic effect. Tolnaftate, miconazole and clotrimazole are all effective. Clayton & Connor (1974) found clotrimazole to be as effective and acceptable as Whitfield's ointment for the treatment of cutaneous ringworm, pityriasis versicolor and erythrasma and as effective and acceptable as nystatin for the topical treatment of candida infection. Similar success was obtained by Spiekermann & Young (1976). Male (1974) found no difference in the efficacy of miconazole and tolnaftate in superficial dermatophyte infections but clotrimazole was superior in mixed dermatophyte and yeast infections.

Candida infections

Numerous local agents are available but most success has been obtained with nystatin or clotrimazole. Nystatin is not absorbed by mouth and is applied locally usually as a cream containing 100 000 units per g. Preparations with added steroids or antibacterial agents are available for use in patients with underlying eczematous conditions or concurrent bacterial infections. Amphotericin B, as a 3 per cent lotion or cream, or other polyene-containing creams sometimes succeed where nystatin has failed.

Tinea capitis and cruris

Fungal infections of the scalp hair due to *Microsporum canis*, *Microsporum audouini* or *Microsporum gypseum* respond well to oral treatment with griseofulvin. *Tinea capitis* rarely affects adults and Pettit (1975) suggests as a dosage for children less than 15 kg body weight, 125 mg per day, from 15–35 kg, 250 mg per day, from 25–40 kg, 375 mg per day and for those more than 40 kg, 500 mg per day. He does not recommend the large once-weekly dose advocated by some authors except where *Tinea capitis* is a public health problem and single dosage has the advantage that its use can be supervised. Treatment should be continued for 2–3 months. For infections of the glabrous skin 3–4 weeks are usually enough.

Griseofulvin is similarly effective in scalp ringworm due to the trichophyton fungi but recognition of carriers and elimination of the source of infection may be more difficult. In Britain at least epidemics occur more frequently with *Trichophyton tonsurans var. sulphureum* than with the microsporum group.

In the management of *Tinea cruris* the whole pubic area as well as the thighs should be treated twice daily for two weeks after the disappearance of all clinical signs. The underwear should be boiled. Successful treatment of severe dermatophyte infections (principally *Tinea cruris*) with topical miconazole was reported by Mandy & Garrott (1974).

Tinea pedis and fungal infection of nails

Although early reports suggested that griseofulvin would cure athlete's foot, this has not been borne out by further experience and the same is true of fungal infection involving nails. Clinical improvement may occur but relapses are frequent and the fungus is rarely eradicated. Although the finger nails may respond to 6–9 month's treatment, some dermatologists doubt whether such prolonged treatment is justified. Local fungicides must be used for these infections whether or not griseofulvin is given.

The immunological factors associated with chronic dermatophyte infections are discussed by Jones et al (1974).

Erythrasma

This is caused by *Corynebacterium minutissimum* which possesses keratolytic properties. The infected skin in erythrasma shows a striking pink fluorescence when viewed in ultra-violet light. In recent years standard treatment has been with oral erythromycin (250 mg 6-hourly for two weeks) but in a controlled trial Seville & Somerville (1970) put benzoic acid ointment and framycetin ointment above erythromycin in order of efficacy. In a later study (Somerville et al, 1971), they found 2 per cent sodium fusidate ointment to be as effective as benzoic acid ointment in clearing the fluorescent lesions and more effective in eliminating the organism, but less effective in de-scaling the lesions. This supports the successful use of sodium fusidate ointment by MacMillan & Sarkany (1970) who were unable to confirm previous claims that *C. minutissimum* is sensitive to tolnaftate or that erythrasma is benefited by treatment with it. Gip (1974) was successful in treating erythrasma with clotrimazole.

Boils

Boils do not require systemic antibiotic therapy, which exerts no significant effect on their rate of resolution (Rutherford et al, 1970). Nevertheless there is a suspicion that antibiotic therapy has contributed to the reduced severity of superficial staphylococcal lesions seen in recent years and it should be instituted if there is evidence of local or lymphatic spread. Local applications of one of the preparations listed on page 307 or of gentian violet paint may be useful in limiting spread to adjacent skin. Infections severe enough to require surgery deserve systemic therapy beginning immediately before operation. Boils on the face should be treated because of the possibility of the grave complication of cavernous sinus thrombosis.

The choice of possible agents is wide. Unless the lesion is sufficiently serious to warrant admission to hospital, oral therapy is obviously desirable. For out-patients, an oral penicillin may well be the drug of choice, although it must be remembered that even outside hospital the staphylococcus is likely to be penicillinase-producing. Erythromycin (250 mg 6-hourly), flucloxacillin (250 mg 6-hourly) and various other anti-staphylococcal agents have all been successfully used. The drugs should be continued until the lesion heals. Failure to respond is an indication for bacteriological and surgical reassessment.

Recurrent boils

The cropping of recurrent boils can usually be stopped only if vigorous and persistent efforts are made to control the carrier state. Swabs from the usual carrier sites should be taken from the patient and all his family. Positive carrier sites should be treated with naseptin or other suitable cream or spray. Where neomycin-resistant strains are prevalent, or sensitization to neomycin proves troublesome, chlorhexidine or chloramphenicol may be used. The patient and carriers in the family should substitute for their normal toilet-soap a soap containing hexachlorophene which they should use for all washing and bathing. The patient's underclothes and sheets should be changed at frequent intervals (initially daily), and boiled. A dusting powder containing hexachlorophene ('Ster-Zac') may also be used with advantage. This process should be continued for two months after the last boil has cleared.

In cases troublesome enough to justify this regimen, systemic antibiotic therapy is usually required initially. The choice of available agents is wide; we have been successful with erythromycin. In particularly troublesome cases it may be worth giving the patient a small supply of the drug to take as soon as signs of a fresh lesion appear. The interesting state of affairs continues where some physicians are convinced of the value of staphylococcal vaccines in the absence of any supporting scientific evidence.

Gas gangrene

This term denotes an acute rapidly spreading myositis with gas formation (detectable by crepitus) caused most often by *Cl. welchii*, and terminating, if unchecked, in a rapidly fatal septicaemia. Darke et al (1977) review their experience with 88 cases. They distinguished clostridial from non-clostridial infections in which anaerobic streptococci are the predominant organisms. It is most likely to result from gross trauma, when the wound is contaminated with soil or dirt, as in battle wounds or farm accidents. It very rarely arises in operation wounds, with one exception: amputation through the thigh for obliterative arterial disease; here the source of infection is the skin in the neighbourhood of the anus, and the low oxygen tension in the tissues resulting from the poor blood supply permits spore germination. Attention has repeatedly been drawn to the dangers of gas gangrene following injection into the buttock of compounds (notably depot adrenaline preparations) which impair the local blood supply. The disease is particularly liable to occur in diabetics in whom gangrene of the extremities is usually of mixed clostridial and non-clostridial origin (Bessman & Wagner, 1975). The unusual variety of the disease which afflicts the gall bladder wall is reviewed by Abengowe & McManamon (1974).

The most important step in preventing clostridial infection of traumatic wounds is surgical debridement with the removal of foreign material and the excision of grossly traumatized tissue, in which alone the initial multiplication of clostridia can occur in the otherwise healthy subject. Any patient seriously at risk (and this includes patients about to undergo amputations through the thigh or orthopaedic operations between the waist and the knees) should also have the benefit of prophylactic penicillin. Darke et al (1977) contrast the value of penicillin for prophylaxis in patients at risk with its unimpressive performance in established infection. Because of the emergence of resistant strains, tetracycline can no longer be relied upon for prophylaxis and several patients given prophylactic ampicillin or cephalothin (to which half the clostridia studied by Mohr et al (1978) were resistant *in vitro*) have developed gas gangrene. Erythromycin (250 mg 6-hourly, if necessary intramuscularly) is generally held to be the best alternative for patients sensitive to penicillin.

Mortality remains high despite aggressive therapy. Of the patients studied by Caplan & Kluge (1976) a quarter of those with infections of the extremities and half of those with infections of the abdominal wall died. It has been repeatedly emphasized that the treatment of clostridial myonecrosis is primarily surgical and that wide excision of the affected tissues or amputation is urgently required. Accumulating experience of hyperbaric oxygen indicates that these mutilating procedures may no longer always be necessary. The treatment is not without dangers, but with its use a number of authors have achieved high survival rates with limited surgery. Fowler et al (1977) are convinced of the value of hyperbaric oxygen and Darke et al (1977) found that in clostridial infection hyperbaric oxygen was life-saving and removed the need for extensive surgery. In mixed infections they found the response to hyperbaric oxygen to be much less impressive and urgent extensive surgery to remain imperative. Treatment with penicillin, 10–20 mega units a day, is still required and local irrigation with antibiotics and hydrogen peroxide is recommended by some.

Many authors side-step the issue of the place of antitoxin in the treatment of gas gangrene by concluding that it is of questionable value, recounting its dangers and then reciting the dose. We have not recommended the use of antitoxin in the few patients we have seen in recent years and there now appears to be general agreement that it is valueless.

Actinomycosis

Although *Actinomyces israeli* is highly sensitive to many chemotherapeutic drugs (Table 14.1) the chemotherapy of actinomycosis can be difficult, because the granulomatous and fibrotic tissue involved is not readily penetrated. Leafstedt & Gleeson (1975) summarize the main features of the disease and Weese & Smith (1975) describe a retrospective analysis of 57 patients seen over 36 years. Intrinsic difficulties in treating the disease were compounded by the fact that only four of the patients were correctly diagnosed on admission to hospital. Cervicofacial actinomycosis is relatively amenable to treatment with oral phenoxymethyl penicillin (2 g per day). At least six weeks' treatment is usually necessary. Successful therapy has also been reported with tetracycline (3 g per day for 28 days; or 3 g per day for 10 days and 2 g per day for a further 18 days) and with erythromycin (300 mg 6-hourly for six weeks).

Thoracic, abdominal, and disseminated actinomycosis (and similar infections with 'anaerobic diphtheroids') can be very difficult to eradicate.

Besides possible involvement of the female genital tract from extension of bowel disease, a number of cases have now been described associated with intrauterine contraceptive devices (Purdie et al, 1977). Lomax et al (1976) review the literature on gynaecological actinomycosis and report four cases involving the uterus and adnexi, two of which were associated with intrauterine contraceptive devices.

Penicillin is generally regarded as the antibiotic of choice, given in doses of 0.5 to 1.0 mega unit procaine penicillin b.d. for periods of two to three months. American authors have tended to give more: Weese & Smith (1975) 1–6 mega units (for 6 weeks to a year) and Leafstedt & Gleeson (1975) up to 40 mega units of benzylpenicillin per day. Because of their powers of penetration, fucidin and clindamycin, both of which are highly active against Actinomyces *in vitro* (Table 14.1), should be considered. Our own experience accords with that of Mohr et al (1970) who obtained rapid improvement in four patients treated with lincomycin but Leafstedt & Gleeson (1975) describe the development of mandibular actinomycosis in a patient receiving 150 mg clindamycin 6-hourly. Weese & Smith (1975) observed one failure on lincomycin treatment and Lomax et al (1976) regard it as less effective than penicillin.

It may be that prolonged therapy is more important than high dosage since there have been several reports of relapse after a few weeks' therapy followed by satisfactory response to further treatment with the same dosage. Surgical treatment is necessary to open and drain abscesses or an empyema and to remove infected bone.

Co-bacteria of actinomyces

In actinomycotic lesions, the Actinomyces is commonly, perhaps regularly, accompanied by small anaerobic Gram-negative bacilli, *Actinobacillus actinomycetem comitans*, and a haemophilus-like organism *Haemophilus aphrophilus*. These may also be found alone as rare causes of endocarditis or of infections arising from the upper respiratory tract (page 296). Their therapeutic interest is that they are relatively insensitive to penicillin, but sensitive to tetracycline. It has occasionally been shown that the actinobacillus persists in actinomycotic lesions after treatment with penicillin. The common presence of penicillin-resistant potential pathogens has been used as an argument for treating actinomycosis with tetracycline.

INFECTION IN BURNS

Advances in fluid and electrolyte therapy and topical treatment of burn wounds have dramatically reduced mortality but sepsis remains the most common cause of death. Chemoprophylaxis has played a major part in preventing burn wound sepsis but it cannot be too strongly emphasised that it is not a substitute for physical methods of controlling access of organisms to the burned site. Immunisation against Pseudomonas infections after thermal injury now appears to be an important adjunctive measure (Jones et al, 1978). The organisms most likely to infect burns are *Str. pyogenes*, *Staph. aureus* or *Ps. aeruginosa*.

From the 1960s Gram-negative bacilli became increasingly important. Mortality from Gram-positive infections was 50 per cent, and from Gram-negative infection 75 per cent. The importance of preventing burn sepsis is obvious. Gram-negative rods are believed to be generally derived from the patient's own faeces and cannot be excluded by isolation techniques. Jarrett et al (1978) argue the value of oral prophylaxis and found that in patients in laminar flow isolation, oral erythromycin, neomycin and nystatin halved the sepsis rate.

Most authors agree that systemic antibiotics, which have led to an increase in fungal infections, should not be given prophylactically although several believe penicillin should be given over the first few hours to prevent the establishment of haemolytic streptococci.

Surface culture techniques correlate poorly with the organisms colonizing deep tissues. Loebl et al (1974) commend full thickness biopsy and quantitative culture of macerated specimens. Antibiotic therapy is indicated on finding 10^4 (or in the view of Jarrett et al, 1978, 10^5) or more organisms per g of tissue.

Antibiotics, with the exception of polymyxin, are generally unsuitable for the topical treatment of burns but it is accepted that a number of topical agents, including silver nitrate, mafenide, silver sulphadiazine and a mixture of silver nitrate and chlorhexidine (Lowbury et al, 1976) are effective in controlling burn sepsis. Silver nitrate is much less effective against miscellaneous Gram-negative organisms than other agents, but as Pseudomonas and Proteus were found less frequently in silver nitrate treated patients, Lowbury et al (1976) commend its use for perineal and genital burns where pseudomonas infection commonly begins.

Cerium nitrate is inhibitory in low concentrations to a variety of bacteria and fungi and is of low toxicity in man. It was used very successfully as a cream or solution for the control of burn wound sepsis by Monafo et al (1976). As the residual flora after silver nitrate applications tend to be predominantly Gram-negative and that after cerium salts predominantly Gram-positive, some patients were treated with a combination of salts of the two metals and this resulted in more efficient reduction in the wound flora (Fox et al, 1977). Clarke (1975) comments on the ease of application of silver sulphadiazine and chlorhexidine and freedom from pain which Harrison et al (1975) found to be the major limitation in the use of mafenide cream. They found the pain was much less when glycerol was omitted from 5 per cent mafenide cream.

Agents are absorbed from extensive burn areas. Both silver nitrate and mafenide have given rise to electrolyte and acid base disturbances in addition to difficulties in application and sensitization. Mafenide and its major metabolite are both potent inhibitors of carbonic anhydrase. In patients with extensive burns, and especially in those with renal failure, local application results in substantial blood levels of the drug with resulting inhibition of red-cell and renal carbonic anhydrase (White & Asch, 1971). The urine becomes persistently alkaline and urinary potassium levels can increase 4–5 fold. Iodophors, usually povidone iodine (pH 2.4), have been used, and Pietsch & Meakins (1976) describe severe metabolic acidosis and high serum iodine concentrations in such patients. They suggest that topical iodophors should not be used for burns of more than 20 per cent of the body's surface or in the presence of renal failure.

As always with topical therapy, superinfection and emergence of resistant strains are foreseeable hazards and may prove uncontrollable. Nash et al (1971) report a tenfold increase since 1964 in the frequency of colonization of burns with fungi. This colonization was not ordinarily of any clinical significance but they point out that the organisms involved—Phycomycetes and Aspergillus—are those responsible for the rare clinical infections which occur. In the study of Bridges & Lowbury (1977) sulphonamide resistance in Klebsiella associated with resistance to a number of antibiotics was plasmid-borne and fell to low levels when silver sulphadiazine was withdrawn, unlike the situation in the same unit where spread of multiply-resistant Pseudomonas was not controlled until all five antibiotics to which the organism was resistant were withdrawn.

The same is true of multiply-resistant *Staph. aureus*, which are common in burns patients in whom cross infection is a major factor. The presence of multiply-resistant strains may be maintained by the use of any agent to which the organisms are resistant even though the use of other agents is strictly limited (Ayliffe et al, 1977).

The application of gentamicin to burns may particularly favour the emergence and subsequent spread of enterobacteria or Pseudomonas with reduced susceptibility not only to gentamicin but to other aminoglycosides (page 143). The level of resistance is relatively small but can be sufficient to compromise treatment. This type of resistance could have been responsible for the behaviour of the strains seen to develop in burned patients by Minschew et al (1977).

Treatment of a burn already infected must depend on the infecting microbe or microbes and its sensitivity to antibiotics. Systemic therapy is required but may be successful only if supplemented by topical application.

Prevention is undoubtedly better than cure and the spread of resistant organisms in burns units can make therapy very difficult as is well illustrated by the experience of Overturf et al (1976) who found that the use of amikacin to treat patients during the course of an outbreak of infection with *Providentia stuartii* resistant to other agents was promptly followed by the emergence of amikacin-resistant strains.

PYOGENIC INFECTIONS OF BONES AND JOINTS

Acute osteomyelitis

Before antibiotic therapy, up to 50 per cent of patients with acute osteomyelitis died and a high proportion of the survivors were left with chronic discharging sinuses. Penicillin dramatically changed that but with the advent of penicillin-resistant staphylococci, the situation to some extent reverted to that of the pre-penicillin era. The incidence of acute osteomyelitis increased, and while the mortality remained low, the complication rate rose. The incidence of chronic infection is substantial and so many treatment regimens have been employed that there is still conflict about the choice of antibiotics, duration of treatment and place of surgery.

The infecting organism is nearly always *Staph. aureus*. Haemolytic streptococci and Salmonella are each responsible for a few per cent, and *Proteus* and other enterobacteria, Haemophilus and other organisms for occasional cases. Children with sickle cell anaemia (and perhaps other haemolytic anaemias) appear to be peculiarly susceptible to salmonella infections (Engh et al, 1971).

Describing *H. influenzae* osteomyelitis in infants Granoff et al (1978) comment that between 2 months and 3 years the humerus is particularly likely to be affected. A rise in antibody was observed in two-thirds of their patients.

Since infection is likely but not certain to be due to staphylococci, attempts should be made to obtain material for bacteriological examination before instituting treatment. In cases not needing surgery this can be obtained by aspiration from the affected metaphysis, from any evident primary focus of infection, often the skin, or blood culture.

If pus is found on needle aspiration of the bone, a drain should be inserted. Antibiotic treatment is instituted in accordance with the Gram film findings. If no organism or Gram-positive cocci are seen, treatment should begin with a mixture of benzyl penicillin (which is the most active agent against penicillinase-negative staphylococci) and an agent active against penicillin-resistant staphylococci. The choice lies between cloxacillin, a cephalosporin, sodium fusidate or clindamycin. Craven et al (1970) treated six severely ill patients infected with penicillin-resistant staphylococci, four of whom had multiple bone lesions, with co-trimoxazole and obtained prompt and satisfactory responses. There has been no extensive direct comparison of different agents and their therapeutic efficacy appears to be so similar that there is at present no reason for preferring one to the others. Clindamycin is more actively bactericidal than the parent lincomycin. Both fusidate and clindamycin have been claimed to have the advantage of unusual penetration into dense tissues but systematically administered β-lactam agents also achieve adequate concentrations in infected bone (Table 16.1).

If the staphylococcus proves to be penicillin-sensitive the other agent should be discontinued. If the staphylococcus proves to be penicillin-resistant, in a patient treated with cloxacillin and penicillin, the penicillin should be discontinued. With clindamycin and fusidate combined treatment with penicillin should continue since this will be effective against any mutants resistant to the second agent which might appear.

If a presumptive Haemophilus is seen on Gram film, treatment is instituted with ampicillin. When aspirate from very young children shows no organisms initial treatment should be with a penicillinase-stable penicillin plus ampicillin.

The work of Engh et al (1971) indicates that Salmonella osteomyelitis should be treated with chloramphenicol. In patients in whom Salmonella appears likely—for example those suffering from Salmonella infections elsewhere or sickle-cell anaemia—chloramphenicol should be given until the bacteriological diagnosis is established. In patients suffering from osteomyelitis of other aetiology the treatment must be guided by the bacteriological findings.

Antibiotics must be given in large doses in order to ensure adequate levels at the site of infection. After the first few days the frequency of injections can be reduced to six- or eight-hourly and after the first week or so oral therapy can be substituted for injections if the response is satisfactory (Nelson et al, 1978).

Tetzlaff et al (1978) begin treatment of proven or presumptive staphylococcal infection with methicillin or cefazolin and continue with penicillin V or cephalexin according to whether the staphylococcus is penicillinase-producing. Proven or presumptive Haemophilus infection is treated with chloramphenicol followed by ampicillin or chloramphenicol depending on whether the Haemophilus is penicillinase-producing or not. Co-trimoxazole is a possible alternative.

If oral treatment is employed, it is essential to ensure that the drug is taken and that absorption is adequate to produce effective serum levels; some require that level to be not less than four times the concentration required to kill the patient's organism.

If treatment is started at the onset of disease the response to penicillin is usually obvious within 24 hours. Therapy is usually continued for a total of three weeks when in the absence of local tenderness or pain on moving the limb treatment may be discontinued. The recommendations of Tetzlaff et al (1978) are generally analagous: 10 days for Haemophilus and streptococcal infections and 3 weeks for all others. If daily examination reveals acute local tenderness or a sense of deep fluctuation, surgery is required.

Chronic osteomyelitis

Chronic osteomyelitis may follow incomplete resolution of acute osteomyelitis or be the sequel to penetrating wounds (West et al, 1970). The treatment is the same in both instances. Most cases are again due to staphylococci but other organisms, including Gram-negative bacilli, are more frequent and mixed infections, sometimes including anaerobes, are not uncommon. Quite apart from complex bacteriology, chemotherapy is difficult because sequestra have no blood supply and the masses of dense fibrous tissue surrounding the affected bone have a very poor blood supply. There is, however, not the same urgency to begin treatment and as surgery is always necessary, antibiotic treatment can be guided by bacteriological examination. Amongst the Gram-negative rods which may superinfect chronic bony lesions or surgical prostheses is Pseudomonas. Good results may be obtained from prolonged gentamicin treatment (with appropriate monitoring of serum levels) as an adjunct to surgery.

Where staphylococci are responsible, sodium fusidate (Heierholtzer et al, 1974) alone or combined with penicillin (Rowling, 1970) may be particularly valuable. Bell (1976) commends long-term oral penicillin in chronic staphylococcal osteomyelitis: 0.5 g cloxacillin or penicillin V (according to whether or not the Staphylococcus is penicillinase-producing) plus probenecid, each dose 1 hour before meals. Treatment and the timing of the doses must be closely supervised and serum levels measured. Treatment should continue for not less than 6 months.

Lewis et al (1978) who review the world literature and their own experience believe anaerobes are much more commonly implicated than is generally supposed. These organisms are usually part of a mixed flora. Raff & Melo (1978) recommend penicillin as the drug of choice in anaerobic osteomyelitis except for *Bacillus fragilis* infections which should be treated with clindamycin, carbenicillin or chloramphenicol; in the U.K. metronidazole would be used.

Infective arthritis

This condition may arise spontaneously, or complicate rheumatoid arthritis or trauma. The primary disease is seen predominantly in the young (Griffin & Green, 1978) but Newman (1976), reviewing 30 years of experience at Oxford, and other authors have found that the disease has become more common in the elderly. Hip and knee joints are most commonly affected. Infections of the bones and joints are reviewed in Symposium (1973) and infection of the sacro-iliac joint by Delbarre et al (1975). *Staph. aureus* accounts for the majority of identified infecting species but streptococci of various kinds, enterobacteria, and mixed infections (sometimes including anaerobes) are all found. In children *H. influenzae* is an important cause. Occasional infections due to Mycoplasma (Verinder, 1978) have been reported as have infections with Candida, for which treatment with flucytosine is commended.

Aspiration of the joint may be necessary to establish the diagnosis, but about half the patients have positive blood cultures—sometimes when aspirate from the joint is negative. About a third of joint aspirates are negative on culture and benign aseptic arthritis of the hip in children cannot be clearly differentiated (Molteni, 1978). By culture of blood, bone, aspirate, joint fluid and wound discharge Dich et al (1975) were able to establish the bacteriological diagnosis in 85 per cent of their cases. The dangers of being misled by the bacteriological findings from sinus tract cultures,

Table 16.1 Reported concentrations of some antibiotics in bone and joint fluid

Drug	Dose	Route	Concentration Per g cancellous bone	Concentration Per ml synovial fluid
ampicillin	50 mg/kg	oral	0–82	4.8–20
benzylpenicillin	25 mg/kg	oral		0.9–2.7
cloxacillin	2 g	i.v.	0–190	1.7–11
dicloxacillin	2 g	i.v.		3.2–23
	50 mg/kg	i.m.	1.8–116	
flucloxacillin	500 mg	i.m.	1.2	1.6
oxacillin	2 g	i.v.	1.1–18	
	25 mg/kg	i.v.	1.4–19	
	50 mg/kg	i.v.	3.4–30	
methicillin	250 mg/kg/d	i.v.	1.2–46	
cephalexin	25 mg/kg	oral		5.3–19
cephaloridine	100 mg/kg/d	i.v.	0.7–6.6	
		i.m.	2.6	
cephradine	1 g	i.v.	4.3–23	
cephalothin	1 g	i.v.	0.3–2.8	
cefamandole	2 g	i.v.	3.0–14	
cefazolin	1 g	i.v.	2.0–36	
	4 g	i.v.	0–48	
	4 g	i.m.	3.1–3.2	
	50 mg/kg/d	i.v.	3.2–5.5	7.1–63
clindamycin	1200 mg/d	i.v.	0.4–4.9	
erythromycin	1 g	i.v.	0.6–12	
fusidate	1.5 g/d	oral	4.8	7
lincomycin	600 mg	i.m.	0–54	2.8–8.1
	1200 mg/d	i.v.	1.7–2.9	

Data from many sources. Concentrations observed in different series and between patients within series vary greatly. Where the ranges are very wide, the average concentrations are often about a quarter of the highest value.

Table 16.2 Recommended dosages for the treatment of bone and joint infection in childhood

Drug	mg/kg/d	Interval hr
benzylpenicillin	100	4
phenoxymethyl penicillin	100	4
cloxacillin	150	4
methicillin	100	6
ampicillin	100	6
cefazolin	100	6
cephalexin	100	6
fusidate	50	6
clindamycin	15	6
chloramphenicol	50	6

particularly if these yield Gram-negative rods, are emphasized by Mackowiak (1978).

There has been such wide variation in the patients studied and the treatment employed that it is impossible to say which regimen is best. For example, in the review by Levine & McCain (1977) of the safety and efficacy of cefamandole, the 30 patients were drawn from 18 institutions and only five were children. The key to success, as so often, is in the early institution of appropriate chemotherapy and in the choice of agent. A Gram stained film of aspirated material can be invaluable. Many would agree with the recommendation of Griffin & Green (1978), who treat with a penicillinase-stable penicillin plus benzylpenicillin except in those between 6 months and 2 years in whom they substitute ampicillin for benzylpenicillin because of the likely involvement of *H. influenzae*. If *H. influenzae* is seen in the Gram film, Harlow et al (1975) recommend ampicillin 150 mg/kg per day in four divided doses intravenously or intramuscularly for three weeks. Chloramphenicol is an excellent alternative. They immobilize the limb for 4–6 weeks. Tetzlaff et al (1978) proceed to oral therapy as soon as the organism is isolated and its identity established—providing compliance and adequacy of absorption is assured (see page 317). Slow response to treatment or rapid reaccumulation of fluid is generally held to be an indication for surgery because tamponade will lead to avascular necrosis of the femoral head (Harlow et al, 1975; Newman, 1976). The prognosis is better in knee than in hip infections in which the prognosis is particularly poor in the very young and in infection secondary to osteomyelitis (Morrey et al, 1976). There has been division of opinion on the value and wisdom of instilling anti-bacterial agents. There are potential dangers (not the least being super-infection with a resistant organism) and it has been shown that the antibiotics useful in this condition reach adequate levels in infected joints on systemic administration (Tables 16.1 and 16.2).

References

Abengowe C U, McManamon P J M 1974 Canad Med Ass J 111: 1112
Albert S, Baldwin R, Czekajewiski S et al 1970 Amer J Dis Child 120: 10
Algra R J, Rosen T, Waisman M 1977 Arch Dermatol 113: 1390
Anthony B F, Kaplan E L, Wannamaker L W, Chapman S S 1976 Amer J Epidemiol 104: 652
August P J 1975 Brit Med J 1: 70
Ayliffe G A J, Green W, Livingston R, Lowbury E J L 1977 J Clin Path 30: 40
Baer R L, Leshaw S M, Shalita A R 1976 Arch Dermatol 112: 479
Basler R S W 1976 Arch Dermatol 112: 383
Bell S M 1976 Med J Aust 2: 591
Bessman A N, Wagner W 1975 J Amer Med Ass 233: 958
Blaney D J, Cook C H 1976 Arch Dermatol 112: 971
Bridges K, Lowbury E J L 1977 J Clin Path 30: 160
Caplan E S, Kluge R M 1976 Arch Intern Med 136: 788
Christie A B 1973 Postgrad Med J 49: 565
Clarke A M 1975 Med J Aust 1: 413
Clayton Y M, Connor B L 1974 Postgrad Med J 50, Suppl 1: 66
Craven J L, Pugsley D J, Blowers R 1970 Brit Med J 3: 201
Darke S G, King A M, Slack W K 1977 Brit J Surg 64: 104
Davis C M, Fulghum D D, Taplin D 1968 J Amer Med Ass 203: 298
Delbarre F, Rondier J, Delrieu F et al 1975 J Bone Jt Surg 57-A: 819
Derrick C W, Dillon J C Jr 1970 J Pediat 77: 696
Dich V Q, Nelson J D, Haltalin K C 1975 Amer J Dis Child 129: 1273
Elias P M, Levy W 1976 Arch Dermatol 112: 856
El Tayeb S H M, Nasr E M M, Attallah A S 1978 Brit J Dermatol 98: 53
Engh C A, Hughes J L, Abrams R C, Bowerman J W 1971 J Bone Jt Surg 53-A: 1
Fowler D L, Evans L L, Mallow J E 1977 J Amer Med Ass 238: 882
Fox C L Jr, Monafo W W Jr, Ayvazian V H et al 1977 Surg Gynaec Obstet 144: 668
Gip L 1974 Postgrad Med J 50, Suppl 1: 59
Granoff D M, Sargent E, Jolivette D 1978 Amer J Dis Child 132: 488
Griffin P P, Green W T 1978 Orthoped Clin N A 9: 123
Harlow M, Chung S M K, Plotkin S A 1975 Clin Pediat 14: 1146
Harrison H N, Shuck J M, Caldwell E 1975 Arch Surg 110: 1446
Hierholzer G, Rehn J, Knothe H, Masterson J 1974 J Bone Jt Surg 56B: 721

Izumi A K, Marples R R, Kligman A M 1970 Arch Dermatol 102: 397
Jarrett F, Balish E, Moylan J A 1978 J Surg Res 24: 339
Jones H E, Reinhardt J H, Rinaldi N G 1974 Arch Dermatol 110: 213
Jones R J, Roe E A, Gupta J L 1978 Lancet 2: 401
Kaminester L H 1978 J Amer Med Ass 239: 2171
Leafstedt S W, Gleeson R M 1975 Amer J Surg 130: 496
Levine L R, McCain E 1978 J Infect Dis 137, May, S119
Lewis R P, Sutter V L, Finegold S M 1978 Medicine (Balt) 57: 279
Leyden J J, Kligman A M 1976 Drugs 12: 292
Loebl E C, Marvin J A, Heck E L, Curreri P W, Baxter C R 1974 Amer J Clin Path 61: 20
Lomax C W, Harbert G M Jr, Thornton W N 1976 Obstet Gynec 48: 341
Lowbury E J L, Babb J R, Bridges K, Jackson D M 1976 Brit Med J 1: 493
MacMillan A L, Sarkany I 1970 Brit J Dermatol 82: 507
Mackowiak P A, Jones S R, Smith J W 1978 J Amer Med Ass 239: 2772
Male O 1974 Postgrad Med J 50 (Suppl 1): 75
Mandy S J, Garrott T D 1974 J Amer Med Ass 230: 72
McSwiggan D A, Hussain K K, Taylor I O 1974 J Hyg (Camb) 73: 151
Melish M E, Glasgow L A, Turner M D, Ullibridge C B 1974 Ann N Y Acad Sci 236: 317
Minshew B H, Pollock H M, Schoenknecht F D, Sherris J C 1977 Antimicrob Ag Chemother 12: 688
Mohr J A, Griffiths W, Holm R et al 1978 J Amer Med Ass 239: 847
Mohr J A, Rhoades E R, Muchmore H G 1970 J Amer Med Ass 212: 2260
Molteni R A 1978 Clin Pediat 17: 19
Monafo W W, Tandon S N, Ayvazian V H et al 1976 Surgery 80: 465
Morrey B F, Bianco A J, Rhodes K H 1976 J Bone Jt Surg 58-A: 388
Nash G, Foley F D, Goodwin M N Jr, et al 1971 J Amer Med Ass 215: 1664
Nelson J D, Howard J B, Shelton S 1978 J Pediat 92: 131
Newman J H 1976 Ann Rheum Dis 35: 198
Noble W C, Presbury D, Connor B L et al 1974 Brit J Dermatol 91: 115
Overturf G D, Zawacki B E, Wilkins J 1976 Surgery 79: 224
Pettit J H S 1975 Drugs 10: 130
Pietsch J, Meakins J L 1976 Lancet 1: 280
Purdie D W, Carty M J, McLeod T I F 1977 Brit Med J 2: 1392
Poulos E T, Tedesco F J 1976 Arch Dermatol 112: 974
Raff M J, Melo J C 1978 Medicine (Balt) 57: 83
Rasmussen J E 1978 Pediat Clin N Amer 25: 285
Ray T, Kellum R E 1971 J Invest Dermatol 57: 6
Report 1975 Arch Dermatol 111: 1630
Rowling D E 1970 J Bone Jt Surg 52-B: 302
Ruby R J, Nelson J D 1973 Pediatrics 52: 854
Rutherford W H, Calderwood J W, Hart D, Merrett J D 1970 Lancet 1: 1077
Seville R H, Somerville D A 1970 Brit J Dermatol 82: 502
Somerville D A, Noble W C, White P M, Seville R H, Savin J A 1971 Brit J Dermatol 85: 450
Spiekermann P H, Young M D 1976 Arch Dermatol 112: 350
Symposium 1973 Clin Orthoped 96: 1
Tetzlaff T R, McCracken G H Jr, Nelson J D 1978 J Pediat 92: 485
Valtonen M V, Valtonen V V, Salo O P, Mäkelä P H 1976 Brit J Dermatol 95: 311
Verinder D G R 1978 J Bone Jt Surg 60-B: 224
Weeks J G, McCarty L, Black T, Fulton J E Jr 1977 J Invest Dermatol 69: 236
Weese W C, Smith I M 1975 Arch Intern Med 135: 1562
West W F, Kelly P J, Martin W J 1970 J Amer Med Ass 213: 1837
White M G, Asch M J 1971 New Engl J Med 284: 1281

17

Meningitis

CAUSES OF MENINGITIS

Primary bacterial meningitis

The common causes of bacterial meningitis, except in the neonate, are *N. meningitidis*, *H. influenzae*, and *Str. pneumoniae*. Their frequency differs in different age groups; in early childhood all three organisms are found, with a predominance of *H. influenzae* and *N. meningitidis*. These two organisms are of approximately equal frequency in Britain. The risk of acute meningococcal infection is estimated as about 1:1000, and of haemophilus meningitis about 1:1500, during the first ten years of life (Goldacre, 1976). Haemophilus meningitis becomes rare by school age, although it is occasionally found even in adults (Eykyn et al, 1974). *N. meningitidis* is the predominant causal organism in school age children and young adults, while in older age groups the pneumococcus becomes predominant.

Neonatal meningitis

In the neonate the situation is completely different. Most cases are caused by enterobacteria, notably *E. coli* and Pseudomonas, and most of the remaining cases are caused by streptococci and staphylococci. Group B streptococci have emerged into prominence in recent years, and, at least in the USA, are about as frequent as coliform meningitis in the newborn (Baker, 1977). An enormous variety of organisms is capable of causing meningitis in the neonate, of which *Listeria monocytogenes* and Salmonella species are especially notable, while the three species commonly found at older ages also occasionally are responsible. Immunosuppressed patients may also suffer from meningitis caused by a large variety of agents, although the usual causes of primary meningitis are also encountered in these patients.

Secondary bacterial meningitis

When meningitis supervenes in chronic ear infection, in association with congenital defects of the central nervous system, or follows trauma, operation or lumbar puncture, the infecting organisms resemble those of neonatal meningitis, with a large proportion caused by staphylococci, streptococci, enterobacteria and pseudomonas, while the pneumococcus is also strongly represented in this group especially in association with meningitis following fracture of the skull. Mixed infections, sometimes including anaerobic organisms, are also found.

Diagnosis

Early diagnosis of bacterial meningitis is essential for successful treatment. The age of the patient is of some value in indicating which of the common bacteria is responsible, but the only sign commonly helpful on physical examination is the characteristic rash found in some patients with severe meningococcal infections. Because of this paucity of clinical evidence, early bacteriological diagnosis is of the utmost importance, and an expert opinion on a Gram-stained film of a specimen of cerebrospinal fluid should be regarded as one of the few bacteriological emergencies.

Other methods to supplement the Gram-stain are now becoming more widely used. Countercurrent immunoelectrophoresis (Coonrod & Rytel, 1972; Editorial (1976) can be used to detect antigen in CSF, blood or urine, and suitably specific sera against the common causal pathogens are available. This method enables a rapid causal diagnosis to be made in some patients, especially those who have received antibiotic treatment before lumbar puncture, in whom no bacteria can be seen in the Gram-stained CSF deposit. Other methods such as immunofluorescent staining (Fox et al, 1969), and a latex agglutination test (Whittle et al, 1974) have also been employed. The limulus test has been used in the diagnosis of Gram-negative meningitis, but cannot of course distinguish between different endotoxin-producing organisms (Ross et al, 1975). If coliform bacilli are seen, although it is impossible to identify the species or even the genus, the observation is nevertheless a guide in the choice of early chemotherapy. As well as cultures of CSF, blood cultures should also be done.

No organisms can be recovered from the CSF in some cases of purulent meningitis; the proportion varies between 12 and 25 per cent in different series. One reason for this shortfall in causal diagnosis, although not the only one, is previous antibiotic treatment (Mandal, 1976; Converse et al, 1973). This has the effect of reducing the number of positive CSF Gram-stained films and cultures and occasionally the changes induced are so great that the CSF findings may simulate those of tuberculous or viral meningitis.

PHARMACOKINETIC FACTORS

Antibiotic concentration in CSF

The factors affecting penetration of antibiotics into the CSF have been reviewed by Norrby (1978) and by Barling & Selkon (1978); chief among them are lipid solubility, ionization, the pH gradient between blood and CSF, protein binding, molecular size and configuration, the presence of active transport systems, and the degree of meningeal inflammation. The available data on CSF levels varies greatly from drug to drug, but it is possible to make a clinical classification into four groups (Table 17.1).

1. Therapeutic CSF concentrations may be reached by standard dosage and routes of administration.
2. A high therapeutic ratio allows adequate CSF concentrations to be achieved by high i.v. or i.m. doses. The CSF concentration is usually higher when the meninges are inflamed.
3. Drug toxicity disallows increase in dose, and CSF concentration may reach therapeutic levels only when the meninges are inflamed.

4. Little or no drug is found in the CSF with or without meningitis. Intrathecal administration may be needed (page 329).

Table 17.1 Penetration of antimicrobial agents into CSF

Therapeutic CSF concn. achieved by standard doses and routes of administration	Therapeutic CSF concn. achieved by high i.v. or i.m. doses, especially in meningitis	Therapeutic CSF concn. *may* be achieved by standard doses and routes in meningitis	Therapeutic CSF concn. cannot be reliably achieved except where intrathecal route is possible
Chloramphenicol	Penicillins†	Clindamycin	Aminoglycosides†
Sulphonamides	Cephalosporins	Vancomycin	Polymyxin†
Trimethoprim		Tetracycline*	
Metronidazole		Erythromycin	Fusidate
Doxycycline*			
Isoniazid			
Rifampicin		Ethambutol	
Pyrazinamide			
Ethionamide			
Amphotericin B		Flucytosine	

* After repeated doses
† Intrathecal preparations available and see Table 17.2

CSF penetration of the penicillins and the cephalosporins is poor. Low CSF/plasma ratios are found with uninflamed meninges and, although better penetration is achieved in meningitis, CSF concentrations still vary widely and unpredictably. The high therapeutic ratio of these compounds does, however, allow large doses to be given by the intravenous route, so that therapeutic levels can be achieved; suitable regimens are described later in this chapter. CSF concentrations can also be increased by the administration of probenecid (Dacey & Sande, 1974). Aminoglycosides, often the appropriate therapy in coliform meningitis, penetrate into the CSF poorly or not at all (Chang et al, 1975). The problem of aminoglycoside therapy in coliform meningitis is discussed on page 329.

The evidence of erratic distribution within the CSF, and that antibiotics injected into the lumbar theca do not easily become distributed throughout the ventricular system, has led many physicians to abandon intrathecal therapy on the grounds that the risks of medullary coning, local toxicity, and the frequency of subdural effusions outweigh the doubtful therapeutic advantage.

There are, nevertheless, a few situations in which intrathecal treatment may be indicated, especially by the ventricular route. In some patients a ventricular reservoir may be needed when injections at this site are easily made. Doses for intrathecal injection are given in Table 17.2.

Antagonism

The evidence that pairs of drugs may operate antagonistically in the treatment of meningitis is derived from the classic observations of Lepper & Dowling (1951) who found that of 43 patients treated with massive doses of penicillin 13 (30 per cent) died; of 14 patients treated with the same dose of penicillin plus chlortetracycline (previously successfully used alone) 11 (79 per cent) died. Similarly, Mathies et al (1968)

Table 17.2 Dose of intrathecal antibiotics

	Single doses in mg except where indicated		
	Adult	Child	Under 2 years
Benzyl penicillin	←	not indicated	→
Ampicillin (sodium)	40	10–20	5–10
Cloxacillin (sodium)	40	10–20	5–10
Carbenicillin (disodium)	40	10–20	5–10
Cephaloridine	50	25	12.5
Gentamicin*	5	2.5	1
Amikacin*	1.5		
Tobramycin*	5		
Colistin sulphomethate	50 000 units	20 000 units	5000 units

*CSF levels should be monitored.

found the fatality rate in patients with bacterial meningitis treated with ampicillin alone to be 4.3 per cent and in those treated with ampicillin plus chloramphenicol and streptomycin 10.5 per cent.

Wallace et al (1966) studied the interaction of penicillin and chloramphenicol against pneumococci and found that, both *in vitro* and in the treatment of experimental pneumococcal meningitis in the dog, penicillin alone or penicillin given before chloramphenicol rapidly killed the pneumococci while chloramphenicol inhibited growth of the organisms and consequently the action of simultaneously or later administered penicillin, the lethal effect of which is only exerted on growing organisms. Antagonistic combinations should therefore be avoided if possible, but this general injunction may sometimes have to be broken, as in the treatment of brain abscess when a combination of penicillin and chloramphenicol may be indicated (page 334). If intrathecal injections are necessary, the irritant effect of introducing a foreign substance into the theca must be remembered. The purest available material must be used: the dose must not be higher than necessary to obtain the appropriate bactericidal effect; and the number of injections must be kept to a minimum.

TREATMENT OF SPECIFIC INFECTIONS

Meningococcal meningitis

Meningococcal meningitis was for many years successfully treated with sulphadiazine. Since 1963, when they first appeared, sulphonamide-resistant meningococci have made rapid strides, so that by 1969, 70 per cent of meningococcal infections in the United States were due to sulphonamide-resistant strains (Artenstein, 1969). Although still uncommon, sulphonamide-resistant strains have been detected in Great Britain and in many other countries, and it must be anticipated that their prevalence will increase. Abbott & Graves (1972) found that 6 per cent of strains isolated from a number of parts of Britain from 1966–71 were resistant. As a result, sulphonamides can no longer be relied upon for the initial treatment of meningococcal meningitis. Treatment should be initiated with benzyl penicillin, two mega units given four-hourly by intravenous injection. The patchy information previously available on CSF levels attained by intravenous injection of benzyl penicillin has been amplified by Hieber & Nelson (1977) who showed that a dose of 250 000 units/kg/day divided into four hourly doses gave CSF concentrations normally adequate for meningococcal and streptococcal meningitis of childhood. In areas where sulphonamide resistance is still rare, a long period of parenteral treatment can be avoided by changing to sulphadiazine, sulphadimidine or sulphafurazole as soon as the isolated strain is reported sensitive to sulphonamide, and when the patient is emerging from the phase of serious illness and can properly be treated by the oral route. The initial dose of sulphonamide should be 50 mg/kg, followed by a dose of 100 mg/kg/day in adults, or 200 mg/kg/day in infants.

The results of penicillin treatment do not appear to be improved by the addition of sulphonamide. In the series treated with penicillin plus sulphonamide by Anglin et al (1965) 10.5 per cent died. Of those treated by Mathies et al (1966) with penicillin alone 9.1 per cent died. It is evident both from the *in vitro* sensitivity of the organism and the poor results of treatment that cephalosporins should not be used for the treatment of meningococcal meningitis (Fisher et al, 1975). Penicillin-allergic patients should be treated with chloramphenicol. Whittle et al (1973) found chloramphenicol as good as penicillin in group A meningococcal meningitis in Nigeria.

Prophylaxis of meningococcal meningitis

Outbreaks of meningococcal meningitis in closed communities, especially of military recruits, are well recognized, but spread within family groups may also occur especially in conditions of overcrowding. If the organism is sulphonamide-susceptible, family contacts should be given 1.0 g sulphadimidine or sulphadiazine three times daily for three days.

Sulphadiazine has been very effective for chemoprophylaxis while many other agents successfully used for the treatment of meningitis are ineffective in prophylaxis. As a result, the emergence of sulphonamide-resistant strains has posed a considerable problem. Rifampicin is much more effective than penicillin, ampicillin, tetracycline or erythromycin in controlling the carriage of sulphonamide-resistant strains. Treatment with rifampicin 600 mg daily for four days produced a reduction in the carrier rate of 84 per cent (Beam et al, 1971) but 73 per cent of the strains isolated just after treatment were resistant, the proportion of resistant strains falling to 30 per cent by the time trainees left camp. In another study 17 of 62 carriers who received rifampicin possessed resistant strains (Guttler et al, 1971). It is clear that widespread use of rifampicin is likely to be followed by an increase in strains resistant to this drug. Rifampicin may, however, be properly used to treat family contacts of sporadic cases of meningococcal meningitis or septicaemia caused by sulphonamide-resistant strains. Moderate success in controlling meningococcal carriage has also been achieved with a tetracycline, minocycline (Guttler et al, 1971; Devine et al, 1971).

Total clearance of carriers was achieved by using a combination of rifampicin and minocycline, but a third of the patients given both drugs experienced unpleasant side effects (Munford et al, 1974).

Pneumococcal meningitis

Despite the extreme sensitivity of *Str. pneumoniae* to the agents commonly used in the treatment of meningitis, the mortality from pneumococcal meningitis remains disappointingly high. In most series treated with massive doses of penicillin, with or without sulphonamide, the mortality rate has been 20–30 per cent (Mathies et al, 1966; Anglin et al, 1965).

Penicillin should be given in doses of 2 mega units 2–4 hourly. This is best achieved by injecting the doses into an intravenous infusion. After the first few days of treatment when the interval between doses can be increased to 4-hourly, it becomes practical to change to the intramuscular route. Treatment should be continued for at least 10 days. Success has also been reported with cephaloridine. Love et al (1970) gave 100 mg/kg/day up to 6 g daily in 8-hourly intramuscular injections, together with daily or alternate daily intrathecal injection (50 mg for adults, 25 mg for children, 12.5 mg for infants): 49 patients were treated of whom seven died (14 per cent), and five showed neurological sequelae.

The emergence of multiply drug-resistant pneumococci (Appelbaum et al, 1977) may necessitate changes in treatment regimens for meningitis caused by this organism.

Haemophilus meningitis

This infection is almost invariably due to *H. influenzae*, type B. For many years chloramphenicol was unquestionably the drug of choice. It inhibits the growth of the infecting organism in a concentration of less than 1 μg/ml and, unlike its action on other species, it is bactericidal in concentrations which can readily be achieved in the CSF and is, indeed, superior to ampicillin in this respect (Turk, 1977).

It then appeared that ampicillin was equally effective (Barrett et al, 1966) and being free from the possible haematological toxicity of chloramphenicol, became the drug most commonly used, especially in the U.S.A. Since then increasing numbers of examples of poor response or relapse have been described after ampicillin treatment, not all of which can be attributed to inadequate dosage. Many of the patients then recovered after subsequent treatment with chloramphenicol (Young et al, 1968; Sanders & Garbee, 1969). It is clear that if ampicillin is to have the best results in haemophilus meningitis, it must be given parenterally, and in high dosage, for the whole course of treatment. The tendency to reduce the dose as treatment progresses must be resisted, since ampicillin passage into the CSF is likely to be impaired as meningeal inflammation subsides. The minimum dose is 150 mg/kg/day, given by intravenous injection at 4-hour intervals for the first 48 hours, and then continuing by intravenous or intramuscular injection to a total of at least 10 days. Many workers favour doses as high as 400 mg/kg/day. This need for prolonged intravenous therapy or the frequent i.m. injection of large volumes of antibiotics is a serious disadvantage of ampicillin treatment in the group of infants and small children who experience this variety of meningitis. Chloramphenicol treatment is much easier to administer. It is given by intravenous or intramuscular injection for the first 48 hours, after which oral therapy can be started if the patient's condition allows it. The dose is 75 mg/kg/day (but see page 449 for dose in younger children).

As regards efficacy there is little to choose between the two methods. Direct comparisons (Schulkind et al, 1971; Feigin et al, 1976) gave very similar results except for a longer average duration of fever with ampicillin therapy. Shackelford et al (1972) found ampicillin inferior to chloramphenicol both as to duration of fever and liability to relapse, which was noted in six of 136 ampicillin-treated patients, but in none of 116 treated with chloramphenicol. The only serious disadvantage of chloramphenicol, the rare possibility of marrow aplasia, must be set against those of ampicillin, namely the psychological and technical difficulties of prolonged injection treatment, and failure of response in a small proportion of cases. Prolonged intravenous therapy is itself not without risk, and i.v. catheters are a common cause of prolonged fever in meningitis (Balagtas et al, 1970).

Despite these disadvantages of ampicillin therapy, fear of chloramphenicol-induced marrow aplasia resulted in the predominance of ampicillin as treatment for haemophilus meningitis until, in 1974, strains of *H. influenzae* type B resistant to ampicillin were first described. Although not yet of any great frequency these strains, associated with the possession of a TEM plasmid conferring transferable drug resistance, have been described in many countries (Katz, 1975; Smith, 1976). The resistance is of a high order, and life-threatening infections, such as meningitis and acute epiglottitis caused by these strains, fail to respond to ampicillin even in large doses. This epidemiological trend has led to a return to chloramphenicol as the drug of choice for haemophilus meningitis. The American Academy of Pediatrics (Committee on Infectious Diseases, 1976) favour the use of chloramphenicol together with high dose penicillin or ampicillin until the susceptibility of the causal strain is known. We feel, in view of the great rarity of chloramphenicol resistance (Kinmonth et al, 1978), that this makes for an unnecessarily complicated scheme of treatment, and recommend chloramphenicol as the treatment of choice in normal circumstances.

If resistance to chloramphenicol and to ampicillin becomes more prevalent, treatment of *H. influenzae* meningitis will present a difficult problem. Tetracycline has a good record of success (Nelson et al, 1972) but resistant strains are not uncommon, and resistance to co-trimoxazole, another possible choice, is also encountered. Carbenicillin, which is much less rapidly degraded than is ampicillin by type IIIa β-lactamase, is certainly effective, given in a dose of 400 mg/kg/day, in ampicillin-sensitive *H. influenzae* meningitis (Overturf et al, 1977), but its efficacy in meningitis caused by ampicillin-resistant *H. influenzae* is not known. The newer β-lactamase resistant cephalosporins and cephamycins may prove effective, in suitable doses, for this purpose, although their CSF penetration is generally poor.

Cephaloridine should not be given for the treatment of *H. influenzae* meningitis. The organism is relatively resistant to the agent *in vitro* and Walker & Collins (1968) treated three cases with intravenous cephaloridine in doses up to 600 mg/kg daily without sterilizing the CSF.

Initial treatment when bacteriological diagnosis is unknown

Treatment begins as soon as the gram-stained smear of the CSF deposit has been examined. If no bacteria are seen or the findings are uncertain, initial treatment must cover as far as possible the likely infecting species. The best method of treating patients with pyogenic meningitis of uncertain cause is in dispute. Until recently a common policy was to initiate treatment with penicillin, chloramphenicol and a sulphonamide ('triple therapy') and good results have been obtained with such a scheme (McKendrick, 1968). On the other hand, the patient is thus exposed to the unwanted effects of three drugs, and the antagonism between penicillin and chloramphenicol (page 324) is also a potential disadvantage. All the three common bacterial causes are susceptible to chloramphenicol, and it is possible to use this drug alone for meningitis of unknown cause. The other method, which has gained favour in recent years, is to give large doses of ampicillin intravenously although, since *H. influenzae* is rare after early childhood, school age children and young adults can just as well be given penicillin. The advantages and disadvantages of ampicillin and chloramphenicol have been discussed in the section on haemophilus meningitis and the same considerations apply to patients with undiagnosed pyogenic meningitis. There is little evidence that the addition of a sulphonamide will enhance the response to either chloramphenicol or ampicillin.

Patients who are allergic to penicillin suffering from any of the three common causes of bacterial meningitis should be treated with chloramphenicol, or, in the case of sulphonamide-sensitive meningococcal infection, by sulphonamide. A decision analysis scheme for meningitis is shown in Figure 17.1.

NEONATAL MENINGITIS

Meningitis is a frequent accompaniment of neonatal septicaemia, and carries a high mortality and a high incidence of residual neurological damage (Gotoff & Behrman, 1970). The variety of organisms which may be responsible has been described on page 322. Factors predisposing to neonatal meningitis (Overall, 1970) are low birth weight, complications during labour, and maternal puerperal infection, while other cases are associated with meningomyelocoele or other neurological defects. The Gram-negative organisms often responsible have a wide variety of antibiotic sensitivity patterns, and it is particularly important in this group to obtain guidance from the laboratory as soon as possible with CSF and blood cultures. The variety of possible causal organisms in neonatal meningitis has led to the widespread use, pending bacteriological diagnosis, of a penicillin, usually ampicillin and an aminoglycoside, usually gentamicin, as initial treatment. In view of the poor penetration of aminoglycosides into the CSF, treatment has normally been supplemented by daily intrathecal injections of gentamicin. The erratic distribution of drugs introduced into the lumbar theca has been recognized for some time and Rieselbach et al (1962) had shown that material injected into the lumbar theca becomes widely distributed through the ventricular system only if the injection volume is large, about 25 per cent of the estimated CSF volume. The introduction of venticular reservoirs allowing repeated CSF sampling enabled Kaiser & McGee (1975) to carry out a detailed series of studies which showed clearly that lumbar intrathecal injection gives high concentrations of gentamicin or tobramycin in the lumbar but not in the ventricular fluid, while intraventricular injection leads to high concentrations in both ventricular and lumbar fluids. To these doubts about the efficacy of lumbar intrathecal injections must be added the technical problems of repeated intrathecal injection in the neonate and the possibility that repeated injections can sometimes be shown to have been placed subdurally rather than into the subarachnoid space. Nor is the achievement of adequate ventricular concentrations of antibiotic merely a theoretical requirement since ventriculitis is established as an important cause of treatment failure in neonatal meningitis, and addition of intraventricular treatment has been shown to sterilize the CSF when conventional treatment has failed (Moellering & Fischer, 1972). McCracken & Mize (1976) have shown, in a collaborative trial of 118 infants with meningitis, that the group treated with additional intrathecal gentamicin by the lumbar route fared no better than those treated with parenteral gentamicin and

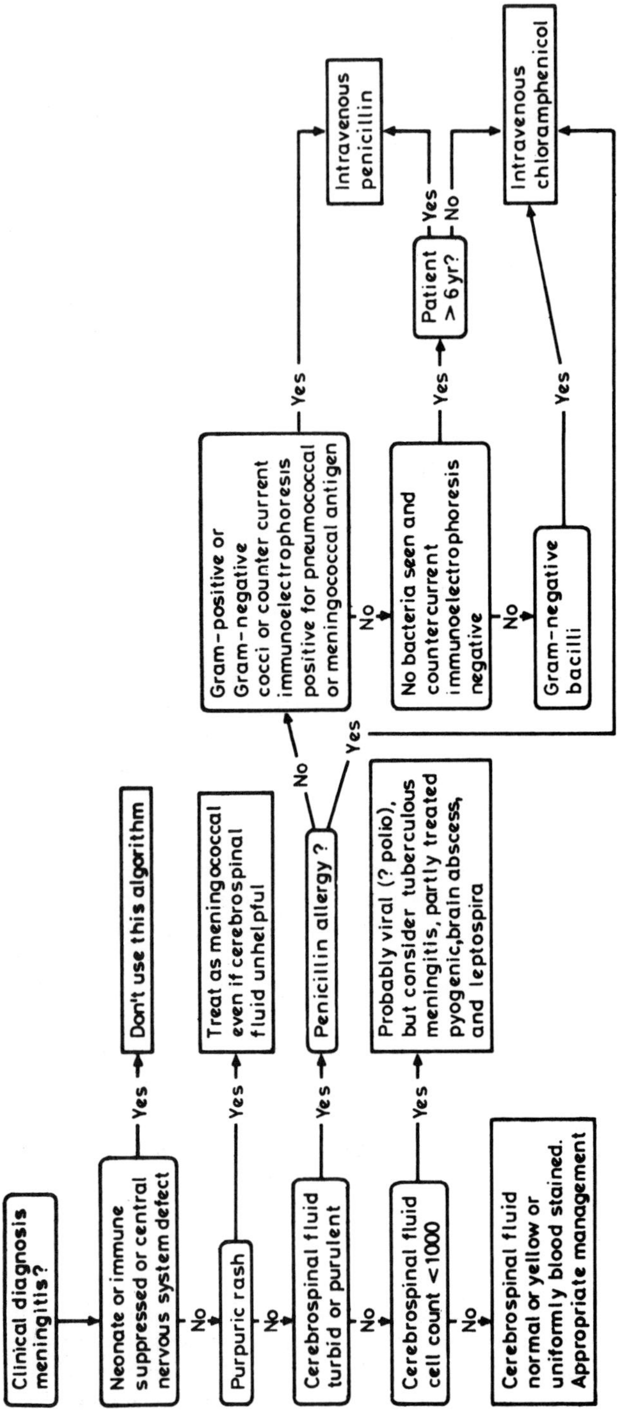

Fig. 17.1 Decision pathway for meningitis (H. P. Lambert Brit Med J 1978 2: 259. Reproduced with kind permission of the Editor)

ampicillin alone, but a later trial (McCracken et al, 1980) showed a high mortality in infants whose treatment included intraventricular gentamicin, in contrast to the good results obtained by Corbeel et al (1979).

A difficult dilemma is thus posed. It cannot now be denied that ineffective antimicrobial treatment may be one cause of the poor results of treatment in neonatal meningitis. On the other hand, repeated intraventricular injections or insertion of a ventricular reservoir is risky and some patients do recover without the need for these measures. We therefore suggest that treatment is initiated with a combination suitable for the control of neonatal septicaemia of which the meningitis is a component, but which includes a drug giving adequate CSF concentrations after i.v. or i.m. administration. A combination of gentamicin with either chloramphenicol or high dose ampicillin fulfils these conditions, although many would favour giving penicillin in addition if a streptococcal origin is suspected. Later treatment can be altered if necessary in the light of bacteriological findings, and intraventricular treatment may need to be added if ventriculitis develops (judged by failure to sterilize the CSF after three or four days of apparently adequate treatment).

The great difficulties in treating neonatal enterobacterial meningitis warrants further study of the value of cotrimoxazole, especially under conditions in which parenteral treatment and intrathecal injections are impracticable. Favourable results have been reported both in *E. coli* neonatal meningitis and in other forms of purulent meningitis at various ages (Sabel & Brandberg, 1975).

Group B streptococcal infections in the neonate

Neonatal infections by this group of organisms have come into prominence in recent years, especially in the U.S.A. and much is now known of their epidemiology and pathogenesis (Baker, 1977). Two syndromes are seen. An early septicaemic variety of rapid course and high mortality (50 per cent) closely simulating the respiratory distress syndrome, and a meningitic syndrome developing somewhat later in the neonatal period. Group B streptococcal meningitis carries a high mortality (20 per cent), as do other forms of neonatal meningitis. The median MIC of benzyl penicillin and ampicillin is 0.02 μg/ml and 0.04 μg/ml with conventional inocula (10^5), but rises appreciably with larger inocula. Since the CSF may contain 10^6–10^8 bacteria per ml, treatment by high doses of penicillin, in excess of 250 000 units /kg/day by i.v. injection, is recommended. Penicillin with an aminoglycoside may kill group B streptococci more effectively than penicillin and is sometimes used in treatment, although poor aminoglycoside penetration of the CSF makes it unlikely that more effective control of meningitis would be achieved in this way.

Whether this form of meningitis can be prevented is as yet uncertain but success has been claimed by giving penicillin to infants with criteria indicating a higher than normal risk of streptococcal disease (Lloyd et al, 1979).

Listeria meningitis

Listeria meningitis is probably less uncommon than was previously thought. It occurs in the newborn when it appears to result from latent genital tract infection in the mother. It is also encountered in adults; some patients have no underlying disease, but listeria meningitis is especially associated with lymphoreticular disease, immune suppression, as with transplant recipients, and with pregnancy, diabetes and alcoholism. Strains of Listeria are in general susceptible to most of the main groups of antimicrobial drugs except the polymyxins, but variation among individual strains has been recorded, especially in relation to penicillins and sulphonamides (Buchner & Schneierson, 1968), and it is important to establish the sensitivity pattern of the isolated strain. A number of schemes of treatment have been used successfully. Seeliger et al (1967) and Buchner & Schneierson (1968) regard tetracycline as the drug of choice, but its lack of bactericidal effect and, in children, its effects on the teeth and bones, are disadvantages. Erythromycin, to which the organism is usually susceptible, has also been used, sometimes in combination with penicillin (English & McCafferty, 1965). Ampicillin is effective against a greater number of strains than is benzylpenicillin and good results have been reported from its use. Lavetter et al (1971) treated 19 patients with penicillin alone or in combination, of whom 17 survived, and Weingartner & Ortel (1967) treated 57 infants with ampicillin with nine deaths (16 per cent). Visintine et al (1977) obtained good results with ampicillin in 29 children, 24 of them neonates.

Mohan et al (1977) have shown *in vivo* bactericidal synergy with a combination of procaine penicillin and gentamicin, confirming similar *in vitro* findings, giving doses in goats equivalent to those used in man.

The treatment of choice appears at present to be ampicillin alone, given in large doses intravenously in the manner described for haemophilus meningitis. In adults the clinical syndrome may be that of meningo-encephalitis or brain abscess rather than one of acute meningitis; treatment may need to be continued for a prolonged period. Other antibiotic schemes may be chosen on the basis of the resistance pattern of the isolated strain.

Cryptococcal meningitis

This form of meningitis is associated especially with immune suppression from lymphoreticular disease and its treatment, or from sarcoidosis, but is also encountered in some areas in patients with no preceding ill health. Amphotericin B remains the mainstay of treatment, although its value is often limited by toxicity (page 241). The introduction of flucytosine enabled an oral treatment, of lower toxicity, to be used but flucytosine treatment too sometimes fails and resistance is encountered both in pretreatment isolates and during the course of treatment. The work of Medoff et al (1971) showed synergy between amphotericin B and flucytosine and this was later demonstrated also in experimental animals. The possibility of using this synergic action to allow lower doses of amphotericin B has been exploited by several workers. Utz et al (1975) treated 20 patients with disseminated cryptococcosis with 20 mg of amphotericin B intravenously and 150 mg/kg of flucytosine orally, daily for six weeks. Of 15 patients whose CSF or blood cultures grew the organism, three died early and four later from other causes. The other eight remained well 8–34 months later, and little drug toxicity was encountered. Tobias et al (1976) treated two patients successfully with this combination together with intrathecal amphotericin B.

Candidal menigitis should probably also be treated by the same drug combination. The value of miconazole in fungal meningitis has been demonstrated in a number of patients.

Amoebic meningo-encephalitis

The causative agent of the fulminant variety seen mainly in children and young adults after swimming in inland water in hot weather is usually of the genus Naegleria, which is sensitive *in vitro* to amphotericin B and possibly to chloroquine but not to the common antimicrobials, to emetine or to metronidazole. The syndrome caused by Acanthamoeba-Hartmanella is more variable and sometimes subacute; although inactive *in vitro*, sulphonamides may possibly have a role in treatment (Marino, 1975).

If a diagnosis of amoebic meningo-encephalitis is established or suspected, amphotericin B should be given, and the report from Apley et al (1970) provides suggestive evidence that such treatment may have been effective in a patient developing the disease. Recovery from the fully established infection seems to be extremely rare.

DURATION AND RESPONSE TO TREATMENT

The response to treatment in cases of acute meningitis is usually extremely rapid. Except with coliform infections and tuberculous meningitis (page 405), if uncomplicated cases are treated early, the cerebro-spinal fluid is often sterile within 24 hours of the onset of treatment and almost invariably within a week. It is rarely necessary for treatment to exceed 10 days. Whittle et al (1973) found a five day course of penicillin or chloramphenicol fully effective in meningococcal septicaemia.

Difficulties are often encountered in judging the progress of treatment in meningitis. In particular, fever may be prolonged, and neurological signs or disturbance of consciousness may persist for a variable time during treatment. If progress is unsatisfactory, it is essential to review the evidence for the initial diagnosis, the basis on which the antibiotic regimen was chosen, and the dose and route of administration of the drugs. But prolonged fever seldom results from antibiotic failure, and it is rare to recover organisms from the CSF within 48 hours of starting treatment. Repeat lumbar punctures are therefore unnecessary if progress is satisfactory. The most common cause of prolonged fever in patients receiving intravenous treatment is phlebitis at injection sites (Balagtas et al, 1970) and similarly patients receiving intramuscular injections may have fever associated with inflamed areas of muscle. Occasionally fever may be associated with metastatic foci of infection, such as arthritis in meningococcal septicaemia, while focal neurological complications such as subdural effusion, sinus thrombosis or brain abscess must be considered. The fever of infection may be supplanted by that of drug hypersensitivity, and very rarely a second organism may be introduced at lumbar puncture. Once antibiotic failure has been excluded, it is often best to stop treatment after 10–14 days, and to observe the patient's progress and temperature thereafter. Once therapy is established on a rational basis it is unnecessary and confusing to make frequent changes of treatment because fever persists. It is often found that the temperature returns to normal as soon as chemotherapy is discontinued.

BRAIN ABSCESS

The mortality from brain abscess is high and has changed little if at all in the antibiotic era. The reasons for this are certainly complex, but especially important among them is the dangerously rapid rise of intracranial pressure which so often accompanies the development of brain abscess during the early stage of suppurative cerebritis. Our discussion is confined to antimicrobial aspects of treatment, but early drainage or excision of abscesses is as important in the brain as elsewhere. As in other forms of abscess, bacteria may often be found in the abscess contents after many days of systemic chemotherapy.

The causal organisms differ to some extent in their order of frequency with the origins of the abscess, but several recent studies have amply confirmed the importance of anaerobic Gram-negative bacteria, especially of the Bacteroides and Fusiformis groups and of aerobic and anaerobic streptococci. Enterobacteriaceae of various genera are commonly also found, and staphylococci are important in infection associated with trauma, and in spinal epidural abscess. Several species are often isolated from a single specimen when suitable selective techniques are used, especially in abscesses of middle ear origin.

An appropriate first choice antimicrobial drug regimen must take into account not only this diverse flora, but also the characteristics of potentially effective drugs in penetrating brain tissue, CSF and abscess cavities. Data on these aspects may be found in the work of Kramer et al (1969), Black et al (1973), Picardi et al (1975) and de Louvois et al (1977a,b). Of special interest in relation to isolates of *Bacteroides fragilis* are the good results in otogenic abscess reported by Ingham et al (1977), who found that metronidazole, given orally or intravenously, achieved high concentration in pus or ventricular fluid. They used this drug in combination with penicillin or ampicillin, and gentamicin, although chloramphenicol with its generally good CNS penetration might be more suitable than gentamicin. We generally favour a combination of metronidazole, high dose ampicillin or penicillin, and chloramphenicol pending additional bacteriological information on which further decisions can be based. In Garfield's (1969) retrospective study of 200 supratentorial abscesses, high dose penicillin appeared to give the greatest success, perhaps reflecting the susceptibility of streptococci and Gram-negative anaerobic rods other than *B.fragilis* to this antibiotic. We agree with Black et al (1973) that local instillation of penicillin into the abscess cavity is best avoided, since the procedure has potential dangers and failure to sterilize the abscess contents is not usually attributable to a deficiency of antibiotic in the pus.

References

Abbott J D, Graves J F R 1972 J Clin Path 25: 528
Anglin C S, Fujiwara M W, Hill D, et al 1965 Appl Ther 7: 1091
Apley J, Clarke S K R, Roome A P C H, et al 1970 Brit Med J 1: 596
Appelbaum P C, Bhamjee A, Scragg J N et al 1977 Lancet 2: 995
Artenstein M S 1969 New Engl J Med 281: 678
Baker C J 1977 J Infect Dis 136: 137
Balagtas R C, Levin S, Nelson K E, Gotoff S P 1970 J Pediat 77: 957
Barling R W A, Selkon J B 1978 J Antimicrob Chemother 4: 203
Barrett F F, Eardley W A, Yow M D, Leverett H A 1966 J Pediat 69: 343
Beam W E, Newberg N R, Devine L F, Pierce W E, Davies J A 1971 J Infect Dis 124: 39
Black P, Graybill J R, Charache P 1973 J Neurosurg 38: 705
Buchner L H, Schneierson S S 1968 Amer J Med 45: 904
Chang M J, Escobedo M, Anderson D C, Hillman L, Feigin R D 1975 Pediatrics 56: 695
Committee on Infectious Diseases 1976 Pediatrics 57: 417
Converse G M, Gwaltney J M, Strassburg D A, Hendley J O 1973 J Pediat 83: 220
Coonrod J D, Rytel M W 1972 Lancet 1: 1154
Corbeel L, De Boeck K, Logghe N et al 1979 Lancet 1: 663

Dacey R G, Sande M A 1974 Antimicrob Agents Chemother 6: 437
de Louvois J, Gortvai P, Hurley R 1977a,b Brit Med J 2: 981, 985
Devine L F, Johnson D P, Hagerman C R et al 1971 Amer J Epidem 93: 337
Editorial 1976 Lancet 1: 1277
English J C, McCafferty J F 1965 Med J Aust 2: 332
Eykyn S J, Thomas R D, Phillips I 1974 Brit Med J 2: 463
Feigin R D, Stechenberg B W, Chang M J et al 1976 J Pediat 88: 542
Fisher L S, Chow A W, Yoshikawa T T, Guze L B 1975 Ann Intern Med 82: 689
Fox H A, Hagen P A, Turner D J, Glasgow L A, Connor J D 1969 Pediatrics 43: 44
Garfield J 1969 Brit Med J 2: 7
Goldacre M J 1976 Lancet 1: 28
Gotoff S P, Behrman R E 1970 J Pediat 76: 142
Guttler R B, Counts G W, Avent C K, Beatty H N 1971 J Infect Dis 124: 199
Hieber J P, Nelson J D 1977 New Engl J Med 297: 410
Ingham H R, Selkon J B, Roxby C M 1977 Brit Med J 2: 991
Kaiser A B, McGee Z A 1975 New Engl J Med 293: 1215
Katz S L 1975 Pediatrics 55: 6
Kinmonth A-L, Storrs C N, Mitchell R G 1978 Brit Med J 1: 694
Kramer P W, Griffith R S, Campbell R L 1969 J Neurosurg 31: 295
Lavetter A, Leedom J M, Mathies A W, Ivler D, Wehrle P F 1971 New Engl J Med 285: 598
Lepper M H, Dowling H F 1951 Arch Intern Med 88: 489
Lloyd D J, Belgaumkar T K, Scott K E et al 1979 Lancet 1: 713
Love W C, McKenzie P, Lawson J H et al 1970 Postgrad Med J 46 (Suppl. Oct.): 155
Mandal B K 1976 Scand J Infect Dis 8: 185
Marino J T 1975 J Pediat 86: 160
Mathies A W Jr, Leedom J M, Ivler D et al 1968 Antimicrob Agents Chemother 1967, p 218
Mathies A W Jr, Leedom J M, Thrupp L D et al 1966 Antimicrob Agents Chemother 1965, p 610
McCracken G H, Mize S G 1976 J Pediat 89: 66
McCracken G H, Mize S G, Threlkeld N 1980 Lancet 1: 787
McKendrick G D W 1968 J Neurol Neurosurg Psychiat 31: 528
Medoff G, Comfort M, Kobayashi G S 1971 Proc Soc Exp Biol Med 138: 571
Moellering R C, Fischer E G 1972 J Pediat 81: 534
Mohan K, Gordon R C, Beaman T C, et al 1977 J Infect Dis 135: 51
Munford, R S, de Vasconcelos Z J, Phillips C J, et al 1974 J Infect Dis 129: 644
Nelson K E, Levin S, Spies H W, Lepper M H 1972 J Infect Dis 125: 459
Norrby R 1978 Scand J Infect Dis, Supplement 14: 296
Overall J C 1970 J Pediat 76: 499
Overturf G D, Steinberg E A, Underman A E, et al 1977 Antimicrob Ag Chemother 11: 420
Picardi J L, Lewis H P, Tan J S, Phair J P 1975 J Neurosurg 43: 717
Rieselbach R E, DiChiro G, Freireich E J, Rall D P 1962 New Engl J Med 267: 1273
Ross S, Rodriguez W, Controni G, et al 1975 J Amer Med Ass 233: 1366
Sabel K G, Brandberg A 1975 Acta Paed Scand 64: 25
Sanders D Y, Garbee H W 1969 Amer J Dis Child 117: 331
Schulkind M L, Altemeier W A, Ayoub E M 1971 Pediatrics 48: 411
Seeliger H P R, Laymann U, Finger H 1967 Dtsch Med Wschr 92: 1095
Shackelford P G, Bobinski J E, Feigin R D, Cherry J D 1972 New Engl J Med 287: 634
Smith A L 1976 New Engl J Med 294: 1329
Tobias J S, Wrigley P F M, Shaw E 1976 Postgrad Med J 52: 305
Turk D C 1977 J Med Microbiol 10: 127
Utz J P, Garriques I L, Sande M A, et al 1975 J Infect Dis 132: 368
Visintine A M, Oleske J M, Nahmias A J 1977 Amer J Dis Child 131: 393
Walker S H, Collins C C 1968 Amer J Dis Child 116: 285
Wallace J F, Smith R H, Garcia M, Petersdorf R G 1966 Antimicrob Agents Chemother 1965, p 439
Weingartner L, Ortel S 1967 Dtsch Med Wschr 92: 1098
Whittle H C, Davidson N McD, Greenwood B M, et al 1973 Brit Med J 3: 379
Whittle H C, Tugwell P, Egler L J, Greenwood B M 1974 Lancet 2: 619
Young L M, Haddow J E, Klein J O 1968 Pediatrics 41: 516

18

Infections of the alimentary tract

ENTERIC FEVER

Typhoid fever is the disease *par excellence* in which *in vitro* antibiotic activity is no guarantee of therapeutic success. Many agents, for example, cephaloridine, gentamicin, and polymyxin E, although bactericidal against *S. typhi*, have no effect on the disease (Dawkins & Hornick, 1967). Those agents effective both *in vitro* and *in vivo* must all be compared with chloramphenicol as the treatment for which the greatest experience is available.

The advantages of chloramphenicol are relative speed of action with a period of defervescence averaging 3–4 days, a low incidence of side effects and cheapness in developing countries. Its disadvantages are the risk of marrow damage, the emergence of chloramphenicol resistance in *S. typhi*, and the frequency of relapse; indeed, short courses may be followed by a greater frequency of relapse than the untreated disease, and it is for this reason that treatment is maintained for 10–14 days.

Ampicillin, even in large doses, proved a disappointing alternative to chloramphenicol, as the response was markedly slower and some patients failed to show any benefit (earlier studies are reviewed in the 4th edition). Combined treatment, however, using ampicillin 4 g daily together with chloramphenicol 2 g daily, were more successful, giving a 29 per cent reduction of fever (de Ritis et al, 1972).

Much more promising are the results obtained with co-trimoxazole and with amoxycillin. The earliest large report was that of Kamat (1970) who treated 220 patients, all having positive blood cultures, with chlorampenicol or with co-trimoxazole, mean periods of defervescence were 4.3 and 4.0 days respectively, but there were no 'toxic crises' in the co-trimoxazole group. Other series were similarly favourable except that of Scragg & Rubidge (1971) who, while confirming rapid symptomatic improvement in children treated with co-trimoxazole, noted persistence of fever, a higher relapse rate, more frequent subsequent stool carriage, and sometimes evidence of bone marrow depression. From the same centre has been reported favourable results using amoxycillin for children with typhoid. Scragg (1976), using chloramphenicol 50 mg/kg/day or amoxycillin 100 mg/kg/day, found a more rapid response from amoxycillin. Of 185 children given this drug in the course of two studies, two had relapsed and one become a convalescent carrier. This compared with two failures to respond, one relapse and 11 carriers in 170 children given chloramphenicol.

Amoxycillin has been compared with chloramphenicol in adults by Pillay et al

(1975) with very similar rates of improvement, usually striking within 72–96 hours with both drugs, and only one failure to respond in each group of 61 and 63 patients. Defervescence was somewhat more rapid in the patients given amoxycillin. Both drugs were given for 14 days, amoxycillin in a dose of 1 g six hourly by mouth. Co-trimoxazole has been compared with amoxycillin in an important study which included both chloramphenicol-sensitive and chloramphenicol-resistant typhoid fever (Gilman et al, 1975). The mean duration of fever was significantly shorter in patients infected with sensitive strains treated with co-trimoxazole (83 hours) than in those treated with amoxycillin (136 hours). This advantage of co-trimoxazole was lost in the chloramphenicol-resistant group. Since the responsible plasmid also confers resistance to sulphonamide and synergy with trimethoprim could not be detected, this group of patients presumably showed the effect in treatment of trimethoprim alone. The rate of stool clearance was about the same in all groups.

A series of comparative trials of parenteral chloramphenicol, oral chloramphenicol, ampicillin and co-trimoxazole by Snyder et al (1976) showed little to choose between the groups, but confirmed the poor absorption of chloramphenicol by the intramuscular route, blood concentration being about half those following oral administration of the same dose (see also page 159).

Lacking from most clinical trials in typhoid is any sizeable information about relapse rates following different regimens. All that can be said is that relapses do occur with all currently available treatments. The most recent addition to antimicrobial treatment in typhoid is mecillinam. Geddes & Clarke (1977) found that 13 of 15 patients responded well, with a mean duration of fever of five days, but Mandal et al (1979) found that drug notably ineffective, despite full *in vitro* sensitivity. Oxolinic acid, also very active *in vitro*, was also found ineffective in the treatment of typhoid in American soldiers in Vietnam (Sanford et al, 1976).

We conclude that co-trimoxazole or chloramphenicol are equally suitable as first choice treatments for typhoid fever, but that co-trimoxazole will be preferred in the knowledge or suspicion of chloramphenicol resistance. Amoxycillin is also effective, but its use also will be limited if ampicillin resistant plasmids become prevalent in *S. typhi.*

Treatment of carriers

Here ampicillin has had much more success. Whereas tetracyclines or large doses of penicillin have in the past cleared only about 25 per cent of cases, ampicillin has been successful in 80 per cent or more. Christie (1964) cleared seven out of eight by 3 months' treatment with initially large doses reduced to 3 g orally daily, together with probenecid and continued for 12 weeks. Münnich et al (1965/6) succeeded in 11 out of 12 cases by giving ampicillin parenterally (500 mg four times a day) together with oral probenecid for up to 6 weeks. Simon & Miller (1966) gave 75–100 mg/kg daily for 4 weeks or more to 15 cases, clearing 13. Scioli et al (1972) cleared every one of 19 longstanding cases (all followed up for 16–24 months), five of whom had gall stones and eight non-functioning gall bladders, by giving 1 g intravenously 8-hourly for 15 days. These findings confirm that success may sometimes be achieved regardless of gall bladder abnormalities, and suggest that parenteral administration may enable the course to be shortened.

The modest success with ampicillin leads naturally to the use of amoxycillin for chronic typhoid carriage. Farid et al (1975) treated 12 patients with *S. typhi* or *S. paratyphi A* bacteriuria and recurrent bacteraemia associated with schistosomiasis with amoxycillin 250 mg four times daily for four weeks. Urine and blood cultures became negative within a week and remained so during a four week follow-up.

Co-trimoxazole has also been employed in the treatment of chronic carriers. Pichler & Spitzy (1972) treated six *S. typhi* and nine *S. paratyphi B* carriers, and 14 of the 15 remained clear during the following year in which 24 stools were examined for each patient.

As strains of *S. typhi* emerge resistant to chloramphenicol and possibly other drugs in the existing armamentarium, other as yet untried chemotherapeutic methods may come to be used. For example, Shanson & Leung (1976) have shown synergy between rifampicin and novobiocin in 17 of 18 strains of *S. typhi*, with optimal concentrations of both drugs which are easily obtainable in bile.

Other salmonella infections

The treatment of paratyphoid fever is the same as that for typhoid. Salmonella enteritis of the food-poisoning type is usually a self-limited disease of short duration, and treatment with antimicrobial drugs is unnecessary. On the other hand salmonella gastroenteritis tends to be particularly severe in patients who are achlorhydric by reason of previous gastric surgery, pernicious anaemia or other reasons, and in infancy. If a systemic infection has been demonstrated by blood culture or is suspected from the clinical condition, chemotherapy should be given.

There is strong evidence that unnecessary antibiotic treatment of mild salmonella enteritis actually prolongs the subsequent carrier state. This was originally observed by Dixon (1965) and was confirmed in an extensive epidemic reported by Aserkoff & Bennett (1969) in which treatment with various antibiotics not only delayed elimination of the organism but in some cases led to its becoming resistant to one or more drugs, this resistance usually being transferable. In a controlled study of the action of oral neomycin, its only effect was to increase the frequency of the subsequent carrier state (Report, 1970).

BACILLARY DYSENTERY

The average mild infection due to *Sh. sonnei* does not require specific treatment, and it seems inadvisable that routine reports of the isolation of this organism should include information about drug sensitivities, since this may seem to encourage such treatment. Moreover, *Sh. sonnei* is now frequently drug-resistant. This is a species in which multiple transferable resistance has been studied for years, and the great majority of strains isolated in London have for some years been resistant not only to sulphonamides but to ampicillin (Davies et al, 1970). The spread of antibiotic resistance in *Shigella* has been noted in other countries: 23 of 24 strains of *Sh. sonnei* in Auckland were ampicillin resistant (Smith et al, 1974), and in Houston, Texas, 55 per cent of *Sh. sonnei* strains were ampicillin resistant (Byers et al, 1976). In the latter study, all 173 strains (mostly *Sh. sonnei* or *Sh. flexneri*) were susceptible to quinoline drugs and to trimethoprim-sulphamethoxazole.

Specific treatment may be required for more severe infections by Shigella species, and the choice of an antibiotic should depend on laboratory tests either of the patient's own strain or of previous isolates in an epidemic. Ampicillin did provide satisfactory treatment before resistance became widespread (Haltanin et al, 1972; Tong et al, 1970), but cephalexin gives poor results, 76 per cent of patients having positive stool cultures after five days of treatment (Nelson & Haltanin, 1975). When the causal strain is susceptible, co-trimoxazole provides effective treatment (Freiberg, 1971; Lexomboon et al, 1972; Nelson et al, 1976) and will usually be agent of first choice for acute shigellosis pending identification of the actual species and its drug susceptibility.

AMOEBIASIS

A full discussion is beyond the scope of this book but, as in giardiasis, older treatments are now yielding to less toxic agents. Emetine and chloroquine are now rarely used in the treatment of invasive amoebiasis including liver abscess. Metronidazole in a dose of 400 mg t.d.s. for five days provides satisfactory treatment for most liver abscesses and aspiration as an additional measure is often unnecessary. Paradoxically a larger dose of metronidazole is needed for the eradication of chronic intestinal carriage (800 mg daily for 5–10 days), since low concentrations of the drug may be found in the colon. Alternative methods of treatment for chronic intestinal carriage include di-iodohydroxyquinoline (diodoquine) 650 mg t.d.s. for three weeks, diloxanide furoate 500 mg t.d.s. for 10 days, paromomycin sulphate 25 mg/kg/day for 5 days, and tetracycline. The latter three drugs are also effective in acute intestinal amoebiasis but diodoquine is ineffective for this purpose.

Tinidazole, mentioned in the discussion of giardia infestations, has also been used in amoebiasis. Scragg et al (1976) and Ahmed et al (1976) achieved excellent results in amoebic infections in childhood, with cures in 28 of 30 children and 39 or 40 children respectively.

GIARDIASIS

This infection is an important cause of acute diarrhoea, and of chronic diarrhoea associated with intestinal malabsorption. Although problems of diagnosis are not the subject of this book, it must be emphasised that giardiasis (and amoebiasis) is easily missed, for two reasons. Culture of the stool without microscopy will, of course, fail to indicate its presence; moreover, stool microscopy detects only about half the number of infestations found in the duodenal aspirate (Kay et al, 1977).

Several drugs are available for treatment. Perhaps the most effective is mepacrine (known as quinacrine in the U.S.A.) which, in a dose for adults of 100 mg t.d.s. for seven days, gives cure rates of at least 95 per cent (Wolfe, 1975). Unfortunately, this drug is associated with a formidable number of unwanted effects, including serious skin reactions, toxic psychosis, gastrointestinal disturbances and yellow skin. For this reason, mepacrine is now recommended only in infestations which have proved resistant to less toxic therapy with metronidazole or tinidazole. Metronidazole in a dose of 200 mg t.d.s. for seven days results in cure rates of 70–90 per cent, and good results have also been achieved by the administration of 1 g once a day for three days. The more recently developed anti-flagellate drug tinidazole, given in a dose of 150 mg b.d. for seven days, cured all 24 students of a group who had acquired giardiasis on a journey to Leningrad (Andersson et al, 1972), whereas a comparable course of metronidazole cleared only 71 per cent of a similarly infested group. Tinidazole can be given as a single dose treatment of 2 g, with overall cure rates of over 90 per cent (Pettersson, 1975). Another moderately effect agent in giardiasis is furazolidone; 22 of 27 children were cured by this agent (Wolfe 1975).

CHOLERA

Recognition that chemotherapy can be effective in cholera came late. Carpenter et al (1964) in India and Greenough et al (1964) in Pakistan have shown that tetracycline in moderate doses, the first few intravenous and thereafter oral, rapidly eliminates *V. cholerae* from the bowel, greatly reduces both stool volume and the requirement for intravenous fluid, and enables patients to be discharged in three days instead of seven. The economy in intravenous fluids and in bed occupancy is important in enabling more patients to be treated in an epidemic. Furazolidone (Chaudhuri et al, 1968; Pierce et al, 1968) is a cheaper and apparently effective alternative.

Since these observations other agents have also been found effective. Pastore et al (1977) found co-trimoxazole as effective as tetracycline and chloramphenicol in ridding the stool of cholera vibrio, and Rahaman et al (1976) found doxycycline as effective as tetracycline in reducing the fluid requirement in acute cholera. The stools became culture-negative in two days on tetracycline, in three days on doxycycline. Tetracycline has also been used successully in preventing cholera in family contacts (McCormack et al, 1968). As with other bowel infections, however, resistance to tetracycline and other antimicrobial agents may emerge rapidly. In an epidemic in Tanzania (Mhalu et al, 1979) all the strains were at first sensitive to tetracycline, but after five months 76 per cent of them were resistant to this drug. Resistance to other agents also increased, although at a slower pace.

CAMPYLOBACTER ENTERITIS

Recent advances in isolation techniques (Skirrow, 1977) have made for easier recognition of this common form of gastrointestinal infection. In patients with mild forms of the illness, isolation of the pathogen coincides with clinical improvement and antibiotics are not indicated. Some patients suffer more prolonged and severe illnesses with abdominal pain, fever and bloody diarrhoea. For these patients, erythromycin, which may be given by mouth as the stearate, is the drug of choice.

TRAVELLER'S DIARRHOEA

The prevention and management of the common and distressing disorder has long been a matter of controversy. It is now evident that the syndrome is of multiple aetiology and that, at least in some areas, enterotoxigenic strains of *E. coli* are responsible for a substantial proportion of attacks. Other identified pathogens include salmonellae, shigellae, *Vibrio parahaemolyticus*, invasive strains of *E. coli*, *Giardia lamblia* and rotaviruses (Gorbach et al, 1975; Merson et al, 1976). The widely variable results of antibiotic trials in traveller's diarrhoea may thus be attributable to the variety of agents at different times and at different places.

Perhaps the drug most extensively used for many years was iodochlorhydroxyquinoline (enterovioform). Its efficacy was dubious even before it was withdrawn because of its relationship to subacute myelo-optic neuropathy. Kean & Waters (1959) found it ineffective in a placebo controlled study and Loewenstein et al (1973) also found it ineffective. Occasional successes have been reported using neomycin or sulphonamides. Turner (1967) found both the attack-rate and severity of attacks to be reduced by a combination of streptomycin and triple sulphonamide, although the sulphonamides with a larger dose of neomycin only had the second of these effects. Some large surveys have tended to show an inverse relationship between attempted chemoprophylaxis and the development of diarrhoea. Kean (1963) found that 52 per cent of those who took 'preventive' medicines developed diarrhoea while only 15 per cent of those who took no drugs became ill. The same trend was evident in lesser degree in the questionnaire survey conducted by Loewenstein et al (1973) among participants at the 10th International Congress of Microbiology. Although these results may only mean that people who feel themselves liable to this disorder take drugs to try and prevent it, they certainly do not suggest much success for chemoprophylaxis as a general preventive measure, nor did this survey show much agreement between the attending microbiologists as to the appropriate drug to take, since in their replies they named 39 different medicinal preparations.

We consider that, although the idea of preventing new bacterial colonisation of the bowel by diarrhoeal organisms is soundly based, its execution in practice has so far proved disappointing, and that no general antibiotic policy for traveller's diarrhoea can be recommended. If chemoprophylaxis is attempted, it should, if possible, be based on the known prevalence of particular pathogens in the area. Where, as is usually the case, no such information is available, it is preferable to rely on normal hygienic precautions. If doctor or patient feel strongly in favour of using antimicrobial drugs for this purpose, streptomycin and triple sulphonamide is a reasonable choice.

ACUTE INFANTILE GASTRO-ENTERITIS

Correction of fluid and electrolyte imbalance are the essential features of treatment, and the rôle of antimicrobial agents has remained uncertain, both for *E. coli* gastroenteritis and for syndromes of uncertain cause. Antimicrobials have been used in gastroenteritis for three different purposes and much confused discussion has resulted from failure to distinguish them.

Antibiotics are used systemically in ill infants because it is often hard to distinguish parenteral infection from gastroenteritis and this mode of use, initiated after taking blood and CSF cultures, constitutes an entirely justifiable provisional treatment of presumed septicaemia.

Second, antibiotics, especially non-absorbable forms, are sometimes used in the attempted control of cross-infection in nurseries. Although this procedure is sometimes successful (Wheeler & Wainerman, 1954), it often fails in serious outbreaks (Ironside et al, 1971) and is certainly no substitute for other recognized methods of cross-infection control.

Finally, absorbable and non-absorbable antibiotics have been used in infantile gastroenteritis as a measure of treatment, and here analysis is bedevilled by a paucity of valid controlled trials, and by the known diversity in aetiology and in severity of this group of conditions. Evidence of benefit in gastroenteritis associated with enteropathogenic strains of *E. coli* has been obtained for both absorbable and non-absorbable antibiotics, when the causal strain is susceptible to the antibiotic given.

Haltanin et al (1972) for example, found, in a controlled trial of ampicillin versus placebo in *E. coli* gastroenteritis, that one of seven of those given ampicillin were still culture positive at five days and one of nine still had diarrhoea; the corresponding numbers in the control groups were six of ten, and seven of eleven. Other studies (Nelson, 1971; Coetzee & Leary, 1971) suggested the value of non-absorbable antibiotics. The results obtained are likely to depend on the precise pathogenic mechanism of diarrhoea in the patients studied, about which little is known in ordinary clinical circumstances. A study by Boyer et al (1975) of a prolonged nursery outbreak by a strain of *E. coli* (0142/K86/H6) known to produce enterotoxin, provided valuable information that for this type of infection, non-absorbable antibiotics might have a useful rôle, presumably by reducing the concentration of toxin-producing organisms in the bowel lumen. Thorén et al (1980) obtained good clinical and bacteriological results in *E. coli* gastroenteritis of infants with co-trimoxazole and with mecillinam. These and other results do suggest that suitable antibiotics may have some rôle in the treatment of gastroenteritis caused by organisms whose pathogenic action is analogous to that of cholera.

Antimicrobial agents would not, however, be expected to provide a benefit in many other forms of diarrhoea and, in particular, in those numerous instances for which a viral causation is now established.

What policy should be adopted for the use of antibiotics in the large number of diarrhoeal illnesses of uncertain cause found in infancy? In recent years the near automatic use of antimicrobials has greatly declined in most centres, without detriment to the patients' progress, and antibiotics are rarely given except in the situation of diagnostic doubt already outlined. What is less certain is how far this policy can be applied generally in all countries. Doctors have been naturally reluctant to withhold antibiotics in developing countries in which diarrhoeal disease has so large an impact on child health, but where the expense and problems of delivery of these drugs make them difficult to use. Rohde (1976), working in Indonesia, found no evidence of benefit between 100 children given antibiotics and 100 who were not, and has virtually abandoned their use. Medical and nursing attention can then be concentrated on water and electrolyte repletion, with much improved results.

In summary, antimicrobial agents are not recommended for general use in diarrhoeal disease of infancy, but only for specific indications, especially diagnostic doubt between a primary bowel infection and a septicaemic illness, invasive salmonellosis, severe shigellosis, cholera, giardiasis and amoebiasis.

PREVENTION OF POST-OPERATIVE INFECTION IN ABDOMINAL SURGERY

The high rate of infection following operations on the lower bowel and pelvic organs, and to a lesser extent on the upper bowel and biliary tree, have long been a source of concern. Post-operative infection may take the form of wound infections of widely varying severity, deep abscesses, or septicaemia sometimes accompanied by the bacterial shock syndrome. At the best, post-operative infections are distressing and prolong post-operative stay; at worst, bacterial shock carries a high mortality.

The source of most post-operative infections after bowel and pelvic surgery is the indigenous flora of the bowel and in recent years much has been done to show the importance of the numerically dominant anaerobic component, as well as that of the aerobes, in the genesis of these infections.

The most effective barrier against infection is provided by skilled surgery, when tissue damage is minimized, suture lines are sound, and accumulations of blood and tissue fluid prevented. Nevertheless, certain operations, for example elective colectomy, are often followed by infection even when surgery has been impeccably performed. Various forms of mechanical cleansing of the bowel are in common use and many experienced surgeons use no local or systemic antimicrobials. Cleansing technique is important as inadequate methods may lead to a worse situation with the bowel full of liquid faeces. The most thorough form of bowel cleansing, based on fluid repletion in cholera, consists of whole gut irrigation with an electrolyte/neomycin solution for 2–3 hours using 9–13 litres of solution. The clear fluid passed from the rectum still contained Bacteroides (against which neomycin is, of course, inactive) but was free of *E. coli* and *Str. faecalis*. Patients found the irrigation method less tiring and unpleasant than the previous four-day enema regimen (Hewitt et al, 1973).

Apart from cleansing, a variety of methods have been used in an attempt to reduce post-operative sepsis. Until recently, these mainly consisted in the combination of mechanical cleansing with pre-operative oral administration of neomycin and/or an unabsorbable sulphonamide. These methods are falling out of favour, partly because the results of controlled trials have been disappointing and partly because of increased consciousness of the danger of emerging antibiotic resistance. Shorter periods of oral pre-operative bowel preparation, systemic administration of antibiotics in the peri-operative period, and intra-incisional instillation of antiseptics or antimicrobials have all found their advocates, and have been subject to controlled trials. No general comparison can be made between the large numbers of recent trials because criteria for inclusion and definitions of post-operative sepsis vary widely.

Gilmore and Martin (1974) and Gilmore and Sanderson (1975), in trials of appendicectomy and of general abdominal surgery reduced post-operative infection rates by half by instilling a powder aerosol of povidone iodine into the wound before closure. Povidone iodine was superior to an antibiotic spray and to a control of propellant spray alone. Pollock & Evans (1975) however, claimed superior results by instilling 1g cephaloridine in 2 ml water into the wound. Local use of antibiotics is difficult to evaluate since the extent of systemic absorption as well as local action needs to be considered, but Galland et al (1977) making a direct comparison in 113 abdominal operations, found the post-operative infection rate unchanged (42 per cent) in the controls compared with those receiving local povidone iodine, but reduced to 8.1 per cent in patients receiving 160 mg tobramycin and 600 mg lincomycin by intramuscular injection with the pre-medication and eight hours later. The idea of a short period of systemic antibiotic use during the expected time of bacterial implantation, well based in experimental infections, was successfully implemented by Polk & Lopez-Mayor (1969) using three doses of intramuscular cephaloridine. The methods used since then have been based on attempts to inhibit anaerobic as well as aerobic infections and to reduce to a minimum the period of antibiotic prophylaxis. Other trials have studied combined parenteral and enteral regimens or short course oral schemes of prophylaxis. Very short courses have been shown effective in reducing wound infection rates in general surgery. Stokes et al (1974) used two doses of lincomycin with gentamicin or tobramycin, at operation and eight hours later, reducing the infection rate from 8 per cent to 1 per cent and the trial of Galland et al (1977) has already been noted. Griffiths et al (1976) reduced the infection rate after gastrointestinal operations from 34 per cent to 5 per cent with the use of a single intravenous dose of tobramycin and lincomycin given at the beginning of surgery. Feathers et al (1977) using a five day course of gentamicin and lincomycin, reduced sepsis from 48 per cent to 4 per cent. Two of 14 patients, however, developed psuedomembranous enterocolitis on this regimen, and for this reason they substituted metronidazole for lincomycin. The possible value of inhibiting strict anaerobes only was shown by Willis et al (1977); 11 of 19 control patients undergoing elective colonic surgery developed anaerobic infections, whereas none developed in 27 patients who received prophylactic metronidazole. Other successful attempts at short course oral chemophrophylaxis for bowel surgery are those of Washington et al (1974), using a neomycin-tetracycline combination, and of Nichols et al (1973) who, basing their use of neomycin-erythromycin on a careful preliminary study of the effect of this combination on aerobic and anaerobic bowel flora, showed that this regimen combined with mechanical cleansing, effectively controlled sepsis following colon surgery. These short courses of prophylactic chemotherapy carry little risk of toxic effects. Prolonged treatment with neomycin with the aim of suppressing the bowel flora, as is sometimes used in hepatic failure, may be dangerous since small amounts of antibiotic can be absorbed especially but not exclusively in patients with renal failure, with resulting oto-toxicity (Berk and Chalmers, 1970).

It must be concluded that the incidence of post-operative sepsis has been successfully reduced by a number of different methods. The methods have in common the idea of reducing the bacterial load in the bowel at the time of operation, or of ensuring an effective antibacterial blood level at the time when organisms are likely to be implanted in the wound. The importance of bacterial numbers at the time of operation was shown in the case of gastric surgery by Gatehouse et al (1978). The incidence of infection was as high as 93 per cent if the pre-operative specimen of gastric fluid had a count of more than 5×10^6 per ml, but only 16 per cent when the count was less than this.

As regards the choice between attempting to control the aerobic or the anaerobic flora preferentially, both methods have succeeded in individual trials, and, for high risk operations, it is probably best to combine both anti-aerobe and anti-anaerobe drugs as in many of the trials quoted. In at least one study of post-appendicectomy wound sepsis (Morris et al, 1979) although peri-operative cefazolin or metronidazole each reduced the sepsis rate from 30 per cent to about 20 per cent, combining the two agents was much more effective, with an incidence of post-operative infection of only 3 per cent. As to the other main choice, between systemic peri-operative chemoprophylaxis and oral bowel preparation, it is again clear that both methods have succeeded. Oral preparation is not, however, applicable in emergency surgery, and workers in Birmingham have observed an increase in post-operative infections by kanamycin-resistant organisms when this drug was given orally in a pre-operative regimen. The risk of antibiotic-colitis would also be less if systemic administration is used (Keighley et al 1979).

The high rates of infection after lower bowel and pelvic surgery and after certain gastric and biliary operations (q.v.) make the use of one or other of these methods entirely justifiable, and we consider that short-term systemic chemoprophylaxis is generally preferable for high-risk operations. Antibiotic prophylaxis in surgery is extensively discussed in a recent monograph (Keighley & Burdon, 1979).

INFECTION OF THE BILIARY TRACT

Bile is a medium congenial to some bacteria, notably the typhoid bacillus, and highly inimical to others, notably the more virulent of the pyogenic cocci, *Str. pyogenes* and *Str. pneumoniae*. Hence most infections in this area are due to coliform bacilli, which are in general bile-resistant: the only Gram-positive organism likely to be found is *Str. faecalis*. Anaerobic organisms including clostridia and anaerobic streptococci are also found in the infected biliary tract.

From the point of view of concentration in the bile, the available drugs are sharply divisible into two classes. Sulphonamides, chloramphenicol, and aminoglycosides are excreted only in low concentrations, usually less than those occurring at the same time in the blood. Others are concentrated in the bile, some of them owing the maintenance of the blood level after an individual dose to reabsorption after excretion by this route. Antibiotics excreted in larger amounts in the bile but nevertheless mainly via the kidney are tetracyclines and penicillins (Harrison & Stewart, 1961), particularly ampicillin (Acred et al, 1962): it should be noted that the very high ampicillin bile levels found in experimental animals are not equalled by those in man, and when any obstruction is present they are further reduced even to *nil* (Mortimer et al, 1969). Cephalexin, according to Sales et al (1972) attains substantial levels in the bile, which can be increased by also giving probenecid. They point out that although some bacteria implicated in biliary tract infections are resistant to this antibiotic, *S. typhi* is highly sensitive, and suggest a trial in the treatment of typhoid carriers. Erythromycin and novobiocin are also excreted mainly in the bile. Much the highest biliary concentrations (Acocella et al, 1968) are attained by derivatives of rifamycin, but this antibiotic has only moderate activity against enterobacteria.

These differences between antibiotics in their ability to achieve high concentrations in bile have been used as a method of examining the relative importance of serum and biliary concentration in the control of post-operative infections. Keighley et al (1975), using a peri-operative course of gentamicin in a randomised trial, found the incidence of bacteria in the bile reduced from 42 per cent to 25 per cent by this method. One patient in the treated and five in the control group developed bacteraemia. In a subsequent comparison (Keighley et al, 1976) of rifamide and gentamicin, the former drug achieving high concentrations in bile, failed to reduce postoperative sepsis; gentamicin, despite the low concentrations in bile, reduced the rate of postoperative wound infection from 22 per cent to 6 per cent and of septicaemia from 14 per cent to 2 per cent. The importance of tissue levels of antibiotic in preventing postoperative infection is also shown by the work of Chetlin & Elliott (1973), who, using a two dose peri-operative regimen of cephaloridine, reduced the incidence of invasive infections without affecting the incidence of positive bile cultures. Other methods successfully used to prevent infection after biliary surgery include cefazolin (Strachan et al, 1977) and parenteral co-trimoxazole given immediately before operation (Morran et al, 1978).

The treatment of acute cholecystitis and of acute cholangitis must include agents active against the majority of isolates found in infected bile and which achieve systemic concentrations in excess of their MIC for these organisms. On this basis, three main choices are available. Co-trimoxazole by intravenous infusion followed by oral administration at a later stage makes a suitable choice as also does a cephalosporin. If gentamicin or another aminoglycoside is used, however, it is best combined with a penicillin in view of the low activity of aminoglycosides against streptococci. Ampicillin and the tetracyclines, formerly commonly used for acute infections of the biliary tree are now less suitable because of the increasing number of coliforms resistant to these agents.

Pseudomembranous and antibiotic colitis

In recent years this dangerous condition has been associated chiefly with the administration of broad spectrum antibiotics, lincomycin and clindamycin, but identical appearances have long been recorded in patients with severe general illnesses and as a sequel of colonic obstruction. A unifying hypothesis has now emerged with the identification of a clostridial toxin, thought to be produced by *Cl. difficile*, in the faeces of patients with this condition (Larson & Price, 1977; Bartlett et al, 1978). Treatment includes careful fluid and electrolyte control, and a number of antibiotic regimens have been used.

At present, oral vancomycin appears to have much to recommend it. Tedesco et al (1978) treated nine patients with this drug in a dose of 2 g daily, showing a favourable clinical and sigmoidoscopic response. The mean vancomycin concentration in stools was 3100 μg/g, and serum levels were undetectable or very low. The concentration of clostridial toxin in the faeces rapidly diminished. A much smaller dose of vancomycin, 125 mg six-hourly, was also shown effective in a randomized placebo-controlled trial (Keighley et al, 1978).

Necrotising enterocolitis

This dangerous infection of special care baby units (Leading article, 1977) is of multiple and uncertain aetiology. Enterobacteria of various species are often found in blood cultures but a possible rôle of clostridia at some stage in the pathogenesis is suggested by an outbreak in which *Cl. butyricum* or its products were found in the blood of nine of 12 infants (Howard et al, 1977). Pig bel and 'Darmbrand' show similar pathological changes and are associated with *Cl. perfringens* infection of the affected bowel. At present it is probably wise to use a broad spectrum antibiotic approach in necrotising enterocolitis with a combination of penicillin and an aminoglycoside. Prevention of this complication in pre-term infants has been attempted by Egan et al (1976) using oral kanamycin in a dose of 15 mg/kg/day but the numbers involved were too small to justify a firm conclusion.

Peritonitis

Antimicrobial aspects of the treatment of peritonitis are discussed in Chapter 15 in which the management of septicaemia of various origins is outlined.

References

Acocella G, Mattiussi R, Nicolis F B, Pallanza R, Tenconi L T 1968 Gut 9: 536
Acred P, Brown D M, Turner D H, Wilson M J 1962 Brit J Pharmacol 18: 356
Ahmed T, Ali F, Sarwar S G 1976 Arch Dis Child 51: 388
Andersson T, Forssell J, Sterner G 1972 Brit Med J 2: 449
Aserkoff B, Bennett J V 1969 New Engl J Med 281: 636
Bartlett J G, Chang T W, Onderdonk A B 1978 Lancet 1: 338
Berk D P, Chalmers T 1970 Ann Intern Med 73: 393
Boyer K M, Petersen N J, Farzaneh I, et al 1975 J Pediat 86: 919

Byers P A, DuPont H L, Goldschmidt M C 1976 Antimicrob Ag Chemother 9: 288
Carpenter C C J, Sack R B, Mondal A, Mitra P P 1964 J Indian Med Ass 43: 309
Chaudhuri R N, Neogy K N, Sanyal S N et al 1968 Lancet 1: 332
Chetlin S H, Elliott D W 1973 Arch Surg 107: 319
Christie A B 1964 Brit Med J 1: 1609
Coetzee M, Leary P M 1971 Arch Dis Child 46: 646
Davies J R, Farrant W N, Uttley A H C 1970 Lancet 2: 1157
Dawkins A T, Hornick R B 1967 Antimicrob Ag Chemother 1966 p. 6
deRitis F, Giammanco G, Manzillo G 1972 Brit Med J 4: 17
Dixon J M S 1965 Brit Med J 2: 1343
Egan E A, Mantilla G, Nelson R M, Eitzman D V 1976 J Pediat 89: 467
Farid Z, Bassily S, Mikhail I A, et al 1975 J Infect Dis 132: 698
Feathers R S, Lewis A A M, Sagor G R et al 1977 Lancet 2: 4
Freiberg T 1971 Arzneimittel-Forsch 21: 599
Galland R B, Saunders J H, Mosley J G, Darrell J H 1977 Lancet 2: 1043
Gatehouse D, Dimock F, Burdon D W et al 1978 Brit J Surg 65: 551
Geddes A M, Clarke P D 1977 J Antimicrob Chemother 3 (suppl. B): 101
Gilman R H, Terminel M, Levine M M et al 1975 J Infect Dis 132: 630
Gilmore O J A, Martin T D M 1974 Brit J Surg 61: 281
Gilmore O J A, Sanderson P J 1975 Brit J Surg 62: 792
Gorbach S L, Kean B H, Evans D G et al 1975 New Engl J Med 292: 933
Greenough W B III, Gordon R S, Rosenberg I S et al 1964 Lancet 1: 355
Griffiths D A, Shorey B A, Simpson R A et al 1976 Lancet 2: 325
Haltalin K C, Kusmiesz H T, Hinton L V, Nelson J D 1972 Amer J Dis Child 124: 554
Harrison P M, Stewart G T 1961 Brit J Pharmacol 17: 420
Hewitt J, Rigby J, Reeve J, Cox A G 1973 Lancet 2: 337
Howard F M, Flynn D M, Bradley J M et al 1977 Lancet 2: 1099
Ironside A G, Brennand J, Mandal B K, Heyworth B 1971 Arch Dis Child 46: 815
Kamat S A 1970 Brit Med J 3: 320
Kay R, Barnes G L, Townley R R W 1977 Austral Paediat J 13: 98
Kean B H 1963 Ann Intern Med 59: 605
Kean B H, Waters S R 1959 New Engl J Med 261: 71
Keighley M R B, Alexander-Williams F, Arabi Y et al 1979 Lancet 1: 894
Keighley M R B, Baddeley R M, Burdon D W, et al 1975 Brit J Surg 62: 275
Keighley M R B, Burdon D W 1979 Antimicrobial prophylaxis in surgery. Pitman Medical, Tunbridge Wells, Kent
Keighley M R B, Burdon D W, Arabi Y et al 1978 Brit Med J 2: 1667
Keighley M R B, Drysdale R B, Quoraishi A H et al 1976 Gut 17: 495
Larson H E, Price A B 1977 Lancet 2: 1312
Leading Article, Lancet 1977 1: 459
Lexomboon U, Mansuwan P, Duangmani C et al 1972 Brit Med J 3: 23
Loewenstein M S, Balows A, Gangarosa E J 1973 Lancet 1: 529
Mandal B K, Ironside A G, Brennand J 1979 Brit Med J 1: 586
McCormack W M, Chowhury A M, Jahangir N 1968 Bull WHO 38: 787
Merson M H, Morris G K, Sack D A et al 1976 New Engl J Med 294: 1299
Mhalu F S, Mmari P W, Ijumba J 1979 Lancet 1: 345
Morran C, McNaught W, McArdle C S 1978 Brit Med J 2: 462
Morris W T, Innes D B, Ellis-Pegler R B 1979 Abstract of 2nd International Metronidazole Conference, p 21
Mortimer P R, Mackie D B, Haynes S 1969 Brit Med J 3: 88
Münnich D, Békési I, Uri J 1965/6 Chemotherapia 10: 253
Nelson J D 1971 Pediatrics 48: 248
Nelson J D, Haltalin K C 1975 Antimicrob Ag Chemother 7: 415
Nelson J D, Kusmiesz H, Jackson L H, Woodman E 1976 J Amer Med Assoc 235: 1239
Nichols R L, Broido P, Condon R E, Gorbach S L, Nyhus L M 1973 Ann Surg 178: 453
Pastore G, Rizzo G, Fera G, Schiraldi O 1977 Chemotherapy 23: 121
Pettersson T 1975 Brit Med J 1: 395
Pichler H, Spitzy K H 1972 Dtsch Med Wschr 97: 1401
Pierce N F, Banwell J G, Mitra R C, et al 1968 Brit Med J 3: 277
Pillay N, Adams E B, North-Coombes D 1975 Lancet 2: 332
Polk H C, Lopez-Mayor J F 1969 Surgery 66: 97
Pollock A V, Evans M 1975 Brit Med J 3: 436

Rahaman M H, Majid M A, Jamiul Alam, K M, Rafiqul Islam M 1976 Antimicrob Ag Chemother 10: 610
Report 1970 Joint Project by Members of the Association for the Study of Infectious Diseases Lancet 2: 1159
Rohde J E 1976 Ciba Foundation Symposium, 42
Sales J E L, Sutcliffe M, O'Grady F 1972 Brit Med J 3: 441
Sanford J P, Linh N N, Kutscher E et al 1976 Antimicrob Ag Chemother 9: 387
Scioli C, Fiorentino F, Sasso G 1972 J Infect Dis 125: 170
Scragg J N 1976 Brit Med J 2: 1031
Scragg J N, Rubidge C J 1971 Brit Med J 3: 738
Scragg J N, Rubidge C J, Procter E M 1976 Arch Dis Child 51: 385
Shanson D C, Leung T 1976 J Antimicrob Chemother 2: 81
Simon H J, Miller R C 1966 New Engl J Med 274: 807
Skirrow M B 1977 Brit Med J 2: 9
Smith J T, Bremner D A, Datta N 1974 Antimicrob Ag Chemother 6: 418
Snyder M J, Perroni J, Gonzalez O et al 1976 Lancet 2: 1155
Stokes E J, Waterworth P M, Franks V, Watson B, Clark C G 1974 Brit J Surg 61: 739
Strachan C J L, Black J, Powis S J A et al 1977 Brit Med J 1: 1254
Tedesco F, Markham R, Gurwith M et al 1978 Lancet 2: 226
Thorén A, Wolde-Mariam T, Stintzing G et al 1980 J Infect Dis 141: 27
Tong M J, Martin D G, Cunningham J J, Gunning J-J 1970 J Amer Med Ass 214: 1841
Turner A C 1967 Brit Med J 4: 653
Washington J A, Dearing W H, Judd E S, Elveback L R 1974 Ann Surg 180: 567
Wheeler W E, Wainerman B 1954 Pediatrics 14: 357
Willis A T, Ferguson I R, Jones P H et al 1977 Brit Med J 1: 607
Wolfe M S 1975 J Amer Med Ass 233: 1362

19

Infections of the respiratory tract

Antimicrobial drugs are prescribed with enormous frequency in acute respiratory infections, but in no part of medicine is rational chemotherapy more difficult. The syndromes of respiratory infection are of widely varied aetiology, and clinical and laboratory evidence often offer limited guidance about the causal organism in a particular patient. For example, acute sore throat may have viral, mycoplasmal or a number of bacterial causes, but only occasionally can the cause be accurately deduced from the clinical findings. Moreover, the frequency and significance of secondary bacterial infection in syndromes of primary viral origin are often quite uncertain.

INFECTIONS OF THE UPPER RESPIRATORY TRACT

The great majority of colds are viral in origin, and are not at present susceptible to any direct form of chemotherapeutic attack. The possible role of secondary bacterial infection in prolonging and worsening the effects of the illness has been in dispute for many years; so too has the value of antimicrobial drugs in mitigating these effects. Ten double-blind trials, mostly involving the use of a tetracycline, were reviewed by Davis & Wedgewood (1965) and a further survey by Soyka et al (1975) confirmed their conclusions. Many trials gave negative results, but in a few the average duration of illness was shortened with small doses of tetracycline taken in lozenge form.

Antibiotics are especially widely used in respiratory infections in children who, in Britain, receive on average one course of antibiotics a year in the first six years of life. The clinician's problem is a difficult one, especially in general practice. The general tendency for these infections to recover rapidly without specific treatment favours a restrictive antibiotic policy, but much parental pressure and a natural fear of bacterial complications tends to lead to non-selective prescribing. Howie et al (1971) have shown that in Scotland the use of antibiotics for new episodes of respiratory illness varies greatly between practitioners, especially when the clinical diagnosis is one of 'influenza'. Most practitioners (90 per cent) gave antibiotics on a diagnosis of tonsillitis and 18 per cent did so when the diagnosis was 'coryza'. Recent attempts to define the role of antibiotics in respiratory infections of childhood include those of Gordon et al (1974) who detected no difference between placebo treatment and a variety of antibiotics in children attending a Casualty Department in Brisbane, and that of Taylor et al (1977) from New Zealand, who completed a double-blind randomized controlled trial of amoxycillin, co-trimoxazole and placebo in 197 children with presumed viral respiratory infections. The pattern of resolution in each syndrome, which they categorized as nasopharyngitis, pharyngo-tonsillitis and bronchitis, was the same in all three groups, but seven children from the placebo group were withdrawn from the trial because of presumed bacterial complications, four of them with otitis media. Two were withdrawn from the antibiotic groups. By other criteria recovery proceeded at a similar pace in all three groups except that nasal discharge cleared up more quickly in the antibiotic groups. They concluded that the benefits of antimicrobial treatment were marginal, and that routine prescription for this type of illness was not indicated. The common belief that prescribing antibiotics saves the general practitioner from extra work has been disproved by Howie & Hutchison (1978).

The evidence of benefit derived from a few of the trials is on the whole outweighed by the likelihood of promoting, by widespread use, an increased incidence of pathogens resistant to the agents. This policy applies to patients with normal chests; by contrast the use of an antimicrobial agent, usually tetracycline or co-trimoxazole, is indicated at the onset of a cold in patients with chronic bronchitis. Exacerbations of bronchitis are often induced by viral infection (Lambert & Stern, 1972), but in this susceptible group it is best to assume the likelihood of secondary bacterial infection, difficult as it is to provide clear evidence of this.

Drugs not normally classified as antimicrobial agents have also been employed in minor infections of the upper respiratory tract. The publicity about Vitamin C and the common cold is scarcely justified by the lack of, or marginal benefit evident from clinical trials, many of which are reviewed in an Editorial (1976) (see also Chapter 25).

Levamisole, thought to act on the cellular immune system, was found by Van Eygen et al (1976) to reduce the number, duration and severity of illnesses experienced by 70 children with a record of relapsing upper respiratory tract infections during the winter. Although no drug related unwanted effects were reported in this study, the many reports of drug toxicity from levamisole do not encourage its use for this purpose.

Acute sore throat (see Fig. 19.1)

Many acute sore throats are caused by virus infection, but an important group is caused by *Str. pyogenes*, which accounts for a quarter to one-third of acute sore throats seen in many studies in general practice (Everett, 1975). In some countries diphtheria remains important, while Vincent's angina is found especially, but not exclusively, in association with gingival sepsis. Clinical signs are often unreliable as a guide to aetiology. Haemolytic streptococci are more likely to be found in association with high fever, follicular tonsillitis, tender anterior cervical glands and neutrophilia in the peripheral blood, but may be grown profusely from patients with mild sore throat or, indeed, from symptomless carriers. Conversely, bad sore throat even with pharyngeal exudate, may be viral in origin. For these reasons antibiotic treatment of acute sore throat is most satisfactory if based on examination of a throat swab. The use of suitable transport medium makes this practicable in the community as well as in hospital.

The most appropriate treatment for streptococcal sore throat is penicillin. This can be given orally as phenoxymethyl penicillin 250 mg four times daily. Because of erratic taking of medicine, especially by children, more satisfactory results may be achieved by initiating treatment with one injection of procaine penicillin or fortified procaine penicillin (containing 300 mg of procaine penicillin and 60 mg benzyl penicillin per unit volume), continuing treatment thereafter with phenoxymethyl penicillin by mouth. Treatment makes little difference to the rate at which symptoms subside and the aim of therapy is eradication of streptococci from the nasopharynx. In order to ensure this in a high proportion of patients, it is necessary to continue penicillin for 10 days (Peter & Smith, 1977). This is rarely achieved in practice, since patients feel well again in a few days and do not complete the course. Patients hypersensitive to penicillin can be treated by erythromycin. Cephalosporins have also been used for this purpose but since there are some examples of cross allergy with the penicillins, they should not be given when the history of penicillin allergy is well-documented or one of severe reaction. Stillerman et al (1972) found that treatment by oral cephalexin was followed by a lower relapse rate than treatment with phenoxymethyl penicillin but Matsen et al (1974) found no difference in effectiveness between 10-day courses of cephalexin or phenoxymethyl penicillin or one injection of benzathine penicillin. Co-trimoxazole has also been used successfully for streptococcal sore throat. For those working in circumstances which do not allow examination of swabs in cases of sore throat, it is useful to have a policy for the use of penicillin which, while including most patients likely to have streptococcal infection, avoids its widespread use in predominantly viral syndromes. In these circumstances penicillin can be given on the following indications:

1. Scarlet fever. Its exact aetiology is implicit in the diagnosis, so that penicillin is indicated.
2. Follicular tonsillitis with fever and tender anterior cervical glands.
3. Bacterial complications of acute pharyngitis such as peritonsillar abscess (quinsy), otitis media, and suppurative cervical lymphadenitis.
4. Acute sore throat in a patient with rheumatic heart disease.
5. Acute sore throat in a family or community in which there is known to be a high prevalence of streptococcal infection.

Streptococcal carriage

The prevention of streptococcal throat infections in patients subject to rheumatic fever is best achieved with penicillin. The most successful method is a monthly injection of benzathine penicillin. Two disadvantages of this method are the need for repeated injections, albeit infrequently, and the likelihood that any allergic reactions will be of long duration. In this country the most widely used method is oral phenoxymethyl penicillin 250 mg twice daily.

Diphtheria

Antibiotics are an essential part of treatment but do not obviate the need for antitoxin. *C. diphtheriae* is moderately sensitive to penicillin, and is also sensitive to ampicillin, erythromycin and clindamycin. As judged by clearance of the carrier state soon after treatment, McCloskey et al (1974) found a variety of regimens effective. Benzathine penicillin 600 000 units or 1.2 mega units (for those under or over 5 years old respectively) by intramuscular injection cleared 125 of 149 carriers (84 per cent), erythromycin estolate for seven days was effective in 82 of 89 (92 per cent) and clindamycin for seven days in 52 of 56 (93 per cent). Miller (1975) has confirmed the finding, familiar when diphtheria was common, that some carriers will later relapse and that cultures should be repeated two or three weeks after treatment.

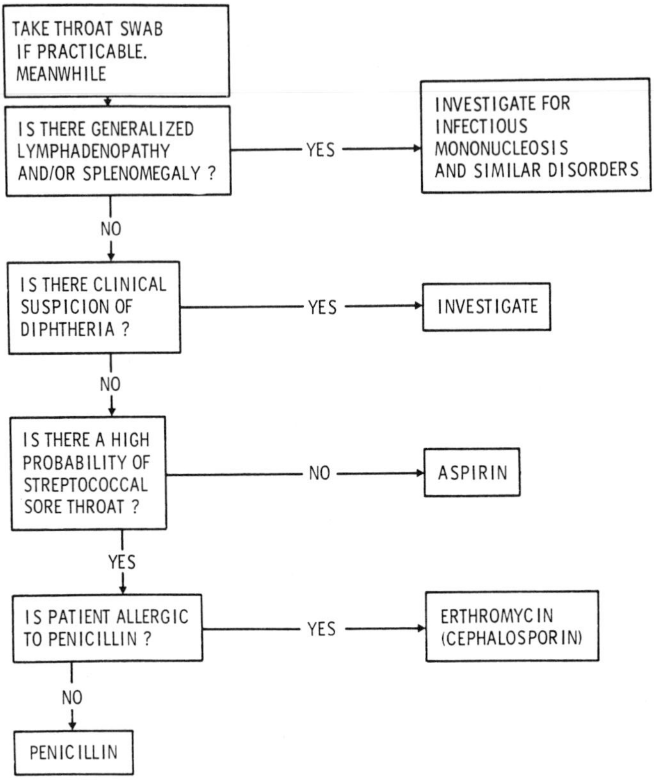

Fig. 19.1 Decision tree for management of acute sore throat

Acute epiglottitis

This rapidly progressive and life-threatening cause of croup is encountered mainly in children, but has also been increasingly recognized in adults. It is caused by infection with *H. influenzae* type B which may often be cultivated from the blood as well as from the local lesion. Treatment is as much concerned with maintaining the airway as with control of the infection (Branefors-Helander & Jeppsson, 1975). Chloramphenicol and ampicillin have both been used on different occasions, and the relative rarity of the condition does not allow an objective judgment between them. Since, however, ampicillin acts more slowly and less certainly than chloramphenicol in a number of acute infections in which they have been compared, we agree with Addy et al (1972) that parenteral chloramphenicol is the drug of choice. The general practitioner may more probably have intramuscular ampicillin to hand, and he should administer this on suspicion of acute epiglottitis without attempting to take throat cultures or to delay until the patient reaches hospital.

Acute otitis media

The milder catarrhal forms often resolve without chemotherapy. The predominant organisms found in otitis media severe enough to need myringotomy are *Str. pneumoniae*, *Haemophilus influenzae* and *Str. pyogenes*. The proportion of cases caused by the latter organism varies greatly in different series. *H. influenzae* was thought to affect mainly children less than 5 years old, but it is evident (Howie et al,

1971) that this organism can cause otitis at all ages. *Staph. aureus* is found more commonly, as are coliforms and less common organisms, in discharge from the ear contaminated by organisms in the external meatus. An interesting observation in many series is the cultivation of *Branhamella (Neisseria) catarrhalis* in pure culture in a small (1.3–5 per cent) but significant number of exudates, taken directly from the middle ear with careful technique to avoid contamination: in such cases intracellular gram-negative diplococci may sometimes be seen in the exudate (Kamme, 1970).

A number of large scale trials of antibiotic treatment have been mounted in recent years, in which regimens have been correlated with bacteriological findings at myringotomy, and sometimes with the results of measurements of antibiotic concentration in the middle ear exudate.

Howard et al (1976) in a double-blind trial in 383 children, in whom the causal organism was the pneumococcus in 31 per cent and *H. influenzae* in 22 per cent found the initial response best with amoxycillin. For *H. influenzae* infections an erythromycin triple sulphonamide combination did as well, but the other two regimens, phenoxymethyl penicillin and erythromycin alone were less successful. Other notable clinical trials are those by Bass et al (1967) and by Nilson et al (1969).

Otitis media often resolves without specific treatment, and in antibiotic trials much depends on the initial selection of patients. We conclude that amoxycillin is the agent of choice for otitis media. Phenoxymethyl penicillin, despite its relatively low activity against *H. influenzae*, also gives satisfactory results provided that full dosage is given; children often receive inappropriately low doses and may not swallow the whole dose. Alternatives to penicillin are erythromycin, and co-trimoxazole (Cooper et al, 1976). Cephalexin too has given generally satisfactory results in a comparative trial with ampicillin in 179 children (Stechenberg et al, 1976,) but 7 of 14 children with *H. influenzae* infections responded poorly to cephalexin. The problem of ampicillin-resistant *H. influenzae*, although still rare in the U.K., has been encountered in otitis media as well as in other infections by this organism. Syriopoulou et al (1976) found nine resistant strains in 984 isolates from middle ear exudate, the incidence increasing from 0.6 per cent in 1973 to 2.4 per cent in 1976.

A decision tree for the management of acute otitis media is shown in Figure 19.2.

Acute sinusitis

Str. pneumoniae and *Str. pyogenes* are usually regarded as the most common isolates in acute sinusitis, but recent studies have shown a greater variety of potential pathogens, especially *H. influenzae* and anaerobes, and a relative dearth of *Str. pyogenes* isolates. A thorough quantitative study made at the University of Virginia of 65 needle punctures in 81 adults with acute infections of the antrum (Hamory et al, 1979) showed *H. influenzae* and *Str. pneumoniae* as the most common isolates, with occasional high counts of staphylococci, *N. catarrhalis*, alpha-haemolytic streptococci, anaerobes and viruses. Ampicillin, amoxycillin and co-trimoxazole were all effective in treatment. Anaerobic isolates are common in chronic sinus infections; heavy pure cultures of anaerobes were found in 23 of 83 specimens removed aseptically at operation (Frederick & Braude, 1974). As with otitis media, results of treatment have generally correlated well with antibiotic concentrations in the sinus secretion; even with high concentrations as judged by conventional tests of MIC, eradication of bacteria in the paranasal sinuses is not easily achieved, perhaps because

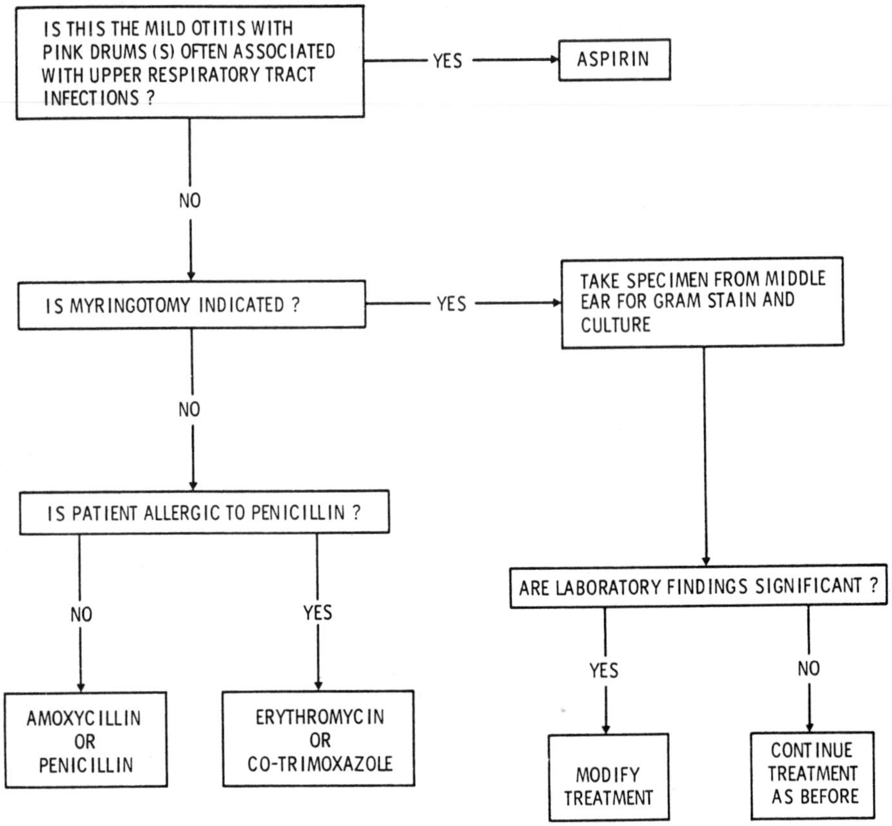

Fig. 19.2 Decision tree for the management of otitis media

of the low pO_2 and high pCO_2 of purulent sinus secretions (Carenfelt et al, 1975; Carenfelt & Lundberg, 1976), conditions often associated with increased bacterial resistance to antimicrobial agents.

Optimal treatment of acute sinusitis is probably best achieved by initial parenteral administration of penicillin or ampicillin followed by oral amoxycillin. Erythromycin is a satisfactory alternative achieving adequate concentrations in the sinus fluid for inhibiting pneumococci and *Str. pyogenes* but reaching the MIC for only 15–30 per cent of strains of *H. influenzae* (Kalm et al, 1975). Co-trimoxazole may also be used.

Influenza

Antiviral chemotherapy is discussed on page 436. As with the common cold, anti-bacterial chemotherapy is not indicated in previously healthy subjects. In those at special risk treatment should be given and should take account of secondary bacterial invaders known to be prevalent in the particular epidemic. If no special information is available, a penicillinase-resistant penicillin should be included, since staphylococci are especially dangerous in association with influenza virus. Other organisms such as *H. influenzae* may also be important in patients with chronic respiratory disease who develop influenza, so a suitable scheme of treatment for such patients is provided by ampicillin and cloxacillin. Those at special risk, for whom antibiotics should be given during an attack of influenza, include patients with chronic bronchitis, those with chronic heart disease, the elderly, and pregnant women. The use of amantadine is discussed on page 439.

PNEUMONIA

A wide variety of organisms may cause pneumonia, but the causal diagnosis is only occasionally evident at the time when the clinical and radiological diagnosis is made. Florid illness, lobar distribution, and a neutrophilia favour a bacterial cause but antibiotic treatment before admission to hospital often mutes the features of a bacterial pneumonia, while viruses and *Mycoplasma pneumoniae* may cause severe illnessess and lobar consolidation. Examination of sputum may be disappointing but a sputum smear should be gram-stained and examined soon after admission. Blood as well as sputum cultures should be taken, since an appreciable number of patients with pneumococcal pneumonia have positive blood cultures. Transtracheal aspiration, used especially in patients with lowered resistance in whom a correct antibiotic choice is especially important, often provides useful information about the flora of the lower tract. Although a large number of bacteria can cause pneumonia, many of them do so only rarely, and in special circumstances, and it is most useful to consider the likely bacterial pathogens in relation to the patient's age and to the setting in which the pneumonia occurs. For example, Gram-negative aerobic bacteria such as *Klebsiella pneumoniae* are rarely encountered in developed countries in previously healthy patients, but are important in pneumonia of the immune suppressed. Table 19.1 gives suitable first and second choices of specific treatment for each pathogen.

Table 19.1 Chemotherapy of pneumonia of known cause

Organism	First choice	Second choice
Strep. pneumoniae	Penicillin	Erythromycin
Mycoplasma pneumoniae	Erythromycin	Tetracycline
Staph. aureus	Flucloxacillin + Penicillin	Sensitivity testing
H. influenzae	Ampicillin/ Amoxycillin	Cotrimoxazole Chloramphenicol
Klebsiella	Gentamicin	Sensitivity testing
Pseudomonas	Gentamicin + Carbenicillin	Sensitivity testing
Anaerobes	Penicillin	Clindamycin Metronidazole
Coxiella burneti	Tetracycline	
Chlamydia psittaci	Tetracycline	
Legionella pneumophila	Erythromycin	

Pneumonia in previously healthy adults and children

The predominant bacterial pathogen is *Str. pneumoniae*. Although less commonly isolated than formerly, it is still by far the most common isolate (Table 19.1), and benzyl penicillin is therefore the drug of choice. Treatment should be by injection initially, but oral penicillin can be given after the first day or two. High penicillin dosage has become customary but Brewin et al (1974) showed no difference in response between 59 patients with pneumococcal pneumonia given a high dose of 20 mega units daily by intravenous infusion and 64 who received the moderate dose of 600 000 units of procaine penicillin 12-hourly. Colonization by potential pathogens was more common in the high dose group. Similarly McHardy & Schonell (1972) found little to choose between ampicillin doses of 1 g or 2 g daily in the treatment of patients with pneumonia who were not desperately ill.

Penicillin treatment for pneumococcal pneumonia is now threatened by the emergence of resistant pneumococci. Relatively insensitive strains, with MICs in the range of 0.1–1.0 μg have been identified in New Guinea and Australia for several years (Hansman et al, 1974); these strains remain susceptible to ampicillin. More threatening are the strains of greater resistance (ca. 4 μg/ml) to penicillin and resistant also to other antibiotics including cephalothin and chloramphenicol, recently found in S. Africa (Appelbaum et al, 1977; Jacobs et al, 1978). Careful surveillance for pneumococcal drug resistance is now necessary.

Tetracycline is no longer suitable as a universal treatment for all pneumonias, since strains of pneumococci resistant to this drug as well as to erythromycin and to lincomycin have emerged. These drugs should now be reserved for patients hypersensitive to penicillin. Resistance to co-trimoxazole has also been reported (Howe & Wilson, 1972). Anderson et al (1968) showed that lincomycin was as effective as penicillin in mild or moderately severe pneumonia.

Table 19.2 Efficacy of different antibiotics against organisms concerned in bronchopneumonia

Species of organism	Antibiotic: Penicillins					
	Benzyl	Ampicillin	Cloxacillin	Cephalosporin	Tetracyclines	Erythromycin
Str. pneumoniae	+	+	+	+	±	+
Str. pyogenes	+	+	+	+	±	+
Staph. aureus	±	±	+	+	±	±
H. influenzae	±	+	–	–	+	±
Kl. pneumoniae	–	–	–	±	+	–
C. psittaci	–	–	–	–	+	–
R. burneti	–	–	–	–	+	–
Mycoplasma pneumoniae	–	–	–	–	+	+

+ = full therapeutic effect.
± = variable therapeutic effect.
– = no therapeutic effect.

The other common agent in this group is *Mycoplasma pneumoniae*. It may be suspected in patients with atypical pneumonia associated with other similar cases within a family or residential institution, and about half the patients show cold agglutinins in their serum. The definitive diagnosis rests on serological tests or cultivation of the organism from the sputum or naso-pharynx. Appropriate antimicrobial treatment shortens the duration of illness and the period during which the chest radiograph is abnormal, but results in civilian communities have been less impressive than in Army camps, possibly because treatment is begun earlier in the latter group. Several tetracyclines or macrolides show a beneficial effect compared with controls who receive penicillin or no antimicrobial drug. If the initial evidence leaves the clinician in doubt between a bacterial and mycoplasmal cause for pneumonia, it is best to ensure that the likely bacterial causes are treated, since bacterial pneumonia is a much greater hazard than mycoplasmal. While pneumococcal strains resistant to it remain rare, erythromycin is suitable to treat both pneumococcal and mycoplasmal pneumonia. The sensitivities to seven antibiotics of a variety of causal organisms in pneumonia are given in Table 19.2. The treatment of pneumonia caused by gram-negative aerobic rods is discussed in the section on pneumonia developing in hospital or in patients with lowered resistance (page 358).

The role of *Haemophilus influenzae* in bronchitis has been studied extensively (page 360) but its importance as a cause of pneumonia has proved more difficult to evaluate. With increasing use of transtracheal aspiration and of blood culture as diagnostic methods in pneumonia, it is evident that both capsulated and non-capsulated strains of *H. influenzae* can cause pneumonia. Wallace et al (1978), describing 41 adult patients with *H. influenzae* pneumonia, found that pneumonia with bacteraemia was nearly always associated with capsulated strains, but either capsulated or non-capsulated strains were found in pneumonia without bacteraemia.

The widespread use of transtracheal aspiration in hospital practice, especially in the U.S.A. has also led to the rediscovery of primary meningococcal pneumonia, first described 60 years ago. Found especially in young adults in Army camps, it is not accompanied by positive blood cultures or rash or meningitis, and may occur as a primary pneumonia (Irwin et al, 1975) or as a complication of measles (Olson & Hodges, 1975).

Q fever and psittacosis are both treated by tetracycline. A dose of 2 g daily continued for 10 days or for three days after the fever subsides is usually recommended but it might be wiser to continue treatment for a longer period in the hope of preventing chronic infections. The causal organism of Legionnaires disease (Fraser et al, 1977) is susceptible to erythromycin, which is at present the treatment of choice for known or suspected infections of this origin. Serious pneumonia of uncertain cause is usually treated, pending the results of bacteriological investigation, by a combination of cloxacillin and an aminoglycoside. If the organism of Legionnaires disease proves, on serological surveys, to be a not uncommon cause of pneumonia in widespread populations, it will become prudent to add erythromycin to this scheme, given preferably by the i.v. route. Frequencies as high as 4–10 per cent have been reported (Symposium, 1979) but only 5 of 500 patients treated for pneumonia in Seattle in 1963–75 had serological evidence of Legionnaires disease (Foy et al, 1979)

Pneumonia in infancy

Most pneumonias in infancy are viral in origin, but a possible bacterial cause must be assumed in the absence of specific evidence to the contrary, since the bacterial pneumonias may be life-threatening. In addition to the pneumococcus, *Staph. aureus* must be considered as a now uncommon but potentially serious cause. Pertussis is considered elsewhere (page 359). Precise evidence of aetiology is especially hard to establish in this group, since children rarely produce sputum except in pertussis, and organisms cultivated from throat swabs poorly represent the bronchial flora. For these reasons it is customary to treat infants with pneumonia by broad spectrum as well as anti-staphylococcal drugs; a combination of ampicillin and cloxacillin is widely used. In the neonate, subject also to serious infections by enterobacteriaceae and pseudomonads, broad spectrum chemotherapy is especially important. Neonatal pneumonia caused by *Chlamydia trachomatis* has also been identified (see Ch. 24).

Acute bronchitis in infancy is commonly caused by respiratory syncytial virus without evidence of additional bacterial infection. Antimicrobial drugs are not indicated if this diagnosis is established by the typical clinical picture, or by identification of the agent by immunofluorescent microscopy of pharyngeal aspirate or material from the throat swab. Controlled trials have shown no benefit from antibiotics in this condition.

Acute laryngotracheobronchitis in infancy is also commonly viral in origin and antimicrobial drugs are not necessary, but other causes of croup, especially acute epiglottitis and diphtheria (q.v.) must always be considered since they demand urgent treatment including antibiotics.

Pneumonia developing in hospital or in patients with lowered resistance

Patients developing pneumonia while in hospital are at special risk of infection with unusual organisms. They are often also in a state of lowered resistance by reason of their underlying disease and of the treatment with drugs such as corticosteroids and antimetabolites which they may be receiving. Antibiotic choice in this group must take account of pneumonia caused by staphylococci, and by a variety of gram-negative organisms including Klebsiella and Pseudomonas. These organisms, although commonly isolated from the sputum of patients who have received antimicrobial drugs, are rarely established as significant pathogens in previously healthy patients. In nosocomial pneumonia they attain great importance. Graybill et al (1973) found that 37 per cent of 224 episodes of pneumonia acquired in hospital, mostly by patients with serious underlying disease, were caused by gram-negative rods. Pneumococci remain important, however, even in hospital-acquired pneumonia, and initial treatment must be guided by these possibilities and by knowledge of the prevalent hospital flora. Treatment is initiated in seriously ill patients by a combination of cloxacillin and gentamicin (or tobramycin).

Patients often develop pneumonia in association with neutropenia and/or depression of cell-mediated immunity. These illnesses, often developing with great rapidity in patients under treatment for leukaemia or lymphoma, or in transplant recipients, present great difficulties in management (see Chapter 15). A wide range of organisms may cause pneumonia, none of them produce absolutely characteristic clinical or radiological features, and a causal diagnosis can rarely be achieved without invasive investigations. A list of causal organisms of pneumonia in the immune suppressed is given in Table 19.3. A reasonable policy for management is to take all appropriate specimens at the first sign of respiratory infection and to begin treatment in the way suggested for a wide range of bacterial pathogens. If the patient's condition continues to deteriorate or fails to improve, more invasive investigations should be undertaken and treatment changed in the light of what is found.

The treatment for pneumonia caused by these opportunistic pathogens is considered in appropriate chapters. Fungal pneumonias are treated with amphotericin B with or without flucytosine, and favourable reports have resulted from the use of miconazole (Chapter 11). Antiviral drugs are discussed in Chapter 25. As regards the treatment of pneumonia caused by *Pneumocystis carinii*, it is now clear that co-trimoxazole in high dosage (trimethoprim 20 mg/kg/day with sulphamethoxazole 100 mg/kg/day, i.e. 12–15 tablets daily for an adult) gives recovery rates of about 70 per cent, as good as those achieved by pentamidine isethionate but with much lower toxicity. Of those who fail to recover with co-trimoxazole, about half will do so if given pentamidine (Lau & Young, 1976; Hughes, 1976). Co-trimoxazole has also been used as a successful long term prophylactic against *Pn. carinii* pneumonia in children under treatment for acute leukaemia. Pulmonary infection in the compromised host is extensively reviewed by Williams et al (1976).

Table 19.3 Causes of pneumonia in patients with immune suppression

Bacteria	*Str. pneumoniae*
	Staph. aureus
	Gram-negative bacteria
	M. tuberculosis
	Other mycobacteria
	Nocardia
Viruses	Cytomegalovirus
	Herpes simplex
	Varicella-zoster
	Adenovirus
Fungi	*Candida albicans*
	Cryptococcus
	Aspergillus
Protozoa	*Pneumocystis carinii*
	Toxoplasma gondii

Aspiration pneumonia and lung abscess

Renewed interest in anaerobic bacteriology has confirmed the well-recognized importance of a variety of anaerobes, together with *Staph. aureus* and gram-negative aerobic rods, in the causation of lung abscess and aspiration pneumonia (Bartlett et al, 1974). Recent studies generally support the tradition of treating lung abscess by long courses of high-dose penicillin, since most of the organisms found—usually several species in each specimen—are susceptible to penicillin, and response to this treatment is often satisfactory even in the patient from whom *Bacteroides fragilis* is isolated. Bartlett & Gorbach (1975) found penicillin and clindamycin equally effective, and suggest reserving the latter drug for patients who are penicillin allergic or with hospital acquired aspiration pneumonia. Whether penicillin or clindamycin is chosen it is reasonable, however, to administer an aminoglycoside in addition in the early phase of treatment. An alternative method is suggested by the work of Tally et al (1975) who successfully treated 10 patients with metronidazole. All of them had bacteroides or fusobacterial species as components of the infecting flora.

Pertussis

Antibiotic treatment of pertussis is generally disappointing, although *Bordetella pertussis* is susceptible *in vitro* to the penicillins, chloramphenicol, tetracyclines, and polymyxin. An early M.R.C. trial (1953) showed some benefit from chloramphenicol and chlortetracycline in patients treated early in the disease, but the advantages were not dramatic even in this group, and it is difficult to make a firm diagnosis of pertussis during its early stages. Bass et al (1969) treated and carefully observed ten cases each with ampicillin, chloramphenicol, erythromycin, oxytetracycline and no antibiotics. No effect was observed on the course of the disease by any of the antibiotics and ampicillin failed to eliminate the organism, whereas erythromycin achieved this rapidly. Strangert (1969) compared ampicillin and chloramphenicol in 148 children with pertussis, finding that cultures were more often negative, and that the number of coughing bouts was somewhat fewer, following treatment with chloramphenicol.

There is probably little to be gained by the use of antibiotics in children with mild pertussis. Children with more severe attacks should be given erythromycin as a relatively non-toxic agent for which benefit has sometimes been claimed and which will eliminate naso-pharyngeal carriage of the organism (Baraff et al, 1978). Children whose lives are threatened by severe pertussis bronchopneumonia would best be treated by chloramphenicol.

Acute bronchitis

In a previously normal subject acute bronchitis is most commonly viral in origin. If the illness is severe, secondary bacterial infection must be assumed and tetracycline or ampicillin given. The former drug, or erythromycin, will be preferred if there is any reason to believe the bronchitis is caused by *Mycoplasma pneumoniae*. Despite its name this organism more often causes bronchitis or upper respiratory tract infection than pneumonia (page 356). An interesting randomized controlled trial by Stott & West (1976) of 212 adults with cough and purulent sputum but without chronic chest disease or abnormal chest signs on clinical examination revealed no difference in recovery rates between those given doxycycline or a placebo except that, oddly enough, runny nose was less persistent and subsequent upper respiratory infections less common in the group receiving the antibiotic. The identical rate of improvement in sputum purulence is notable, since this feature is commonly used as a positive indication for the prescription of an antibiotic.

Chronic bronchitis

The role of antimicrobial drugs in chronic bronchitis has been especially difficult to assess since the disease varies so greatly in its rate of progress, and especially in its propensity to acute exacerbations. *H. influenzae* and the pneumococcus are the most common bacterial isolates from sputum; staphylococci may be found and Klebsiella, Pseudomonas and other gram-negative species may become predominant after antibiotic treatment. *Bramhanella (Neisseria) catarrhalis*, as in otitis and sinusitis, may possess pathogenic capabilities in patients with chronic bronchitis; Ninane et al (1978) found significant infection by this organism using transtracheal puncture in 15 of 193 miners with acute exacerbations. Some strains produce a β-lactamase.

Antibacterial drugs have been given in chronic bronchitis with three main objects; the treatment of exacerbations when they occur, long term prophylaxis aimed at preventing exacerbations and suppressive treatment in advanced cases with constantly purulent sputum.

The benefits attained by long term treatment throughout the winter have been explored in a number of trials, the results of which were reviewed in previous editions of this book and by Stuart-Harris (1968). Tetracyclines have been used most commonly for this purpose, but ampicillin and penicillin V have also been employed. In most studies a reduction in time of work was achieved, usually by a diminution in the duration rather than the number of exacerbations, but little or no change in the rate at which respiratory function deteriorated was demonstrated in three 5-year trials of tetracycline treatment (M.R.C., 1966; Calder et al, 1968; Johnston et al, 1969). Two of these studies gave convincing evidence to support the common view that long term treatment was beneficial in that group of patients, representing only a small proportion of those with chronic bronchitis, who suffer frequent acute exacerbations during the winter. Treatment throughout the winter is now prescribed for few patients, but the early treatment of acute exacerbations is widely practised. In summary, tetracyclines, ampicillin or amoxycillin, and co-trimoxazole have all been shown effective in the home treatment of exacerbations, with little to choose between them on grounds of efficacy. Co-trimoxazole was found superior to ampicillin in respect of most criteria of improvement by Chodosh et al (1973), and by Pines et al (1972a). Molla (1974) found amoxycillin somewhat superior to oxytetracycline. In many trials, the recorded differences between treatment groups have been slight, and the choice between them will depend on the patient's previous treatment, his experience of unwanted effects of the different drugs, and occasionally on the results of laboratory tests.

Treatment by injection is often used in severe exacerbations requiring treatment in hospital and in advanced cases commonly with injections of ampicillin, or by cloxacillin with ampicillin if staphylococcal infection is suspected. Cephaloridine is not very effective against *H. influenzae*, the MIC for most strains being about 8μg/ml, and often fails to eliminate this organism from the sputum. These reasons, together with the large number of injections required, limit the value of this drug in severe purulent bronchitis but the role of newer cephalosporins and cefoxitin has yet to be fully established. The role of chloramphenicol, often considered by clinicians to be a valuable drug in severe purulent chest infections, has been usefully defined in a group of patients with advanced disease. Chloramphenicol given by injection (500 mg 8 hourly) for 2 days followed by oral treatment (500 mg 6 hourly) for 12 days gave significantly better results than ampicillin (500 mg by injection 8 hourly for 2 days followed by 1 g 6 hourly by mouth for 12 days) in severely ill patients with purulent exacerbations of bronchitis (Pines et al, 1972b). For moderately ill patients chloramphenicol was compared with tetracycline, both given orally, and were found equally effective, although chloramphenicol was the better tolerated (Pines et al, 1972c). Another point emerging from this last trial was the outstanding superiority of either antibiotic over the placebo. The value of antibiotics in bronchitis is often held in doubt, which may be justified of mild virus-induced exacerbations treated at home; but the results of these and other trials leave no doubt of the importance of bacterial infection in exacerbations bad enough to lead to hospital admission.

The factors which influence treatment of pneumonia in patients with chronic bronchitis are the same as in severe exacerbations, and are not greatly influenced by whether or not the patient has areas of pulmonary consolidation.

Results of treatment for acute exacerbations of bronchitis are not easily related to antibiotic levels in serum or bronchial secretion, but the work of Stewart et al (1974) with amoxycillin, and of Maesen et al (1976) using bacampicillin, indicates the possible importance of adequate concentration in bronchial secretion. Penetration of antibiotics in bronchial secretion varies greatly between different agents and, in some cases, in relation to sputum purulence; the clinical significance of these properties is reviewed by Lambert (1978).

Bronchiectasis

Treatment follows the same principles as in purulent chronic bronchitis, especially as *H. influenzae* may be a dominant pathogen and treatment should be directed against this organism. In other cases the sputum contains a mixed flora which includes anaerobes, and antibiotic sensitivity tests should be used to guide treatment.

Staphylococcal infection in children with cystic fibrosis poses a difficult and long-term problem since antibiotic-resistant strains are commonly present. Oral cloxacillin, to which flucloxacillin is now preferred, has been given for very long periods starting from the time of diagnosis. Superinfection by *Ps. aeruginosa* is very common, especially as the patient begins to deteriorate, and evidence of infection by *H. influenzae* is also commonly found.

References

Addy M G, Ellis P D M, Turk D C 1972 Brit Med J 1: 40
Anderson R, Bauman M, Austrian R 1968 Amer Rev Resp Dis 97: 914
Appelbaum P C, Scragg J N, Bowen A J et al 1977 Lancet 2: 995
Baraff L J, Wilkins J, Wehrle P F 1978 Pediatrics 61: 224
Bartlett J G, Gorbach S L 1975 J Amer Med Ass 234: 935
Bartlett J G, Gorbach S L, Finegold S M 1974 Amer J Med 56: 202
Bass J W, Cohen S H, Corless J D, Mamures P 1967 J Amer Med Ass 202: 697
Bass J W, Klenk E L, Kotheimer J B, Linnemann C C, Smith M H D 1969 J Pediat 75: 768
Branefors-Helander P, Jeppsson P-H 1975 Scand J Infect Dis 7: 103
Brewin A, Arango L, Hadley W K, Murray J F 1974 J Amer Med Ass 230: 409
Calder M A, Lutz W, Schonell M E 1968 Brit J Dis Chest 62: 93
Carenfelt C, Eneroth C-M, Lundberg C, Wretlind B 1975 Scand J Infect Dis 7: 259
Carenfelt C, Lundberg C 1976 Scand J Infect Dis Suppl 9, 78
Chodosh S, Eichel B, Ellis C, Medici T C, Faling L J 1973 J Infect Dis 128: S710
Cooper J, Inman J S, Dawson A F 1976 Practitioner 217: 804
Davis S D, Wedgewood R G 1965 Amer J Dis Child 109: 544
Editorial 1976 Brit Med J 1: 606
Everett M T 1975 J Roy Coll G P 25: 317
Foy H M, Broome C V, Hayes P S et al 1979 Lancet 1: 767
Fraser D W, Tsai T R, Orenstein W et al 1977 New Engl J Med 297: 1189
Frederick J, Braude A I 1974 New Engl J Med 290: 135
Gordon M, Lovell S, Dugdale A E 1974 Med J Austral 1: 304
Graybill J R, Marshall L W, Charache P et al 1973 Amer Rev Resp Dis 108: 1130
Hamory B H, Sande M A, Sydnor A, Seale D L, Gwaltney J M 1979 J Infect Dis 139: 197
Hansman D, Devitt L, Miles H, Riley I 1974 Med J Austral 2: 353
Howard J E, Nelson J D, Clahsen J, Jackson L H 1976 Amer J Dis Child 130: 965
Howe J G, Wilson T S 1972 Lancet 2: 184
Howie J G R, Hutchison K R 1978 Brit Med J 2: 1342
Howie J G R, Richardson I M, Gill G, Duono D 1971 J Roy Coll G P 21: 657
Hughes W T 1976 New Engl J Med 295: 726
Irwin R S, Woelk W K, Coudon W L 1975 Ann Intern Med 82: 493
Jacobs M R, Koornhof H J, Robins-Browne R M et al 1978 New Engl J Med 299: 735
Johnston R N, McNeill R S, Smith D H et al 1969 Brit Med J 4: 265
Kalm O, Kamme C, Bergstrom B, Lofkvist F, Norman O 1975 Scand J Infect Dis 7: 209
Kamme C 1970 Scand J Infect Dis 2: 117

Lambert H P 1978 Scand J Infect Dis Suppl 14: 262
Lambert H P, Stern H 1972 Brit Med J 3: 323
Lau W K, Young L S 1976 New Eng J Med 295: 716
McCloskey R V, Green M J, Eller J, Smilack J 1974 Ann Intern Med 81: 788
McHardy V U, Schonell M E 1972 Brit Med J 4: 569
Maesen F P V, Beeuwkes H, Davies B I et al 1976 J Antimicrob Chemother 2: 279
Matsen J M, Torstenson O, Siegel S E, Bacaner H 1974 Antimicrob Agents Chemother 6: 501
Medical Research Council 1953 Lancet 1: 1109
Medical Research Council 1966 Brit Med J 1: 1317
Miller L W 1975 Ann Intern Med 82: 720
Molla A L 1974 Practitioner 212: 123
Nilson B W, Poland R L, Thompson R S et al 1969 Pediatrics 43: 351
Ninane G, Joly J, Kraytman M 1978 Brit Med J 1: 276
Olson R W, Hodges G R 1975 J Amer Med Ass 232: 363
Peter G, Smith A L 1977 New Engl J Med 297: 311, 365
Pines A, Greenfield J S B, Raafat H, Siddiqui G 1972b Brit J Dis Chest 66: 116
Pines A, Raafat H, Greenfield J S B et al 1972a Practitioner 208: 265
Pines A, Raafat H, Greenfield J S B et al 1972c Brit J Dis Chest 66: 107
Soyka L F, Robinson D S, Lachant N, Monaco J 1975 Pediatrics 55: 552
Stechenberg B W, Anderson D, Chang M J et al 1976 Pediatrics 58: 532
Stewart S M, Anderson I M E, Jones G R, Calder M A 1974 Thorax 29: 110
Stillerman M, Isenberg H D, Moody M 1972 Amer J Dis Child 123: 457
Stott N C H, West R R 1976 Brit Med J 2: 556
Strangert K 1969 Scand J Infect Dis 1: 67
Stuart-Harris C H 1968 Abstr Wld Med 42: 649
Symposium 1979 International symposium on Legionnaires disease. Ann Intern Med 90, 489
Syriopoulou V, Scheifele D, Howie V et al 1976 J Pediat 89: 839
Tally F P, Sutter V L, Finegold S M 1975 Antimicrob Ag Chemother 7: 672
Taylor B, Abbott G D, Kerr M McK, Fergusson D M 1977 Brit Med J 2: 552
Van Eygen M, Znamensky P Y, Heck E, Raymaekers I 1976 Lancet 1: 382
Wallace R J, Musher D M, Martin R R 1978 Amer J Med 64: 87
Williams D M, Krick J A, Remington J S 1976 Amer Rev Resp Dis 114: 359

20

Antibiotics in obstetrics

The vaginal and cervical canal contain a varied bacterial flora which, in normal circumstances, fails to gain access to the amniotic fluid, placenta or fetus. Aerobes include a variety of streptococci including, in some women, group B haemolytic streptococci, coagulase-negative staphylococci, diphtheroids, and coliforms. The normal anaerobic flora includes peptococci, peptostreptococci, Veillonella, Bacteroides and Fusobacteria. The most thorough study of the bacteriology of cervix and uterus, involving multiple biopsies of 50 specimens taken at hysterectomy (for menorrhagia) showed conclusively that the uterus is normally sterile, as was the cervical canal in half the subjects. The lower half of the cervical canal showed organisms similar to those of the vaginal vault, while 90 per cent of cultures from the ectocervix showed vaginal organisms (Sparks et al, 1977).

Infection of the uterus is prevented by potent antibacterial defences in the cervix which include lysozyme and IgA (Schumacher et al, 1977). The amniotic fluid too has an antibacterial action by virtue of a number of mechanisms, including a recently described zinc-protein complex. Schlievert et al (1976) claim that this effect of amniotic fluid depends greatly on the ratio of inorganic phosphate to zinc, and that fluids with a ratio of less than 100 are strongly bactericidal.

Ascending infection is favoured by inflammatory conditions of the lower genital tract, by premature rupture of membranes, and by repeated vaginal examinations. An additional factor in modern obstetrics which may be conducive to intra-uterine infection is the practice of intra-uterine monitoring. Hagen (1975) reported a great increase in maternal infection after Caesarean section in patients who were monitored in this way, but Gassner & Ledger (1976), while acknowledging an increase of infection in monitored patients pointed out that these patients constituted a high risk group, and that infection rates were not related to the duration of monitoring.

Infection rates rise steadily with increasing interval between rupture of membranes and onset of labour, mainly because premature labour is often prolonged, and prematurity is itself strongly associated with a higher risk of sepsis (Ledger, 1978).

Both fetus and mother may suffer the consequences of ascending infection and there is a sharp rise in perinatal mortality and maternal morbidity when the membranes have been ruptured for more than 24 hours (Still & Adamson, 1967). Uterine sepsis may develop insidiously, with no evidence of infection beyond a foul or foetid vaginal discharge for as long as 48 hours. The result of untreated sepsis may be a foul-smelling still-birth and, in the mother, bacteraemia with a 30–60 per cent incidence of septic shock.

With such potentially serious consequences, it generally continues to be the practice in premature rupture of the membranes to protect the fetus, as far as possible, by maternal antibacterial prophylaxis. Although convincing evidence is lacking that either systemic treatment of the mother, or the instillation of topical antibacterial agents into the genital tract, significantly reduces the incidence of infections in the amnion or fetus, there is no doubt about the need and efficacy of antibiotic protection of the mother.

Choicc of agent

In selecting the appropriate antibiotic its antibacterial spectrum and its capacity to pass into the liquor amnii and into the fetal circulation must be borne in mind. Only negligible amounts of streptomycin, the tetracyclines and chloramphenicol reach the liquor amnii, whereas with penicillins and cephalosporins high and prolonged levels result from excretion by the foetal kidneys. Benzyl penicillin has been found to produce levels up to 32 times those in the blood and Blecher et al (1966) have shown that after three 500 mg doses of ampicillin to the mother, the liquor amnii usually contains 2.5 μg per ml or more. Barr & Graham (1967) found that doses of 1 g of cephaloridine produced levels of 1–8 μg/ml in both the amnion and the cord serum of the majority of babies, but in 5–10 per cent, the levels were less than 1 μg/ml.

Penetration of antibiotics into the fetal circulation

The transport of antimicrobial drugs across the placenta and their distribution within the fetus are affected by a number of factors; concentration in the infant circulation are also naturally affected by dose, route and frequency of administration. For these reasons, and because the information available is often scanty, only general guide lines can be established, and the administration of antimicrobial agents, as of other drugs, in pregnancy should be restricted as far as possible. In general, penicillins, aminoglycosides, sulphonamides, and tetracyclines readily cross the placental barrier, as do some cephalosporins. Chloramphenicol concentrations reached in the infant after maternal administration are also high enough to ban its use in pregnancy, since the fetal liver is unable to inactivate the drug by glucuronidation. Erythromycin and clindamycin, by contrast, achieve only low infant/maternal serum ratios. Despite these caveats fetal damage following antibiotic administration to the mother has been established for only a few agents. The most notable are the deposition of tetracycline in fetal bone and teeth (see Ch. 7), occasional instances of fetal hyperbilirubinaemia after sulphonamide administration, and the relationship of streptomycin administration to defects of auditory nerve function (Conway & Birt 1965). Since other aminoglycosides are transported across the placenta in a similar manner to streptomycin, it would be wise to avoid the use of these agents in pregnancy if possible. The pharmacology of the placenta is reviewed by Juchau & Dyer (1972) and placental transport of antibiotics is fully discussed by McCracken (1976).

MANAGEMENT OF PREMATURE MEMBRANE RUPTURE

A policy for the management of premature membrane rupture outlined by MacVicar (1978) is to induce labour if the patient is more than 38 weeks pregnant. In patients whose membranes rupture at less than 36 weeks he recommends admission to hospital. Vaginal examination is omitted or done only under strict aseptic precautions. Antibiotics are not given routinely but are started if more than 24 hours has elapsed between membrane rupture and the onset of labour. Ledger (1978) too recommends a selective approach to antibiotic use after membrane rupture, advocating the use of ultrasound and amniotic sampling as guides to the onset of infection. Evidence of maternal infection at any time following membrane rupture demands the use of antibiotics after taking the necessary specimens for culture. Cover is best provided, in the absence of specific evidence of aetiology, by ampicillin or a cephalosporin.

CAESAREAN SECTION

The increasing trend towards Caesarean section has been accompanied by an increased risk of hospital acquired uterine infection. Gassner & Ledger (1976) made a prospective survey of 5240 deliveries in a hospital serving patients of lower socio-economic classes in Los Angeles, finding a maternal infection rate of 40 per cent in patients undergoing Caesarean section with intra-uterine monitoring, 20 per cent after Caesarean section without monitoring, 2.7 per cent after vaginal delivery with monitoring and 1.4 per cent after vaginal delivery without monitoring. Prophylactic antibiotics are not generally recommended for uncomplicated Caesarean section, but are indicated when risk factors such as preceding membrane rupture are present (Hilliard & Harris, 1977). Gibbs et al, (1973) achieved a significant reduction of endometritis and wound infection using a three dose regimen of ampicillin and kanamycin (together with methicillin in the early part of the trial). Since the importance of anaerobic infections has been newly recognized, it has become customary to include an anti-anaerobe agent, so that in Britain ampicillin or penicillin together with metronidazole are often used. Elsewhere clindamycin is employed, and Hirsch (1977) also showed a significant reduction of wound sepsis and endometritis with a four dose regimen of clindamycin and ampicillin. Several cephalosporins have also been used successfully for this purpose (Moro & Andrews, 1975). Timing should follow the principles discussed for abdominal operations generally in Chapter 18, i.e. the antimicrobial drugs should be given immediately before operation and for 24–48 hours after.

PUERPERAL PYREXIA

Slight fever in the puerperium without clinical signs should be observed and not treated with antibiotics in the absence of positive findings. Observation should include examination of the urine and high vaginal or cervical swabs.

Patients with severe pyrexia of more than 24 hours' duration or with clinical signs of genital tract infection should always be given antibiotic treatment. The bacteriological investigation of puerperal infection of the genital tract is not very satisfactory. In most hospitals reliance is placed on the high vaginal swab, which is perfectly adequate if the infecting agent is *Str. pyogenes* but in other cases may give misleading results, either because the infecting agent is not isolated or because the organism isolated is so frequently present in the vagina of apparently healthy women in the puerperium that its pathogenic significance is doubtful.

These cases arise in the same way as the ascending infection which may complicate premature rupture of the membranes. Cervical swabs and blood and urine cultures should be taken and treatment started, in patients not seriously ill, with amoxycillin or a cephalosporin. In patients with more severe illnesses, it is proper to aim at a wider cover of possible infecting organisms using the principles described below in the section on infection following abortion. Removal of retained products of conception, and the treatment of concomitant shock, are both very important aspects of treatment. If β-haemolytic streptococci are isolated, high dose penicillin is the drug of choice. Other organisms of uncertain significance in puerperal pyrexia are the genital mycoplasmas. *M. hominis* has been associated with a few cases of post-partum septicaemia (Tully & Smith, 1968) and puerperal sepsis associated with the isolation of a T-strain mycoplasma from blood, urine and vagina has also been reported (Sompolinski et al, 1971).

Puerperal bacteraemia in patients with heart disease

It has been claimed that bacteraemia can be demonstrated in up to 5 per cent of women during delivery and that there is a corresponding risk of endocarditis in those with heart disease. Baker & Hubbell (1967) found the incidence to be only a tenth of this, with no bacteriaemia after the first 24 hours. They doubt the necessity of giving prophylactic antibiotics during the uncomplicated delivery of women with heart disease.

INFECTION FOLLOWING ABORTION

Infection is liable to occur in cases of incomplete abortion, where all or part of the placenta is retained, or in cases where abortion is illegally performed by the inexpert use of unsterile instruments.

Organisms most commonly isolated in relation to abortion are β-haemolytic streptococci, bacteroides, anaerobic streptococci, enterococci and *Cl. perfringens* (Smith et al, 1970). Although isolation of the latter organism is not uncommon, the severe picture of clostridial post-abortal sepsis accompanied by intravascular haemolysis and a high mortality rate, is now fortunately rare. (Decker & Hall 1966.) *N. gonorrhoeae* is also sometimes identified in these patients.

Antibiotic therapy depends in practice on the severity of illness. Burkman et al (1977), describing endometritis in 228 women following elective abortion, obtained a good response with penicillin or ampicillin for those treated as outpatients, adding an aminoglycoside for those ill enough to be admitted. As with other forms of abdominal and pelvic sepsis, although anaerobes are commonly identified, the importance of including antibacterial cover against those strains, mainly *Bacteroides fragilis*, which are insensitive to the penicillin, is still uncertain. While this issue remains uncertain, it is proper to include an anti-anaerobic agent, metronidazole in Britain or clindamycin in the U.S.A., for patients with severe post-abortal infections. All obstetricians agree that evacuation of retained products is an important component of treatment, and should be carried out as soon as the patient's condition allows. The treatment of pelvic inflammatory disease not related to recent pregnancy is discussed on page 428.

The frequency and severity of post-abortal infections is closely related to the stage of pregnancy, the method of induction and skill with which the procedure is performed, and severe infection is now uncommon in countries whose laws permit early termination. Hodgson & Portmann (1974) reported a prospective study of more than 10 000 abortions performed in the first trimester by the vacuum aspiration method. 25 pelvic infections were recorded in a 65 per cent follow-up, an incidence of 0.37 per cent.

Trichomoniasis in pregnancy

Despite the efficacy of oral metronidazole in trichomoniasis, there has been reluctance to prescribe it for pregnant patients for fear of fetal toxicity. Rodin & Hass (1966) review the previously published results of treatment during pregnancy and add 78 patients of their own, including ten treated during the first eight weeks with the conventional dose of 200 mg metronidazole 8-hourly for seven days. In no instance was any congenital malformation attributable to the drug. This is supported by Sands (1966) who gave 750 mg metronidazole daily for only three days. Only 2/113 patients failed to respond. There was no fetal abnormality and no maternal disturbance other than a rash in one patient and vomiting in another.

An alternative is nimorazole, given as a single dose of 2 g. This is found in effective concentrations in blood, vaginal and salivary secretions, but no specific information is available on its use in pregnancy.

Vaginal candidiasis

This is common both in pregnant and non-pregnant women. It may be controlled by the use of nystatin vaginal pessaries inserted twice daily and nystatin cream is often used additionally. Persistent or recurrent infection may be associated with intestinal candidiasis for which oral nystatin is given in a dose of 500 000 units three times daily. Infection in a sexual partner may also be a cause of persistent infection.

Nystatin may not always succeed and many other anti-fungal agents have been successfully employed, pimaricin (Don, 1967), candicidin (Cameron, 1969) and, more recently miconazole, econazole and clotrimazole. Wallenburg & Wladimiroff (1976) treated 94 pregnant patients, obtaining a cure rate of 83 per cent with miconazole vaginal cream applied for 10 days and 68 per cent with nystatin vaginal tablets used for seven to nine days. Balmer (1976) reported a cure rate of 93·4 per cent in 996 women treated with two courses of econazole vaginal suppositories. Prophylactic treatment for recurrent vaginal candidiasis has also been attempted; Davidson & Mould (1978) found no relationship between symptoms and the isolation of candida, although the group receiving clotrimazole had fewer symptoms after the trial period.

BREAST ABSCESS

Breast abscess in the puerperium is invariably due to *Staph. aureus* and the general principles of chemotherapy are the same as those outlined for staphylococcal infection generally in Chapter 15. Treatment should be started with cloxacillin or flucloxacillin pending a bacteriological report, since penicillin resistance is common among staphylococci in and out of hospital. It is impossible to say how often surgery is avoided by the use of antibiotics in incipient breast abscess, but Goodman & Benson (1970) found no evidence of benefit from their use once surgery had become necessary. In their series 59 of 115 abscesses arising in hospital were caused by penicillin-sensitive strains of staphylococci, as were five of nine developing after home delivery.

NEONATAL INFECTIONS

Babies born to mothers receiving chemoprophylaxis because of premature rupture of the membranes should continue on treatment especially if the membranes have been ruptured for some time or if the mother's temperature has risen during labour. It is also generally felt that because of the high risk and danger of respiratory infection, prophylactic antibiotics should also be given to babies asphyxiated at birth or with the respiratory distress syndrome, or those requiring tracheal intubation or assisted respiration.

Generalised infection

If an infant is seriously ill with no obvious cause, cultures of blood and urine and swabs from any local lesions, nose, throat and umbilicus should be examined bacteriologically: a lumbar puncture may also be indicated.

Difficulty of localizing infection and rapid deterioration of the newborn not infrequently demand the institution of treatment before the nature of infection is fully established. Choice of antibiotics in these circumstances is difficult, since it must provide cover for a variety of enterobacteria, Pseudomonas, streptococci of various types, and staphylococci; some guidance may be obtained by the local prevalence of strains of known resistance pattern, or the known presence of a nursery outbreak caused by a particular organism. Combinations of ampicillin and cloxacillin, or a cephalosporin alone, have been widely used for generalized neonatal infection of uncertain cause, but neither method is suitable if Pseudomonas infection is likely, and a number of other enterobacteria are now resistant to these drugs. Gentamicin has now been used quite extensively in neonates (Klein et al, 1971) and dose limits for this age group well defined. A combination of gentamicin with a penicillin provides cover against most Gram-negative pathogens as well as against streptococci and penicillin-resistant staphylococci. Septicaemia in neonates is often accompanied by meningitis, and further discussion of this topic will be found on page 329. Once the identity of the invading organism is known, other drugs than those used to initiate treatment may prove more suitable.

Local experience in a particular hospital may indicate other lines of initial treatment, for example, use of amikacin if gentamicin-resistant enterobacteria are prevalent, or the inclusion of carbenicillin as well as an aminoglycoside if pseudomonas infection is prevalent. Much valuable guidance on the use of antimicrobials in the newborn is to be found in a monograph by McCracken & Nelson (1977).

Thrush

This is usually confined to the mouth and can be treated by local application of gentian violet or nystatin. The lesions sometimes extend down the alimentary tract, in which case nystatin should be given orally in a dose of 100 000 units every six hours. If the infant is having a broad spectrum antibiotic, this should if possible be stopped.

Antibiotics and breast milk

The passage of drugs into breast milk is reviewed by Savage (1977), Catz & Giacoia (1972) and Knowles (1965). A few low molecular weight water soluble compounds like sulphonamides and isoniazid achieve concentrations in breast milk similar to those in the maternal plasma. Erythromycin, tetracycline and chloramphenicol are also easily transported into milk, with concentrations approximately half that of maternal plasma. Penicillins, by contrast, are found in milk in very low concentration. Aminoglycosides, too, are not transported readily unless the mother has renal failure. Although adverse effects on breast fed infants resulting from antibiotics given to their mothers are apparently uncommon, it would be sensible to avoid sulphonamides, tetracycline and chloramphenicol if possible. Sulphamethoxazole is unlikely to affect bilirubin binding appreciably, so an exception could be made in using co-trimoxazole for post-partum urinary infections. Penicillins will not achieve a significant antibacterial action in ingested breast milk, but may still sensitize by this route. The small amount of antibiotic likely to be administered in breast milk can be illustrated by an example. The concentration of tetracycline in breast milk averages 1 μg/ml (range 0.65–3.0) after a maternal dose of 2 g daily. A 3 kg baby receiving 600 ml of milk daily will receive a daily dose of 0.6 mg, or 0.2 mg per kg, approximately 1 per cent of the therapeutic level.

References

Baker T H, Hubbell R 1967 Amer J Obstet Gynec 97: 575
Balmer J A 1976 Amer J Obstet Gynec 126: 436
Barr W, Graham R 1967 Postgrad Med J 43: (Suppl Aug) 101
Blecher T E, Edgar W M, Melville H A H, Peel K R 1966 Brit Med J 1: 137
Burkman R J, Atienza M F, King T M 1977 Amer J Obstet Gynec 128: 556
Cameron P F 1969 Practitioner 202: 695
Catz C S, Giacoia G P 1972 Pediat Clin N Amer 19: 151
Conway N, Birt B D 1965 Brit Med J 2: 260
Davidson F, Mould R F 1978 Brit J Vener Dis 54: 176
Decker W H, Hall W 1966 Amer J Obstet Gynec 95: 394
Don R A 1967 Med J Aust 1: 382
Gassner C B, Ledger W J 1976 Amer J Obstet Gynec 126: 33
Gibbs R S, Hunt J E, Schwarz R H 1973 Amer J Obstet Gynec 117: 419
Goodman M A, Benson E A 1970 Med J Aust 1: 1034
Hagen D 1975 Obstet Gynec 46: 260
Hilliard G D, Harris R E 1977 Obstet Gynec 50: 285
Hirsch H A 1977 In: Gynecology and obstetrics. Proceedings of the VIII World Congress. Excerpta Medica, Amsterdam, p 227
Hodgson J E, Portmann K C 1974 Amer J Obstet Gynec 120: 802
Juchau M R, Dyer D C 1972 Pediatr Clin N Amer 19: 65
Klein J O, Herschel M, Therakan R M, Ingall D 1971 J Infect Dis 124: Suppl 224
Knowles J A 1965 J Pediat 66: 1068
Ledger W J 1978 Clin Obstet Gynaec 21: 455
MacVicar J 1978 Practitioner 221: 885
McCracken G H 1976 In: Remington J S, Klein J O (eds) Infectious diseases of the fetus and newborn infant. W B Saunders, Philadelphia
McCracken G H, Nelson J D 1977 Antimicrobial therapy for newborns. Grune and Stratton, New York
Moro M, Andrews M 1975 Obstet Gynec 44: 688
Rodin P, Hass G 1966 Brit J Vener Dis 42: 210
Sands R X 1966 Amer J Obstet Gynec 94: 350
Savage R L 1977 J Hum Nutr 31: 459
Schlievert P, Johnson W, Galask R P 1976 Amer J Obstet Gynec 125: 899
Schumacher G F B, Kim M H, Hosseinian A H, Dupon C 1977 Amer J Obstet Gynec 129: 629

Smith J W, Southern P M, Lehmann J D 1970 Obstet Gynec 35: 704
Sompolinsky D, Solomon F, Leiba H et al 1971 Israel J Med Sci 7: 745
Sparks R A, Purrier B G A, Watt P J, Elstein M 1977 Brit J Obstet Gynaecol 84: 701
Still R M, Adamson H S 1967 J Obstet Gynaec Brit Cwlth 74: 412
Tully J G, Smith L G 1968 J Amer Med Ass 204: 827
Wallenburg H C S, Wladimiroff J W 1976 Obstet Gynec 48: 491

21

Urinary tract infections

The presence of urinary infection and the efficacy of its treatment cannot be established without bacteriological examination of the urine. Many infections, particularly in pregnancy, in the elderly or the later infections of a series, are asymptomatic. Conversely, sometimes in the child and frequently in the adult, typical symptoms, notably frequency and dysuria, are unaccompanied by infected urine. About half the symptomatic women seen in general practice fall into this category and are said to be suffering from the 'urethral syndrome'. This is almost certainly a complex of disorders of which one major variety is associated with subsequent urinary infection and may be very clearly related to sexual activity. In a minority of persistently symptomatic patients some underlying gynaecological, intestinal or other disorder can be demonstrated which may respond to appropriate measures (O'Grady et al, 1973a). The treatment of the remainder is generally very unsatisfactory. Some patients respond to treatment as for urinary infection, to local antibacterial or other applications, to a single dose of an antibacterial agent taken prior to intercourse, or to urological procedures. Rees et al (1978) claim considerable success in managing this generally intractable condition by a 'multifactorial approach' which employs spasmolytic and psychotropic agents, psychiatric support and where necessary urethral dilatation or urethrotomy.

Initial treatment

Most reviews of the treatment of urinary tract infection emphasize the complexity and difficulty of the subject. In fact the majority of sufferers are non-pregnant women most of whom respond readily to treatment. The problems arise with the minority of women who develop intractable infection, pregnant women, men and children. The management difficulties of these groups are such that they must be considered separately.

WOMEN

About 80 per cent of acute urinary tract infections are caused by *E. coli*; *Proteus* species (almost all *Pr. mirabilis*) account for another 8–12 per cent. The remainder are other enterobacteria, *Strep. faecalis* and a certain type of coagulase negative Staphylococcus which has several times been renamed. The name now settled on, *Staphylococcus saprophyticus*, biotype 3, seems a singularly unfortunate choice for an organism held by some authors to be responsible for as many as 30 per cent of acute urinary infections in women under the age of 25 (Gillespie et al, 1978). In chronic infections, Escherichia are much less common and various other enterobacteria, notably Proteus, Klebsiella, and *Ps. aeruginosa* are found.

Another important difference is that acute infection is almost always caused by a single bacterial species. In chronic infection, particularly in patients with gross structural or functional abnormalities of the urinary tract, more than one kind of organism is frequently present. Escherichia—responsible for the great majority of infections—are naturally sensitive to a great variety of agents excreted in the urine (Table 21.1) all of which have been successfully used for treatment.

Table 21.1 Sensitivity to drugs of bacteria causing urinary infections

Drug	Concentration attained in urine (μg/ml)	Minimum inhibitory concentration (μg/ml)					
		Esch. coli	*Proteus mirabilis*	*Kl. aerogenes*	*Ps. aeruginosa*	*Staph. aureus*	*Str. faecalis*
Sulphonamides	1000	8	8	R	50	4–16	R
Nitrofurantoin	125	16	200	100	R	4	25
Ampicillin	250+	8	4	R	R	0.04	2
Cycloserine	250	64	250	64	128	16	128
Cephalexin	500+	4	4	32	R	4	128
Nalidixic acid	250+	4	4	16	R	64	R
Trimethoprim	100	0.5	2	2	R	0.5	0.5
Penicillin	250+	20–>100	8	R	R	0.02	4
Carbenicillin	2000	5	2.5	250	50	0.5–50	25
Cephaloridine	300	4	4	4–R	R	0.1–5	16
Streptomycin	1000	5	50	5	50	10	100
Kanamycin	300	2	4	2	64	0.5	64
Gentamicin	50	1–4	2–8	1–2	1–8	0.1–1	8–16
Tetracyclines	300	5	R	100	10	200	0.5
Polymyxin	50	1	R	1	1	R	1

R = resistant to concentrations attainable.

However, strains resistant to the widely used agents sulphonamides and ampicillin are now common. Table 21.2 shows the species isolated from domicilary practice urines over a three month period in one of our laboratories and the proportions sensitive to commonly used agents. Differences in antibacterial spectra and prevalence of resistance combine to produce little overall difference in the applicability of several of the agents but geographical differences in the distribution of resistant strains are often so marked that prescribers will be wise to consult the local laboratory about the suitability of their favourite agent for that particular community.

Some comparative studies—for example that of Gower & Tasker (1976)—have shown clear benefits of one agent over another but generally it appears that there is little to choose between them providing the organism is sensitive *in vitro* (Brumfitt & Pursell, 1972; Slade & Crowther, 1972). Claims that patients commonly respond to agents to which the infecting organism is said by the laboratory to be resistant may be due to several things: sensitivity tests on organisms recovered from poorly collected specimens and having no relation to the patient's condition, spontaneous resolution of infection, or to an erroneous sensitivity report. False reports of Escherichia resistant to sulphonamides or Proteus resistant to ampicillin are prominent amongst errors made in routine sensitivity tests. Gleckman (1977) showed that about 80 per cent of patients infected with sulphonamide-sensitive strains responded to sulphonamide therapy—a result similar to that obtained with other agents—while of the patients infected with sulphonamide-resistant strains about 50 per cent resolved—a result consistent with other estimates of spontaneous resolution rates.

Table 21.2 Percentage of all urinary pathogens and of the principal infecting species, resistant to common antibacterial agents

	Percent resistant to				
	Ampicillin	Sulphonamide	Trimethoprim	Nalidixic acid	Nitrofurantoin
E. coli	28	34	6	1	3
Klebsiella spp.	100	34	14	5	22
Proteus spp.	15	15	1	1	100
Staph. saprophyticus	80	2	13	100	0
Enterococcus	0	89	6	100	0
All species	36	38	17	23	26

Figures from Nottingham Area Public Health Laboratory, 1979

Dosage regimens

It has been customary to treat patients with acute infection with three or four doses of drug daily for 7–10 days or even for two weeks. About 80 per cent of patients respond to these regimens but so far, the evidence accumulated from the copious use of all these agents has failed to establish with any certainty the optimum dosage and duration of therapy. A substantial number of acute infections resolve spontaneously (Brumfitt, 1972) or respond to minimum treatment. Brumfitt et al (1970) cured a proportion of their patients with a single dose of cephaloridine and Williams & Smith (1970) a proportion of theirs with a single dose of streptomycin. Such ready response strongly suggests that this is a clear example of the use of antibiotic to support the natural defences. This being so, it is sensible to plan treatment in such a way as to offer this support as efficiently as possible.

Intrinsic clearance mechanisms

It is now generally conceded that in the genesis of bladder infection, faecal organisms first colonize the anterior urethra and are transferred to the bladder (Stamey, 1972).

In the urine enterobacteria are able to grow freely but are normally soon eliminated by dilution with incoming ureteric urine and discharged at the next voiding—a process which is enhanced by the frequent micturition naturally excited by urinary infection. Organisms which remain in the normally very small volume of residual urine will be disposed of by cellular or humoral mechanisms. During the overnight period, the rate of ureteric urine flow naturally falls and there is a long period without micturition during which organisms have a special opportunity to establish themselves. In the same way, where bladder emptying is impaired infection is particularly likely to occur and especially difficult to treat. Shand et al (1970) showed that patients in whom the residual volume was increased by only a few ml were more difficult to treat and more liable to recurrent infection than patients whose bladder emptying was completely normal.

This suggests that optimum results will be obtained by encouraging patients to drink copiously, and to empty the bladder completely (if necessary by double or triple micturition) at frequent intervals.

It may be objected that fluid loading will exert a detrimental effect on antibacterial therapy by diluting the agent in the urine. In fact, agents used for the treatment of urinary infection normally appear in the urine in very high concentrations (Table 21.1) and the degree of dilution which can be achieved by increased drinking still leaves a concentration greatly in excess of that required to inhibit sensitive organisms. Moreover, many antibacterial agents exert less effect on high concentrations of bacteria and the beneficial effect of diluting the culture greatly outweigh any detrimental effect of diluting the agent (Fig. 21.1).

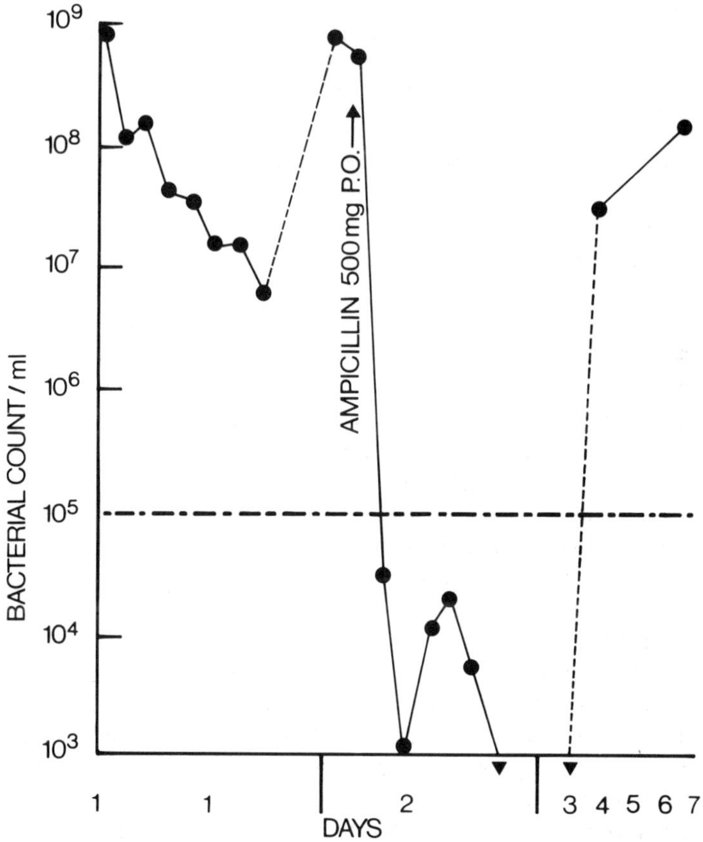

Fig. 21.1 Poor wash-out effect on day 1, followed by prompt response to a single dose of ampicillin, but reappearance of infection on day 4. Reproduced from Cattell W R et al (1968) in Urinary tract infection, Oxford University Press, p. 212

In patients given a single dose of a drug to which the organism is sensitive the concentration of bacteria in successive samples of urine frequently falls below detectable levels within a few hours and does not reappear for several days (Fig. 21.1). This suggests that patients are customarily given far more drug than is necessary for the treatment of acute infection and several studies have now shown that a large proportion of patients with acute infection respond to a single dose. Several agents have been used. Bailey & Abbott (1978) and Fang et al (1978) used a 3 g oral dose of amoxycillin but whether a large dose of a rapidly excreted agent represents the optimum presentation of the drug has not been established. Charlton et al (1976) showed that in patients receiving conventional dosages the results of three days' or ten days' therapy were indistinguishable. It is possible that even less drug over two or three days would provide the most economical and least toxic regimen. Whatever the regimen, the last dose should be given immediately before retiring, having emptied the bladder completely, since the overnight period provides the longest time for uninterrupted bacterial growth when urine flow and frequency of micturition are at their lowest.

Failure of initial therapy

In a proportion of patients infection is not controlled or promptly returns on cessation of therapy, or quickly recurs. Much effort has been expended on trying to identify before the event those patients who will prove to be intractable to treatment and particularly those who are at risk from the development of renal failure. One clue to the identity of patients likely to prove therapeutically difficult is provided by the species of the infecting organism. Since patients with chronic infections are more commonly infected with organisms other than *Escherichia coli* the presence of such organisms should arouse the suspicion that infection will recur.

Relapse and re-infection

In some patients whose infections rapidly reappear after treatment the organisms prove to be identical with those responsible for the original infection. It is reasonable to conclude in such cases that therapy succeeded only in suppressing growth of the organisms which somehow hid in the urinary tract and quickly re-established infection when treatment was withdrawn. Such recrudescence of the original infection is described as *relapse*. In other patients, and typically after a longer interval, bacteriuria reappears but is shown to be due to *re-infection* with a different organism.

In practice, it is not always easy to distinguish relapse from re-infection in the individual patient, but much has been made of the distinction because of the belief that relapse indicates persistence of infection within the kidney, with the attendant danger of renal damage while re-infection indicates simply susceptibility to bladder infection which is easily treated and carries little risk to the upper urinary tract.

Cattell et al (1973) confirmed that a greater proportion of patients whose disease involved the upper tract relapsed and a greater proportion of those whose disease involved the lower tract became re-infected, but the difference was not great. In addition, the methods for distinguishing upper from lower tract infection, which include ureteric catherization, tests of renal function, biochemical evidence of renal damage and the demonstration of antibody response are far from infallible. In

Rumans & Vosti's (1978) hands the most recent test for renal involvement, the appearance of antibody-coated bacteria in the urine, succeeded in identifying only 60 per cent of patients they believed from other observations to have renal infection. In the management of the individual patient, therefore—as distinct from elucidation of the many remaining mysteries of urinary tract infection—currently available localization studies are not helpful, particularly as distinctive forms of therapy for sub-groups of patients with intractable infection have not been defined.

Treatment of relapse

Patients whose infection quickly reappears should be questioned for compliance and re-treated for two weeks ideally with an agent chosen on the basis of *in vitro* sensitivity tests. Emergence of a resistant mutant is a very uncommon cause of failure except with streptomycin and, in some series, nalidixic acid. Fluid loading and frequent complete micturition with the last of the daily doses given just before retiring to bed should be continued.

If relapse again occurs there is a high chance that radiography will show some abnormality of the urinary tract which may be surgically correctable, and uro-radiography is essential at this stage. The most important example of renal infection uncontrollable before and controlled after surgery is that associated with stones.

Persistence in the form of spheroplasts (page 259) is most likely to be a feature of infection with Proteus in which eradication may be achieved by sequential treatment with a cell-wall-inhibiting agent, such as ampicillin or cephalexin, followed by a spheroplast inhibitor such as erythromycin. We have confirmed the success of this regimen, but it is much less likely to be useful in relapsing infection due to Escherichia since only the minority of its survivors from exposure to cell-wall-inhibiting agents are in the form of spheroplasts.

It might reasonably be hoped that failure to achieve adequate agent concentration at the site of infection following oral treatment would be overcome by intensive parenteral therapy. This certainly sometimes succeeds but must obviously be done in hospital using agents chosen on the basis of *in vitro* sensitivity tests. Ampicillin and other penicillins and kanamycin and other aminoglycosides have been principally used for this purpose. Dosage should be given frequently, preferably by rapid intravenous infusion. The effect of the penicillins or cephalosporins should be enhanced by probenecid and that of aminoglycosides by alkalinization of the urine. Administration of the antibiotic should not be started until the pH is at least 7.0, and it should be verified that this reaction is being maintained. If surgery is undertaken (for example for the removal of renal stones) intensive therapy should begin at the time of operation. Harrison et al (1977) gave ticarcillin 200 mg per kg per day (adjusted for renal function) as four to six 30-minute infusions or up to 60 000 000 units benzylpenicillin a day to patients with infected renal calculi. They eradicated infection from all patients infected with *Proteus mirabilis* and most of those infected with other species but relapse and reinfection were common.

There is no evidence that patients who relapse after two weeks' therapy will respond to similar treatment continued for 6–8 weeks but they may ultimately be controlled by much longer low-dose therapy (see below).

Treatment of re-infection

Irrespective of the ease with which infection is eradicated some patients become re-infected with a new organism. In some women the onset of frequency and dysuria is clearly related to sexual intercourse. Not all of these episodes are accompanied by bacteriuria but it is not difficult to believe that deformity of the urethra could introduce organisms into the bladder and Buckley et al (1978) found a rise (usually transient) in the count of bladder bacteria following intercourse on at least one occasion in half the women they studied. The management of patients subject to re-infection depends on the frequency with which infections occur. If new infections occur infrequently (not more than 2 or 3 a year) and respond readily to treatment, each episode is probably best treated as a first infection as described on page 374. If, on the other hand, attacks occur frequently, or if infection, once established, is difficult to eradicate, then such patients are probably better managed on long-term prophylaxis. Infection should be eradicated, if necessary by intensive therapy, and chemoprophylaxis instituted as soon as the initial treatment has been shown to be successful, in order to prevent the establishment of fresh exogenous infection.

As with patients who repeatedly relapse, full uro-radiological examination of patients who suffer frequent re-infection may reveal correctable abnormalities.

Long-term therapy

Much disagreement about the place and efficacy of long-term therapy results from failure to recognize that such treatment may be used for three distinct purposes: (1) cure, (2) suppression (3) prophylaxis. Patients who relapse even after extended or intensive therapy may benefit from prolonged treatment which keeps the urine 'sterile' as long as sufficient antibacterial agent is present. Such suppressive treatment may provide symptomatic relief and prevent fresh acute attacks but since it is not curative there is a possibility that resolution of symptoms may conceal the progression of urinary tract disease. There are undoubtedly, however, a significant number of patients in whom therapy may be discontinued after six months or more without infection re-appearing (O'Grady et al, 1973b). Successful long-term therapy has been described with a number of agents, including mandelamine, cycloserine, sulphonamides, nitrofurantoin and co-trimoxazole. Once control has been established patients can often be maintained on a single nightly dose. In the case of co-trimoxazole, adults with persistently relapsing infection or with frequent re-infections have been successfully maintained for years (O'Grady et al, 1973b) on a dosage which was halved at fortnightly intervals (from 12-hourly to nightly then alternate nightly) as long as control was maintained. We have argued that it is important to give the single daily dose of agent immediately before retiring to bed, having emptied the bladder completely, in order to control regrowth of organisms overnight (page 375). Others have attached considerable importance to sexual intercourse in the initiation of urinary infection and have recommended a single dose of agent (nitrofurantoin has been generally used) to prevent the overgrowth of organisms introduced into the bladder (Vosti, 1975).

Long-term therapy has two main foreseeable disadvantages: toxicity and super-infection with resistant organisms. These hazards may be minimized by choosing the least toxic agent and progressively reducing the dose to the effective minimum; and by accepting only the most compelling reasons for bringing patients into hospital where the most undesirable organisms live. Long-term toxic effects on these regimens must, of course, be constantly watched for, and only time will tell whether such protracted medication is completely safe.

The particular success of nitrofurantoin and co-trimoxazole in these regimens is probably due to the absence of resistant flora in the gut of patients receiving nitrofurantoin and to the virtual abolition of organisms colonizing the urethra by co-trimoxazole (Stamey et al, 1977).

SPECIAL GROUPS

Women suffering from relapsing infection, possibly representing persisting renal infection, or from abnormalities of the urinary tract, are most effectively recognized by their failure to respond to sequential therapy. In addition to this minority group special attention is required by pregnant women, children and men.

PREGNANCY

On screening, about five per cent, in some series more, of pregnant women are found to have asymptomatic bacteriuria. The condition is important because about a quarter or a third of the patients develop clinical pyelonephritis and a number of studies have shown that bacteriuric patients are more likely to suffer abortion or premature labour and to deliver small or dead babies.

It is generally agreed that adequate treatment will prevent the development of acute pyelonephritis but a good deal of controversy has raged about the claims that uncontrolled urinary infection in pregnancy exerts detrimental effects on the fetus which can be prevented by adequate antibacterial therapy (Williams et al, 1973). Whether or not entirely satisfactory statistical evidence for these claims can be produced it may still be argued that both mother and fetus must be better off if continuing maternal infection can be eradicated. The issue (rather like that of the treatment of trichomonas vaginitis in pregnancy: page 368) turns largely on whether the fetus is likely to suffer more from the drug used in treatment than from maternal infection.

Some patients respond readily to treatment with ampicillin or with nitrofurantoin which reaches the fetus with such difficulty (page 47) that it is hard to see how conventional doses could be injurious. As in the non-pregnant patient, some do not respond to short-term therapy and bacteriuria may persist after the pregnancy. In some series a high proportion of such patients show urological abnormalities. It appears that pregnancy may effectively advertise the existence of long-standing renal disease but a history of childhood infection and reflux does not necessarily result in infective complications or further renal damage in pregnancy (MacGregor & Freeman, 1975).

Since some patients respond readily to treatment it seems reasonable to give them the chance to do so, thereby avoiding the disadvantages of prolonged medication. Patients who fail to respond may require suppressive therapy throughout pregnancy, and should undergo urological investigation post-partum. Safe and successful therapy throughout pregnancy has been described with a variety of agents including sulphamethoxydiazine (0.5 g per day) changing after the 13th week to sulphadimidine (1 g 8-hourly); sulphamethoxypyridazine (0.5 g per day); ampicillin (500 mg, 8-hourly) and nitrofurantoin (100 mg nightly: Bailey, 1970).

CHILDREN

In children, the danger of renal damage is very real (Smellie, 1970). In the very young the still developing defence mechanisms often fail to localize infection and where this involves the urinary tract there may be grave damage to the kidney. In the older child, urinary infection, especially if repeated, can lead to the distortion and scarring of the kidney identified radiologically as 'chronic pyelonephritis', and to ultimate loss of renal function, but the course may well be benign. It is important to recognize that the infecting organisms and the nature of abnormalities is different in the two sexes (Bergström, 1972). The effect of age is well brought out by Cohen (1976) who found that boys under ten years of age usually had fever and a high proportion (76 per cent) proved to have urinary tract abnormalities. Over the age of 10 they suffered frequency and dysuria but generally without fever and few (15 per cent) had radiological abnormalities. As in the adult with recurrent infection *E. coli* accounted for a considerably smaller proportion (62 per cent) of infections than is the case with simple acute infection in the adult female.

Scarring of the kidney is commonly associated with cystoureteric reflux which plays an important part— some, for example Shah et al (1978), believe the dominant part — in the genesis of the renal damage. This has led to emphasis on control of the mechanical defect rather than the infection and as a result there has been frequent and elaborate endoscopic and radiological examination of some children and many antireflux operations have been performed.

With increasing experience, it appears that, as in the adult, children with urinary infection are not equally at risk.

Treatment should be along the lines already discussed: short term initial therapy, repeated if necessary, followed where this fails by more intensive or prolonged treatment. As in the adult (page 378), long-term co-trimoxazole or nitrofurantoin is very successful for this purpose (Smellie et al, 1978). Just as in the adult, if infection cannot be eradicated or there is frequent re-infection, surgically remediable abnormalities may be demonstrable and long-term therapy may be required.

ADULT MALE

Spontaneous uncomplicated infection occurs in the adult male but it is a very rare condition compared with that seen in the adult female. Underlying abnormalities of the urinary tract are common in the infected male and early recourse to investigation is necessary. In the series studied by Freeman et al (1975) 84 per cent had IVP abnormalities, only 36 per cent were infected with *E. coli* and mixed infections were found in 21 per cent. In the majority of these patients (85 per cent) the urine was sterile during initial treatment but the recurrence rate was high and the long-term results on prolonged therapy disappointing. On continuous therapy there was a progressive rise in recurrence rate until after two years it reached the level observed in patients receiving placebo. It appears, therefore, that men generally correspond with the minority of women in whom intractable infection is predominantly due to species other than Escherichia, is not infrequently due to mixed infection and is associated with abnormalities of the urinary tract.

In addition, recurrent urinary infection may arise from a focus in the prostate. Unfortunately the existence of such a focus is difficult to demonstrate unequivocally and difficult to eradicate. Stamey and his colleagues have described how the diagnosis can be made and its bacterial aetiology established (Meares & Stamey, 1972) but frequency, dysuria and perineal pain believed to be of prostatic origin appears to have much in common with the 'urethral syndrome' in that only in a minority of patients can the symptoms be confidently ascribed to infection. *Escherichia coli* is usually responsible with enterococci the second most frequently isolated species. The possible role of chlamydia is discussed in Chapter 24.

Failure to eradicate prostatic organisms may result from the fact that the concentration of most agents active against Gram-negative organisms is considerably less in the prostate than it is in the plasma. To be concentrated in the acid secretion of the prostate, a drug must be basic and lipid-soluble (Stamey, 1972). Trimethoprim behaves in this way and co-trimoxazole has been successfully used in treatment, although the other component of the mixture, sulphamethoxazole, is not concentrated in the prostate and there has been some disagreement about the special efficacy of this treatment (Paulson & White, 1978).

INFECTION IN THE GROSSLY ABNORMAL URINARY TRACT

Urinary infections in patients with grossly impaired bladder emptying or with obstructive uropathy are frequently distinguished from those in patients with radiologically normal tracts in being caused by more than one bacterial species, often including resistant organisms such as *Pr. vulgaris*, Klebsiella, and particularly *Ps. aeruginosa*, or by resistant strains of otherwise sensitive species such as *E. coli*. By using selective media it is often possible to show, even when infection appears to be with only one organism, that other species are present in small numbers (Slade & Linton, 1965). These minor members of the bacterial population inevitably come to predominate if they are resistant to an agent effective in suppressing initially more numerous organisms. Better results of treatment are sometimes obtained if these minor species are isolated and an agent chosen for therapy which is active also against them or if suitable combined therapy is instituted.

In many such patients instrumentation in hospital for diagnostic or therapeutic purposes is unhappily responsible for the introduction of resistant organisms. The importance of avoiding such infections, which enormously increase the difficulty of managing these patients, is obvious.

Therapeutically, these patients present a series of difficulties which tend to compound one another. The abnormalities of their urinary tracts greatly impair both natural resolution and response to treatment. The resulting need for repeated therapy (plus instrumentation) facilitates the emergence of organisms sensitive only to a few agents, the more potent of which are toxic—the kidney itself being one of the organs affected. Impaired kidney function results both in poor concentrations of administered agents in the renal tract, and where dosage is not scrupulously regulated, to their accumulation in the blood with increased remote toxic effects and perhaps further impairment of renal excretion.

Because of the extreme resistance of some of the organisms and the need to monitor dosage, these patients cannot be managed without full bacteriological surveillance. As much as possible should be done to rectify anatomical and functional abnormalities. Patients with large residual volumes should be encouraged to empty their bladders at frequent and regular intervals, practising double or, if necessary, triple micturition. Systemic antibacterial therapy in such patients is seldom successful and should be avoided (particularly if the organisms prove to be sensitive only to toxic agents) unless there is evidence of systemic upset. Control may sometimes be established by washing out the bladder two or three times a day and instilling 50 ml of a 0.1 per cent solution of an appropriate antibiotic (for example polymyxin or neomycin) or antiseptic (for example chlorhexidine or noxytiolin) which is allowed to remain until the bladder refills. Once the urinary bacterial count has been substantially reduced, recurrent symptoms and even re-emergence of high counts of urinary bacteria can sometimes be prevented by long-term suppressive therapy.

In patients with renal calculi, short-term therapy even if intensive is seldom successful but a proportion of patients can be controlled by long-term suppressive therapy (O'Grady et al, 1973b). Eradication of infection is very unlikely unless the stones are removed. Once this has been achieved it is important to maintain the patient on long-term low dose prophylaxis in order to prevent re-accumulation of calculi.

INSTRUMENTAL INFECTION

Where there is obstructive uropathy or bladder emptying is expected or known to be impaired, for example in obstetric patients or in prostatic obstruction—especially where the natural male anatomical advantage is set aside by catheterization—the importance of avoiding infection is obvious. Short-term catheterization can be successfully 'covered' by giving the patient nitrofurantoin, or washing out the bladder with neomycin, plus polymyxin if pseudomonas infection is at large.

After prostatectomy many urologists still seem to take infection for granted, and minimize its importance. The patients themselves, overjoyed at having cleared the most dangerous hurdle in later male life, make light of discomfort and accept it as a natural consequence of what they have gone through. They would surely be better off if their urine could be kept sterile. Nitrofurantoin has been successfully used to prevent infection after transurethral resection of the prostate, for example, by Matthew et al (1978) but it should be noted that Berger & Nagar (1978) from a review of 31 studies found the topic of chemoprophylaxis in urology in some disarray and were impressed mostly by the little effect exerted by the lessons of the past 30 years. Over the long-term, with the use of indwelling catheters, the inevitable result of continuous medication—as with other forms of prolonged prophylaxis for endogenously acquired infections—is superinfection with resistant organisms and the one lesson which must not be forgotten is the importance of aspects of the management other than the use of antibacterial agents, particularly closed drainage.

References

Bailey R R 1970 NZ Med J 71: 216
Bailey R R, Abbott G D 1978 Canad Med Ass J 118: 551
Berger S A, Nagar H 1978 J Urol 120: 319
Bergström T 1972 Arch Dis Child 47: 227
Brumfitt W 1972 J Roy Coll Physcns Lond 6: 194
Brumfitt W, Faiers M C, Franklin I N S 1970 Postgrad Med J 46: (Suppl Oct), 65
Brumfitt W, Pursell R 1972 Brit Med J 2: 673
Buckley R M Jr, McGuckin M, MacGregor R R 1978 New Engl J Med 298: 321
Cattell W R, Charlton C A C, Fry I K, McSherry D A, O'Grady F 1973 In: Brumfitt W, Asscher A W (eds) Urinary tract infection. Oxford University Press, London, p 206
Charlton C A C, Crowther A, Davies J G, et al 1976 Brit Med J 1: 124
Cohen M 1976 Amer J Dis Child 130: 810
Fang L S T, Tolkoff-Rubin N E, Rubin R H 1978 New Engl J Med 298: 413
Freeman R B, Smith W McF, Richardson J A, et al 1975 Ann Intern Med 83: 133
Gillespie W A, Sellin M A, Gill P, et al 1978 J Clin Path 31: 348
Gleckman R 1977 J Urol 117: 757
Gower P E, Tasker P R W 1976 Brit Med J 1: 684
Harrison L H, Whitehurst A W, Boyce W H 1977 J Urol 118: 233
MacGregor M E, Freeman P 1975 Quart J Med 44: 481
Matthew A D, Gonzalez R, Jeffords D, Pinto M H 1978 J Urol 120: 442
Meares E M Jr, Stamey T A 1972 Brit J Urol 44: 175
O'Grady F, Charlton C A C, Fry I K, McSherry A, Cattell W R 1973; In: Brumfitt W, Asscher A W (eds) Urinary tract infection. Oxford University Pres, London, p 81
O'Grady F, Fry I K, McSherry A, Cattell W R 1973b J Infect Dis 28 Suppl: 652
Paulson D F, White R D 1978 J Urol 120: 184
Rees D L P, Wickham J E A, Whitfield H N 1978 Brit J Urol 50: 524
Rumans L W, Vosti K L 1978 Arch Intern Med 138: 1077
Shah K J, Robins D G, White R H R 1978 Arch Dis Child 53: 210
Shand D G, O'Grady F, Nimmon C C, Cattell W R 1970 Lancet 1: 1305
Slade N, Crowther S T 1972 Brit J Urol 44: 105
Slade N, Linton K B 1965 Brit J Urol 37: 73
Smellie J M 1970 Brit Med J 4: 97
Smellie J M, Katz G, Grüneberg R N 1978 Lancet 2: 175
Stamey T A 1972 Urinary infections, Williams & Wilkins, Baltimore
Stamey T A, Condy M, Mihara G 1977 New Engl J Med 296: 780
Vosti K L 1975 J Amer Med Ass 231: 934
Williams J D, Reeves D S, Brumfitt W, Condie A P 1973 In: Brumfitt W, Asscher A W (eds) Urinary tract infection. Oxford University Press, London, p 103
Williams J D, Smith E K 1970 Brit Med J 4: 651

22

Infections of the eye

The treatment of serious ocular infections is a highly specialised task, and a full account of it would be out of place in a work of this kind. The following is no more than an outline of the underlying principles and of the more important methods employed. Sabiston (1977), Baum (1978) and Furgiuele (1978) have reviewed the treatment of eye infections.

Superficial infections respond readily to various forms of local treatment, and few of them present any problems. Those involving the interior of the eye do present a special problem, that of penetration of the affected area by anti-bacterial drugs. Since adequate concentrations may only be obtainable there by the method of sub-conjunctival injection of a substantial dose in a small volume, the choice is limited by solubility and local tolerance.

Local applications

Superficial application may take the form of drops or ointment. The former may need very frequent application, and neglect of this is probably the commonest cause of failure. Alternatives are small capsules placed in the upper fornix which continuously release antibiotic or antibiotic-impregnated soft contact lenses. Ointments, which obscure vision, are convenient for application last thing at night. Newer types of base form a gel in the conjunctival sac and do not interfere with vision. Continuous irrigation of the cornea can be achieved by a scleral contact lens adapted for perfusion or by a conjunctival catheter. Among the sulphonamides, sulphacetamide, as 10 per cent drops or 2.5–6 per cent ointment, has been chiefly used for local application because of its high solubility: it is doubtful whether there is any purpose for which an antibiotic is not more effective. Penicillin is also used in the form of drops containing up to 10 000 units (6 mg) per ml. Despite the commonly expressed fear of allergic reactions, such local applications of penicillin are generally well tolerated.

In ointments the antibiotic can be incorporated in the base in solid form, which ensures stability, and a slow process of solution in the lachrymal secretion gives a persistent effect. Penicillin can be used in this way in almost any desired concentration, and an ointment containing 50 000 units (30 mg) per g even gives some penetration into the interior of the eye. Ointments containing streptomycin, neomycin, tetracyclines or chloramphenicol are usually made up to contain one per cent. Ointment containing 10 000 and 4 000 units of polymyxin and bacitracin respectively per g has been found satisfactory for a variety of purposes. Magnuson & Suie (1970) have confirmed their previous finding that gentamicin (0.3 per cent) ophthalmic drops and ointment are highly effective in the treatment of conjunctivitis, blepharitis or meibomianitis. In a double-blind, bacteriologically monitored comparison, Gordon (1970) found gentamicin at least as effective as a mixture of neomycin, bacitracin and polymyxin.

Intra-ocular concentrations after systemic administration

Systemic administration is seldom used in the treatment of intra-ocular infection but some anti-bacterial drugs diffuse into the aqueous humour in therapeutic concentrations after administration by the ordinary route: the levels attained in the vitreous are much lower and often undetectable (Table 22.1). This penetration has been studied extensively in both animals and man, employing a variety of doses including some very large ones. This and other variables discourage any too concise and quantitative expression of the results. With the uveal blood flow of about 0.2 ml per min it takes a week for the blood volume to perfuse the eye. Hence prolonged rather than transiently high blood levels are necessary if systemic treatment is to be used to control intraocular infection.

Sulphonamides

The concentration of sulphadimidine attained in the aqueous is about 30 per cent of that in the blood in the rat, and about 60 per cent in the rabbit, 30 minutes after the intravenous administration of a large dose. Experimentally, sulphonamides will control intra-ocular infections due to a fully sensitive organism such as *Str. pyogenes*. No other drugs penetrate with this facility.

Penicillin

Benzyl penicillin is useful, despite poor penetration, because of the large doses which can be given and its great intrinsic activity. An intramuscular dose of 1 000 000 units (0.6 g) produces a concentration in the aqueous of about 0.5 unit per ml.

Ampicillin

Unless the drug is given 4 to 6-hourly, or in very large doses, intra-ocular concentrations adequate for the treatment of any other than the most sensitive organisms are unlikely to be achieved.

Cephalosporins

In patients about to undergo cataract operations who were given 1 g cephalothin by rapid intravenous infusion, Records (1968) found concentrations in the aqueous of 0–2.5 μg/ml at 15 min and 0–1.0 μg/ml after 30 min, the corresponding serum levels being 22–100 and 10–14 μg/ml. Cephaloridine, given in the same way and in the same dose produced considerably higher levels between 1 and 2 hours which persisted to give 2.5–17 μg/ml after 8 hours (Records, 1969).

Fusidate

Williamson et al (1970) found aqueous levels around 1.2 μg/ml with serum levels of 52–72 μg/ml. After only two days' preoperative treatment, the aqueous and serum levels were 1.2 and 18–64 μg/ml, and after one day's treatment, 0.1–0.84 and 4–36 μg/ml. Fusidate was present in the vitreous of three patients whose eyes were enucleated; in two the levels were 2 to 3 times as high as those in the aqueous. In one patient, presumably as the result of prolonged inflammation, the vitreous level was 28.8 (aqueous 12.8) μg/ml and in another patient the vitreous level was still 0.32 (aqueous 0.1) μg/ml 4 days after the last dose.

The concentrations obtained by treatment of rabbits with various agents are shown in Table 22.1.

Table 22.1 Concentrations of various agents achieved in normal rabbits' eyes after systemic injection

Agent	Dose	Route	Interval after Last Dose	Concentration, μg per ml: Aqueous	Vitreous	Serum
Chloramphenicol	50 mg/kg	i/v	15 min	12	≤6	48
Erythromycin	6.5 mg/kg 8 hrly × 4	i/v	2½ hr	0.1	0	0.36
Tetracycline	20 mg/kg 12 hrly × 3	i/v	2½ hr	0.5	0	2–4
Kanamycin	50 mg/kg	i/v	1 hr	8–16	0	128–256
	50 mg/kg hrly × 2	i/m	15 min	1.6	0	26
Ampicillin	1 g 2 g	Oral	6 hr	0.96 1.6	0	—
	250 mg 8 hrly	Oral	1 hr	0.08	0	—
Methicillin	20 mg/kg 40 mg/kg	i/m	1 hr	0.8 0.2	0	—
Vancomycin	45 mg/kg 12 hrly × 3	i/v	2½ hr	1.5	0	23

Furgiuele F P 1964 Amer J Ophthal 58: 443
Green W R, Leopold I H 1965 Amer J Ophthal 60: 800
Kurose Y et al 1965 Arch Ophthal (Chicago) 73: 366

Sub-conjunctival injection

There are several ways of introducing anti-bacterial substances locally, apart from application to the lids or conjunctiva. Injection into the orbit gives poor penetration, and direct injections into the chambers of the eye are not often indicated. The method of choice is sub-conjunctival injection, a fine needle being inserted between the anaesthetized conjunctiva and the sclera usually below the cornea since the injections are often painful and the patient tends to roll the eyeball up. Up to 1 ml of solution can be injected. Trapped in this situation, the substance diffuses into the cornea and the chambers of the eye, where concentrations are attained far higher than any to be achieved by systemic administration, and maintained above the therapeutic minimum for as long as 48 hours. It should not be forgotten that antibiotics will be absorbed from this site and there is the possibility of remote toxic effects with such agents as neomycin—which can be given by this route in substantial doses—especially in patients with impaired renal function. The addition of adrenaline to the solution prolongs the effect.

Table 22.2 Dosage for infections in the eye

	Sub-conjunctival	Intra-vitreal
Benzyl penicillin	0.5–1 mega unit	1000–4000 units
Ampicillin	100 mg	—
Methicillin	100–150 mg	1–2 mg
Carbenicillin	100 mg	2 mg
Cephaloridine	100 mg	0.25 mg
Chloramphenicol	1 mg	1–2 mg
Tetracycline	2.5–5 mg	—
Erythromycin	2.5–5 mg	1–2 mg
Streptomycin	50 mg	—
Kanamycin	10–20 mg	—
Gentamicin	20–40 mg	0.5 mg
Tobramycin	20–40 mg	0.5 mg
Neomycin	100–500 mg	2.5 mg
Bacitracin	10 000 units	500–1000 units
Polymyxin	5–10 mg	0.1 mg
Vancomycin	15–25 mg	—

Based on Leopold I H 1964 Invest Ophthalmol 3: 504
Furgiuele F P 1978 Drugs, 15: 310

Doses recommended for sub-conjunctival and intra-ocular injection are given in Table 22.2. The intra-ocular concentrations of various agents achieved in the rabbit by the sub-conjunctival route are shown in Table 22.3.

Table 22.3 Concentrations of various agents achieved in normal rabbits' eyes after subconjunctival injection

			Concentration μg (or units) per ml	
Agent	Dose	Interval after Injection	Aqueous	Vitreous
Penicillin	50 000 units	1 hr	>32 units	17 units
Methicillin	20 mg	1 hr	13	0
	40 mg		20	
Streptomycin	10 mg	3 hr	8–20	—
Kanamycin	10 mg	1 hr	8	0–4
	20 mg		10	0
Neomycin	500 mg	4 hr	240	33
Colistin	250 000 units	1–3 hr	10–200 units	20–200 units
Sulphomethyl-polymyxin B	500 000 units	45–120 min	95–750 units	—

Sorsby A, Ungar J 1947 Brit J Ophthal 31: 517
Gadiner P A et al 1948 Brit J Ophthal 32: 449
Ainslie D, Smith C 1952 Brit J Ophthal 36: 352
Ainslie D 1965 Brit J Ophthal 49: 98
Green W R, Leopold I H 1965 Amer J Ophthal 60: 800

Treatment of superficial infection

The minutiae of the treatment of various conditions of the eyelids and conjunctiva and of the lachrymal system, which include measures other than the application of antibacterial agents, are outside the scope of this book. Apart from the fact that staphylococci, which are responsible for most infections involving the eyelids, may be resistant to penicillin or tetracyclines, the organisms concerned are sensitive to most of the antibiotics mentioned. Even the two Gram-negative species causing conjunctivitis, *Haemophilus aegyptius* and *Moraxella lacunata*, are sensitive to penicillin, as well as to other antibiotics more usually thought of in connection with Gram-negative infections.

Lid infections rarely require antibiotic treatment. Simple measures such as removal of lash or encrusted exudate, and expression of pus from a blocked tear duct, are essential to success and may be the only therapy necessary. The possibility that continuing or recrudescent inflammation is a reaction to locally applied antibacterial agent must be considered. Troublesome conjunctivitis not responsive to antibiotics may be allergic or viral in origin or associated with lachrymal duct obstruction or infection. Wilson et al (1975) warn that mascara and its applicators can become contaminated during use and may be responsible for the maintenance of staphylococcal blepharitis. Chronic blepharitis involving the meibomian glands may be a disorder similar to acne and respond to prolonged tetracycline treatment (Sabiston, 1977).

Gonococcal ophthalmia Treatment of this condition is discussed in Chapter 24.

Infected corneal ulcer The commonest organism isolated from traumatic corneal ulcer is *Staph. aureus*, but infections with enterobacteria and Pseudomonas, as in other situations, are becoming more prevalent. Baum (1978) recommends the use of topical and sub-conjunctival cefazolin plus gentamicin. Various regimes have been used (Furgiuele, 1978) and probably gentamicin alone would suffice.

Pseudomonas ophthalmia

This dangerous condition has received publicity through outbreaks traced to contamination of solutions used for ophthalmic medication. The danger of contamination of eye medicaments and the importance of avoiding multidose containers for this reason has several times been emphasized.

Colistin sulphate by irrigation (1 mg per ml) or by continuous lavage (0.5 mg per ml) or gentamicin given both topically and by daily sub-conjunctival injection (Table 22.1) are effective. Treatment is continued for 7–10 days.

Fungus infections of the eye

In recent years there has been considerable interest in these infections and in the role of broad-spectrum antibiotics and corticosteroids in encouraging their emergence. A great variety of fungi have been identified (sometimes only on morphological grounds) in mycotic keratitis and endophthalmitis. They include both organisms normally regarded as saprophytic, such as Cephalosporium and Mucor, and some which are conceded more general pathogenic roles such as Sporotrichum, Aspergillus and Candida. It appears to be the consensus of opinion on both experimental and clinical grounds that broad spectrum antibiotics do not predispose to fungus infections of the eye but corticosteroids do, and numerous warnings have been issued against the indiscriminate use of corticosteroids in the eye. Fungus infection should be suspected wherever purulent corneal ulceration cannot be explained by bacterial infection. Most authors believe that any applications of corticosteroid must be stopped (even though this may result in initial apparent deterioration), but that antibiotics should be continued in order to limit, as far as possible, secondary bacterial invasion. Candida ophthalmitis has been seen as a complication of candidaemia arising from infected intravenous infusion sites.

Until recently, the only agents of proven value in keratitis were the polyenes (page 238). Nystatin is irritating but reasonably safe as ointment (100 000 units per g). Amphotericin is more effective and can be given as drops containing up to 3 mg per ml of the colloidal suspension for injection, in distilled water (not saline) which can be supplemented by subconjunctival injections of 125 μg. Local treatment with amphotericin B is unpleasant and irritating, has often to be supplemented with debridement and must be continued for months. Newmark et al (1970) obtained good visual results in seven patients suffering from Cephalosporium or Fusarium keratitis treated with pimaricin. At hourly intervals, they instilled alternately a 5 per cent suspension of pimaricin and 1 per cent potassium iodide drops. They originally used potassium iodide in the belief that it exterted an antifungal effect but suggest that the benefit is due to the potassium which helps to maintain the physiological state of the cornea and reduce the chance of intra-ocular sequelae. Treatment was continued for two to four weeks. The pimaricin suspension was non-irritant and sufficiently viscous to remain in the cul-de-sac for long periods.

The results of treatment of fungal endophthalmitis with polyenes are very unsatisfactory. There is little intra-ocular penetration of nystatin or amphotericin from subconjunctival injection, and intra-ocular injections are not well tolerated so that the final visual result even if the fungus is eliminated is likely to be poor.

Intra-ocular levels of amphotericin are obtained by systemic therapy, but the dangers of this (page 241) are such that the treatment should only be undertaken in proven cases of fungal infection. Intra-ocular injections of amphotericin are exceedingly irritating but doses of 35–40 μg in 0.05 ml distilled water are tolerated. Injections of 200 units nystatin directly into the aqueous or vitreous are tolerated, but produce inhibitory levels (6–12 μg per ml) for only 24 hours. Larger or repeated injections cause vitreous degeneration. Encouraging results have been obtained by combined topical and oral treatment with flucytosine (150 to 200 mg/kg).

Trachoma

Inclusion conjunctivitis, inclusion blenorrhoea and trachoma are caused by the TRIC agent which belongs to the group of *Chlamydia* (page 428). It has also been suggested that in the trachoma-infected eye, commensal bacteria may function as opportunist pathogens and partly determine the severity of the lesions. In keeping with the sensitivity of the causal organism and the possible role of bacterial super-infection, trachoma has been shown to respond either to prolonged systemic sulphonamide treatment or to the local application of ointment containing tetracycline. There has been considerable disagreement about the efficacy of this treatment, particularly in the long term—partly, no doubt, because of reinfection—but Tarizzo (1972) warns that 'a hypercritical approach may hinder positive action'. He believes that currently available treatment, while not wholly effective, can do much to control the disease. Schachter (1978), in his extensive review of chlamydial infections concedes that the ideal drug for treatment of trachoma has not yet been developed. Hope that rifampicin might prove to be that drug has faded somewhat with the demonstration of the ease with which resistance developed. Inclusion conjunctivitis responds well to tetracycline ointment 4–6 times daily for three weeks.

Herpes simplex keratitis

Treatment of this condition, which resolves spontaneously in about 10 per cent of patients, is discussed on page 441.

Acute orbital cellulitis

Watters et al (1976) reviewed the predisposing conditions, clinical diagnosis, course and complications of acute orbital cellulitis, an uncommon and potentially lethal disease which usually occurs in children and young adults. They found bacteriaemia in a third of their patients who were not receiving antibiotics at the time of admission and in nearly half of those aged less than two years. About 80 per cent of the patients yielded *Haemophilus influenzae* type B and the rest pneumococci. Conjunctival or nasopharyngeal cultures were of some help in non-bacteriaemic patients but because of the common presence of potential pathogens can be misleading. They successfully treated their patients with ampicillin in doses approaching those used in meningitis but the comments and warnings related to the use of that agent for the treatment of severe haemophilus infections on page 328 should be borne in mind.

Post-operative endophthalmitis

Pre-operative prophylaxis

Opinions differ on the advisability of performing cultures before such operations as cataract extraction when there is no sign of infection. Even when secretion is obtained, as it should be, with a loop from the depths of the lower conjunctival sac, a few *Staph. albus* from the lid may be cultivated, and *C. xerosis* is a normal inhabitant. Okumoto and Smolin (1974) report that pneumococci are the second commonest organism after *Staphylococcus aureus* recovered from the eye and Okumoto et al (1976) confirmed previous observations that Proteus species (85 per cent *Proteus mirabilis*) can be recovered from 2–3 per cent of uninflamed eyes. If a pathogenic organism such as *Staph. aureus* is found, pre-operative treatment with antibiotic drops is indicated and Allen & Mangiaracine (1974) conclude from a very large series in which the post-operative infection rate over the last 15 000 patients was 0.02 per cent, that pre-operative antibiotic prophylaxis with chloramphenicol (0.4 per cent) plus polymyxin (0.1 per cent) eye drops and erythromycin ointment (0.5 per cent) at night contributed materially to this success. They do not recommend routine pre-operative culture except in patients suspected of having local infection or a generalized condition predisposing to infection.

Post-operative prophylaxis

The majority view appears to be against routine antibiotic administration, whether systemic or subconjunctival, after clean operations but the evidence is equivocal. Some studies evidently show benefit but others indicate that such prophylaxis delays the recognition of infection with poorer ultimate visual results. The position is different after removal of an intra-ocular foreign body: the infection which may follow this is usually staphylococcal, and subconjunctival neomycin or cephaloridine is indicated.

Treatment of established infection

Bacterial endophthalmitis after clean surgery is an unusual and serious complication occurring in most series in about 0.1 to 0.3 per cent of cases. The results of treatment are poor with loss of useful vision in 70–80 per cent of affected patients. The principal organisms are now *Staph. aureus* and *Pseudomonas aeruginosa* followed by Klebsiella, Proteus and Escherichia. The classical causes of eye infection, pneumococci and streptococci, appear now to be of much less importance. A bacteriological diagnosis is urgent in such a case. Conjunctival swabs can be misleading by yielding organisms other than those responsible for intra-ocular infection and several pleas have been made for early anterior chamber or vitreous aspiration. Gram-stained smears of this material may offer the most valuable guide to therapy since even where organisms are seen they may prove impossible to cultivate; but Forster (1974) found the results in his series equivocal.

Table 22.4 Minimum inhibitory concentrations (μg/ml) of antibiotics administrable by subconjunctival injection for bacterial species causing ocular infections

	Penicillin	Gentamicin	Neomycin	Polymyxin
Staph. aureus	0.03–R	0.12–1	1	R
Str. pyogenes	0.015	16	R	R
Str. pneumoniae	0.015	16–32	128	R
Ps. aeruginosa	R	1–8	50	0.12
Proteus spp.	5–R	1–8	5–50	R
Klebsiella spp.	R	0.5–4	2	0.25
Escherichia	R	1–4	8	0.25

The choice of an antibiotic for subconjunctival injection must take account of the properties of the four principal antibiotics available as stated in Table 22.4. Penicillin is clearly indicated for pneumococcal and streptococcal infection, but staphylococci responsible for hospital-acquired infection are almost certain to be resistant. Polymyxin is active, and to a high degree, against *Ps. aeruginosa*, Klebsiella, and Escherichia; but not against Proteus or the Gram-positive cocci. Neomycin and gentamicin on the other hand, have satisfactory activity against all these problem organisms: staphylococci, whether penicillin-resistant or not, and both *Ps. aeruginosa* and Proteus.

Kanski (1970) successfully treated 13 out of 20 patients with subconjuctival injections of a mixture of gentamicin, framycetin and methicillin. Intravenous, intramuscular and subconjunctival injections fail to maintain minimum effective levels in the vitreous (Table 22.3) and intravitreal injections are required. Recommended doses are given in Table 22.2.

References

Allen H F, Mangiaracine A B 1974 Arch Ophthalmol 91: 3
Baum J L 1978 New Engl J Med 299: 28
Forster R K 1974 Arch Ophthalmol 92: 387
Furgiuele F P 1978 Drugs 15: 310
Gordon D M 1970 Amer J Ophthalmol 62: 300
Kanski J J 1970 Brit J Ophthalmol 54: 316
Magnuson R, Suie T 1970 Amer J Ophthalmol 70: 734
Newmark E, Ellison A C, Kaufman H E 1970 Amer J Ophthalmol 69: 458
Okumoto M, Smolin G 1974 Amer J Ophthalmol 77: 346
Okumoto M, Smolin G, Belfort R, Kim H B, Siverio C E 1976 Amer J Ophthalmol 81: 495
Records R E 1968 Amer J Ophthalmol 66: 441
Records R E 1969 Arch Ophthalmol (NY) 81: 331
Sabiston D W 1977 Drugs 14: 207
Schachter J 1978 New Engl J Med 298: 540
Tarizzo M L 1972 WHO Chronicle 26: 99
Watters E C, Wallar H, Hiles D A, Michaels R H 1976 Arch Ophthalmol 94: 785
Williamson J, Russell F, Doig W M, Paterson R W W 1970 Brit J Ophthalmol 54: 126
Wilson L A, Julian A J, Ahearn D G 1975 Amer J Ophthalmol 79: 596

23

Tuberculosis and leprosy

TUBERCULOSIS

Chemotherapy has radically transformed the outlook in this disease. A mortality rate which had been falling by only 3 per cent per annum from 1900 to 1948, fell thereafter by 15 per cent per annum and this reduction was even steeper in the lower age groups. The significance of the year 1948 is that it marks the general introduction of streptomycin for treating the disease: since then many other antibiotics and synthetic drugs have followed, the introduction of isoniazid in 1952 being of particular importance.

During the 1970s methods of chemotherapy have again greatly changed with the introduction of rifampicin and the development of regimens of intermittent and short course chemotherapy. Tuberculosis remains, nevertheless, a common disease in all countries. Eight thousand notifications were recorded in England and Wales in 1974 (Fig. 23.1) with wide regional variations between 6 per 100 000 in East Anglia to 27 per 100 000 in the North West Thames Region, with its large population of Asian immigrants.

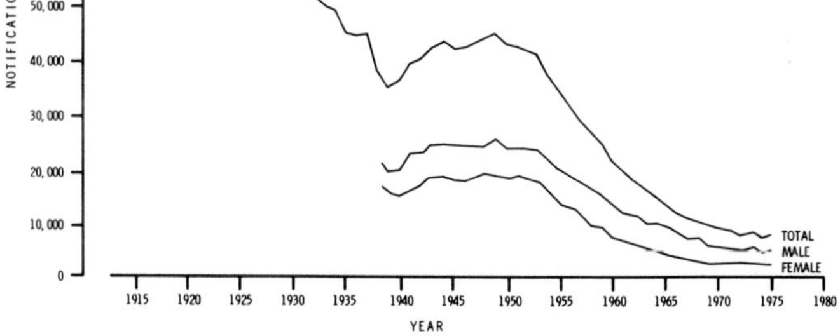

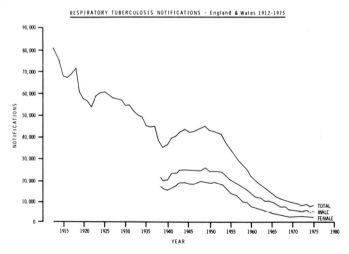

Fig. 23.1 Respiratory tuberculosis notifications—England and Wales 1912–1975. Reproduced from: On the state of the public health 1976, with kind permission of HM Stationery Office and the Chief Medical Officer of the DHSS

In this chapter the properties of antituberculous drugs are described, followed by an account of the main methods of treatment.

Streptomycin is discussed on page 118, kanamycin on page 130, and the use of rifampicin in conditions other than tuberculosis on page 229. The structures of some important antituberculous drugs are given in Figure 23.2.

Para-aminosalicylic acid (PAS)

The antituberculous activity of PAS was discovered in Sweden in 1946 in the course of a systematic study of analogues of salicylic acid and benzoic acid. The activity of PAS is highly specific to *M. tuberculosis*, against which it is active at a concentration of about 1 μg/ml. Its *in vivo* activity is bacteristatic and not very great, and PAS had its main rôle in preventing the development of resistance to the major compounds given at the same time. It is well absorbed from the gastro-intestinal tract, but large daily doses, 10–12 g, have to be given.

PAS is well distributed through the tissues except the CSF, has a serum half life of about one hour, and is eliminated mainly in the urine, as the acetyl derivative, the compound itself and as several other minor metabolites.

Side effects

Gastric discomfort and nausea, with or without diarrhoea, occur in nearly all patients treated with large doses of the drug. These effects often subside in the first weeks of treatment, but an appreciable proportion of patients are unable or unwilling to continue taking PAS (Stradling & Poole, 1970). Many preparations have now been evolved with the aim of reducing gastro-intestinal side-effects and, by combining PAS with isoniazid, ensuring that the patient receives either appropriate combined chemotherapy or none at all.

Allergic reactions in the form of rashes with or without fever are unfortunately common and may be severe. Other reactions such as hepatitis, a syndrome resembling infectious mononucleosis, and rarely an encephalitis-like syndrome may occur. These reactions are usually dealt with by replacing PAS with another drug, but desenitization can be achieved, at least after the milder reactions. An initial dose of 0.5 g is given, and this increased by 0.5 g daily. Severe reactions are treated by corticosteroids.

PAS causes slight interference in the metabolism of iodine in the thyroid gland and after six months or more of treatment some patients may develop a goitre and occasionally signs of myxoedema. These symptoms can be relieved by giving thyroxine, without stopping PAS.

Isoniazid

Isoniazid or 1-isonicotinyl hydrazide was synthesized as long ago as 1912 but its antituberculous properties were first announced in the American press in February 1952. Its activity against *Myco. tuberculosis in vitro*, in experimental infection in laboratory animals and in human infection was soon established, and in 1952, the Medical Research Council launched a large controlled clinical trial, which established the value of isoniazid in the treatment of tuberculosis (Report, 1952).

Isoniazid has an active bactericidal action on *Myco. tuberculosis* and inhibits the growth of most pre-treatment strains in a concentration as low as 0.2 μg/ml. It has the advantage over streptomycin that it is readily absorbed from the intestinal tract, diffuses well into the body tissues and fluids, including the cerebro-spinal fluid, and penetrates into macrophages, so that it is effective against intracellular tubercle bacilli. It is effective clinically in small doses (e.g. 200–300 mg daily) and with this dosage toxicity is very low. It has the disadvantage that tubercle bacilli very readily develop resistance to it.

Metabolism

Human populations show genetically determined differences in the speed with which isoniazid is inactivated by acetylation. Rapid inactivators achieve plasma concentrations of <0.2 μg/ml six hours after an oral dose of 4 mg/kg, whereas in slow inactivators the concentration is >0.8 μg/ml at this interval after ingestion. Rapid acetylators have the dominant genotype, in homozygous or heterozygous form, while the slow acetylators are homozygous recessives. Concentration of free isoniazid in the plasma is a little higher if the patient is also receiving PAS, which is also acetylated. Isoniazid inactivator status has an important effect on the results of intermittent chemotherapy for tuberculosis (page 402).

Isoniazid is excreted in the urine in three forms, free drug, its acetyl derivative and hydrazones. The proportion in the latter form is constant: that in the free form is higher in slow inactivators, and that in the form of acetyl isoniazid is higher in rapid inactivators. Isoniazid levels are little affected in renal failure (see Ch. 26).

Adverse reactions

Toxic effects are unusual on the standard dosage of 200–300 mg but are significantly more frequent among slow inactivators when larger doses are used when the most common side-effects are restlessness, insomnia, muscle twitching and difficulty in starting micturition. More serious effects are peripheral neuritis and psychotic upsets. The incidence of toxic symptoms is reduced by the simultaneous administration of pyridoxine.

Hypersensitivity reactions to isoniazid, although uncommon, are well recognized, with fever, rashes and sometimes abnormalities in the blood such as eosinophilia. Various forms of joint pain and swelling, especially 'frozen shoulder', have been ascribed to isoniazid.

Liver damage was reported early but considered a rare complication of isoniazid until schemes of widespread chemoprophylaxis provoked a re-examination of the problem. Maddrey & Boitnott (1973) described 14 patients with isoniazid hepatitis, of whom three died of fulminant hepatic failure. The biopsies of eight of the 11 survivors showed bridging or multilobular necrosis or both, and some relapsed when isoniazid was again administered. The severity of this complication of treatment is also shown in a series of 114 patients with isoniazid hepatitis, of whom 13 died (Black et al, 1975). Liver damage is mainly hepatocellular and is best detected by warning the patient of the characteristic prodromal symptoms of hepatitis, rather than by serial liver function tests, since liver enzymes may often be raised in patients receiving isoniazid who do not develop hepatitis.

The risk of isoniazid hepatitis, estimated overall at 5.2 per 1000 patients treated for one year, rises with age, and the benefits of chemoprophylaxis for patients over 35 are probably outweighed by the risk of hepatitis. Girling (1978) in an extensive survey of hepatic toxicity of various antituberculous regimens, concluded that the incidence of hepatitis during standard chemotherapy containing isoniazid is about 2 per cent and, that, contrary to current belief, the risk is not increased in rapid acetylators, nor when rifampicin is used in combination with isoniazid.

Rifampicin

Earlier derivatives of rifamycin had little success in the treatment of tuberculosis, but rifampicin (see also page 229) represents an enormous advance on them in two directions. It can be administered orally, attaining high and well sustained blood levels, and it has greatly enhanced antibacterial activity. Apparent activity against *Myco. tuberculosis* varies with the medium used, but in a Tween-albumin medium the mean MIC is only about 0.02 μg/ml. As with all rifamycin derivatives, bacterial populations contain a minute proportion of resistant cells which grow out unless this is prevented by the presence of another active drug.

Numerous experimental studies in mice show the efficacy of rifampicin alone, and in various combinations with other drugs, in sterilizing organs of mice infected with *M. tuberculosis*, (Batten, 1970; Grumbach et al, 1969), and these studies, reviewed by Grosset (1978) form one of the bases of the clinical use of rifampicin in tuberculosis, discussed later in this chapter. Widespread use is still limited by the high cost of the drug. Rifampicin is active against *M. kansasii* and *M. marinum*.

Rifampicin is fully absorbed from the gastro-intestinal tract, absorption being diminished by simultaneous administration of PAS. Meals also delay absorption slightly (Siegler et al, 1974) with peak serum levels of 8.8 μg/ml two hours after a 600 mg dose in the fasting state, and 6.6 μg, usually at four hours when given post-prandially. The length of time for which effective antimycobacterial serum levels are maintained is little affected by this phenomenon, and patients who prefer to take the drug with or after meals may do so.

After absorption, rifampicin undergoes an enterohepatic circulation, the deacetylated form being excreted in the bile. The drug is well distributed through body tissues including the CSF, and is excreted in both bile and urine. Patients should be warned of the orange colour imparted to urine and secretions during rifampicin therapy. Its biological half-life varies between one and a half and five hours, and is prolonged in patients with liver disease. Hepatic uptake of rifampicin in rats and in man is depressed by administration of probenecid, and the serum levels are about doubled (Kenwright & Levi, 1973).

Adverse reactions

Rifampicin-containing antituberculous regimens are of generally low toxicity, although a large number of unwanted effects have been associated with its use. In an extensive review, Girling (1977) classifies adverse reactions into those associated with daily or intermittent administration, and those found only with intermittent therapy.

The former group includes skin reactions, mostly flushing with or without rash, often transient even when therapy is continued, and most common in the early weeks of treatment, gastro-intestinal disturbances, which are usually mild, and disturbance of hepatic function. Transient abnormalities of liver function, especially a rise in serum transaminases and less commonly a raised bilirubin level, are common during rifampicin treatment, and clinical hepatitis, usually of mild degree also occurs (Scheuer et al, 1974). The large number of patients involved in clinical trials of rifampicin-containing regimens has enabled the clinical significance of rifampicin hepatitis to be fully assessed. Whereas hepatitis was commonly recorded in some earlier studies, the incidence in short course regimens appears to be low, e.g. eight of 802 patients in the trials conducted by the British Thoracic and Tuberculosis Association (Report 1975a). Earlier suggestions that hepatic damage was more common in rapid acetylators, and when given in combination with isoniazid, are not borne out by more recent studies (Girling, 1978).

Thrombocytopenia, associated with complement fixing serum antibody, is an uncommon adverse reaction. The platelet count falls within a few hours, returning to normal within a day or two. Rifampicin administration should at once be discontinued. Thrombocytopenia is more common with intermittent schemes (Poole et al, 1971) but is also encountered in patients receiving daily treatment.

Other adverse effects of rifampicin are confined to patients receiving intermittent therapy. The most important is the 'flu' syndrome, with fever, chills and malaise usually developing after three to six months' treatment. Its incidence is less with frequent than infrequent dosage, less with lower than higher doses, and less when intermittent therapy is preceded by an initial phase of daily treatment. It is not, however, prevented by a daily supplement of 25 mg in an intermittent regimen (Report 1975b). Circulating IgM antibodies to rifampicin are formed in the serum, and the 'flu' syndrome may be caused by complement activation mediated by them.

Other rare syndromes associated with intermittent administration of rifampicin are acute renal failure, sometimes associated with acute haemolysis. Intermittent therapy preceding these complications may result from irregular drug taking or even self-prescribing rather than from an intentionally intermittent regimen (Flynn et al, 1974). Shortness of breath, wheezing and fall of blood pressure have occasionally been recorded.

In addition to these unwanted effects, certain drug interactions involving rifampicin are of some importance. The drug is a potent inducer of hepatic microsomal enzymes and this effect leads to more rapid elimination of some agents metabolized in the liver. The most important are warfarin, the anticoagulant effect of which is thereby diminished and oral contraceptives, with possible breakthrough bleeding and unwanted pregnancy (Bolt et al, 1974). Adjustments to steroid dose in patients with Addison's disease may also become necessary (Edwards et al, 1974).

Finally, a considerable body of evidence, summarised by Sanders (1976) has accumulated to show that rifampicin has immunosuppressive properties demonstrable in a number of experimental systems, but no ill effects in man resulting from these properties have yet been established.

Rifampicin must always be used in combination with one or more other drugs to which the patient's organisms are susceptible since resistant strains emerge rapidly if it is used alone.

Ethambutol

This compound inhibits the growth of human and bovine strains of *Myco. tuberculosis* in a concentration of 1–5 μg/ml and is effective in the treatment of experimental infection in mice and guinea-pigs (Thomas et al, 1961; Karlson, 1961a and b).

About 80 per cent of the dose is absorbed after oral administration, a dose of 25 mg per kg body weight giving peak serum concentrations of about 5 μg per ml at two hours. The half life in man is long, about eight hours, and the drug is mainly excreted in the urine, partly as unchanged compound and partly as an aldehyde and a dicarboxylic acid derivative. A small amount is lost in the faeces.

The use of ethambutol has until recently been restricted because it can cause impairment of vision, due to a retrobulbar neuritis, of which the first signs are blurred vision and inability to distinguish colours. Recovery from this is usual and it can be prevented by regulating the dose: 25 mg per kg for 60 days should then be reduced to 15 mg. This scheme of dosage has now become widely accepted and ocular toxicity is now rare. For example, only one of 72 patients treated with this dose by Lees et al (1971) developed optic neuritis. Routine tests of colour vision and of the visual fields should precede treatment and patients should be warned to stop treatment if they have visual symptoms. Routine eye tests are not, however, useful in anticipating toxic effects (Citron, 1969).

Thiacetazone

Thiosemicarbazones were used for the treatment of tuberculosis in Germany as long ago as 1946. The most active was 4-acetylaminobenzaldehyde thiosemicarbazone which was given the name thiacetazone; *in vitro* and in experimental infection in laboratory animals, thiacetazone in large doses appears to have an activity greater than that of PAS and similar or slightly inferior to that of streptomycin.

Earlier pharmacokinetic and bacteriological studies were greatly amplified by a thorough study, using newer analytical methods, by Ellard et al (1974). The peak serum concentration after the standard 150 mg oral dose averaged from 1.2 to 2.3 μg/ml in different groups and rose proportionately in the dose range 150 to 600 mg. Urinary excretion averaged 20 per cent of the dose administered. Strains from Kenya were considerably more susceptible than strains from Hong Kong, a concentration of 0.4 μg per mg completely preventing multiplication of the former and partially inhibiting 77 per cent of the latter.

Thiacetazone is a reliable companion drug, and excellent results have been reported from its use with isoniazid, especially when treatment is initiated with a phase of additional daily streptomycin (Report 1970). Its value is somewhat limited by adverse reactions, especially by rashes: other side-effects include nausea, vomiting and dizziness. An international investigation showed that 16.1 and 17.6 per cent of patients on two thiacetazone-containing regimens developed rashes compared with 7.7 per cent of patients receiving streptomycin and isoniazid (Ferguson et al, 1971). The incidence of rashes varies greatly in different areas. In E. Africa adverse effects are uncommon. In Chinese patients in Hong Kong, and in all the three racial groups in Singapore, the incidence of rashes is unacceptably high, and daily thiacetazone-containing regimens cannot be generally used (Report 1971b). Intermittent doses ranging from 150 to 600 mg twice weekly gave a lower incidence of side-effects, 2.3 per cent (Fox et al, 1974).

Ethionamide

This compound, like isoniazid, is a derivative of isonicotinic acid. In spite of the structural similarity between isoniazid and ethionamide, tubercle bacilli do not show cross-resistance and ethionamide is fully active against isoniazid-resistant tubercle bacilli with an average MIC of about 2.5 μg per ml. The activity of ethionamide *in vitro* and in experimental infection is about twice that of streptomycin but inferior to that of isoniazid. Like streptomycin and isoniazid the action of ethionamide on tubercle bacilli is bactericidal (Rist et al, 1959). As with isoniazid, ethionamide-resistant tubercle bacilli emerge rapidly, and there is cross-resistance between thioacetazone and ethionamide (Rist et al, 1959).

Ethionamide is well distributed in body tissues, including the CSF. Excretion is largely in the form of various metabolites, especially dihydropyridines.

The full dose, a total of 1 g daily, is liable to cause nausea and anorexia, and may on that account have to be somewhat reduced: neurotoxic effects may also occur (Brouet et al, 1959). Prothionamide is somewhat less likely to provoke severe gastro-intestinal symptoms, at least in males, and may therefore be preferred to ethionamide, with which there is complete cross-resistance.

Pyrazinamide

Following the discovery of the anti-tuberculous activity of nicotinamide a number of nicotinic acid derivatives were synthesized, of which pyrazinamide was the most active.

The activity against *M. tuberculosis* is highly pH-dependent. Pyrazinamide is almost inactive at neutral pH, with an MIC of 15–20 μg per ml at pH 5.5. Serum concentrations achieved at different times with three different regimens are given in a study by Ellard (1969). A serum concentration of 25 μg/ml is necessary to achieve maximal therapeutic effect.

In experimental animals, the combination of pyrazinamide and isoniazid is highly effective in killing tubercle bacilli (McCune et al, 1966). Although early trials in human tuberculosis carried out in the 1950s also gave promising results, a high incidence of hepatitis was reported in several studies and for this reason use of the drug was abandoned except in re-treatment therapy of drug-resistant disease. It was later recognized that hepatic toxicity varied greatly in different studies and was dose-related. In earlier studies dosage was often 3 g daily, whereas with doses of the order of 1.5 g daily evidence of hepatic damage was uncommon. A low incidence of disturbance of liver function, mostly symptomless, has also been established with intermittent pyrazinamide-containing regimens, 6–8 per cent with 1.5 or 2.0 g daily, 9 per cent with 2.0 or 2.5 g three times weekly, and 6 per cent with 3.0 or 3.5 g twice weekly (Report 1976e).

The hepatic toxicity of regimens containing isoniazid, rifampicin and pyrazinamide is fully reviewed by Girling (1978).

Pyrazinamide is now established as an important component of many successful short-course regimens, and its rôle in therapy is considered later in the chapter.

Capreomycin

Capreomycin is a peptide derived from *Streptomyces capreolus* and is available as the sulphate. It has little action on species other than mycobacteria. Streptomycin-resistant tubercle bacilli are sensitive to it, but there is some cross-resistance with viomycin and kanamycin. Intramuscular injection of 1 g gives peak serum concentrations of 20–35 μg per ml, and half the dose is excreted unchanged in the urine. Hesling (1969) described adverse reactions in 34 patients treated with 1 g daily, 14 of whom completed two years' treatment. The drug was stopped because of renal damage in eight patients, because of hearing loss in three, and because of an allergic reaction in one. Its use in drug-resistant tuberculosis is described by Donomae (1968).

Viomycin

This is another antibiotic isolated from a species of Streptomyces and similar in many ways to streptomycin, both in its anti-bacterial activity and its pharmacokinetics. It also has to be given by intramuscular injection. Unfortunately, its anti-bacterial activity is lower than that of streptomycin and its toxicity is higher. With daily treatment for long periods giddiness, deafness and renal damage are frequent, but the incidence of side-effects is greatly reduced by giving the drug on only two days of the week, and 1 g twice a day on each of the two days is the usually recommended dose. There is cross-resistance between viomycin and both streptomycin and kanamycin, but once again it is usually one-way, so that strains which have become resistant to streptomycin and kanamycin are often still sensitive to viomycin, but viomycin-resistant strains are usually resistant to both the other two.

Cycloserine

This is a broad spectrum antibiotic, sometimes used for other purposes (see Chapter 10). It has a relatively weak action on the tubercle bacillus *in vitro*, but is effective *in vivo*; resistance to it develops only slowly and its inclusion in combinations deters the development of resistance to other drugs. The usual dose is 0.25 g twice daily, and toxicity is reduced if the serum concentration is less than 30 μg per ml. Confusion, excitability, hallucinations and depression have all been reported, and treatment should be stopped promptly if any mental or neurological signs develop.

ANTITUBERCULOUS TREATMENT

During the 1950s a number of regimens of antituberculous treatment were established as effective by extensive clinical trials. The essential features were the need to employ more than one drug in order to prevent the emergence of bacterial drug resistance, and to continue treatment for a long period in order to reduce to a low level the incidence of relapse after chemotherapy had been terminated. In the U.K. the most commonly used scheme was to begin treatment with streptomycin, isoniazid and PAS, and provided sensitivity tests on the original isolates showed fully sensitive bacilli, treatment was then continued with isoniazid and PAS alone. In practice this meant that most patients received three drugs for two or three months, but the initial intensive phase was often longer for patients with extensive disease. It was essential to continue treatment for at least 18 months, and for two years in those with extensive disease, since relapse rates were high with shorter courses.

Although 'standard' chemotherapy of this sort was shown to achieve near 100 per cent success rates when operated by enthusiastic and efficient chest clinic staff, results were often far from ideal under conditions which normally prevail during treatment both in wealthy and in developing countries. The last decade has seen great changes in methods of antituberculous chemotherapy, made possible by the introduction of rifampicin, the re-introduction of pyrazinamide and a powerful combination of experimental studies and extensive new clinical trials (see reviews by Fox & Mitchison, 1975; Fox, 1977) (Table 23.1). The major changes can be

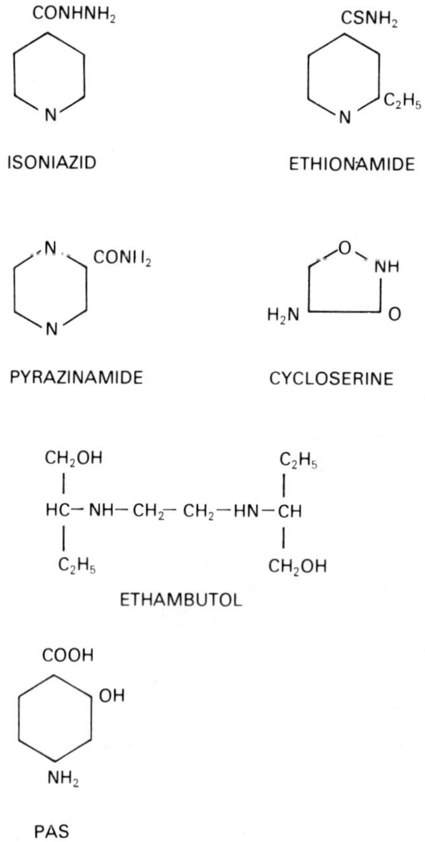

Fig. 23.2 Structures of some important anti-tuberculous drugs.

summarized as the introduction of new regimens of intermittent chemotherapy, short course chemotherapy and combinations of the two methods, the virtual abandonment of sanatorium treatment and of surgery in the treatment of tuberculosis, the shorter length of follow-up now thought necessary after completion of chemotherapy, and more rational use of radiography and sputum examinations in assessing the results of treatment. In parallel with these major developments, the last few years have seen a tendency to abandon the use of PAS in favour of ethambutol or, in developing countries where cost of chemotherapy is especially important, thiacetazone.

Resistance to standard drugs

Primary drug resistance (i.e. resistance in newly diagnosed patients who have had no treatment) has remained uncommon in advanced countries. Most surveys naturally relate to the three drugs first introduced, and successive studies in Britain have shown resistance to streptomycin, isoniazid or PAS in about 5 per cent of strains. The proportion of resistant strains is much higher in Africa and the Far East and countries with mixed populations occupy an intermediate position. A co-operative study by the

U.S. Public Health Service (Kopanoff et al, 1978) recorded the antibiotic sensitivity of 3146 cultures examined in 1975–7. The incidence of primary resistance varied from 3.4–18.7 per cent (average 8.6 per cent) in different areas, and was higher in patients of Hispanic (15.0 per cent) or Asian (20.7 per cent) origin. The resistance rates for different drugs were streptomycin 5.1 per cent, isoniazid 4.4 per cent, PAS 1.3 per cent, rifampicin 0.3 per cent and ethambutol 0.7 per cent. Of cultures yielding resistant strains, 67 per cent showed single drug resistance, 17 per cent were resistant to two drugs and 14 per cent to three.

INTERMITTENT CHEMOTHERAPY

A number of schemes of intermittent chemotherapy have now been tried and shown to be at least as good, and sometimes better, than standard chemotherapy. These methods, which are of great theoretical interest, have important practical advantages because they can be closely supervised and because, in some cases, the incidence of adverse drug reactions is less than that encountered with daily chemotherapy. The first step towards intermittent chemotherapy followed an investigation in Madras (Gangadharam et al, 1961) which showed that a dose of 400 mg of isoniazid administered once a day (as part of a standard scheme of combined treatment) was more effective than 200 mg given twice daily, although the latter scheme produced continuous levels of isoniazid in the plasma while the former did not. Since then a number of trials have been completed in which standard chemotherapy has been compared with various schemes of intermittent treatment. For example, in one closely supervised trial standard or intermittent treatment followed an intensive phase in which all patients received three months' treatment with daily streptomycin, PAS and isoniazid. All 233 patients on twice-weekly streptomycin and high-dose isoniazid achieved quiescence, as did 163 of the 165 patients receiving conventional daily PAS and low dose isoniazid (Reports 1971a, 1976f). It would clearly be of great advantage if treatment could be given even less often than twice weekly, but the individual dose of isoniazid cannot be much increased over about 15 mg/kg because of the risk of acute toxic effects. Trials of once-weekly streptomycin and high dose isoniazid have given clearly inferior results in the rapid inactivators of isoniazid. For example, in a later trial from Czechoslovakia twice weekly streptomycin and isoniazid gave excellent results after an intensive daily phase lasting either six or 13 weeks, but a once weekly scheme gave satisfactory results only for slow inactivators, with a favourable response in 97 per cent comparing with 78 per cent in rapid inactivators (Report 1977c). The satisfactory results of a twice weekly continuation phase of streptomycin and isoniazid was also clearly shown in a large trial in the U.K., which also included continuation phases of daily isoniazid with PAS, isoniazid with ethambutol and isoniazid with rifampicin (Report 1973a). The poor results of once weekly chemotherapy for rapid inactivators of isoniazid can be overcome neither by the addition of pyrazinamide nor by an initial intensive phase of one month's daily treatment with streptomycin and isoniazid. Several slow release preparations of isoniazid have been devised and one of them, given in a dose of 30 mg/kg, is suitable for a once weekly scheme (Parthasarathy et al, 1976). Intermittent chemotherapy would be much easier to apply if injections of streptomycin could be avoided. Schemes involving only drugs administered by mouth have now been successfully used, following an initial intensive phase of treatment including daily streptomycin. A comparison has been made in Madras of standard daily PAS and isoniazid with twice weekly PAS and high dose isoniazid both continued for 50 weeks following two weeks of daily streptomycin, isoniazid and PAS. Both schemes were equally effective, with a favourable response rate at the end of the year of 87 per cent and 88 per cent for the two regimens. PAS toxicity was, however, much less serious in the twice weekly scheme (Report 1973b).

Intermittent chemotherapy with rifampicin and isoniazid has been used effectively in Singapore (Report 1975b). After two weeks of daily streptomycin, isoniazid and rifampicin, patients received twice weekly or once weekly rifampicin with isoniazid, using either 900 mg or 600 mg of rifampicin with 15 mg/kg isoniazid. All four regimens gave good results, but adverse reactions were frequent (25 per cent) in the once weekly high dose rifampicin scheme. The twice weekly scheme was somewhat more effective than the once weekly; nevertheless the results of the latter regimen were notably good, with a total of only 64 doses of chemotherapy.

SHORT COURSE CHEMOTHERAPY

Effective standard chemotherapy leads to rapid radiological and clinical improvement, and to the disappearance of cultivable tubercle bacilli from the sputum, but a long total period of chemotherapy, at least 18 months, is essential to ensure a low risk of relapse after treatment is discontinued. The introduction of new and powerful antituberculous drugs raises the possibility that shorter regimens of chemotherapy might be devised which would nevertheless be followed by an acceptably low relapse rate.

The first short course trial in East Africa compared four six-month regimens with one of the standard 18-month schemes (Report 1972). All the methods gave immediately favourable results, but significant differences between them emerged in the six months after chemotherapy was completed. Daily streptomycin, isoniazid and rifampicin, and daily streptomycin, isoniazid and pyrazinamide were followed by low rates of relapse, 4 per cent and 6 per cent respectively. The other two methods, daily streptomycin, isoniazid and thiacetazone, and daily streptomycin and isoniazid only, were followed by high relapse rates of 21 per cent and 18 per cent. The standard 18-month scheme of daily isoniazid and thiacetazone, with daily streptomycin in addition during the first eight weeks of treatment, had a relapse rate of 2 per cent. It is notable that the rate at which cultures became negative during the first three months of treatment was more rapid in the rifampicin- and the pyrazinamide-containing regimens, and that all bacilli cultivated during relapses were fully drug-sensitive. These results were maintained during a two-year follow-up period, with a final relapse rate of 3 per cent after the rifampicin-containing scheme, and 8 per cent following the regimen with pyrazinamide (Report 1974).

The next East African study used the six months streptomycin-isoniazid-rifampicin regimen, now of proven efficacy, with three other methods. One consisted of isoniazid and rifampicin alone, which was also highly effective but somewhat less so than the three drug scheme with relapse rates of 7 per cent and 2 per cent respectively in a two-year follow-up period. The other two regimens employed an initial intensive phase of two months in which streptomycin, rifampicin, isoniazid and pyrazinamide, followed by four months either of daily isoniazid-thiacetazone, the standard E. African continuation treatment, or twice-weekly streptomycin, isoniazid and pyrazinamide (Report 1976c). These two were very effective with relapse rates of 7 per cent and 4 per cent respectively. The importance of the initial intensive phase was shown by the good results with relatively weak continuation therapy (isoniazid and thiacetazone), and by the greater speed at which negative cultures were achieved in the first two months with all four drugs than in the three drug regimen omitting pyrazinamide.

Even shorter courses have now been authenticated. A recent study (Report 1978a) compared five regimens of chemotherapy lasting only four months. Those in which rifampicin was continued throughout (streptomycin, isoniazid, rifampicin, and pyrazinamide for eight weeks followed by isoniazid, rifampicin and pyrazinamide or by isoniazid and rifampicin for nine weeks), were followed by relapse rates of only 8 per cent in the first six months after completion of chemotherapy, while the relapse rate was high when rifampicin was discontinued after two months. Streptomycin seemed to provide a small contribution to the efficacy of treatment, but the relapse rate was as high (24 per cent) when the continuation phase consisted of isoniazid and pyrazinamide as with a continuation phase of isoniazid alone (26 per cent), raising the possibility that the bactericidal rôle of pyrazinamide is mainly operative in the first two months of chemotherapy whereas that of rifampicin acts over a longer period.

This suggestion, that the early bactericidal action of pyrazinamide is its most important function in the treatment regimen, is supported by a study from Singapore of four and six months regimens, in which streptomycin, isoniazid, rifampicin and pyrazinamide followed by isoniazid and rifampicin for four months gave very good results which were not improved by including pyrazinamide in the continuation phase. A continuation phase of only two months gave a high relapse rate (Report 1979b).

Antituberculous therapy in the U.K. has tended, in recent years, to follow the short course regimens explored by the British Thoracic and Tuberculosis Association (Reports 1975a, 1976a). Patients received treatment for six, nine, 12 or 18 months with daily rifampicin and isoniazid supplemented in the first two months of treatment by daily streptomycin or ethambutol. Six hundred and ninety-six patients were included in the trial; dosages were rifampicin 600 mg, or 450 mg for patients weighing less than 50 kg, isoniazid 300 mg, streptomycin 0.75 g intramuscularly on six days a week, and ethambutol 25 mg/kg/day. Comparisons were made of six and 12-month courses for patients with less extensive disease, and of nine or 18-month courses for those with cavities larger than 2 cm in diameter. Follow-up showed a relapse rate of 5 per cent following the six months course but there were no relapses in patients who had received the nine months regimen, and only two relapses in 155 patients who received the 12-month course. Adverse effects were encountered in 8 per cent of patients receiving streptomycin in the initial phase of treatment, but in none receiving ethambutol. The 9-month scheme of treatment is that most commonly employed in the U.K. An alternative and less expensive scheme was proposed by Lees et al (1977) who treated 126 patients with isoniazid, rifampicin and ethambutol for an average of three and a half months, thereafter completing one year of chemotherapy with either rifampicin and isoniazid or with ethambutol and isoniazid. The latter scheme was as effective as the former and much less costly.

Short course and intermittent chemotherapy using pyrazinamide but not rifampicin has been explored in Hong Kong. A combination of streptomycin, pyrazinamide and isoniazid was given daily or three times weekly or twice weekly, each regimen being given for six or for nine months (Report 1977a). The nine months regimen either with daily or three times weekly dosage, gave good results when assessed up to 30 months and no serious toxicity problems were encountered. Initial results with strains resistant to isoniazid or streptomycin or both were poor, with 30–39 per cent failures. By contrast, relapse rates following treatment were not influenced by pre-treatment sensitivity to isoniazid and streptomycin, again suggesting the important rôle of pyrazinamide in the sterilizing activity of these regimens.

Another method of solving the economic and social problems of delivering effective anti-tuberculous treatment in developing countries is to select groups of patients expected to derive most benefit from short courses of treatment. Chinese patients considered to have radiographic evidence of active disease, with negative sputum smears and whose first sputum culture proved negative showed only a 1 per cent relapse rate after either two or three months' treatment with daily streptomycin, isoniazid, rifampicin and pyrazinamide. Those with positive pre-treatment cultures, by contrast, had relapse rates of 14 per cent and 7 per cent, showing that these very short courses were inadequate for control in smear-negative but culture-positive patients (Report 1979a).

An important point established by trials of short course chemotherapy is that most relapses occur early, within the first six months of stopping chemotherapy, and that in the great majority of these relapses, the organisms remained fully drug-susceptible. It has been shown, both in East Africa and in Hong Kong, that these patients who relapse with drug-susceptible strains can be satisfactorily re-treated with standard regimens (Report 1976d).

Table 23.1 summarizes a number of major trials of short course and/or intermittent chemotherapy for pulmonary tuberculosis.

TUBERCULOUS MENINGITIS

The continued severity of the disease can be gauged by the report of Freiman & Geefhuysen (1970) who treated 131 African children with tuberculous meningitis. Two-thirds of them were unconscious on admission, 40 per cent had died within a year, and half the survivors showed serious sequelae. No recent controlled clinical trials have been done which would provide guidance for the optimal management of this condition of the type available for pulmonary tuberculosis. Treatment policy is therefore based on the results of older trials together with knowledge of the pharmacokinetics and antituberculous activity of the newer drugs. Isoniazid penetrates well into the CSF, as does pyrazinamide, for which CSF concentrations in one study were identical with those in serum (Forgan-Smith et al, 1973). Rifampicin concentration in the CSF is about 10 per cent of that in serum representing efficient penetration of the non-protein bound fraction of the drug (D'Oliviera, 1972). Ethambutol achieves modest concentrations in the CSF in tuberculous meningitis although not in normal subjects (Place et al, 1969; Pilheu et al, 1971), while streptomycin also, like other aminoglycosides, penetrates the CSF poorly. Ethionamide, by

Table 23.1 Some important trials of short course and intermittent chemotherapy in pulmonary tuberculosis

Source	Regimens	Duration in months*	Relapse rate %	Comments
Report 1974	Streptomycin/Isoniazid	6	29	Most relapses within 12 months of end of treatment,
	Streptomycin/Isoniazid/Thiacetazone	6	22	and with drug-susceptible organisms.
	Streptomycin/Isoniazid/Rifampicin	6	3	
	Streptomycin/Isoniazid/Pyrazinamide	6	8	
Report 1976c	Streptomycin/Isoniazid/Rifampicin	6	2	36 relapses, 32 of them within 6 months of end of
	Isoniazid/Rifampicin	6	7	course, 35 of them with drug-susceptible organisms.
	Streptomycin/Isoniazid/Rifampicin/Pyrazinamide			
	→ Isoniazid/Thiacetazone daily	2 + 4	7	
	or → Strep/Ison/Pyrazinamide			
	twice weekly	2 + 4	4	
Report 1976a	Isoniazid/Rifampicin/Streptomycin	2 + 4	5	8% adverse effects with streptomycin, none
	or	2 + 7	0	with ethambutol
	Isoniazid/Rifampicin/Ethambutol	2 + 10	1	
	→ Isoniazid/Rifampicin	2 + 15	0	
Report 1978a	Streptomycin/Isoniazid/Rifampicin/Pyrazinamide			Poor results when rifampicin given for 2 months only
	→ Isoniazid/Rifamp/Pyrazinamide		8	No apparent effect of continuing pyrazinamide in
	→ Isoniazid/Rifampicin		8	second 2 months
	→ Isoniazid/Pyrazinamide	2 + 2	24	Possible contribution of streptomycin in first
	→ Isoniazid		26	2 months.
	Isoniazid/Rifampicin/Pyrazinamide			
	→ Isoniazid			
Report 1977a	Streptomycin/Isoniazid/Pyrazinamide	6	21	Twice weekly regimen slightly inferior to others.
	Daily or 3× weekly or 2× weekly			
	Daily or 3× weekly or 2× weekly	9	6	

Report 1977b	Isoniazid/Rifampicin → Isoniazid/Streptomycin or Isoniazid/Ethambutol	3 + 6	5.6	Drug susceptible strains in all relapses.
	Isoniazid/Streptomycin/Ethambutol → Isoniazid/Streptomycin or Isoniazid/Ethambutol All given twice weekly	3 + 6	8.9	
Report 1975b	Streptomycin/Isoniazid/Rifampicin Daily → Isoniazid/Rifampicin 900 or Isoniazid/Rifampicin 600 Twice weekly or Isoniazid/Rifampicin 900 or Isoniazid/Rifampicin 600 Once weekly	½ + 12 or ½ + 18		Favourable response at 12 months in all 2× weekly group, less good (97 and 93%) in once weekly. Adverse effects common only in once weekly high dose rifampicin group.
Lees et al, 1977 Lancet i: 1232	Isoniazid/Rifampicin/Ethambutol → Isoniazid/Rifampicin or Isoniazid/Ethambutol	3½ + 8½	0 0	

*Where 2 figures are given in this column, the first is the duration of the initial intensive phase, and the second of the continuation phase of chemotherapy.

contrast, passes into the CSF well even in the absence of meningitis (Hughes et al, 1962).

We consider that, in the initial intensive phase of treatment, two possible courses can be adopted. Isoniazid (10 mg/kg/day, with pyridoxine supplement) with rifampicin and pyrazinamide would constitute a logical choice for this intensive phase, now that the toxicity of pyrazinamide has been re-assessed (q.v.). Alternatively, isoniazid and rifampicin could be given together with streptomycin and ethambutol. After an initial phase of about two months, treatment can then be continued with isoniazid and rifampicin for another eight or ten months. Evidence of drug resistance, either direct or because a contact is known to be excreting drug-resistant organism, would necessitate modification of this scheme.

Whether intrathecal treatment should be given or not is still in dispute; reports from many centres suggest that intrathecal injections of any kind are now unnecessary and possibly undesirable because of their irritant effect and because it is evident that lumbar intrathecal injections of aminoglycosides cannot be relied upon to penetrate throughout the CSF circulation (see Chapter 17). Intrathecal treatment for tuberculous meningitis is not now given in most centres, although the evidence of possible benefit from this mode of treatment before the newer antituberculous drugs were introduced should not be forgotten (Lorber, 1960).

Additional treatment with corticosteroids may be helpful in severe cases. Lorber (1960) recommends this for patients unconscious on admission or for children under one year of age. The dose must be adequate and the duration rarely needs to exceed one month. If intrathecal injections of hydrocortisone are contemplated, special precautions must be taken to prevent secondary infection. Freiman & Geefhuysen (1970), whose experience is quoted above, believe that their results have been improved by the addition of intrathecal streptomycin and hydrocortisone.

OTHER FORMS OF TUBERCULOSIS

The principles of treatment established for pulmonary tuberculosis can be applied to other forms of the disease, although, as with tuberculous meningitis, few controlled trials have been done in other forms of non-pulmonary disease. One exception is the notable series of studies of management of spinal tuberculosis, made in Nigeria, Korea, Rhodesia, Hong Kong and S. Africa, which have established that, for uncomplicated disease of the thoracic spine, the good results of standard chemotherapy are improved neither by bed rest, nor by wearing a plaster jacket, nor by surgical débridement.

In Hong Kong a radical operation with bone grafting gave identical results with those of simple débridement except that healing with bony fusion was more common in patients undergoing the radical operation (Editorial, 1974), a finding confirmed in a more recent comparison of the two operations in S. Africa (Report 1978b).

The success rate in these trials, with or without operation, varies from 81–88 per cent, as judged by clinical and radiological recovery, absence of signs in the central nervous system, and the healing of abscesses and sinuses. These results were achieved with standard chemotherapy of the early 1970s, that is, 18 months of daily isoniazid and PAS, usually supplemented by daily injections of streptomycin during the first three months. It is possible that even better results could be achieved by the newer regimens. Surgery is still sometimes necessary, to establish a diagnosis, drain large abscesses, and, of course, for decompression of the spinal cord.

Treatment of genito-urinary tuberculosis can now also follow modern regimens of chemotherapy. Streptomycin should be avoided if renal function is impaired. Corticosteroids are often given in the early phases of treatment in an attempt to avoid stricture formation, and surgery is indicated mainly, after some weeks of preliminary chemotherapy, for removal of a non-functioning kidney or for the relief of stricture by plastic repair.

Lymph node tuberculosis

The belief that surgical treatment without chemotherapy is appropriate treatment for tuberculosis of lymph nodes was widely prevalent until recent years. Iles & Emerson (1974), however, recorded 10 relapses in 12 patients treated by local excision alone, and it is evident that this form of tuberculosis requires efficient chemotherapy as the basis of management. Precisely which regimen is most effective in glandular tuberculosis, which tends to run an indolent course with a low bacillary population in the caseous material, is not certain, but conventional modern regimens can certainly be applied.

In a trial under the auspices of the British Thoracic and Tuberculosis Association (Campbell & Dyson, 1977) daily rifampicin with isoniazid was compared with daily ethambutol with isoniazid, both given for 18 months with supplementary streptomycin by intramuscular injection for the first two months in both groups. The rate of resolution was the same in both groups, with a final good result in nearly all the patients. Nodes commonly appear, enlarge or even break down during what is ultimately successful chemotherapy and these events should not deter the physician from continuing chemotherapy by established methods. The rôle of surgery has not been studied in controlled trials, but since biopsy is usually necessary, a reasonable approach is to excise smaller nodes for biopsy, to drain established abscesses, but not to undertake extensive node excision.

TREATMENT OF PATIENTS WITH DRUG-RESISTANT INFECTION

The introduction of new drugs has widened the effective choices for these difficult problems, and lessened the need for multiple regimens including drugs with high toxicity. In particular, earlier reports of the value of daily ethambutol with rifampicin in drug-resistant tuberculosis (Lees et al, 1971; Somner et al, 1971) have been confirmed. In one extensive study, 329 patients with isoniazid-resistant organisms, were treated in this way, using daily administration for the first 12 weeks, and then once or twice weekly for a total of 12, 18 or 24 months (Report 1976b). All bacteriological failures (5 per cent) had occurred by 12 months and only six patients relapsed during the two-year period of follow-up. As with other trials, unwanted effects were more common with once-weekly rifampicin-containing regimens.

Complex and often toxic regimens are still occasionally needed for patients with multi-resistant strains, and these are a matter for expert guidance. Combinations of ethionamide, pyrazinamide and cycloserine were widely used before the introduction of rifampicin and ethambutol, and Donomae (1968) reported some success with the use of capreomycin, ethambutol and isoniazid. Seventy-five per cent of the patients had negative cultures at six months, but resistance to ethambutol and to capreomycin often emerged in those whose cultures remained positive.

Treatment of drug-resistant tuberculosis should be distinguished from re-treatment of patients who relapse, mostly with drug-susceptible organisms, during the year after the end of short course chemotherapy. These can be successfully re-treated with standard regimens. Daily streptomycin with isoniazid and either PAS or pyrazinamide followed by twice weekly streptomycin and isoniazid or by daily isoniazid and PAS has been used for these patients in Hong Kong, while in E. Africa daily isoniazid with thiacetazone, with supplementary streptomycin in the first few weeks, was employed. Twelve months after starting treatment all 28 Chinese (whose treatment was fully supervised) and 40 of 45 Africans re-treated by these methods showed favourable responses (Report 1976d).

CHEMOPROPHYLAXIS

Recent contacts should in the first place have a tuberculin test and a chest X-ray. Those with positive tuberculin tests and X-ray changes should be investigated and treated on the usual principles as presumed cases of tuberculosis. Child contacts with normal X-ray but positive tuberculin tests should be treated for one year. The upper age limit for prophylactic chemotherapy of contacts with positive tuberculin test will vary with the prevalence of infection in the community and will rise as the prevalence declines.

Patients with known recent tuberculin conversion, or in whom a strongly positive tuberculin test is accompanied by erythema nodosum or phlyctenular conjunctivitis, should also be given prophylactic chemotherapy. Preventive therapy in children with subclinical infection is very effective. Hsu (1974) recorded six cases of tuberculosis in the follow-up of 1881 children who received isoniazid prophylaxis.

The use of chemoprophylaxis on a larger scale is discussed below. A special case among contacts is the infant of a tuberculous mother. If the disease has been diagnosed and adequately treated during pregnancy, so that it is quiescent at term, the infant is vaccinated with BCG at birth and need not be separated from the mother. A serious problem arises if the disease is diagnosed late in pregnancy, or even after delivery. If the infant is vaccinated with BCG, segregation is necessary until the tuberculin test has converted, but in many communities this is impracticable and itself dangerous to the infant. In these circumstances the infant should be given oral isoniazid for a year, and then vaccinated with BCG. The production of immunity by BCG is impaired by simultaneous administration of isoniazid, but chemoprophylaxis and vaccination can be combined by using an isoniazid-resistant strain of BCG (Gaisford & Griffiths, 1961). If this preparation is available, vaccination need not then be delayed until after the period of isoniazid prophylaxis.

Apart from the use of chemoprophylaxis in infant and child contacts of patients with tuberculosis, isoniazid has also been used on a much larger scale in attempting to prevent infection and to lessen the incidence of tuberculous disease in infected subjects.

The U.S. Public Health Service has carried out extensive controlled trials in children with asymptomatic primary tuberculosis, in household contacts, among Alaskan villages in which 'the disease was so widespread that for all practical purposes everyone could be regarded as a close contact of an active case of tuberculosis', in patients in mental institutions and in people with inactive lesions compatible with healed tuberculosis. These and other controlled trials have been extensively reviewed by Ferebee (1970). The degree of protection afforded by one year's treatment with isoniazid varied greatly with the different trials. At its best, among the good pill takers in the trial of household contacts, the tuberculosis morbidity was reduced by 88 per cent during the treatment year. Of great interest is the finding that these beneficial effects are maintained in lesser degree during the following years, suggesting that chemoprophylaxis has a long-term effect on the risks of endogenous breakdown. In the trial quoted, morbidity was reduced by 60 per cent in the post-treatment phase, with a follow-up of 5–10 years.

Smaller doses are evidently less effective than daily administration of about 5 mg/kg, as shown by a trial in Greenland in which isoniazid on two consecutive days a week for two periods of three months each with an interval of three months gave a reduction of morbidity of only 30 per cent, with no difference between treated and placebo groups in the latter half of a 12-year follow-up (Horwitz & Magnus, 1974).

Adverse reactions do not present a serious problem with the dose used, 5 mg/kg/day, but 1.9 per cent of contacts, and 6 per cent of those with inactive lesions, discontinued treatment because of reactions, mainly gastro-intestinal upsets and rash. Unwanted effects are more common in older patients, and in a prospective study in the U.S. Army (Byrd et al, 1972) 16 of 160 men were unable to complete one year of chemoprophylaxis.

Enthusiasm for the results of controlled trials has led to discussion of even more widespread use of these schemes, which might in theory be extended to the whole tuberculin-positive section of the population. The logistics of schemes for chemoprophylaxis have been examined by Katz & Kunofsky (1971), who confirm that a useful reduction of tuberculosis morbidity can be expected by treating special groups, namely patients with inactive tuberculosis who have received inadequate or no chemotherapy in the past, certain patients at special risk, contacts of cases, and known recent tuberculin converters.

By contrast, the general use of isoniazid in large groups such as all tuberculin reactors would require enormous numbers to be treated for a low yield of cases prevented. The useful limits of programmes of chemoprophylaxis will, of course, vary with the tuberculosis morbidity of the population. Enthusiasm for isoniazid prophylaxis has been greater in the U.S.A. than in Britain, and the American Thoracic Society (1974) recommends this measure for people less than 35 years of age who are tuberculin positive, as well as for those in special risk categories already discussed. The special clinical situations for which chemoprophylaxis is recommended for tuberculin reactors include prolonged treatment with corticosteroids, other immunosuppressive therapy, lymphomas and other haematological malignancies, diabetes, silicosis or previous gastrectomy. Chemoprophylaxis is not used in Britain on indications as widespread as this.

LEPROSY

The treatment of leprosy can only briefly be discussed here. Its study has been facilitated by two discoveries which circumvent to some extent the grave handicap imposed by the non-cultivability of *Myco. leprae*.

The first is a method for producing a transmissible infection by the human bacillus in animals. Shepard (1962) inoculated the footpads of mice intradermally with suspensions of bacilli from human lesions. Slow multiplication followed (50–1000 fold in up to 10 months) and serial transmission succeeded. This technique has now been widely applied in studying the effects of different treatments, and the incidence and significance of bacillary resistance to anti-leprosy drugs. The second observation is that bacilli showing irregular staining by Ziehl-Neelsen are probably dead, corresponding as they do with bacilli showing degenerative changes on electron microscopy (Rees & Valentine, 1962). Estimation of the proportion of bacilli in skin biopsies showing irregular staining (morphological index) is used as a method of assessing the results of treatment.

Dapsone

For many years dapsone (diaminodiphenylsulphone, DDS) has been the mainstay of treatment. The very low minimal inhibitory dose found for this drug in the mouse footpad (0.003 μg per ml) led to many trials of reduced dosage since lepra reactions were thus diminished. It is now evident, however, that low dosage favours the development of dapsone resistance. Pearson et al (1975), reviewing one hundred proven examples of dapsone resistance, found that this emerged only in lepromatous leprosy and that clinical evidence of resistance appeared five to 24 years after treatment with dapsone had started. They favour full dosage treatment (100 mg daily) which should continue despite erythema nodosum leprosum reactions. Regular treatment is difficult to achieve in leprosy, as in tuberculosis, without full supervision, and long-acting preparations have been developed. Acedapsone (4-4 diacetyl-diaminodiphenylsulphone, DADDS) can be given by intramuscular injection in a dose of 225 mg every 11 weeks with maintained plasma concentrations well in excess of the MIC and with good therapeutic effect (Shepard et al, 1972).

Rifampicin

Of the other drugs active in leprosy, rifampicin is especially important, although its use is limited by high cost in most areas where leprosy is found. It acts in the mouse footpad with a speed unequalled by any other agent. In human infection also rifampicin induces rapid improvement, so that within a month of beginning treatment, bacilli can scarcely be found in skin biopsies, a much more rapid rate of progress than that induced by dapsone (Report 1975c). Waters et al (1978) found, however, that despite the rapid effect of rifampicin, a few persistent viable *M. leprae*, could still be detected even after five years of treatment in seven of 12 patients. Moreover rifampicin resistance in *M. leprae* has already been reported in a patient under treatment (Jacobson & Hastings, 1976).

Clofazimine

This orally administered drug is a fat soluble phenazine dye, with activity in experimental systems against a number of mycobacteria (Vischer, 1969). Its efficacy in leprosy appears to be of the same order as that of dapsone (Karat et al, 1971). Clofazimine possesses anti-inflammatory as well as antibacterial properties. Patients who receive it appear to develop erythema nodosum leprosum less often than do patients on dapsone, and it is more effective than prednisone (Karat et al, 1970) and than a placebo (Helmy et al, 1972) in controlling lepra reactions. A disadvantage of clofazimine is the red-brown pigmentation produced in the skin and conjunctivae, and the darkening of the lesions themselves. Apart from this, the only adverse effects have been, in a few patients, abdominal discomfort and mild diarrhoea. Earlier reports of its value in tropical ulcers caused by infection with *Mycobacterium ulcerans* were denied by a controlled trial in which clofazimine was found ineffective in this condition (Revill et al, 1973).

Thiambutosine

This is slightly less effective than dapsone but also less toxic, and has been used in patients intolerant of dapsone. The dose is gradually increased to 2 g daily in divided doses and a parenteral compound has been formulated, suitable for once weekly administration. Resistance tends to develop after about two years' treatment.

Other diphenylthioureas, and thiacetazone, are also active against *M. leprae* in the mouse footpad and in human infection, but, as with thiambutosine, drug resistance emerges easily with subsequent clinical relapse.

Long-acting sulphonamides

Sulphadoxine, sulphadimethoxine, and sulphamethoxypyridazine show a modest degree of activity against *M. leprae*, but they are inactive against dapsone-resistant strains and are much more expensive than dapsone.

Ethionamide and prothionamide

These drugs show a similar and substantial degree of bactericidal activity in leprosy and may come to take an important rôle in treatment. Their use is however limited by the nausea and vomiting which they frequently induce (page 399).

Combined treatment

It is evident that, as in tuberculosis but on a longer time scale, success in the treatment of leprosy may be threatened by the development of drug resistance after single drug treatment, and by the problem of persistent drug-sensitive bacilli. Monotherapy with dapsone is still appropriate for tuberculoid leprosy since the bacillary population is low in this form of disease. In lepromatous and borderline lepromatous leprosy, combined treatment should if possible be given at least in the initial phase of treatment. Waters et al (1978) could barely detect persisters in patients with dapsone-susceptible organisms treated for six months with both drugs, and persisters were much less common than after treatment with dapsone alone. The possibilities of an initial phase using several anti-leprosy drugs have not yet been fully explored. Dapsone-resistant patients can also receive two bactericidal drugs by using rifampicin in combination with clofazimine, ethionamide or prothionamide; combinations of rifampicin and thiambutosine or rifampicin and thiacetazone have also been proposed (Waters, 1977) for sulphone-resistant leprosy.

In leprosy, again as in tuberculosis, clinical advances have stemmed from newer work in experimental chemotherapy and in pharmacology. The mouse footpad technique, in its original form, was unsuited to the analysis of bactericidal versus bacteristatic effects but a modification by Colston et al (1978b) has enabled drugs to be evaluated in this way. Dapsone appears to show a slow bactericidal effect, while ethionamide, prothionamide and clofazimine have activity intermediate in degree between that of rifampicin and dapsone, although this property of clofazimine is hard to demonstrate in experimental systems. Some bacteriological and pharmacological properties of anti-leprosy dugs are summarized in Table 23.2, and pharmacological aspects of leprosy chemotherapy are reviewed by Ellard (1975). It is still uncertain whether this remarkably persistent infection can be fully eradicated by chemotherapy alone, or whether chemotherapy will need to be combined with immunotherapy to achieve complete success.

Prophylaxis

The possibility of preventing leprosy has attracted much attention in recent years. As well as trials of BCG vaccine, which have given widely variable results, other workers have used chemoprophylaxis by dapsone or by repository dapsone (DADDS) in epidemic areas (Sloan et al, 1971). Results so far suggest that leprosy can be prevented by treatment of contacts, but the effect of long-term low-dose dapsone on the incidence of drug resistance has already been noted.

Table 23.2 Properties of some anti-leprosy drugs (adapted from Colston, Ellard and Gammon 1978a)

	MIC μg per ml	Ratio peak serum conc./MIC	Duration of serum conc. exceeding MIC in days	Bactericidal activity
Dapsone	0.003	500	10	+
Acedapsone	0.003	15	200	NT
Rifampicin	0.3	30	1	+++
Long-acting Sulphonamides	20–35	3–7	3–14	NT
Thiambutosine	0.5	1	<1	—
Thiacetazone	0.2	8	1	—
Ethionamide } Prothionamide }	0.05	60	1	++

NT = not tested

References

American Thoracic Society 1974 Amer Rev Resp Dis 110: 371
Batten J 1970 Tubercle 51: 95
Black M, Mitchell J R, Zimmerman H J, Ishak K G, Epler G R 1975 Gastroenterology 69: 289
Bolt H M, Kappus H, Bolt M 1974 Lancet 1: 1280
Brouet G, Marche J, Rist N, Chevallier J, LeMeur G 1959 Amer Rev Tuberc 79: 6
Byrd R B, Nelson R, Elliott R C 1972 J Amer Med Ass 220: 1471
Campbell I A, Dyson A J 1977 Tubercle 58: 171
Citron K M 1969 Tubercle 50: (Suppl) 32
Colston M J, Ellard G A, Gammon P T 1978a Lepr Rev 49: 115
Colston M J, Hilson G R F, Banerjee D K 1978b Lepr Rev 49: 7
D'Oliviera J J G 1972 Amer Rev Resp Dis 106: 432
Donomae I 1968 Amer Rev Resp Dis 98: 699
Editorial 1974 Brit Med J 4: 613
Edwards O M, Courtenay-Evans R J, Galley J M, Hunter J, Tait A D 1974 Lancet 2: 549
Ellard G A 1969 Tubercle 50: 144
Ellard G A 1975 Lepr Rev 46: (Suppl) 41
Ellard G A, Dickinson J M, Gammon P T, Mitchison D A 1974 Tubercle 55: 41
Ferebee S H 1970 Adv Tuberc Res 17: 28

Ferguson G C, Nunn A J, Fox W et al 1971 Tubercle 52: 166
Flynn C T, Rainford D J, Hope E 1974 Brit Med J 2: 482
Forgan-Smith R, Ellard G A, Newton D, Mitchison D A 1973 Lancet 2: 374
Fox W 1977 Proc Roy Soc Med 70: 4
Fox W, Mitchison D A 1975 Amer Rev Resp Dis 111: 325
Fox W, Stark A J, Tall R et al 1974 Tubercle 55: 29
Freiman I, Geefhuysen J 1970 J Pediat 76: 895
Gaisford W, Griffiths M I 1961 Brit Med J 1: 1500
Gangadharam P R J, Devadatta S, Fox W, Nair C N, Selkon J B 1961 Bull WHO 25: 793
Girling D J 1977 J Antimicrob Chemother 3: 115
Girling D J 1978 Tubercle 59: 13
Grosset J 1978 Tubercle 59: 287
Grumbach F, Canetti G, Le Lirzin M 1969 Tubercle 50: 280
Helmy S H, Pearson J M H, Waters M F R 1972 Lepr Rev 42: 167
Hesling C M 1969 Tubercle 50: (Suppl) 39
Horwitz O, Magnus K 1974 Amer J Epidem 99: 333
Hsu K H K 1974 J Amer Med Ass 229: 528
Hughes I E, Smith H, Kane P O 1962 Lancet 1: 616
Iles P B, Emerson P A 1974 Brit Med J 1: 143
Jacobson R R, Hastings R C 1976 Lancet 2: 1304
Karat A B A, Jeevaratnam A, Karat S, Rao P S S 1970 Brit Med J 1: 198
Karat A B A, Jeevaratnam A, Karat S, Rao P S S 1971 Brit Med J 4: 514
Karlson A G 1961a & b Amer Rev Resp Dis 84: 902, 905
Katz J, Kunofsky S 1971 Chest 59: 600
Kenwright S, Levi A J 1973 Lancet 2: 1401
Kopanoff D E, Kilburn J O, Glassroth J L et al 1978 Amer Rev Resp Dis 118: 835
Lees A W, Allan G W, Smith J, Tyrrell W F, Fallon R J 1971 Tubercle 52: 182
Lees A W, Smith J, Allan G W, Tyrrell W F 1977 Lancet 1: 1232
Lorber J 1960 Brit Med J 1: 1309
McCune R M, Feldmann F M, Lambert H P, McDermott W 1966 J Exper Med 123: 445
Maddrey W C, Boitnott J K 1973 Ann Intern Med 79: 1
Parthasarathy R, Devadatta S, Fox W et al 1976 Tubercle 57: 115
Pearson J M H, Rees R J W, Waters M F R 1975 Lancet 2: 69
Pilheu J A, Maglio F, Cetrangolo R, Pleus A D 1971 Tubercle 52: 117
Place V A, Pyle M M, de la Huerga J 1969 Amer Rev Resp Dis 99: 783
Poole G, Stradling P, Worlledge S 1971 Brit Med J 3: 343
Rees R J W, Valentine R C 1962 Int J Lepr 30: 1
Report 1952, Medical Research Council Brit Med J 2: 735
Report 1970, East African/British MRC Tubercle 51:353
Report 1971a, Czechoslovakian Tuberculosis Service/WHO/British MRC Cooperative Investigation Bull WHO 45: 573
Report 1971b, Singapore Tuberculosis Services/Brompton Hospital/British MRC Investigation Tubercle 52: 88
Report 1972, East African/British MRC Lancet 1: 1079
Report 1973a, British Medical Research Council Cooperative Study Tubercle 54: 99
Report 1973b, Tuberculosis Chemotherapy Centre, Madras Brit Med J 2: 7
Report 1974, East African/British Medical Research Council Lancet 2: 237
Report 1975a, British Thoracic and Tuberculosis Association Lancet 1: 119
Report 1975b, Singapore Tuberculosis Service/British Medical Research Council Lancet 2: 1105
Report 1975c, United States Leprosy Panel/Leonard Wood Memorial Amer J Trop Med Hyg 24: 475
Report 1976a, British Thoracic and Tuberculosis Association Lancet 2: 1102
Report 1976b, Cooperative Tuberculosis Chemotherapy Study in Poland Tubercle 57: 105
Report 1976c, East African/British Medical Research Council Amer Rev Resp Dis 114: 471
Report 1976d Hong Kong Tuberculosis Treatment Services/East African and British Medical Research Council Lancet 1: 162
Report 1976e, Hong Kong Tuberculosis Treatment Services/British Medical Research Council Tubercle 57: 81
Report 1976f, World Health Organization Collaborating Centre for Tuberculosis Chemotherapy, Prague Tubercle 57: 45
Report 1977a, Hong Kong Chest Service/British Medical Research Council Amer Rev Resp Dis 115: 727

Report 1977b, Tuberculosis Research Institute, Bucharest Tubercle 58: 1
Report 1977c, World Health Organization Collaborating Centre for Tuberculosis Chemotherapy, Prague Tubercle 58: 129
Report 1978a, East African/British Medical Research Council Lancet 2: 334
Report 1978b, Medical Research Council Working Party on Tuberculosis of the Spine, 7th Report, Tubercle 59: 79
Report 1979a, Hong Kong Chest Service, Tuberculosis Research Centre. Madras and British MRC Lancet 1: 1361
Report 1979b, Singapore Tuberculosis Service/British MRC Amer Rev Resp Dis 119: 579
Revill W D L, Pike M C, Morrow R H, Ateng J 1973 Lancet 2: 873
Rist N, Grumbach F, Libermann D 1959 Amer Rev Tuberc 79: 1
Sanders W E 1976 Ann Intern Med 85: 82
Scheuer P J, Lal S, Summerfield J A, Sherlock S 1974 Lancet 1: 421
Shepard C C 1962 Int J Lepr 30: 291
Shepard C C, Levy L, Fasal P 1972 Amer J Trop Med Hyg 21: 440
Siegler D I, Burley D M, Bryant M, Citron K M, Standen S M 1974 Lancet 2: 197
Sloan N R, Worth R M, Jano B, Fasal P, Shepard C C 1971 Lancet 2: 525
Somner A R, Selkon J B, Walton M, White A B 1971 Tubercle 52: 266
Stradling P, Poole G W 1970 Tubercle 51: 44
Thomas J P, Baughn C O, Wilkinson R G, Shepherd R G 1961 Amer Rev Resp Dis 83: 891
Vischer W A 1969 Lepr Rev 40: 107
Waters M F R 1977 Lepr Rev 48: 95
Waters M F R, Rees R J W, Pearson J M H et al 1978 Brit Med J 1: 133

Antimycobacterial agents. Pharmaceutical preparations and dosage

Name	*Dosage*	*Preparation*	*Common international proprietary names*	
Capreomycin	*Adult* i.m.: 1 g daily with a maximum of 20 mg/kg.	Injection	Capastat Ogostal	(UK) (Ger)
Ethambutol	*Adult* 15–25 mg/kg as a single daily dose.	Tablets	Myambutol Dexambutol	(UK) (Fr)
Ethionamide	*Adult* Oral: 500 mg–1 g daily maximum. *Children* (under 10 yrs.) 10 mg/kg body weight daily, initially, with a gradual increase to 20 mg/kg in 15 days if it is tolerated.	Tablets	Trescatyl Trecator	(UK) (Fr, USA)
Isoniazid	*Adult* Oral, i.m.: 300–600 mg daily. Intrathecal: 25–50 mg daily. *Children* Oral, i.m.: 10–30 mg/kg body weight daily to a maximum of 500 mg a day. Intrathecal: 10–20 mg daily.	Tablets Syrup Injection Also combinations with Sodium aminosalicylate	Rimifon (= injection) Cedin, Isozid INH, Nydrazid Inapasade	(UK) (Ger) (USA) (UK)
Sodium aminosalicylate	*Adult* Oral: 8–15 g daily in divided doses, with a maximum of 20 g a day. *Children* Oral: 200–300 mg/kg body weight daily in divided doses.	Powder Also combinations with Isoniazid.	Paramisan Pamisyl Sodium, Teebacin PAS Sodique Elbiol Solu—PAS Elbiol	(UK) (USA) (Fr) (Ger)
Prothionamide	*Adult* Oral: 500 mg–1 g daily.	Tablets	Trevintix Ektebin, Petama	(UK) (Ger)
Pyrazinamide	*Adult* Oral: 20–35 mg/kg a day The maximum daily dose should not exceed 3 g	Tablets	Zinamide Pyrafat	(UK) (Ger)

Antimycobacterial agents. Pharmaceutical preparations and dosage

Name	*Dosage*	*Preparation*	*Common international proprietary names*	
Rifampicin Rifampin (USP)	*Adult* Oral: 8–12 mg/kg body weight as a single daily dose. *Children* Oral: 10–20 mg/kg body weight, with a maximum daily dose of 600 mg. An injectable form is available on special request	Capsules Suspension Tablets in combination with Isoniazid.	Rifadin, Rimactane Rifa	(UK) (Ger)
Streptomycin	See Chapter 5			
Thiacetazone	*Adult* Oral: 2 mg/kg body weight daily in divided doses.	Tablets		
Viomycin	*Adult* i.m.: 1 g twice daily on two days a week	Injection	Viocin No longer available in the UK	(Ger)
Thiambutosine	*Adult* Oral: 1–2 g daily with a maximum of 4 g a day. *Children* Oral: 500 mg–1.5 g daily depending on age.	Tablets	Ciba 1906	(UK)
Clofazimine	*Adult* Oral: 100 mg three times a week.	Capsules	Lamprene	(UK)
Dapsone	*Adult* Oral: 100 mg daily.	Tablets Injection	Dapsone	(UK)
Ditophal	By inunction 5 ml 2–3 times weekly	Application	Ditophal	(UK)

24

Sexually transmitted infections, chlamydial infections and non-venereal spirochaetoses

It is a remarkable fact that the most sensitive of all microorganisms to penicillin are those causing the two principal forms of venereal disease. Their treatment is now within the capacity of anyone, but because clinical skill and special laboratory facilities are necessary to verify cure and sometimes even to make a diagnosis, the subject must remain a speciality.

SYPHILIS

The degree of sensitivity of *Treponema pallidum* to antibacterial agents cannot be measured in the ordinary way *in vitro* since the organism cannot be cultured artificially, but the results of curative tests in rabbits are highly significant. Early experiments showed that four days after the intratesticular or intracutaneous inoculation of rabbits a very small dose of penicillin sufficed to abort the infection, even though administered in a long-acting form giving very low blood levels. At two weeks a dose about seven times larger was required to produce the same effect. These findings indicated the possibility of aborting the disease in man by a single dose of a long-acting preparation administered at an early stage (see below).

The use of penicillin in the treatment of syphilis over three decades is fully described by Idsøe et al (1972). In the U.S.A., methods of treating syphilis are reviewed from time to time by a Venereal Diseases Control Advisory Committee, and published by the Center for Disease Control (C.D.C.). Regimens in the U.K. follow generally similar policies, except that less reliance is placed on one dose schemes in Britain than in the U.S.A. Current recommendations may be summarized as follows:

Early syphilis, i.e., of less than one year's duration

Either benzathine penicillin 2.4 mega units by intramuscular injection at a single session

or procaine penicillin 600 000 units by intramuscular injection daily for eight days. (Procaine penicillin in oil with 2 per cent aluminium monostearate, PAM, is no longer used either in the U.K. or the U.S.A.)

Patients allergic to penicillin are treated either with tetracycline 500 mg four times daily by mouth for 15 days, or by erythromycin in the same dose and for the same length of time.

Syphilis of more than one year's duration

Either benzathine penicillin 2.4 mega units by intramuscular injection weekly for three successive weeks.

or procaine penicillin 600 000 units daily by intramuscular injection for 15 days.

If cerebrospinal fluid examination provides evidence of neurosyphilis, benzathine penicillin should not be used, since the CSF levels achieved may be inadequate. Tramont (1976), for example, demonstrated persistence of viable *T. pallidum* in the CSF of a patient who had received 1.2 mega units of benzathine penicillin three times weekly for three weeks and in another patient who had received 2.0 g of tetracycline daily for ten days. Many physicians use benzyl penicillin in high dosage for 14 days in the treatment of neurosyphilis.

Patients with neurosyphilis who are allergic to penicillin may be given tetracycline or erythromycin in the doses already stated for 30 days. Regular follow-up examination, always indicated after treatment of syphilis, is especially important in patients treated with drugs other than penicillin.

Syphilis in pregnancy

Patients are given penicillin in the schedule appropriate for the stage of syphilis in the same way as non-pregnant patients and, if allergic to penicillin, are given erythromycin as stearate, ethyl succinate or base, but this may not protect the fetus (p. 188). Tetracycline or erythromycin estolate are not given to pregnant women according to the Center for Disease Control (C.D.C., 1976).

Congenital syphilis

Although now fortunately rare in many countries, congenital syphilis presents a difficult problem, since the infant may show no clinical signs of infection and may be seronegative if maternal infection occurs in late pregnancy. Assessment of CNS involvement may also be difficult in the neonate. The C.D.C. therefore recommends that infants should be treated at birth if maternal treatment was inadequate, unknown, with drugs other than penicillin, or if proper follow-up cannot be ensured. If the CSF is abnormal, benzyl penicillin is given by intramuscular or intravenous injection, 50 000 units/kg daily in two divided doses for at least 10 days. As an alternative procaine penicillin 50 000 units/kg can be given daily by intramuscular injection for at least ten days. McCracken & Kaplan (1974) have measured CSF penicillin levels in infants with congenital syphilis demonstrating the need for high dosage. Although C.D.C. recommendations include cautious endorsement of a previous regimen of single dose benzathine penicillin (50 000 units/kg) if the CSF is normal, its efficacy is unproved and procaine or aqueous penicillin should if possible be used in congenital syphilis.

Treatment of contacts

The tracing of contacts is rigorously pursued by efficiently run clinics for sexually transmitted diseases. If untreated, 5–20 per cent of sexual contacts of patients with syphilis will develop the disease within three months, and these cases can be completely prevented by prophylactic or 'epidemiological' treatment with one of the regimens employed in early syphilis, such as a single injection of benzathine penicillin, 2.4 mega units (Pirozzi, 1973).

Jarisch-Herxheimer reaction

Many patients develop fever, malaise and headache, sometimes with exacerbation of existing syphilitic lesions, within a few hours of starting penicillin treatment. The reaction is accompanied, it has recently been established (Editorial, 1977), by the release of endotoxin from the spirochaetes and by evidence of complement consumption. The reaction is not dangerous when it is most common, in primary and secondary syphilis, but the focal reaction can be dangerous in certain cases of gummatous, cardiovascular or neurosyphilis.

The traditional method of attempting to avoid reactions by starting treatment with injections of bismuth was shown to be ineffective by Knudsen & Aastrup (1965), who, in a direct comparison of 149 patients treated with penicillin with 184 patients treated with bismuth and organic arsenicals, found no difference in the course or frequency of Jarisch-Herxheimer reactions in the two groups.

Although the risks of a focal reaction in late syphilis have been much disputed and serious reactions are certainly rare, it is now normal practice to give prednisolone, in a dose of 40 mg daily for 3–4 days beginning two days before the penicillin, during penicillin treatment of late syphilis, although its effectiveness in this respect remains unproved. Jarisch-Herxheimer reactions are common and dangerous during the treatment of relapsing fever, and are further discussed on page 432.

Persistence of treponemes in treated syphilis

Several investigators have claimed that treponemes are recoverable from the tissues of some penicillin-treated patients long after the disease was believed to have been eradicated (Collart et al, 1962). In patients believed to have been adequately treated, Rice et al (1970) demonstrated by darkground and immunofluorescent microscopy the persistence in the aqueous humour and CSF of forms at least some of which were *Treponema pallidum*. It is generally felt, however, that as the clinical results of treatment are excellent and only the moist early lesions are infectious, there is no reason to modify the present treatment regimens.

The importance of achieving adequate CSF levels of penicillin in the treatment of neurosyphilis has already been stressed.

Penicillin allergy

Venereal diseases clinics have provided the largest source of information about the incidence and severity of reactions to penicillin. Rudolph & Price (1973), reviewing experience in the U.S.A., note reactions in 183 of 27 673 patients (6.61/1000) in recent years, compared with a rate of 9.71 per 1000 in 1959. Urticaria and maculopapular rashes were most common, 11 patients developed anaphylaxis and three serum sickness, but none of these reactions was fatal. It appears, therefore, that although still an important factor in treatment, penicillin allergy does not pose an increasing threat to the control of syphilis.

Patients allergic to penicillin are treated with tetracycline or erythromycin in the manner already described. Although cephalosporins have been used successfully in the treatment of syphilis, they are no longer recommended for patients with an authentic history of penicillin allergy, in view of the appreciable incidence of cross allergy between penicillins and cephalosporins (page 99). The general problem of penicillin allergy is discussed in Chapter 3.

Other treponematoses

Yaws. T. pertenue is highly penicillin-sensitive, and this disease has commonly been treated with a single dose of PAM (procaine penicillin in oil with 2 per cent aluminium monostearate), the dose being 0.6 and 1.2 mega units in children and adults respectively. Benzathine penicillin in a single treatment of 2.4 mega units, or procaine penicillin 600 000 units daily for eight days, are also effective. For adults with palmar and plantar hyperkeratosis and those with late lesions, Gentle (1965) recommends 4–6 mega units aqueous procaine penicillin spread over a period of several weeks. Contacts and latent cases can be treated with 0.6 mega unit benzathine penicillin and active cases with 1.2 mega units benzathine penicillin (children under 10 should receive half these amounts). Nicol (1962) emphasizes the difficulty of distinguishing with certainty between yaws and syphilis and recommends that where there is any doubt treatment should be with procaine penicillin 0.6 mega unit intramuscularly daily for 10 days. Reports on yaws eradication campaigns emphasize the necessity for treating the entire population of an area, and not merely overt cases, since others may be latent or in the stage of incubation.

Bejel and *Pinta* are reported to respond well to a single large dose of a repository penicillin preparation.

GONORRHOEA

The treatment of gonorrhoea has been transformed twice in the past 30 years. The first success, that of sulphonamides, was relatively short-lived, resistant strains of gonococci becoming common within a few years. That of penicillin has been both more dramatic and more prolonged, but is threatened by the emergence of several forms of drug resistance.

The gonococcus is the most sensitive to penicillin of all ordinary bacteria. It disappears from the exudate within two hours of a moderate dose being given, and that single dose is usually curative. This rapid destructive action, leaving the organism no time to adapt itself, was believed to be the reason why no resistant strains appeared, although it was very early shown that by careful training resistance could be increased *in vitro* several thousand-fold.

The first unequivocal evidence of the existence of resistant strains was obtained in 1958, when it was evident that treatment failures were becoming rather more frequent. Whereas the normal inhibitory concentration is <0.01 μg/ml, an increasing proportion of strains was inhibited only by higher concentrations, the least sensitive showing MICs of up to 1 μg/ml. This form of relative resistance to penicillin was closely linked to tetracycline resistance. Moreover, it was clearly shown that these strains of higher resistance are associated with treatment failure.

Penicillin resistance of this type increased in frequency until the early 1970s, becoming a serious threat to the use of penicillin for gonorrhoea in certain areas, notably in South-East Asia (Willcox, 1970). Penicillin treatment could still be achieved by increased dosage and by other modifications of regimen discussed in the following pages, but in 1976 a new problem emerged with the identification of strains showing highly inoculum-dependent resistance to penicillin characteristic of β-lactamase-producing organisms. At least two different plasmids coding for penicillinase production have been identified, linked with the two epidemiological sources of these strains in the Far East and in West Africa. Many of the widespread but as yet infrequent infections with penicillinase-producing gonococci have been associated with sexual contacts in these areas (Perine et al, 1977). Other strains of *N. gonorrhoeae*, highly resistant to penicillin but not producing β-lactamase are also being identified.

Penicillinase-producing strains are resistant to other penicillins and to cephaloridine and some of them are relatively resistant to tetracycline, but are inhibited by cefuroxime and by spectinomycin and can be sucessfully treated by these agents (Arya et al, 1978; Berg, et al 1979). Gonococci isolated from patients whose treatment has failed must now be tested for production of penicillinase.

Treatment of gonorrhoea

The rising incidence in gonorrhoea observed in most countries during the last two decades is perhaps only now beginning to level off, and this infection, together with non-gonococcal urethritis, has become the most common sexually transmitted disease in North America and Western Europe. The problems of controlling the epidemic are daunting and arise from several causes. Slowly and rapidly emerging forms of antibiotic resistance have already been discussed and require alert and skilled laboratory services for their detection. The prevalence of subclinical infection, now thought to be somewhat more common in men (although less common in women) than was formerly supposed (Handsfield, 1978) underlines the importance of contact tracing, a control measure only achievable by efficient and well staffed clinics. A further problem is the high incidence of defaulters after a first attendance, resulting in a strong tendency to favour regimens which are completed at one visit and which have a very high success rate. These aims have been to some extent achieved by magnified penicillin therapy and by the use of a number of other antimicrobial agents. Fortunately, most gonococcal strains isolated in Britain can still be eradicated by easily achievable penicillin regimens, but other methods are necessary for penicillin-allergic patients, while penicillinase-producing strains cannot be eliminated by any form of penicillin treatment. It must be emphasized that, as regards the smaller degrees of penicillin resistance which have developed over the course of 20 years, there is copious evidence that therapeutic success is directly related to the *in vitro* sensitivity of the strain and the dose and method of penicillin treatment.

Standard penicillin treatment

The common range of penicillin resistance in gonococci can be overcome by giving larger and more frequent doses, or by adding probenecid and this last modification is now commonly used. Most clinics employ procaine penicillin by intramuscular injection together with oral probenecid in the manner summarized on Table 24.1, although benzyl penicillin, or a mixture of benzyl and procaine penicillin (fortified procaine penicillin) may also be used successfully together with probenecid. Triplopen, a mixture of benethamine, procaine and benzyl penicillins, is also widely used. Preparations yielding prolonged but low plasma penicillin levels, such as benzathine penicillin, although effective in treating syphilis, are not suitable for the treatment of gonorrhoea.

Other penicillins

Successful one-session treatment has been well documented with oral ampicillin and probenecid (Table 24.1) and the more recently developed comparable compounds have also been widely used. Wise & Neu (1974), reviewing experience with amoxycillin in the U.S.A., showed cure rates of at least 96 per cent in both men and women given a total dose of 3.0 g either as a single dose or over four days, but doses of 1.0 or 1.5 g gave cure rates in the range of 80–92 per cent. In one of the few double blind trials recorded in the treatment of gonorrhoea, Thin et al (1977) noted 43 cures in 50 patients given 1.0 g amoxycillin and 1.0 g probenecid (86 per cent), and 51 cures of 54 patients given 3.0 g amoxycillin and 1.0 g probenecid. Although the difference did not achieve significant levels, they felt the smaller antibiotic dose was unsuitable, since the MIC for *N. gonorrhoeae* was less than about 0.05 μg per ml in only 60 per cent of the isolates.

Table 24.1 Treatment of gonorrhoea

Regimen	C.D.C. recommended dose	Clinics in England + Wales		
		Common dose used	% of clinics using method	
* Aq. Procaine penicillin	4.8 mega units	1.2–2.4 mega units	22	
with Probenecid	yes			50
† Triplopen		1.2–2.5 mega units	11	
with Probenecid	no			0
* Ampicillin	3.5 g	0.5–2.5 g	33	
with Probenecid	yes			97
* Amoxycillin	3.0 g	2.0–2.5 g		
with Probenecid	yes			
* Tetracycline	0.5 g q.i.d. 5 days	0.25–0.5 g q.i.d. 5 days	2.3	
Co-trimoxazole		2 tabs b.d. 2–8 days	9	
* Spectinomycin (treatment failures and resistant strains)	2.0 g			

* C.D.C.-recommended treatment schedules
† Triplopen is a mixture of benethamine penicillin, procaine penicillin and benzyl penicillin

Based on
Centre for Disease Control 1979 and Adler 1978a

Oral talampicillin has similarly been used for gonococcal urethritis and cervicitis. Price et al (1977) record four failures of 245 patients given a single dose of 1.48 g together with 1.0 g of probenecid. It is worth noting that gonococcal strains show a narrower range of sensitivity to ampicillin than to benzyl penicillin. Although the MIC of ampicillin for sensitive strains is higher than that of benzyl penicillin, penicillin-resistant strains are more sensitive to ampicillin than to benzyl penicillin (Johnson et al, 1970).

Other agents

Numerous other agents have been tried. Oral treatments which need to be continued for several days are at a disadvantage because of defaulting by an appreciable proportion of patients, and several one-dose oral treatments have shown a high failure rate. On the other hand, several oral drugs have proved effective when given as two doses at an interval of five hours. These methods have been reviewed by Willcox (1971); it is hoped that a higher proportion of patients might be relied upon to take one additional dose of a drug a few hours after leaving the clinic than could be expected to complete a five- or seven-day course. There is also the problem that a proportion of strains more resistant to penicillin are also more resistant to other agents, possibly as the result of previous alternative treatment (Waterworth et al, 1979; Phillips et al, 1970), so that treatment with an alternative regimen may again fail.

Spectinomycin (page 117). This aminocyclitol antibiotic has emerged as a safe and effective parenteral treatment for gonorrhoea. The sulphate first used was soon replaced by the dihydrochloride pentahydrate, which is more soluble and requires a smaller volume for injection. Most gonococci are inhibited by concentrations of spectinomycin of 8–16 μg per ml. Although *in vitro* sensitivities to spectinomycin and to penicillin are correlated, response to spectinomycin treatment does not relate closely to *in vitro* susceptibility (within the sensitive range) as with penicillin (McCormack & Finland, 1976). Spectinomycin-resistant strains have been detected (Thornsberry et al, 1977) but are so far rare, although tolerance can easily be induced *in vitro*. Earlier clinical studies showed that single intramuscular doses of 2.0 g or 4.0 g were equally effective in uncomplicated gonorrhoea. Duncan et al (1972) obtained cure rates of over 90 per cent in 353 men and 314 women with culture-proven gonorrhoea with either dose. More recent series have confirmed the value of spectinomycin. Porter & Rutherford (1977), for example, who treated 110 patients, succeeded in obtaining follow-up examination in 75 of them, in only one of whom treatment failed. In the treatment of complicated gonorrhoea, spectinomycin is apparently effective in gonococcal proctitis. Fiumara (1978) obtained negative cultures in 127 patients at one week follow-up after a single dose of 4.0 g, but poor results in pharyngeal gonorrhoea have been described. Karney et al (1977) obtained, in a very large series, a minimum cure rate of 94 per cent in anogenital gonorrhoea but failed to eradicate pharyngeal infection in six of 11 men and one of 13 women.

Streptomycin is no longer a suitable treatment for gonorrhoea because of wide-spread resistance.

Kanamycin, as a single intramuscular injection of 2.0 g, gives good results with failure rates of about 5 per cent, and is used in some clinics for patients with penicillin sensitivity (Farrell, 1969).

Cephalosporins. Starting with cephaloridine, the efficacy of a number of these compounds has been established. Shapiro & Lentz (1970) obtained 94.3 per cent of cures in female patients after a single dose of 2.0 g cephaloridine by intramuscular injection. A high cure rate may be obtained by cefazolin as a single injection of 2.0 g combined with 1.0 g probenecid in a single oral dose, but smaller doses give unsatisfactory results (Karney et al, 1973).

The newer cephalosporins and cefoxitin may become important if penicillinase-producing gonococci become widespread (see below) but their effectiveness in ordinary gonorrhoea is also being tested. Price & Fluker (1978) treated 110 patients with uncomplicated urethral gonorrhoea with cefuroxime. Eighteen patients who returned for re-examination after 1 g by intramuscular injection together with probenecid (1.0 g) were all cured, as were 66 of 67 after a dose of 1.5 g, also with probenecid. Cefamandole is apparently satisfactory as a single 3.0 g injection, curing 39 of 42 patients, but a 2.0 g dose succeeded in only 44 of 54 patients, oral probenecid being given in both schemes (Tennican et al, 1979). Platt et al (1979) found cefoxitin 2.0 g together with probenecid as effective as a conventional penicillin-probenecid scheme, curing 57 of 59 patients and Berg et al (1979) cured all of a group of 21 patients infected with penicillinase-producing strains with the same regimen.

Tetracyclines. Tetracycline is well established as alternative treatment for penicillin-allergic patients. It has two limitations, that single dose treatment is ineffective, and that strains relatively resistant to penicillin tend also to be tetracycline-resistant, so that tetracycline is unsuitable for use in treatment failures on penicillin or ampicillin. On the other hand, tetracycline used in gonorrhoea acts also against the most common causes of post-gonococcal urethritis, *Chlamydia trachomatis* and *Ureaplasma urealyticum.*

Co-trimoxazole. Trimethoprim and sulphamethoxazole are strongly synergic in their action on *N. gonorrhoeae* (page 28), but results in practice are somewhat conflicting. Rahim (1975) used single dose treatment in 1223 patients, giving eight tablets with milk. Of the 1069 patients who were seen again 46 (4 per cent) failed to respond, and post gonococcal urethritis developed in 6 per cent. Different dose schemes were studied by Elliott et al (1977) in 271 men with gonococcal urethritis, with random allocation of treatment. Whereas only 4 per cent failed on a conventional procaine penicillin-probenecid scheme, 23 per cent failed to respond to nine tablets of co-trimoxazole as a single dose, and 19 per cent to 12 tablets given as two doses with a six hour interval. Isolates from treatment failures showed increased resistance to sulphamethoxazole and to the combination. As with tetracycline, resistance to the components and the combination shows a general correlation with penicillin resistance, so that co-trimoxazole is probably unsuitable for the re-treatment of penicillin failures.

Drugs for gonorrhoea and simultaneous infection with syphilis

Concern has often been expressed that the use of other agents and the increased dose of penicillin necessary to treat less sensitive gonococci will mask the development of concurrent syphilis. It goes without saying that every patient treated for gonorrhoea should undergo serological tests for syphilis six months later. Provided that this is done, cannot the possible effect on incubating syphilis be disregarded? The ordinary dose of penicillin might only be suppressive: larger doses will probably cure early syphilis. Tetracyclines and erythromycin are also active against *T. pallidum*: streptomycin and kanamycin are not.

Spectinomycin has some degree of activity against *T. pallidum* and it is possible that the incubation period of syphilis might be prolonged, or subclinical infection made more likely, after treatment of gonorrhoea by this drug. Co-trimoxazole is said not to mask incubating syphilis (Rahim, 1975). The role of tetracyclines, and the difficult problem of attempting to reconcile optimal treatment for gonorrhoea with control of non-gonococcal urethritis and cervicitis, are discussed in the following section on chlamydial infection.

Common treatment regimens

As regards comparative effectiveness of the commonly used regimens, several studies have already been described in the account of individual agents. Two very large scale trials are especially notable. Kaufman et al (1976), in a randomly assigned study of the main 1972 recommendations of the U.S. Public Health Service, note the results of three schemes in a total of 9000 patients of whom, however, only 3871 could be re-examined. For ampicillin (3.5 g with probenecid 1.0 g) the cure rate was 92.8 per cent, for tetracycline (1.5 g followed by 0.5 g four times daily for four days) 96.2 per cent, and for spectinomycin (2.0 g for men and 4.0 g for women) 94.8 per cent.

Karney et al (1977) compared the results in 4043 patients given tetracycline in the standard regimen with spectinomycin 2.0 or 4.0 g, finding also a minimum cure rate of 94 per cent for both drugs. Post-gonococcal urethritis was less common after tetracycline (5 of 398 patients) than after spectinomycin either in the 2.0 g dose (46 of 659 patients) or the 4.0 g dose (30 of 638 patients). They question the primacy of penicillin treatments for gonorrhoea, considering that tetracycline or spectinomycin provide equally rational choices.

Which regimens should actually be chosen from the large number available and established as effective by soundly based clinical trials? Where penicillin resistance is not a serious problem, one of those based on penicillin, ampicillin or amoxycillin will normally be used for initial treatment, while patients allergic to penicillin can be given tetracycline, co-trimoxazole, kanamycin or spectinomycin (Willcox, 1977). For the reasons given, treatment failures are probably best treated with spectinomycin.

Table 24.1 provides a summary of the main recommendations of the Center for Disease Control (1979), in which they are compared with common clinic practice in England and Wales, as examined by Adler (1978a). Two main differences emerge, the relatively lower doses used in British clinics in comparison with the C.D.C. recommendations, and the relatively wide use of triplopen and of co-trimoxazole in Britain. In both countries once-only dose schemes are favoured but tetracycline cannot be used successfully as a single dose regimen so that compliance presents a problem with this group and with co-trimoxazole.

Epidemiological treatment. Sexual partners of patients with gonorrhoea should be examined and appropriate specimens taken for culture. Whether contacts should then be given routine treatment is much in dispute. Such a course is recommended by the C.D.C. but Barlow & Phillips (1978) have drawn attention to the differences between the U.S.A. and Britain in patterns of presentation and treatment of sexually transmitted diseases, showing that routine epidemiological treatment of contacts in this country would include a large number of uninfected individuals.

Complicated infections

Positive rectal cultures in the absence of proctitis are commonly found in gonorrhoea, and are eliminated by standard treatment. Gonococcal proctitis is more resistant to treatment than urethritis, and procaine penicillin is usually given for 3–5 days rather than as single dose treatment. Spectinomycin gives good results (Fiumara, 1978).

Pharyngeal infection has proved difficult to eliminate; ampicillin-probenecid and spectinomycin have both proved relatively unsuccessful, and procaine penicillin-probenecid or tetracycline should be used.

Pelvic inflammatory disease. N. gonorrhoeae is a major cause of ascending endocervical infection in women and of pelvic inflammatory disease, although the relationships between sexually transmitted infection and the aetiology of non-specific pelvic inflammatory disease—in which aerobes and anaerobes characteristic of normal vaginal flora are found in the peritoneum or tubes—is still obscure. Indications that chlamydia may be a common cause of the syndrome must also be taken into account in planning treatment (page 429). In patients with illnesses mild enough to be treated without admission to hospital, tetracycline and penicillin appear equally effective. Cunningham et al (1977) obtained good results in 197 outpatients, 68 per cent of them with evidence of gonococcal infection, with tetracycline 0.5 g four times daily for 10 days, or with procaine penicillin 4.8 mega units with probenecid followed by ampicillin 0.5 g four times daily for 10 days.

For more seriously ill patients needing in-patient treatment, C.D.C. (1979) recommends benzyl penicillin 20 million units daily intravenously initially, followed by ampicillin orally to complete 10 days' treatment, with parenteral tetracycline as an alternative. Parenteral doxycycline may be preferable if a drug of this group is used (Chow et al, 1975). Excellent results have been obtained in 30 patients given cefoxitin 2 g eight-hourly (Sweet et al, 1979). Sexual partners of patients with gonococcal salpingitis should be examined and treated if necessary and the patients re-examined for evidence of persistent or recurrent infection.

Disseminated gonococcal infection. The common variety of disseminated infection is usually now known as the arthritis-dermatitis syndrome (Holmes et al, 1971). C.D.C. (1979) consider the following regimens equally effective:

Ampicillin 3.5 g or amoxycillin 3.0 g, each with probenecid, followed by 0.5 g of either drug four times daily for seven days.

Tetracycline 0.5 g four times daily for seven days.

Spectinomycin 2.0 g intramuscularly twice for three days (indicated for penicillinase-producing gonococcal infection).

Erythromycin 0.5 g four times daily for seven days.

Benzyl penicillin 10 mega units intravenously daily until the patient improves, followed by ampicillin 0.5 g four times daily to complete seven days' treatment.

Gonococcal meningitis and endocarditis are treated with high dose intravenous penicillin.

CHLAMYDIAL INFECTIONS

Advances in technique of cell culture have led to rapid changes in our knowledge of chlamydial disease. These organisms are now classified in two species, *C. psittaci* causing psittacosis-ornithosis, and *C. trachomatis*. Different serotypes of the latter species are important in the causation of non-gonococcal urethritis and related syndromes (serotypes D-K), of lymphogranuloma venereum (L1, L2 and L3), and of endemic trachoma (A, B, Ba, C). The specific name *C. trachomatis* has now replaced the former term TRIC agent (trachoma-inclusion conjunctivitis).

Chlamydia trachomatis is now established as the main cause of non-gonococcal urethritis, being responsible for 40–50 per cent of cases in a number of studies (reviewed by Schachter, 1978; Handsfield, 1978; Ridgway, 1979). Of the non-chlamydial causes *Ureaplasma urealyticum* (formerly 'T' strain mycoplasma) is probably responsible for some, while *Haemophilus vaginalis, Trichomonas vaginalis*, Candida species, *Herpesvirus hominis* type 2, and other viruses and bacteria may sometimes be involved. *C. trachomatis* has also been implicated in the causation of pelvic inflammatory disease, being isolated from the cervix in 19 of 53 patients with acute salpingitis, and from 1 of 18 with lower genital tract infections but not from 12 women with no signs of genital infection (Mårdh et al, 1977). Other syndromes in which *C. trachomatis* appears aetiologically important are acute epididymitis in young men (Berger et al, 1978), non-gonococcal ophthalmia neonatorum, and a particular variety of infant pneumonia seen mainly so far in the U.S.A. (Beem & Saxon, 1977; Harrison et al, 1978).

Cell culture techniques have also enabled more accurate study of the effect of antimicrobial agents on *C. trachomatis*. These organisms are very susceptible to rifampicin, tetracyclines and erythromycin, moderately susceptible to sulphonamides, resistant to penicillins and highly resistant to aminoglycosides.

Non-gonococcal urethritis

Treatment of NGU presents a difficult problem; spontaneous remission is noted in about 30 per cent of patients, but relapse is also common, and the causal diversity of the syndrome makes definition of the rôle of antimicrobial agents especially hard. Nevertheless recent studies, some of them utilizing the selective effects on putative causes of the syndrome, have enabled treatment policies to be evolved. Bowie et al (1976) showed that patients with chlamydia-positive but ureaplasma-negative NGU responded to a sulphonamide, active against the former organism but not the latter. Streptomycin and spectinomycin were unsuccessful in the chlamydial group, but produced a clinical response in those patients with *U. urealyticum* cultures when the organism was eradicated but not in those patients with persistently positive cultures. Similarly Oriel et al (1977) isolated *C. trachomatis* from 17 of 63 men with gonorrhoea successfully treated with spectinomycin. All these 17 men developed post-gonococcal urethritis, as did eight men from whom *C. trachomatis* had not been isolated.

The treatment of choice for NGU is at present tetracycline in a dose of 0.25 g four times daily. There is some dispute about the optimal duration of treatment, but 14- or 21-day courses at this dose range, or a dose of 2 g daily for seven days, certainly eradicate chlamydial infection and relieve symptoms (Schachter, 1978). The most common regimen in clinics in England and Wales is one or other form of tetracycline, given for five or seven days, with a range of 4–21 days (Adler, 1978b). Minocycline, with some advantage in its less frequent dose schedule, is about as effective as tetracycline (Oriel et al, 1975; Prentice et al, 1976). Pregnant patients or patients intolerant of tetracycline can be given erythromycin, and patients with oculogenital infection should be given 1 per cent chlortetracycline eye ointment four times daily in addition to systemic treatment with tetracycline or erythromycin.

The problem of combining optimal treatment of gonorrhoea with that of NGU is analyzed in a thoughtful review by Richmond & Oriel (1978). When diagnostic facilities for chlamydial infection are available, they recommend that patients treated for gonorrhoea with penicillin, ampicillin or spectinomycin should then receive tetracycline if chlamydia are cultured from the initial specimens. If laboratory facilities for the culture of chlamydia are not available, patients with treated gonorrhoea shown to have NGU at two-week follow-up should also be treated.

Sexual contacts of patients with NGU should be given a full course of tetracycline; where this is not routine practice, screening for chlamydial infection is advisable. Since *C. trachomatis* can be isolated from 30–60 per cent of patients with gonorrhoea, Richmond & Oriel (1978) consider there may be a case for routine treatment following eradication of the gonococcus when culture facilities for chlamydia are not available.

Lymphogranuloma venereum

The serotypes of *C. trachomatis* responsible for LGV differ in a number of respects from other members of the species, notably in greater invasive ability in mice and in other tests. Little recent information is available about treatment. Tetracyclines and sulphonamides are apparently effective, but prolonged treatment is usually advised for at least two weeks in acute inguinal disease, three weeks for rectal disease and longer periods for more chronic infections.

It is uncertain to what extent resolution is attributable to therapy. Fever and pain were promptly relieved by seven-day courses of either tetracycline or co-trimoxazole, in a recent study from Ethiopia, although resolution and healing of buboes was not complete for two or three weeks (Perine et al, 1979).

Ophthalmia neonatorum

Gonococcal ophthalmia neonatorum should be treated by high dose intravenous penicillin (50 000 units/kg/day in two divided doses) for 7–10 days, together with saline cleansing of the eyes when needed.

Chlamydial ophthalmia is treated topically with 1 per cent chlortetracycline eye ointment four-hourly, for at least two weeks and perhaps for as long as 5–6 weeks. Because prolonged local treatment of this type is difficult to achieve, many authorities (Richmond & Oriel, 1978) recommend, in addition to topical treatment, oral erythromycin 6 mg per kg six-hourly for at least two weeks. Both parents should also be treated for chlamydial infection.

Chancroid

Haemophilus ducreyi has similar sensitivities to other species in this genus, and there is therefore a considerable choice of suitable drugs. Streptomycin 1–3 g daily in divided doses for five days or tetracycline 250–500 mg 6-hourly for 4–5 days have been recommended, tetracycline therapy being continued for 12 days if the nodes have suppurated. Some prefer sulphonamides (4 g daily until healing) or streptomycin to tetracyclines because they eliminate the risk of masking syphilis, and on the ground of lesser cost. Among American troops in Saigon, Kerber et al (1969) obtained good results with sulfisoxazole (sulphafurazole) 4 g daily and with this drug together with tetracycline, but very poor results with tetracycline alone; resistance may have emerged because of the large amount of 'bootleg' antibiotics consumed by prostitutes in Vietnam.

The causal organism is also very susceptible to erythromycin and good clinical results have been noted in a small number of patients treated with this agent (Carpenter et al, 1979).

Single dose treatment has also been successful in treating chancroid, Stamps (1974) obtaining healing in 30 of 31 patients within seven days by this method. A good comparison between two regimens was made in a prospective study by Hammond et al (1979) during an outbreak of chancroid. Of 32 patients given a single dose of doxycycline (300 mg), eight showed a poor response of the 30 who returned for follow-up examination. Of 30 patients given sulfisoxazole (1 g four times daily for a week) only 19 were followed and six of them showed poor response. Large buboes and genital lesions healed slowly in both groups.

Trichomoniasis

A variety of nitroimidazole compounds is now available for the treatment of trichomoniasis. Metronidazole is highly effective, and can be given either as a conventional seven-day course or in a single dose of 2 g (Csonka, 1971). Both give good results; a higher incidence of side-effects is seen with single dose treatment, but patients often fail to complete longer courses. Nouira (1978) proposes a compromise regimen of 500 mg twice daily for three days with which he obtained complete success in 52 women with confirmed vaginal trichomoniasis. Their partners were treated in the same way.

The propriety of using the drug early in pregnancy is discussed on page 368. There is no evidence that increased resistance of Trichomonas to metronidazole is a cause of failure, or that the presence in the vagina of numerous bacteria which inactive metronidazole significantly affects the response to treatment.

Nifuratel has been used for vaginal trichomoniasis; when given by combined oral (200 mg three times daily for seven days) and local (250 mg pessaries nightly × 10) administration has been shown as less effective than metronidazole in a comparative trial by Evans & Catterall (1970). Nimorazole, a nitroimidazole derivative formerly known as nitrimidazine, has also been compared with metronidazole and found less effective (Evans & Catterall, 1971), with cure rates of 68 per cent and 89 per cent respectively, although results as good as those with metronidazole were reported by Moffett et al (1971) and by Cohen (1971). Metronidazole emerges as superior to these contenders in the treatment of trichomoniasis. Its continued efficacy where treatment can be rigidly controlled has been established by Keighley (1971) who cured 488 of 496 female prisoners (98.3 per cent) with one seven-day course. Nevertheless, occasional patients are seen who will be cured by, or will be more tolerant of, one of the newer drugs.

Two more recent compounds shown to be effective are tinidazole and secnidazole. Videau et al (1978) obtained a 97 per cent cure rate in 140 patients using a single 2 g dose of the latter compound, comparing well with cure rates of the same order with single dose metronidazole and tinidazole. Single dose treatment of trichomonas infection is also effective in men, who should be treated at the same time as their partners. Kawamura (1978) treated 73 men successfully with a single dose of tinidazole (1 g) or metronidazole (1.5 g); all were cured at careful follow-up examination seven and 14 days later. Difficulty in persuading male consorts to undergo treatment is increased by the fact that only about 10 per cent of male infections produce symptoms. Some observers claim that the male disease is commonly self-limiting if re-infection is prevented by treatment of the female. The organism may, nevertheless, underly some chronic infections in the male, and Catterall (1965) successfully managed 27/38 cases of prostatitis, believed to be of trichomonal origin, with metronidazole.

Granuloma inguinale

This doubtfully venereal disease is due to *Calymmatobacterium granulomatis*. Most authors are agreed that the choice lies between streptomycin (administered for 5 days) or tetracycline (500 mg 6-hourly for 10–15 days). Davis (1970) describes 14 cases, seven of whom also had evidence of syphilis; eight of the 10 males were homosexuals. With one exception, all responded to tetracycline 2 g per day given until the lesions were completely healed (1–4 weeks). Two patients treated over several weeks with ampicillin (up to 4 g per day) failed to respond and were subsequently successfully treated with tetracycline.

Vaginal candidiasis

This is discussed on p. 368.

OTHER SPIROCHAETOSES

Relapsing fever

Borrelia recurrentis (reviewed by Southern & Sanford, 1969) is sensitive to arsenicals and to various antibiotics. Penicillin, which originally replaced arsenicals, is now generally considered inferior to tetracyclines, which are effective in remarkably low dosage. Bryceson et al (1970) found that 250 mg tetracycline given intravenously over 2–3 minutes cleared the blood of spirochaetes within $2\frac{1}{2}$ hours. Two intramuscular injections of 150 mg at an interval of 6 hours were also effective. There was no relapse in 18 patients so treated, nor in 45 patients given a total dose of 4.3–5.5 g over 4–5 days.

Single dose treatment has now been used in both forms of the disease. Perine et al (1974) cured 26 patients with louse-borne relapsing fever using a single dose of 100 mg doxycycline, and de Clercq et al (1975) employed this method successfully in 103 patients with tick-borne disease.

Other single dose treatments were evaluated by Butler et al (1978). Tetracycline 0.5 g by mouth, 0.5 g erythromycin by mouth, tetracycline 0.25 g intravenously and a single injection of procaine penicillin (600 000 units) were all effective, although parenteral penicillin was slower in its action than parenteral tetracycline.

Antibiotic treatment of relapsing fever is bedevilled by the almost universal development of a characteristic Jarisch-Herxheimer reaction showing the prodromal, chill and flush phases of endotoxic fever. Cardiorespiratory disturbance in the flush phase may be so severe that patients die. Correction of extracellular fluid depletion, cardiac failure and hypoxia may prevent fatalities. Hydrocortisone has little effect on the reaction (Warrell et al, 1970; Butler et al, 1978). Bryceson (1970) recommends a small initial dose of penicillin (20 000 units of benzyl with 60 000 units of procaine penicillin) followed by tetracycline on the following day. Butler et al (1978) consider single dose tetracycline or erythromycin optimal therapy and that a saline infusion should accompany treatment in anticipation of a severe J-H reaction.

Rat-bite fever. Roughgarden (1965) describes the clinical manifestations, diagnosis and laboratory investigation of the acute illnesses caused by *Streptobacillus moniliformis* and *Spirillum minus*. Penicillin is the drug of choice for both infections, which respond to as little as 0.6 mega units daily. Treatment should be given for not less than seven days. Streptomycin and tetracycline are also effective, but sulphonamides have uniformly failed. McGill et al (1966) successfully treated two patients in this country with penicillin (0.5 mega units, 6-hourly) plus streptomycin (0.5–1 g, 12-hourly). Bacterial endocarditis due to either organism is said to require 12–15 mega units penicillin per day for three to four weeks.

Leptospirosis

This infection is in a different category, in regard both to the causative organism and its response to treatment. *Leptospira* spp. are susceptible in varying degrees to most of the major antibiotics. Nevertheless the evaluation of their effect presents unusual difficulties in all three spheres, *in vitro*, in the experimental animal and in the clinical field, and their place in the treatment of this disease is still the subject of a controversy which breaks out in print from time to time.

In vitro studies are complicated by the fact that different degrees of anti-leptospiral activity are exerted by antibiotics over a very wide range of concentrations, and any quantitative result depends on the criterion adopted. Very low concentrations of penicillin will inhibit the normally slow growth of the organism, but motility is retained, and very much higher concentrations fail to sterilize a culture. The effective concentrations determined by various authors, using different methods, are therefore not comparable or worth quoting.

Animal studies meet another difficulty: the guinea-pig and hamster, although suitably susceptible to the infection, are also uniquely susceptible to a 'toxic' effect not only of penicillin but of tetracyclines and macrolides, and are liable to succumb to this when adequate doses are given. These drug deaths have interfered with animal studies of the treatment of *L. icterohaemorrhagiae* infection, but a beneficial effect has nevertheless been demonstrated for a number of antibiotics, including penicillin, various tetracycline compounds, streptomycin, erythromycin and cephalothin.

The clinical value of antibiotic treatment is difficult to assess (Heath et al, 1965). It is clearly necessary to distinguish the severe infections caused by *L. icterohaemorrhagiae*, occurring sporadically, the diagnosis of which is often delayed, from those due to other serotypes, which are milder generally. Moreover, most patients with leptospirosis recover spontaneously. For all these reasons, there is a great lack of convincing clinical trials of antibiotic treatment in leptospirosis. Some studies have shown no effect on the course of the disease or on the incidence of complications, but Kocen (1962) showed a shortened duration of fever in patients given penicillin during the first four days of the disease. Most authors favour treatment of at least the more serious forms of leptospirosis with parenteral penicillin or tetracycline, with a preference for the former in view of the risks of renal failure in severe leptospirosis. Ampicillin or amoxycillin are acceptable alternatives, Münnich & Lakatos (1976) quoting good results in 28 patients infected with a variety of serotypes treated with these agents for six days. Prevention may be as difficult as cure, since Broom & Norris (1957) described a laboratory-acquired infection in spite of immediate penicillin administration. Problems of human leptospirosis are extensively reviewed by Feigin & Anderson (1975).

References

Adler M W 1978a Brit J Vener Dis 54: 15
Adler M W 1978b Brit J Vener Dis 54: 428
Arya O P, Rees E, Percival A et al 1978 Brit J Vener Dis 54: 28
Barlow D, Phillips I 1978 Lancet 1: 761
Beem M O, Saxon E M 1977 New Engl J Med 296: 306
Berg S W, Kilpatrick M E, Harrison W O, McCutchan J A 1979 New Engl J Med 301: 509
Berger R E, Alexander E R, Monda G O, et al 1978 New Engl J Med 298: 301
Bowie W R, Alexander E R, Floyd J F, et al 1976 Lancet 2: 1276
Broom J C, Norris T St M 1957 Lancet 1: 721
Bryceson A D M, Parry E H O, Perine P L et al 1970 Quart J Med 39: 129
Butler T, Jones P K, Wallace C K 1978 J Infect Dis 137: 573
Carpenter J, Back A, Gehle D 1979 Abstracts—19th Interscience Conference on Antimicrobial Agents and Chemotherapy
Catterall R D 1965 Brit J Vener Dis 41: 302
Center for Disease Control 1976 J Infect Dis 134: 97
Center for Disease Control 1979 J Infect Dis 139: 496
Chow A W, Malkasian K L, Marshall J R, Guze L B 1975 Antimicrob Ag Chemother 7: 133
Cohen L 1971 Brit J Vener Dis 47: 177
Collart P, Borel L J, Durel P 1962 Ann Inst Pasteur 103: 953
Csonka G W 1971 Brit J Vener Dis 47: 456
Cunningham F G, Hauth J C, Strong J D et al 1977 New Engl J Med 296: 1380
Davis C M 1970 J Amer Med Ass 211: 632
de Clercq A G, Meheus A Z, de Pierpont E, Nyirashema C 1975 E African Med J 52: 428
Duncan W C, Holder W R, Roberts D P, Knox J M 1972 Antimicrob Ag Chemother 1: 210
Editorial 1977 Lancet 1: 340
Elliott W C, Reynolds G, Thornsberry C et al 1977 J Infect Dis 135: 939
Evans B A, Catterall R D 1970 Brit Med J 2: 335
Evans B A, Catterall R D 1971 Brit Med J 4: 146
Farrell L 1969 Brit J Vener Dis 45: 232
Feigin R D, Anderson D C 1975 CRC Crit Rev Clin Lab Sci 5: 413
Fiumara N J 1978 J Amer Med Ass 239: 735
Gentle G H K 1965 Brit J Vener Dis 41: 155
Hammond G W, Slutchuk M, Lian C J et al 1979 J Antimicrob Chemother 5: 261
Handsfield H H 1978 Med Clin N America 62: 925
Harrison H R, English M G, Lee C K, Alexander E R 1978 New Engl J Med 298: 702
Heath C W, Alexander A D, Galton M M 1965 New Engl J Med 273: 857, 915
Holmes K K, Counts G W, Beaty H N 1971 Ann Intern Med 74: 979
Idsøe O, Guthe T, Willcox R R 1972 Bull WHO 47: supplement
Johnson D W, Kvale P A, Afable V L, et al 1970 New Engl J Med 283: 1
Karney W W, Pedersen A H B, Nelson M et al 1977 New Engl J Med 296: 889
Karney W W, Turck M, Holmes K K 1973 J Infect Dis 128: S399
Kaufman R E, Johnson R E, Jaffe H W et al 1976 New Engl J Med 294:1
Kawamura N 1978 Brit J Vener Dis 54: 81
Keighley E E 1971 Brit Med J 1: 207
Kerber R E, Rowe C E, Gilbert K R 1969 Arch Dermatol 100: 604
Knudsen E A, Aastrup B 1965 Brit J Vener Dis 41: 177
Kocen R S 1962 Brit Med J 1: 1181
McCormack W M, Finland M 1976 Ann Intern Med 84: 712
McCracken G H, Kaplan J M 1974 J Amer Med Ass 228: 855
McGill R C, Martin A M, Edmunds P N 1966 Brit Med J 1: 1213
Mårdh P-A, Ripa T, Svensson L, Weström L 1977 New Engl J Med 296: 1377

Moffett M, McGill M I, Schofield C B S, Masterton G 1971 Brit J Vener Dis 47: 173
Münnich D, Lakatos M 1976 Chemotherapy 22: 372
Nicol C S 1962 Practitioner 189: 491
Nouira H 1978 Practitioner 220: 790
Oriel J D, Reeve P, Nicol C S 1975 J Amer Vener Dis Ass 2: 17
Oriel J D, Ridgway G L, Tchamouroff S, Owen J 1977 Brit J Vener Dis 53: 226
Perine P, Andersen A, Krause S et al 1979 Abstracts—19th Interscience Conference on Antimicrobial Agents and Chemotherapy
Perine P L, Krause D W, Awoke S, McDade J E 1974 Lancet 2: 742
Perine P L, Thornsberry C, Schalla W et al 1977 Lancet 2: 993
Phillips I, Rimmer D, Ridley M, Lynn R, Warren C 1970 Lancet 1: 263
Pirozzi D J 1973 Ann Intern Med 79: 447
Platt R, Fiumara N J, McCormack W M 1979 Abstracts—19th Interscience Conference on Antimicrobial Agents and Chemotherapy
Porter I A, Rutherford H W 1977 Brit J Vener Dis 53: 115
Prentice M J, Taylor-Robinson D, Csonka G W 1976 Brit J Vener Dis 52: 269
Price J D, Fluker J L 1978 Brit J Vener Dis 54: 165
Price J D, Fluker J L, Giles A J H 1977 Brit J Vener Dis 53: 113
Rahim G 1975 Brit J Vener Dis 51: 179
Reyn A, Bentzon M W 1969 Brit J Vener Dis 45: 223
Rice N S C, Dunlop E M C, Jones B R, et al 1970 Brit J Vener Dis 46: 1
Richmond S J, Oriel J D 1978 Brit Med J 2: 480
Ridgway G L In: Reeves D, Geddes A (eds) Recent advances in infection. Churchill Livingstone, Edinburgh, 1979 p 183
Roughgarden J W 1965 Arch Intern Med 116: 39
Rudolph A H, Price E V 1973 J Amer Med Ass 223: 499
Schachter J 1978 New Engl J Med 298: 490
Shapiro L, Lentz J W 1970 Amer J Obstet Gynec 108: 471
Southern P M, Sanford J P 1969 Medicine (Baltimore) 48: 129
Stamps T J 1974 J Trop Med Hyg 77: 55
Sweet R L, Biderman A, Hadley W K, Draper D 1979 Abstracts—19th Interscience Conference on Antimicrobial Agents and Chemotherapy
Tennican P O, Leis A A, Strawbridge K M 1979 Abstracts—19th Interscience Conference on Antimicrobial Agents and Chemotherapy
Thin R N, Symonds M A E, Shaw E J et al 1977 Brit J Vener Dis 53: 118
Thornsberry C, Jaffee H, Brown S T et al 1977 J Amer Med Ass 237: 2405
Tramont E C 1976 J Amer Med Ass 236: 2206
Videau D, Niel G, Siboulet A, Catalan F 1978 Brit J Vener Dis 54: 77
Warrell D A, Pope H M, Parry E H O, Perine P L, Bryceson A D M 1970 Clin Sci 39: 123
Waterworth P M, Oriel J D, Ridgway G L, Subramanian S 1979 Brit J Vener Dis 55: 343
Willcox R R 1970 Brit J Vener Dis 46: 217
Willcox R R 1971 Brit J Vener Dis 47: 31
Willcox R R 1977 Brit J Vener Dis 53: 314
Wise P J, Neu H C 1974 J Infect Dis 129: S266

25

Antiviral chemotherapy

The present striking contrast between bacteria and viruses in the availability of effective antimicrobial therapy arises from a number of special difficulties. The metabolism of bacterial pathogens is often sufficiently different from that of the host to make them susceptible to agents which have little or no effect on the host's metabolism. Viral replication, on the other hand, occurs by distortion of normal cellular processes causing the cell to synthesize viral nucleic acids and proteins in place of normal cellular components. This intimate relationship between normal and infected cell processes means that compounds capable of interrupting viral replication will have to show an extraordinary degree of selective toxicity if they are not at the same time to inhibit similar processes crucial to the metabolic needs of normal cells. Nevertheless, any enzymic capacity possessed by the virus itself, for example the RNA-polymerase of the poxviruses, or even host enzymes sufficiently modified to subserve the parasite's needs, may well show (just as bacterial enzymes do) different susceptibility to inhibitors from that of the corresponding mammalian enzyme.

In recent years many differences have been revealed between viral and host systems of genome replication, with a consequent increase in potential forms of selective antiviral chemotherapy. The remarkably low toxicity and wide antiviral range of the interferons also provide evidence of the differences which can be exploited between viruses and mammalian cells. Until very recently it was held that viruses are not susceptible to any of the agents used for the treatment of bacterial diseases. It now appears that some antibacterial agents, albeit in concentrations very much greater than those required to inhibit the growth of sensitive bacteria, exert some antiviral effects. Rifampicin in a concentration about 1000 times that effective against sensitive bacteria has been shown to inhibit the growth of several poxviruses and an adenovirus. It acts, both in bacteria and viruses, by inhibiting DNA-dependent RNA-polymerase, and resistant variants of vaccinia virus arise quickly in experimental systems. Fusidic acid and cephalosporin P_1 in concentrations of 25–50 μg per ml also inhibit some viruses. These are encouraging signs that viruses are perhaps not quite so insusceptible to attack as was once feared, but the very high plasma concentrations of these agents which would be required for treatment makes it unlikely that these findings will have any immediate clinical benefit. The Chlamydia, which were at one time included amongst the viruses but differ from them fundamentally (page 428) are sensitive to tetracyclines and some other agents.

One serious therapeutic difficulty is that the signs and symptoms of virus disease often appear after peak viral growth is over, the clinical manifestations being due to inflammatory and other processes. It may be, therefore, that symptomatic control of such infections is more likely to be obtained with compounds which interfere with the host response than with those which interfere with viral growth. It follows that substances which inhibit viral replication are more likely to be of use in prophylaxis than in treatment.

Large and growing numbers of compounds have been shown to exert antiviral activity both *in vitro* and against experimental infections in animals. How many of these antiviral effects can be put to any clinical use remains to be seen.

In this chapter we will consider only those compounds which have been developed as far as clinical trials in man, or at least in laboratory primates. Many extensive reviews of antiviral chemotherapy are available, see especially that of Stalder (1977), and those edited by Merigan (1976) and Herrmann (1977).

Interferons

First described by Isaacs and Lindemann (1957), interferons are a family of closely related proteins liberated by cells which are actively synthesizing virus and which act on other cells reducing their susceptibility to viral infection. With some exceptions, interferons will protect only the cells of the animal species in which they were manufactured, or those of closely related species. On the other hand, the protection afforded includes not only the inducing virus but a wide variety of unrelated viruses. Interferon production is blocked by actinomycin D which inhibits the synthesis of messenger-RNA and it appears that viral infection of the cell may induce (or derepress) the production of a messenger-RNA which codes the ribosome to produce interferon. They are proteins of molecular weight variously calculated to be between 19 000 and 160 000. They are destroyed by proteolytic but not by other enzymes and are otherwise remarkably stable. Some preparations are said to withstand 72°C for 1 hour but human interferon is considerably less heat-stable. They are active against a wide variety of both DNA and RNA viruses but viral sensitivity differs considerably. Their potency is at least comparable with that of antibacterial antibiotics: partially purified preparations inhibit viral growth in concentrations of about 1 or 2 μg per ml. Interferons are apparently of low toxicity and very poor antigens. Unlike neutralizing antibody, interferons have no effect on extra-cellular virus and do not prevent virus from penetrating cells. They appear to exert their effect very soon after the virus has entered the cell, interfering with the earliest stages of viral replication. Since they have generally little activity in species unrelated to the one in which they were produced, only human or possibly primate interferon is likely to be of any use for therapy in man.

Human leucocytes, and tissue culture lines of human diploid fibroblasts, are at present the chief sources for trials in man, and, long after monkey interferon was first shown to prevent smallpox vaccination from taking (M.R.C., 1962), and to be effective in vaccinial keratitis (Jones et al, 1962), the difficult technical problems of production and purification of human interferon are much nearer solution, and several promising clinical trials now reported. Extensive reviews have been published recently by Tyrrell (1976) and Baron & Dianzani (1977).

Merigan et al (1973) showed that intranasal administration of human leucocyte interferon induced only a small delay in the onset of symptoms of influenza B, but that a larger dose given for four days beginning one day before infection with a rhinovirus did reduce both clinical symptoms and virus shedding.

Interferon therapy has aroused especial interest in hepatitis B virus infections. Rapid reduction has been achieved in several markers of infection, notably in the levels of core antigen, and in two patients 'e' antigen disappeared during treatment. Indices of chronic infection usually returned rapidly once administration was stopped but lasted for nine and 15 weeks respectively in two patients treated for more than one month (Greenberg et al, 1976; Desmyter et al, 1976; Kingham et al, 1978).

The effect of interferon on herpes zoster has been studied in three trials, each of 30 patients, by Merigan et al (1978). Increase in dose, and in purity of the preparations was reflected in improved results, and in the later trials the number of days of pain experienced was almost halved in the group receiving interferon, while post-herpetic neuralgia was recorded in eight of 29 in the placebo groups compared with two of 29 treated with interferon.

Human leucocyte interferon was given, in 12-hourly intramuscular injections for 14 days, to a patient with laboratory acquired Ebola virus infection (Emond et al, 1977). The patient also received convalescent serum, the administration of which was followed by a striking fall in the concentration of virus circulating in his blood.

The concentration of cytomegalovirus in the urine of infants with congenital infection caused by this agent has been reduced by parenteral administration of human leucocyte interferon in large doses, but the effect was transient (Arvin et al, 1976; Emodi et al, 1976).

Interferon from human sources has also been applied locally, and a significant reduction in recurrence rates of dendritic ulcers caused by herpes simplex was reported by Coster et al (1977).

Interferon inducers

Of considerable interest is the possibility of treating systemic infections by stimulating endogenous interferon production.

An assortment of substances has been found to excite the production or release of preformed interferons. It appears that the anti-viral effects of the fungal products helenine (derived from *Penicillium funiculosum*) and statolon (derived from *Penicillium stoloniferum*) are exerted in this way (Rytel et al, 1966) and the mechanism of these effects is of great theoretical interest. Lampson et al (1967) showed that the interferon inducer in helenine is double-stranded RNA. Double- and multiple-stranded RNA is produced in cells infected with RNA viruses and this suggests that the origin of the interferon inducer in statolon and helenine is fungal virus and that the inducer is polystranded RNA (Banks et al, 1968; Kleinschmidt et al, 1968). This raises the possibility of using extracted polystranded RNA or synthetic analogues for therapeutic purposes. Some multi-stranded complexes of synthetic polyisosinic and polycytidinic acids are active inducers of interferons (Field et al, 1967). In man, interferon inducers have been used mainly by local application in attempting to prevent respiratory virus infections in volunteers. Significant effect has been scored in some trials but the benefits have usually been small (Hill et al, 1972; Panusarn et al, 1974; Reed et al, 1976; Stanley et al, 1976). Interferon induction has also been attempted in herpes simplex encephalitis

(Bellantini et al, 1971), and in subacute sclerosing panencephalitis (Leavitt et al, 1971). One of three patients to whom a pyran copolymer was administered in an attempt to influence the course of S.S.P.E. developed a haemolytic uraemic syndrome. More information will doubtless be forthcoming about the properties and potential toxicity of these interesting compounds.

Amantadines

These compounds appear to act by blocking entry of the virion into the host cell or by preventing uncoating of the infecting virus particles. Their main use has been in the prevention and treatment of infections by influenza A viruses, although they are active against some other viruses *in vitro*, including rubella and arenaviruses. Their effect in experimental systems is not profound and cell-to-cell spread of some strains is prevented only if the infecting dose is small. The drug is active against influenza A including H_2N_2 and H_3N_2 strains, and is also active in experimental systems against swine influenza (HSW_1N_1) (Grunert & Hoffmann, 1977), but has no inhibitory effect on influenza B.

Clinical experience with amantadine and its congeners is now extensive, since the parent compound was licensed in the U.S.A. in 1966. Numerous trials, many of them well controlled, in volunteers and in field conditions, have been carried out with somewhat discordant results, so that much uncertainty still prevails about the proper use of the compound. These uncertanties are probably attributable to varying immune state of different study populations, and to the relatively small effect of the compound. Certainly in most studies of attempted prevention of influenza A infection, some reduction in the incidence and severity of infection has been noted. For example, Oker-Blom et al (1970), in a controlled field trial among Finnish students, recorded a modest degree of protection against natural infection with influenza A2/Hong Kong. Serological evidence of infection was obtained in 27 of 192 amantadine-treated students, and in 57 of 199 in the placebo group, a protection rate of 52 per cent.

One especially useful trial was that of Galbraith (1975), carried out in general practice during two seasons when influenza A2 and B were both prevalent. Amantadine effected a mean reduction in the duration of fever of 23 hours in patients with influenza A2 infections, but had no effect in those caused by influenza B.

In terms of the prospects for antiviral chemotherapy, there have been several encouraging reports of the therapeutic use of amantadines. In natural outbreaks of influenza A2, there was more rapid defervescence of illness in patients treated within about 20 hours of the onset of symptoms with amantadine than in those treated with placebo (Hornick et al, 1969; Togo et al, 1970). The results in naturally occurring influenza A2/Hong Kong in Britain were somewhat disappointing (Galbraith et al, 1971). The mean duration of fever was significantly reduced in the treated group, but the duration of a variety of symptoms was no different in the two groups, although in some trials improvement in other features of the illness as well as in the duration of fever has been shown. Virus shedding is, however, usually not reduced with amantadine treatment.

Several allied compounds have been shown to act in a similar way both in prevention and treatment. Rimantadine seems to be about as effective as the parent compound. In a trial during an influenza A2 outbreak in a penitentiary, both compounds induced a more rapid reduction in fever and a shortened duration of fever than that recorded in the placebo group but, as in other trials, the advantage was small, about one day less fever in the treated groups (Wingfield et al, 1969). A number of recent comparative trials of amantadine and rimantadine are reviewed by La Montagne & Galasso (1978).

Another compound, spiroamantadine, was shown effective in mitigating influenza in volunteers when given before challenge with a partly attenuated strain (Beare et al, 1972). A later trial showed no effect when the drug was started 46 hours after virus inoculation, but the titre of virus in nasal washings declined more rapidly in the treated group (Arroyo et al, 1975).

A claim which, if substantiated by further work is of some importance, is that the increased resistance of small airways recorded in patients with influenza resolves more rapidly in patients treated with amantadine (Little et al, 1976).

Since amantadine is about as effective in prevention as influenza vaccine (although only for A strains, whereas influenza B is included in polyvalent vaccine), it is perhaps surprising that the drug has been so little used. Jackson (1977) recommends its use in a variety of circumstances, namely household and hospital contacts of influenza A infection, those in residential institutions, people with chronic chest or heart disease or immune deficiency, vaccinated adults at high risk during periods of unusual exposure, hospital workers when no vaccine is available for the prevalent A strain, and patients with acute influenza A seen in the first 48 hours of illness. Perhaps the most important limitation in applying these recommendations is the unpredictable behaviour of influenza viruses and the poor discriminatory power of clinical diagnosis when many respiratory viruses are prevalent in the community. We believe the drug could be used, in a selective manner, both in prevention and treatment, for groups at special risk from influenza A infection, but that this policy could be implemented only at a time of proven high prevalence of this virus as a cause of acute respiratory disease.

The toxicity of amantadine is low, and has been well documented because of its extensive use in Parkinson's disease. A small proportion of patients suffer mental and neurological symptoms, insomnia, confusion, vertigo or hallucinations, usually in the first 48 hours of treatment, which resolve rapidly when administration is stopped.

Amantadine is excreted unchanged in the urine, and patients with renal failure and high blood levels of the drug may develop confusional states and toxic psychosis. A few patients develop an unusual drug effect, livedo reticularis.

Inhibitors of DNA viral replication

A number of antiviral purine and pyrimidine nucleoside analogues has been synthesized, and several of them have been authenticated for use in human infections caused by herpes viruses.

Idoxuridine

Idoxuridine and the corresponding 2′-deoxy-5-bromouridine are thymidine analogues which inhibit the utilization of thymidine in the rapid synthesis of DNA which normally occurs in herpes-infected cells. The possibility of a similar effect in uninfected cells and the rapid dehalogenation of these compounds in the body makes them unpromising for systemic use, and it has been used principally for the treatment of herpes keratitis and cutaneous herpes. Its use in herpetic eye infections is discussed in the following section on vidarabine. In cutaneous herpes, variable results may be the result of poor contact between the agent and the infected cells. Juel-Jensen and MacCallum (1965) who had previously failed to influence the disease by local applications of idoxuridine ointment, reduced the average duration of lesions from 8.9 to 5.5 days, by injecting 0.1 per cent idoxuridine into the affected skin with a spray-gun.

Idoxuridine in dimethylsulphoxide has been used successfully in recurrent genital herpes. A 20 per cent solution was superior to a 5 per cent solution, which was superior to placebo (Parker, 1977).

Herpes zoster

Juel-Jensen et al (1970) conducted a controlled trial in 20 patients with herpes zoster. The treated group received idoxuridine in the form of a 40 per cent solution in dimethylsulphoxide, continuously applied to the affected area. No new lesions appeared after idoxuridine treatment was started, and pain abated much more quickly than in the controls. In later trials lower concentrations of idoxuridine were used. Dawber (1974) found that duration of vesicular phase, of healing time and of pain were reduced as effectively by four-hourly application of 5 per cent idoxuridine in 100 per cent dimethylsulphoxide (DMSO) as by 25 per cent idoxuridine applied two-hourly, while Simpson (1974) found no difference between 5 per cent and 40 per cent idoxuridine.

These results suggest that 5 per cent idoxuridine in 100 per cent DMSO (Herpid) should be applied to the early erythematous and vesicular lesions of herpes zoster. Unwanted effects include tenderness, local or generalized urticaria, and, if treatment is prolonged beyond three or four days, maceration of the skin.

Herpes simplex encephalitis

This form of encephalitis carries a poor prognosis, with a high risk of death or of residual neurological damage. Idoxuridine has been used in the form of daily intravenous infusions, and occasionally by intra-carotid infusion, in an attempt to mitigate the results of the infection. Although the disease is serious, the course varies greatly and unpredictably in individual patients and, as in other forms of brain damage, the effects of a particular form of treatment are difficult to assess.

Changing opinion about the use of antiviral agents in herpes encephalitis reveals the unreliability of historical comparisons and the need for controlled trials of high quality early in the evaluation of a new compound. Earlier favourable reports such as those of Nolan et al (1970) were contradicted by others such as that of Upton et al (1971). Its use in this condition came to an end with publication of a double-blind randomized trial (Boston Interhospital Virus Study Group, 1975) which showed no reduction of mortality or of concentration of herpes virus in the brain, while significant toxic effects on the bone marrow were recorded.

Cytarabine

Cytosine arabinoside, like the halogenated nucleosides, acts by inhibition of nucleic acid synthesis. It appears to act by depressing the formation of phosphorylated derivatives of deoxycytidine from their ribose-containing precursors. It is active against herpes group viruses and has been used in patients with severe varicella-zoster arising in the course of leukaemia and other malignant diseases, in zoster without underlying malignancy, and in severe herpes simplex infections. Its use in 25 patients including eight of their own, is summarized by Chow et al (1971), who noted dramatic clinical improvement in several instances. Most authors used a dose of 100 mg/m^2/day intravenously but in a later report Hryniuk et al (1972) claim that a response can be achieved with a lesser risk of toxic effects by lower doses, ranging from 10–100 mg/m^2/day for 1½ to 7 days.

Again, the early favourable reports have been tempered by later experience. Davis et al (1973) reported failure in a small controlled trial of varicella-zoster infections in immune-suppressed patients, and Stevens et al (1973), in a larger controlled study, found that no beneficial effect could be detected, and that dissemination of zoster was prolonged in some treated patients with lymphoma, in whom host responses were further impaired by the drug. Schimpff et al (1974) found that cytarabine failed to benefit cancer patients with localized zoster.

In herpes encephalitis also, cytarabine has failed to provide any benefit after a few early apparently favourable reports. In smallpox, a controlled trial of cytarabine was terminated when all nine treated patients died, compared with four of 11 who had received a placebo preparation (Monsur et al, 1975).

Although still used in anti-cancer chemotherapy, cytarabine has now been superseded by other drugs in the chemotherapy of viral disease.

Another interesting possible application for cytarabine has been propounded by Kraybill et al (1972) who administered the drug to two infants with congenital cytomegalovirus infection. Infection was not suppressed in either but the dose used was small.

Vidarabine (Adenine arabinoside, Ara-A, arabinofuranosyladenine)

This compound has actions similar to those of cytarabine, but shows appreciably less toxicity for normal cells and, in men, is less myelosuppressive and immunosuppressive than the earlier compounds. Several favourable reports of its use in systemic viral infections and in local treatment of herpes keratitis are now available.

Whitley et al (1976) gave the relatively low dose of 10 mg/kg/day for five days in 47 immunosuppressed patients with herpes zoster; 40 other patients received placebo infusions. The group receiving active compound showed benefit by several criteria, cessation of new vesicle formation, shorter time before the lesion formed pustules, and accelerated clearing of virus from the lesions. No changes in indices of bone marrow, kidney or liver function were noted even in immune-suppressed patients, but nausea and vomiting were fairly common (16 per cent), and a few patients developed diarrhoea or rashes. Encephalopathy has also been recorded, but usually at the higher dose range of 20 mg/kg/day, and when renal function is impaired; weakness and fatigue, jaw pain, tremor, and quickly reversible granulocytopenia and thrombocytopenia have also been noted (Sacks et al, 1979).

A collaborative study in herpes simplex encephalitis (Whitley et al, 1977) which included brain biopsy in every case and a double-blind placebo procedure, gave results suggestive of benefit from vidarabine. One month after the onset of treatment, five of 18 biopsy-positive patients who received the drug had died, compared with seven of ten in the placebo group. Of the biopsy-negative patients, one of 11 in the treated group, and three of 11 in the placebo group died. Although the difference in mortality between the biopsy-positive groups achieved significant levels ($P = 0.03$) it was unfortunate that the code was broken and the trial terminated at a comparatively early stage, especially as three additional patients in the treated group died in the following six months. It will now scarcely be possible to conduct further placebo-controlled trials in this condition and, until newer antiviral agents can be compared with vidarabine, this drug should be used in herpes simplex encephalitis. The trial dose was 15 mg/kg/day for 10 days.

Vidarabine has been used in other serious systemic viral infections, notably in cytomegalovirus infection (Chi'en et al, 1974; Phillips et al, 1977), and in hepatitis B infection. In two patients with chronic active hepatitis, vidarabine induced rapid decrease in Dane-particle associated DNA polymerase (Pollard et al, 1978), which in one of the patients remained undetectable in the following 12 months. The drug had no beneficial effect in the treatment of smallpox (Koplan et al, 1975), although the adverse effects of cytarabine were not seen.

Vidarabine is available for local treatment of herpetic eye infections in the form of an ointment containing 3 per cent of the active compound. A number of comparisons have been made showing a similar degree of effectiveness to that of idoxuridine in herpetic keratitis (Markham et al, 1977). Travers & Patterson (1978) showed vidarabine ointment and trifluorothymidine drops as highly and equally effective in herpetic keratitis, while in dendritic ulcers these two compounds are apparently somewhat more effective than idoxuridine (Falcon et al, 1977). Vidarabine used locally in the eye causes fewer unwanted effects than idoxuridine, and these are rare in the short-term. Allergic reactions occur, but vidarabine and idoxuridine do not cross-react in this respect.

Acyclovir (Acycloguanosine)

This purine nucleoside is a potent inhibitor of herpes viruses, but is inactive against vaccinia virus, adenovirus type 5 and many RNA viruses. It acts by inhibiting viral DNA polymerase, against which it is at least 30 times more active than against the host cell enzyme. It is highly stable after systemic administration and has low toxicity in mammalian cells and, so far, in man.

An early trial using 3 per cent ointment against placebo showed good results without adverse effects in herpes simplex corneal ulcers. The compound is also under trial for serious systemic herpes virus infections (Jones et al, 1979; Selby et al, 1979).

Ribavirin

This synthetic nucleoside is active *in vitro* against a number of RNA and DNA viruses. A few trials in prevention or early treatment of influenza in volunteers have shown at best marginal benefit, and in one trial four of 14 students receiving the active compound had transient rises in serum bilirubin (Magnussen et al, 1977; Togo & McCracken, 1976). The drug had no effect in chronic hepatitis B infection in chimpanzees (Denes et al, 1976).

Methisazone

This compound (N-methylisatin β-thiosemicarbazone) was shown by Bauer et al (1962) to be active against variola following a number of observations over the years that various thiosemicarbazones would inhibit poxviruses in mice and chick embryos. They appear to act on a late stage of viral protein synthesis, probably by selective inhibition of translation of late viral messenger RNA.

Anorexia, nausea and vomiting are common in those treated with the drug, despite the use of cyclizine or chlorpromazine. Diarrhoea, rashes and thinning of the hair have also been described. Alcohol may exacerbate the side-effects and it is currently recommended that the drug should not be given to pregnant women or to those with liver or kidney disease. By the time the lesions of variola have appeared viral multiplication is rapidly declining, and methisazone has no effect on the course of the disease. The principal use of these compounds has been in the contact prophylaxis of smallpox. Several successful trials have been reported in variola major. Bauer (1965) reported six cases with two deaths amongst 2297 close contacts treated with methisazone and 114 cases with 20 deaths amongst 2842 similar untreated contacts. Similar success has been described in the prophylaxis of variola minor (do Valle et al, 1965). Subsequent trials in West Pakistan in contacts of variola major have given much less favourable results (Heiner et al, 1971) and it appears that methisazone is less valuable in prophylaxis that at first appeared. Using a related compound, M & B 7714 for the prophylaxis of variola major, Rao et al (1966) were successful, finding 40 cases with 7 deaths amongst 197 treated contacts and 80 cases with 12 deaths amongst 201 untreated contacts. Methisazone given at the time of vaccination depresses the local reaction but also possibly impairs the antibody response (Landsman & Grist, 1964). Good results were claimed in 16 patients with ectopic vaccinial lesions, in four with eczema vaccinatum, and two with vaccinia gangrenosa (Jaroszynska-Weinberger, 1970). Established eczema vaccinatum was favourably influenced by methisazone treatment in 14/24 of Adels and Oppé's (1966) patients, some of whom also received anti-vaccinial gamma globulin. Progressive vaccinia (vaccinia gangrenosa) which without treatment is almost invariably fatal has been treated by a number of authors (usually together with anti-vaccinial gamma globulin) and half have recovered (Connolly, 1966).

Methisazone should not be used as a substitute for vaccination, which currently remains the best prophylactic, and treatment should not begin before vaccination lest it interfere with the development of immunity.

Other antiviral compounds

Of the many compounds fully tested in laboratory models, several other than those already discussed have reached clinical trials but for various reasons have not achieved widespread application in human disease. Two isoquinoline derivatives were shown to have suppressive effects on infectivity or replication of several viruses but, in a well controlled trial Stark et al (1970) found that prophylactic use of one of these compounds failed to influence the incidence of respiratory virus infections, including influenza, in a students' residence.

Another compound inosiplex (isoprinosine), a derivative of inosine dimethylaminoisopropanolol, showed moderate activity in therapeutic trials against a rhino virus and against influenza, although, paradoxically, it was ineffective in several prophylactic trials. It may act by immune stimulation rather than by its antiviral action (Hadden et al, 1977; Soto et al, 1973).

The rôle of ascorbic acid in the common cold is discussed in Chapter 19. The subject is fully reviewed by Dykes & Meier (1975).

References

Adels B R, Oppé T E 1966 Lancet 1: 18
Arroyo M, Beare A S, Reed S E, Craig J W 1975 J Antimicrob Chemother 1: Suppl 87
Arvin A M, Yeager A S, Merigan T C 1976 J Infect Dis 133: A205
Banks G T, Buck K W, Chain E B et al 1968 Nature (Lond) 218: 542
Baron S, Dianzani F (eds) 1977 Texas Rep Biol Med vol 35. The interferon system: a current review to 1978
Bauer D J 1965 Ann NY Acad Sci 130: 110
Bauer D J, Dumbell K R, Fox-Hulme P, Sadler P W 1962 Bull Wld Hlth Org 26: 727
Beare A S, Hall T S, Tyrrell D A J 1972 Lancet 1: 1039
Bellantini J A, Catalano L W Jr, Chambers R W 1971 J Pediat 78: 136
Boston Interhospital Virus Study Group 1975 New Engl J Med 292: 599
Ch'ien L T, Cannon N J, Whitley R J et al 1974 J Infect Dis 130: 32
Chow A W, Foerster J, Hryniuk W 1971 Antimicrob Agents Chemother 1970 p 214
Connolly J H 1966 Practitioner 197: 373
Coster D J, Falcon M G, Cantell K, Jones B R 1977 Trans Ophthal Soc UK 97: 327
Davis C M, Van Dersarl J V, Coltman C A 1973 J Amer Med Ass 224: 122
Dawber R 1974 Brit Med J 2: 526
Denes A E, Ebert J W, Berquist K R et al 1976 Antimicrob Ag Chemother 10: 571
Desmyter J, Ray M B, De Groote J et al 1976 Lancet 2: 645
do Valle L A R, de Melo P R, de Salles Gomes L F, Proenca L M 1965 Lancet 2: 976
Dykes M H M, Meier P 1975 J Amer Med Ass 231: 1073
Emodi G, O'Reilly R, Muller A et al 1976 J Infect Dis 133: A199
Emond R T D, Evans B, Bowen E T W, Lloyd G 1977 Brit Med J 2: 541
Falcon M G, Jones B R, Williams H P et al 1977 Trans Ophthal Soc UK 97: 345
Field A K, Tytell A A, Lampson G P, Hilleman M R 1967 Proc Nat Acad Sci (Wash) 58: 1004
Galbraith A W 1975 J Antimicrob Chemother 1 Suppl: 81
Galbraith A W, Oxford J S, Schild G C, Potter C W, Watson G I 1971 Lancet 2: 113
Greenberg H B, Pollard R B, Lutwick L I et al 1976 New Engl J Med 295: 517
Grunert R R, Hoffmann C E 1977 J Infect Dis 136: 297
Hadden J W, Lopez C, O'Reilly R J, Hadden E M 1977 Ann NY Acad Sci 284: 139
Heiner G G, Fatima N, McCrumb F R et al 1971 Amer J Epidem 94: 435
Herrmann E C Jr (ed) 1977 Third conference on antiviral substances. New York, Ann NY Acad Sci 284
Hill D A, Baron S, Perkins J C et al 1972 J Amer Med Ass 219: 1179
Hornick R B, Togo Y, Mahler S, Iezzoni D 1969 Bull Wld Hlth Org 41: 671
Hryniuk W, Foerster J, Shojania M, Chow A 1972 J Amer Med Ass 219: 715
Isaacs A, Lindemann J 1957 Proc Roy Soc B 147: 258
Jackson G G 1977 J Infect Dis 136: 301
Jaroszynska-Weinberger B 1970 Arch Dis Child 45: 573
Jones B R, Coster D J, Fison P N et al 1979 Lancet 1: 243
Jones B R, Galbraith J E K, Al-Hussaini M K 1962 Lancet 2: 875
Juel-Jensen B E, MacCallum F O 1965 Brit Med J 1: 901
Juel-Jensen B E, MacCallum F O, Mackenzie A M R, Pike M C 1970 Brit Med J 4: 776
Kingham J G C, Ganguly N K, Shaari Z D et al 1978 Gut 19: 91
Kleinschmidt W J, Ellis L F, Van Frank R M, Murphy E B 1968 Nature (Lond) 220: 167
Koplan J P, Monsur K A, Foster S O et al 1975 J Infect Dis 131: 34
Kraybill E N, Sever J L, Avery G B, Movassaghi N 1972 J Pediat 80: 485
La Montagne J R, Galasso G J 1978 J Infect Dis 138: 928
Lampson G P, Tytell A A, Field A K et al 1967 Proc Nat Acad Sci (Wash) 58: 782
Landsman J B, Grist N R 1964 Lancet 1: 330
Leavitt T J, Merigan T C, Freeman J M 1971 Amer J Dis Child 121: 43
Little J W, Hall W J, Douglas R G et al 1976 Ann Intern Med 85: 177
Magnussen C R, Douglas D G, Betts R F et al 1977 Antimicrob Ag Chemother 12: 498
Markham R H C, Carter C, Scobie M A et al 1977 Trans Ophthal Soc UK 97: 333

Medical Research Council Scientific Committee on Interferon 1962 Lancet 1: 873
Merigan C (ed) 1976 J Infect Dis 133: (June Suppl) A1
Merigan T C, Hall T S, Reed S E, Tyrrell D A J 1973 Lancet 1: 563
Merigan T C, Rand K H, Pollard R B et al 1978 New Engl J Med 298: 981
Monsur K A, Hossain M S, Huq F et al 1975 J Infect Dis 131: 40
Nolan D C, Carruthers M M, Lerner A M 1970 New Engl J Med 282: 10
Oker-Blom N, Hovi T, Leinikki P et al 1970 Brit Med J 3: 676
Panusarn C, Stanley E D, Dirda V et al 1974 New Engl J Med 291: 57
Parker J D 1977 J Antimicrob Chemother 3: Suppl A 131
Phillips C A, Fanning L, Gump D W, Phillips C F 1977 J Amer Med Assoc 238: 2299
Pollard R B, Smith J L, Neal E A et al 1978 J Amer Med Ass 239: 1648
Rao A R, McFadzean J A, Kamalashki K 1966 Lancet 1: 1068
Reed S E, Craig J W, Tyrrell D A J 1976 J Infect Dis 133: Suppl A128
Rytel M W, Shope R E, Kilbourne E D 1966 J Exper Med 123: 577
Sacks S L, Smith J L, Pollard R B et al 1979 J Amer Med Ass 241: 28
Schimpff S C, Fortner C L, Greene W H, Wiernik P H 1974 J Infect Dis 130: 673
Selby P J, Powles R L, Jameson B et al 1979 Lancet 2: 1267
Simpson J R 1974 Brit Med J 3: 523
Soto A J, Hall T S, Reed S E 1973 Antimicrob Ag Chemother 3: 332
Stalder H 1977 Yale J Biol Med 50: 507
Stanley E D, Jackson G G, Dirda V A, Rubenis M 1976 J Infect Dis 133: Suppl A121
Stark J E, Heath R B, Oswald N C et al 1970 Thorax 25: 649
Stevens D A, Jordan G W, Waddell T F, Merigan T C 1973 New Engl J Med 289: 873
Togo Y, Hornick R B, Felitti V J et al 1970 J Amer Med Ass 211: 1149
Togo Y, McCracken E A 1976 J Infect Dis 133: A109
Travers J P, Patterson A 1978 J Int Med Res 6: 102
Tyrrell D A J 1976 Interferon and its clinical potential. Heinemann, London
Upton A R M, Barwick D D, Foster J B 1971 Lancet 1: 290
Whitley R J, Ch'ien L T, Dolia R et al 1976 New Engl J Med 294: 1193
Whitley R J, Soong S J, Dolin R et al 1977 New Engl J Med 297: 289
Wingfield W L, Pollack D, Grunert R R 1969 New Engl J Med 281: 579

Antiviral agents. Pharmaceutical preparations and dosage

Name	*Dosage*	*Preparations*	*Common international proprietary names*	
Amantadine	*Adult* Oral: 100 mg twice a day. *Children* Oral: (10–15 years) 100 mg daily.	Capsules Syrup	Symmetrel Mantadin PK-Merz, Contenton	(UK) (Fr) (Ger)
Methisazone	*Adult* Oral: Two doses of 3 g at 12 hourly intervals. *Children* Oral: 3–10 years, 1.5 g, then repeated 12 hours later. Under 3 years: 750 mg and repeated 12 hours later.	Suspension	Marboran	(UK)
Idoxuridine	Topical or ophthalmic application.	Eye drops and ointment In solution in DMSO	Herpid, Kerecid Iduridan Iduviran Stoxil	(UK) (Ger) (Fr) (USA)
Vidarabine	*Adult* i.v. infusion: 10–12 mg/kg body weight daily. *Children* i.v. infusion: as for adults.	Sterile suspension for infusion Eye ointment	Vira-A	(UK)
Trifluorothymidine	For ophthalmic application.	Eye drops	Not yet available in the UK	
Cytarabine	*Adult* i.v.: for Herpes infection, 100 mg/m^2 body surface area, daily, for 5 days: or, 2–4 mg/kg body weight.	Injection	Cytosar Alexan Aracytine	(UK) (Ger) (Fr)
Acyclovir	*Adult* i.v.: 5 mg/kg body weight daily in 3 divided doses. *Children* as for adults. Ophthalmic application.	Injection Eye ointment	Not yet available in the UK	

26

Special problems of dosage

Data of normal doses are specified in appendices to earlier chapters, and some indications for increasing these are mentioned in the text. We are here concerned with situations in which normal dosage needs to be modified, and with other problems of administration.

DOSAGE IN CHILDREN

In general, dosage is related to that for the adult on a basis of body weight or of surface area, using one of a number of standard formulas. Although methods based on estimation of surface area are of disputed validity and are little used in Britain in their direct form, the 'Percentage Method' of Catzel (1974) which is a simplified form of a surface area method, is widely used for its convenience. The dose is given as a percentage of adult dose appropriate to the child's age; for example, at birth a child receives 10 per cent of the adult dose, at one year 25 per cent, at seven years 50 per cent. Different considerations apply in premature infants and in the full term neonate during the first week of life, mainly because of the undeveloped state of their hepatic and renal function. Detoxification mechanisms in the liver are inadequate, and deficiency of glucuronyl transferase in particular renders the infant incapable of rapidly detoxifying drugs such as chloramphenicol and novobiocin. Other enzyme systems may be genetically deficient and a low concentration of glucose 6-phosphate dehydrogenase leads to increased likelihood of haemolysis when drugs such as nitrofurantoin and sulphonamides are administered. A number of drugs, such as sulphonamides, may compete for binding sites to albumin in plasma, thus causing a rise in serum bilirubin and a consequent increased risk of kernicterus. Renal function, too, is not fully developed in the first weeks of life and deficient renal excretion accounts for higher blood levels and a slower rate of decline than in older patients.

The low glomerular filtration rate found in early infancy affects especially serum levels of penicillins and aminoglycosides. This slow rate of elimination is an advantage in one respect, since the interval between doses can be increased, but drugs such as aminoglycosides with a low therapeutic ratio require careful dose adjustment. Another factor affecting serum antibiotic concentrations is the relatively large extracellular volume in infancy, about 35 per cent of the body weight at birth, falling rapidly in the first few days of life and then more slowly to reach a near adult proportion of 25 per cent by about nine months. The large ECF volume of infancy affects drug concentrations because agents distributed through the whole ECF will show relatively lower peak levels if the ECF volume is high, and are often excreted slowly.

The difficult task of studying the behaviour of antimicrobial drugs in neonates and premature babies has been tackled with some success in recent years, and Table 26.1 provides guide-lines for the commonly used agents in this age group. As in the older

Table 26.1 Dosage of parenterally administered antimicrobials in newborn

Drug	Single dose	Dose interval in hours at age	
	per kg body wt	0–7 days	>7 days
Benzyl penicillin	25,000 u	12	8
Cloxacillin	25 mg	12	6– 8
Ampicillin	50 mg	12	6– 8
Carbenicillin	100 mg	12	6– 8
Ticarcillin	75 mg	12	4– 8
Cephalothin	20 mg	12	8
Gentamicin	2.5 mg	12	8
Tobramycin	2 mg	12	8–12
Kanamycin	7.5–10 mg	12	8
Amikacin	7.5 mg	12	8–12
Chloramphenicol	12.5 mg	12	6– 8

The dosages given for the first week of life are often also appropriate in somewhat older babies, if they are small (<2000 g) or preterm. By contrast, an 8 hr interval may often be used after the first 48 hours of life in larger, mature babies.

child and adult, administration of aminoglycosides for a prolonged period, or even for a short time when renal function is poor, should be checked by estimation of serum levels. The recrudescence of interest in chloramphenicol which followed the emergence of ampicillin-resistance in *H. influenzae*, has led to increased attention to dose schedules in early infancy and to the realization that chloramphenicol serum levels may need to be estimated in this age group. Further information on the clinical pharmacology of antimicrobial agents in the newborn may be found in a valuable monograph by McCracken & Nelson (1977), and in articles by Davies (1975) and Rhodes (1977), while therapy of infections in infancy and childhood is generally reviewed by Eichenwald & McCracken (1978).

ANTIBIOTICS IN RENAL FAILURE

It is often necessary to administer antibacterial drugs to patients with impaired renal function, either for the treatment of infection of the renal tract itself, or for infection at other sites. The likelihood of accumulation and the consequent chance of toxic effects is influenced by a number of factors, which differ in their relative importance with different drugs. Most important is the mode of elimination of the antibiotic. The risks of toxicity associated with renal failure are in general higher for those drugs, such as the aminoglycosides, of which a high proportion is excreted in the urine than for those, for example the macrolides, in which renal excretion plays a small part in their elimination. An important exception to this rule must be made for some drugs whose metabolites, although antibacterially inactive (and therefore undetectable by assay systems relying on their biological effects) are excreted by the kidneys and therefore accumulate in renal failure. In this situation the possible toxicity of the inactive metabolites must be considered, as well as that of the undegraded antibiotic. Antimicrobial drugs differ greatly in their stability in body tissues, and this factor, together with the ratio between toxic and therapeutic levels, again affects the likelihood of toxic effects. Among the antibiotics, those which are known to be nephrotoxic must be regarded with particular caution in renal failure. An additional factor has to be evaluated when antibacterial drugs are used for the treatment of urinary infection, since the urinary concentration of a drug may be greatly affected by declining renal function. This diversity of factors affecting the relationship between antimicrobial drugs and renal function often leads to practical difficulties of administration in renal failure. At one extreme no limitation is imposed by the presence of renal failure on the dosage of a drug, such as fusidate, which is handled entirely by non-renal mechanisms. For other drugs, renal excretion accounts for a small proportion of the administered dose, and only moderate restriction of dosage is required in renal failure. This is also true for the penicillins because, despite the importance of renal excretion in their elimination, the ratio of therapeutic to toxic concentration is so great.

The serum concentration of most antibiotics, after reaching a peak, usually declines exponentially at a rate characteristic of the particular drug. Thus, although the pharmacokinetics of the different agents vary widely, the serum half-life of the drug is a useful general measure of its duration of action, and is prolonged in renal failure when an appreciable proportion of the drug is eliminated by the kidney. The degree to which the half-life is prolonged offers, for many antibiotics, a useful guide to dosage in renal failure.

The half-life of many antimicrobial drugs has been estimated in different degrees of renal failure and simple dosage formulas, nomograms and computer-based programmes have all been employed to determine dosage of potentially toxic drugs, especially aminoglycosides. While these methods are of great value in initiating therapy they cannot, for a variety of reasons, be employed for more than a short period. A special problem emphasized by Whelton (1974) is that many guide-lines define dose ranges for severe renal failure, including all patients whose glomerular filtration rate is less than about 10 ml per min. At this level of renal function, small changes in clearance cause large shifts in plasma drug concentration, so that a standard dose scheme of gentamicin, for example, might well give toxic levels in an anephric patient, inadequate levels in a patient with a GFR of 10 ml per min, and adequate levels in a patient with an intermediate GFR. Moreover, antibiotics must often be given to patients with conditions such as septicaemic shock, in which renal function is threatened and may decline rapidly during the course of the illness. Serum levels of antibiotics are also influenced by factors other than renal function. These are discussed fully by Barza & Lauermann (1978), and include variable absorption of the drug from sites of intramuscular injection, altered distribution volumes resulting from oedema, inaccurate dosage because of obesity (since calculations should be based on lean body weight), and poor elimination of drug from sites of pathological fluid accumulation. Anaemia and fever also influence drug levels. For all these reasons administration of potentially toxic antibiotics to patients with renal failure must be monitored by assay of plasma concentrations of the drug, and suitable methods are described in Chapter 27.

Table 26.2 Limitations on antibiotic prescribing in renal failure

Normal dose	Slight modification of dose	Major modification of dose	Avoid in renal failure
Erythromycin	Penicillins[3]	Aminoglycosides	Tetracyclines[5]
Sodium fusidate	Cephalosporins[4]	Vancomycin	Cephaloridine
Doxycycline	Lincomycin	Polymyxins	Nitrofurantoin
Chloramphenicol[1]	Clindamycin	Carbenicillin	Nalidixic Acid
	Co-trimoxazole	Ticarcillin	
Rifampicin	Isoniazid	Ethambutol	
		P.A.S.	
Amphotericin[2]		Flucytosine	
Clotrimazole			
Miconazole			
Griseofulvin			

1. Metabolic products of uncertain toxicity accumulate in renal failure
2. But see page 241 for renal toxicity of amphotericin
3. Except carbenicillin/ticarcillin
4. Except cephaloridine
5. Except doxycycline

Table 26.2 categorizes the various antimicrobial drugs in relation to renal failure.

Factors bearing upon the use of individual antibiotics in renal failure are considered in the following sections. Further information on the management of antibacterial chemotherapy in renal insufficiency may be found in extensive reviews by Whelton (1974) and by Hewitt & McHenry (1978), and guide-lines for initial therapy in articles by Bennett et al (1977) and by Van Scoy & Wilson (1977). The nephrotoxicity of antimicrobial agents is thoroughly reviewed by Appel & Neu (1977).

INDIVIDUAL ANTIMICROBIAL DRUGS AND RENAL FAILURE

Penicillins

Penicillins are eliminated by both glomerular filtration and tubular secretion, and the serum half-life is generally much prolonged in renal failure. Isoxazolyl penicillins, however, show little change in half-life in renal failure, since they are partly eliminated by biotransformation, while nafcillin, because of its high biliary excretion, provides another exception (Barza & Weinstein 1976). Even in anuria, however, serum levels do slowly decline by virtue of non-renal elimination. Since the margin of safety in dosage is very great, and penicillin encephalopathy is associated with very high serum levels, only modest adjustments of dosage are required in renal failure, as indicated in Table 26.3.

When penicillins are administered in very high dosage, the possibility of electrolyte disturbance must be considered even in patients with normal renal function. The sodium content of carbenicillin is 5.4 mEq per g, so that with a full dosage of 30 g daily used in the treatment of Pseudomonas infections, the patient receives 162 mEq sodium per day. Dosage should be reduced to 8 g daily in moderate renal impairment and to 4 g daily in severe renal failure. The sodium content of ticarcillin is much the same, 5.3 mmol per g, so that the smaller daily dose involves a correspondingly smaller sodium load. Mezlocillin, which is given in the same dose as ticarcillin, contains only 1.85 mmol per g.

Table 26.3 Dose of penicillins and cephalosporins in renal impairment

	Severity of renal failure					
	Mild		Moderate		Severe	
	Dose		Dose		Dose	
	g	interval hr	g	interval hr	g	interval hr
Benzyl penicillin	NC		NC		0.6	12
Cloxacillin	NC		NC		1.0	8
Ampicillin	NC		NC		1.0	12
Carbenicillin	NC		4.0	12	2.0	12
Mecillinam	0.4	8	0.2	8	0.2	12
Cephaloridine	NR		NR		NR	
Cephalothin	NC		1.0	6	1.0	12
Cephazolin	0.5	12	0.25	12	0.25	24
Cephradine	0.5	6	0.25	6	0.25	12
Cephalexin	0.5	6	0.25	6	0.25	12
Cefamandole	1.0	6	1.0	8	1.0	12
Cefuroxime	NC		0.5	8	0.5	12
Cefoxitin	1.0	8	1.0	12	0.5	12
Cefotaxime*						

NC No change from normal
NR Not recommended

*Dose schedules in renal failure not yet established; probably similar to cefuroxime

Cephalosporins

Serum half-lives of cephaloridine and of cephalexin are greatly increased in renal failure, but that of cephalothin is only slightly prolonged. Cephaloridine is potentially nephrotoxic in doses of 6 g or more daily, and there is danger of renal damage when cephaloridine is given together with aminoglycosides or frusemide (p. 99). Evidence of deteriorating renal function has been obtained occasionally in patients receiving cephalothin, particularly in very large doses, but more recently introduced cephalosporins have not so far been definitely associated with renal damage. If a cephalosporin is indicated in a patient with threatened or established renal failure, cephaloridine should therefore be avoided. Because of their generally low toxicity, blood levels of cephalosporins are not usually estimated and dosage in renal failure is based on known changes in half-life at different degrees of renal failure. Table 26.3 gives appropriate doses and dose intervals for compounds in this group, for cefoxitin, and for the penicillins.

Aminoglycosides

The serum concentrations of these drugs are greatly influenced by renal function, they have relatively low margins of safety, and they may be needed for infections which patients with renal failure may suffer. A number of studies have provided data on the relationship of serum half-life to creatinine clearance for each of these drugs.

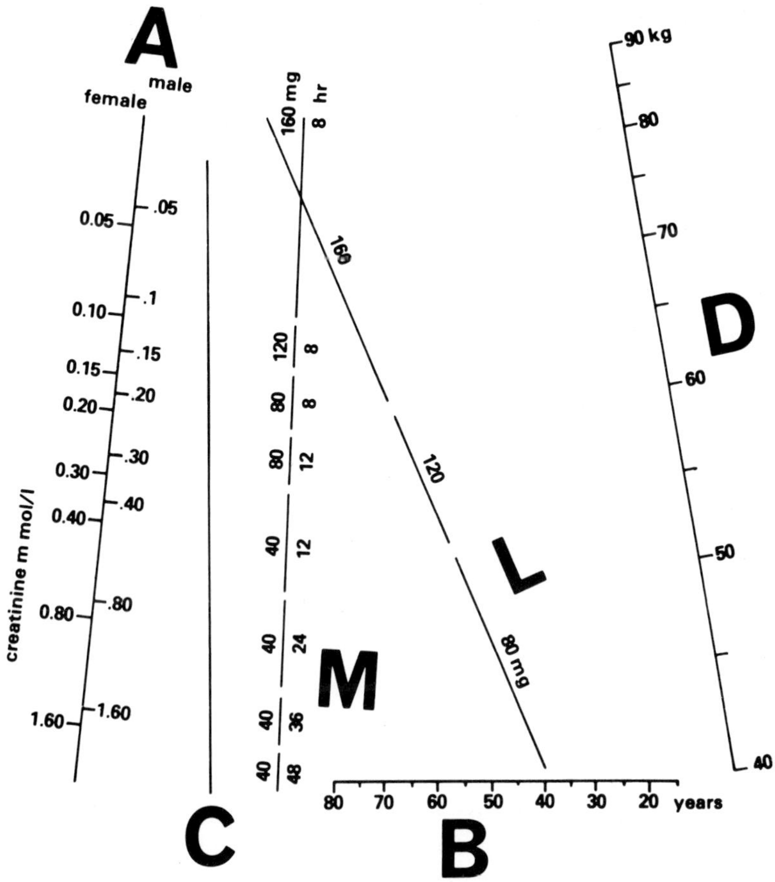

Fig. 26.1 Nomogram for gentamicin dosage. The nomogram provides a loading dose (L), a maintenance dose (M) and a suitable interval between doses for a patient whose serum creatinine concentration (A), age (B) and body weight (D) are known. To use, join A to B with a line which cuts C, then join C to D with a line which cuts L and M. Reproduced from Mawer et al (1974) by kind permission.

In general, aminoglycosides have a serum half-life in the normal subject of two to three hours, which is prolonged greatly in renal failure, sometimes up to a period of days. The $T\frac{1}{2}$ in renal failure in hours is generally found to be three to five times the serum creatinine, in mg, and more precise equations relating the overall elimination rate of each aminoglycoside to the endogenous creatinine clearance have also been established. For treatment in renal failure the same loading dose is given as in the subject with normal renal function; subsequent doses are calculated from a nomogram such as that provided by Mawer et al (1974) for gentamicin (Fig. 26.1), or by the use of simple dose formulas based on the relationships of drug elimination rate to renal function. For example, a dose interval in hours of nine times the serum creatinine in mg for kanamycin (Cutler & Orme, 1969) and amikacin. Table 26.4 provides guide-lines of this sort for gentamicin.

Two methods are employed to adjust aminoglycoside dosage in renal failure; the more commonly used method is to increase the interval between doses after the initial loading dose. The alternative is to reduce the maintenance dose while keeping

Table 26.4 Gentamicin dosage in renal failure. Initial dose 80–160 mg depending on weight

Blood urea mg/100 ml (mmol/l)	Creatinine clearance ml/min	Dose (mg) 8-hourly	Dose interval in hours with constant dose
<40 (<7)	>70	80–160	8
40–100 (7–17)	≤70	40	12
100–200 (18–33)	≤30	20	24
>200 (>33)	≤10	10	48

the same interval as in the normal subject. Since the former method allows wider swings of serum concentration (O'Grady, 1971), long periods of subinhibitory serum concentrations may occur in patients with severe renal failure. In these patients it is preferable to use the dosage reduction rather than the interval extension method.

We must emphasize, however, that these methods should only be used for initiating therapy with aminoglycosides and other potentially toxic agents, pending the results of assay. Noone et al (1978), in monitoring aminoglycoside treatment in 20 patients with severe renal failure, 17 of whom were renal transplant recipients, showed that serum levels in these patients varied widely and could not be related to serum creatinine concentrations.

Tetracyclines

The dangers of tetracyclines in renal failure are well documented (Phillips et al, 1974). Clinical and biochemical deterioration may follow their use in patients with previously well compensated renal failure, and they are generally contraindicated in renal impairment. The effects are caused by the anti-anabolic action of this group of drugs, and it is important to note that the maximal effect is often delayed for some days, so that deterioration of renal function may not be linked with the episode of tetracycline treatment.

The effects are not related in any direct way to prolongation of action of the drug; although the serum half-life of tetracycline and oxytetracycline is prolonged in renal failure, that of chlortetracycline is little affected, but all are potentially dangerous in renal failure. Doxycycline appears to provide an exception, although it must be remembered that the dose of this drug is much smaller than that of other tetracyclines. The long half-life of this drug, about 17 hours, is usually, but not always, unaffected in renal failure. More importantly, a number of patients with renal failure have received this tetracycline without showing ill effects. We conclude that tetracyclines are, in general, contraindicated in renal failure. If it is essential to use this group of drugs, doxycycline should be given (see page 175).

Sulphonamides

Williams et al (1968) found that the renal clearance of sodium sulphadimidine was greater in patients with renal failure than in normal subjects. This was attributable to the lower plasma concentration found in the patients with renal failure, itself presumably related to the increased volume of distribution for the drug. Sharpstone (1969) also found little relationship between the clearance of sulphamethoxazole and creatinine clearance. By contrast Fischer (1972) found the mean clearance of sulphadimidine much reduced in renal failure, with significant prolongation of plasma levels in the uraemic patients. The urinary concentration of sulphonamide in renal failure usually exceeds the MIC for most sulphonamide-sensitive pathogens.

Short-term administration of sulphonamides is probably safe in renal failure, but plasma levels should be monitored if the drug is given for more than a few days.

Trimethoprim

Clearance of this agent, which rises with increasing urinary acidity, is closely correlated with creatinine clearance, but declines at a lesser rate than does creatinine clearance with falling renal function, and even in advanced renal failure concentrations in the urine are greater than those required for urinary pathogens.

Co-trimoxazole

Kalowski et al (1973) observed 16 patients in whom renal function deteriorated in association with treatments by this drug combination. Deterioration continued in some in spite of modification of dose.

Tasker et al (1975) found, however, that this combination was safe in renal failure if appropriate dose adjustments are made. Of 20 patients with renal failure, only three showed deterioration of renal function while receiving co-trimoxazole, and these changes were attributable to factors other than the drug. They recommend normal dosage of two tablets twice daily (each tablet contains 80 mg trimethoprim and 400 mg sulphamethoxazole) in mild renal failure (creatinine clearance >25 ml/min, or plasma creatinine < 3 mg per cent in men or < 2 mg per cent in women), two tablets twice daily for three days, then two tablets daily in moderate renal failure, and two tablets daily in severe renal failure (creatinine clearance <15 ml/min, plasma creatinine >7 mg per cent in men or >4.5 mg per cent in women). Hansen (1978) makes similar recommendations but suggests estimation of plasma sulphamethoxazole levels if treatment is to be continued for more than a few days. As indicated in discussion of the individual components, urinary concentrations in renal failure are adequate for the treatment of infections of the urinary tract.

Nitrofurantoin

The serum half-life of this drug in normal subjects is short, about 20 minutes, no doubt reflecting an important extra-renal component in its metabolism, but peripheral neuropathy as a complication of nitrofurantoin treatment has developed chiefly in patients with renal failure, and for these reasons nitrofurantoin is contraindicated in renal failure.

Nalidixic Acid

Only a small proportion of the administered dose, 4–7 per cent, is found as biologically active drug in the urine, and serum concentrations rise little in renal failure. Nevertheless, adequate concentrations for the inhibition of most urinary pathogens are achieved even in advanced renal failure (Adam & Dawborn, 1971; Stamey et al, 1969). Unfortunately clearance of the inactive conjugates, mainly the glucuronide, is closely related to renal function, and the serum concentration of these compounds rises in renal failure. Their toxic effects are uncertain, but unwanted effects of nalidixic acid are encountered more commonly in renal failure. Nalidixic acid should be avoided if possible in renal failure.

Chloramphenicol

The situation is very similar to that described for nalidixic acid. The duration of action of the active compound is not much changed in renal failure, but the metabolic products accumulate significantly; since their toxicity is unknown, this agent is best avoided in renal failure.

Polymyxins

These drugs accumulate in renal failure, and are potentially nephrotoxic. A high incidence of renal failure has been reported in patients receiving large doses of colistin sulphomethate sodium (Price & Graham, 1970). Serious restriction of dose is imposed by renal failure, and a number of dose schedules have been described, (Curtis & Eastwood, 1968; Goodwin & Friedman, 1968). Polymyxins should be avoided if possible in renal failure.

Antituberculous Drugs

Streptomycin dosage follows the guide-lines already described for aminoglycosides generally.

The half-life of isoniazid is somewhat prolonged in renal failure, but variation of serum isoniazid levels is more dependent on inactivator status than on renal function. Bowersox et al (1973) recommend a dose of 300 mg daily if the serum creatinine is less than 12 mg per 100 ml. Patients with more severe renal failure should also be given an initial dose of 300 mg, but later doses will need to be reduced in slow inactivators.

Rifampicin clearance is somewhat reduced in renal failure but normal dosage can be continued (Acocella, 1978; McGeachie et al, 1970). In contrast, ethambutol is excreted largely by the kidney and dosage in severe renal failure should be reduced to 5–10 mg per kg daily.

PAS is eliminated entirely by the kidney and accumulates in renal failure. If it cannot be avoided in patients with renal failure, assays of plasma concentration should be performed.

Sodium Fusidate

Very little of the administered dose can be found in the urine and normal doses can be given in the presence of impaired renal function.

Erythromycin, Clindamycin, Lincomycin

The elimination rate of erythromycin and clindamycin is not significantly prolonged in renal failure. Dosage of erythromycin need not be changed, while in severe renal failure the dose of clindamycin may be limited to 300 mg every eight hours.

Vancomycin

This agent is eliminated mainly by the kidney, and the serum half-life, about 6–8 hours in the normal subject, is greatly prolonged in renal failure. The dose may need to be reduced to as little as 1 g every ten days, but serum level estimations are essential if vancomycin has to be given to a patient with impaired renal function.

ANTIMICROBIAL AGENTS AND DIALYSIS

Whether or not a drug is eliminated by peritoneal or haemodialysis depends on its molecular size and configuration, and on its degree of protein binding, since only the non-protein bound moiety is available for dialysis. The method of dialysis must also be taken into account, since most artificial kidneys achieve creatinine clearance rates of 100–200 ml per minute, whereas clearance rates with peritoneal dialysis are usually 15–20 ml per minute, so that a much longer dialysis time is needed to achieve the same result. Thus some poorly dialyzable agents may show appreciable reduction of serum levels after haemodialysis but not after peritoneal dialysis, others may be easily removed by either method, while some antimicrobials are not eliminated by any form of dialysis. Among the latter are cloxacillin, clindamycin,

Table 26.5 Antimicrobial drugs in patients on dialysis

	Dosage during peritoneal dialysis	Dose (g) after each haemodialysis
Benzyl penicillin ⎫ Cloxacillin ⎬ Ampicillin ⎭	as in S.R.I.[1]	
Carbenicillin	2 g every 8–12 hours	2
Ticarcillin	1 g every 8–12 hours	3
Cephalothin ⎫		1
Cephazolin		0.5
Cephradine		0.5
Cephalexin ⎬	as in S.R.I.	0.5
Cefamandole[2]		0.5
Cefuroxime		0.5
Cefotaxime		0.5[5]
Cefoxitin[3] ⎭		1
	mg/2.1[4]	mg/kg body wt
Gentamicin	1	1.0–1.3
Tobramycin	1	1.0–1.3
Kanamycin	3–4	5.0–7.5
Amikacin	3–4	7.5
Sissomycin	1	1.0
Vancomycin	as in S.R.I.	
Flucytosine[6]		15–25

1. S.R.I. = severe renal impairment, see Table 26.3.
2. Conflicting data. See Winchester et al (1977) and Czerwinski & Pederson (1979)
3. See Fillastre et al (1978)
4. These doses given i.v. or i.m. to replace estimated losses for each 2 litres of dialysis fluid removed
5. Provisional recommendation on available data
6. See Dawborn et al (1973) and Drouhet (1978)

tetracyclines (which should not, however, with the exception of doxycycline, be used in renal failure), vancomycin and amphotericin. The type of dialyser, and the patient's own residual renal function also greatly influence resultant drug levels so that, as in patients with renal failure who are not receiving this form of treatment, the dose schemes which follow and those summarized in Table 26.5, should be used only as guide-lines for initial management pending frequent estimations of serum antibiotic concentration. A full account is given by Winchester et al (1977).

Aminoglycosides

The serum concentrations of aminoglycosides fall by an average of 50 per cent (range 24–64 per cent) during 6–8 hours of haemodialysis session. The serum half-life, normally 2–3 hours, is greatly prolonged in renal failure; during haemodialysis it falls to about 5–10 hours, but elimination during peritoneal dialysis is much slower. Much variation is found, depending on drug, characteristics of the dialyser membrane, and methods of measurements. Details may be found in surveys by Leroy et al (1978) and Pechere & Dugal (1979). Gentamicin dosage in renal impairment was studied by Gingell & Waterworth (1968) who recommend an 80 mg dose post-haemodialysis (see also McHenry et al, 1971). Christopher et al (1974), agreeing with these general findings, showed that significant plasma clearance (2.2 ml per minute) could be demonstrated even in anephric patients, indicating a small degree of non-renal elimination. Mean gentamicin clearance in 11 patients on Kiil dialysers was 24 ml per minute and the predicted 'top-up' dose varied between 30 per cent of the loading dose in anephric patients to 100 per cent of the loading dose in patients with a residual glomerular filtration rate of 5 ml per minute. The characteristics of tobramycin in dialysis are similar to those of gentamicin. Using amikacin by intravenous infusion in a dose of 300 mg in patients with end-stage renal failure, Madhaven et al (1976) showed a mean serum $T\frac{1}{2}$ of 3.75 hours while on haemodialysis (mean $T\frac{1}{2}$ in normal subjects is 2.8 hours) and of 29 hours while on peritoneal dialysis, not much different from patients not being dialysed. The clearance of amikacin during dialysis varied between 29 and 81 per cent of the administered dose, again emphasizing that monitoring of serum levels is essential. Since only initial guidance can be provided, simple schemes can be used for the first dose or two. Cutler et al (1975) for example, recommend for gentamicin and tobramycin a loading dose of 2 mg/kg, and a post-dialysis dose of 1.3 mg/kg in anephric patients and 1.5 mg/kg in those with residual function. Leroy et al (1978) suggest the slightly lower post-dialysis dose of 1 mg/kg for gentamicin, tobramycin, sissomycin and netilmycin, and 5 mg/kg for streptomycin, kanamycin, and amikacin.

Polymyxins

Contradictory results have been obtained by different workers in estimating the effects of peritoneal and haemodialysis. Little is removed by peritoneal dialysis and the degree of elimination by haemodialysis evidently depends on the type of membrane used. Both forms of polymyxin are nephrotoxic and should be avoided in renal failure if possible.

Vancomycin

Although non-protein bound, this agent, with a molecular weight of about 3300, is dialysed very slowly, a 12-hour haemodialysis reducing the serum level by only 10 per cent. Dosage during dialysis should be as in severe renal failure. Frequent monitoring will be needed, and a dose of 0.5–1 g is likely to be indicated every 7–10 days (Eykyn et al, 1970).

Antituberculous Drugs

Isoniazid is removed by peritoneal and haemodialysis. A daily dose of 150 mg is usually recommended for patients on dialysis, but higher doses may be used if serum concentration is measured (Editorial, 1980)

Acocella (1978) reports that rifampicin, although mainly metabolized in the liver, is cleared by peritoneal and haemodialysis. Normal doses should be given in patients on dialysis. Ethambutol is cleared by peritoneal dialysis, about one-third of the administered dose appearing in the dialysate over a period of 30 hours; the clearance rate on haemodialysis is approximately 35 ml per minute (Winchester et al, 1977). A dose of 5 mg per kg per day may be given, or a larger dose (18–25 mg per kg) before each dialysis. Streptomycin behaves in the same way as other aminoglycosides, requiring similar dose adjustments as kanamycin and amikacin.

INCOMPATIBILITIES AND INTERACTIONS

When a patient receives an antimicrobial drug by intravenous injection it is necessary to ensure its compatibility with the infusion fluid, and with other drugs, including other antimicrobial agents, which may be administered at the same time.

It is important to follow manufacturers' instructions or to take advice from the Pharmacy Department. *The Extra Pharmacopoeia* (Martindale, 1977) is a good source of information, as are the volumes referred to in the ensuing section on drug interactions. An important incompatibility of common relevance to antimicrobial drug administration is the inactivation of gentamicin when mixed with carbenicillin. These drugs should not be mixed in intravenous fluids (McLaughlin & Reeves, 1971; Noone & Pattison, 1971).

Another factor bearing on the use of antibiotics by the intravenous route is the choice of intravenous infusion or bolus injection. As regards efficacy there is little evidence on which to decide which method is superior, but pharmaceutical factors may also be important, and Simberkoff et al (1970) have shown that penicillins lose activity rapidly in solutions containing glucose, sucrose or dextran together with bicarbonate. In general we prefer, when antibiotics are given intravenously, to inject them at intervals into the infusion, but the following antibiotics should be given by continuous slow infusion; amphotericin, diethanolamine fusidate, and the tetracyclines.

The term 'incompatibility' refers to an adverse relationship between two drugs *in vitro*, but increasing attention is now being directed to interactions between different drugs *in vivo*. The forms of interaction between various antimicrobial drugs are referred to in a number of chapters, but interactions between antimicrobial and other drugs must also be considered. These may operate before absorption, for example, the chelating effect of a number of metallic ions tends to diminish

Table 26.6 Interactions of antimicrobial agents with other drugs

Antimicrobial drug	Interacting drug	Effect of interaction
Aminoglycosides	Frusemide	Increased ototoxicity.
	Ethacrynic acid	Increased ototoxicity.
	Skeletal muscle relaxants	Enhancement of neuromuscular blockade.
	Some cephalosporins	Renal toxicity.
Tetracyclines	Antacids Ferrous sulphate	Diminished absorption due to chelation and lowered blood level of tetracycline.
	Oral anticoagulants	Prothrombin utilisation impaired. Reduced dose of anticoagulant may be needed.
	Phenformin	Induction of lactic acidosis.
	Methoxyflurane	A report of fatal renal failure. Avoid this anaesthetic if patient is receiving a tetracycline.
Sulphonamides	Oral hypoglycaemic agents	Serum levels of hypoglycaemic agent may rise giving increased effect.
	Oral anticoagulants	Possible potentiation of anticoagulant by displacement from binding sites and reduced vitamin K in gut.
	Methotrexate	Displacement from plasma binding sites and increased methotrexate toxicity.
Chloramphenicol	Oral hypoglycaemic agents	Enhanced effect as above.
	Oral anticoagulants	Enhanced effect as above.
	Phenytoin	Phenytoin levels rise with possible toxicity.
Ampicillin	Contraceptive pill	Report of failures in women taking ampicillin.
Cephaloridine	Aminoglycosides Frusemide	Enhanced nephrotoxicity.
Rifampicin	Oral anticoagulants	Warfarin metabolism stimulated. Dose may need adjustments when starting or stopping rifampicin.
	Corticosteroids	Enzyme induction by rifampicin causing increased cortisol metabolism and need for increase of steroid dose.
	Contraceptive pill	Enzyme induction by rifampicin causing increase of oestrogen metabolism and consequent failure. Increase to two tablets daily or use another method.
Metronidazole	Alcohol	Disulphiram action in some patients from inhibition of aldehyde dehydrogenase.
	Oral anticoagulants	May inhibit warfarin metabolism.
Nalidixic acid	Oral anticoagulants	Displacement from binding sites may increase anticoagulant effect.
Griseofulvin	Oral anticoagulants	Enzyme induction by griseofulvin reduces anticoagulant effect.
	Barbiturates	Increase of liver microsomal enzymes by barbiturate reduces griseofulvin effect.
Amphotericin	Digoxin	Hypokalaemia induced by amphotericin will potentiate digitalis toxicity.

tetracycline absorption. After absorption, competition for serum binding sites may be important, and has been especially referred to in discussing antibiotic dosage in the neonate (p. 448), while interactions related to inhibition or stimulation of hepatic enzymes responsible for drug inactivation have also assumed growing importance. Again, this form of interaction is especially important in the newborn. Interaction related to competition in the renal tubule may be used to therapeutic advantage, as in the use of probenecid to enhance serum levels of penicillins or some cephalosporins.

A very large number of interactions has been described between antimicrobial and other drugs. Some of them are probably unimportant, but the possibility of adverse drug interaction should always be considered when treatment is initiated or changed. Table 26.6 gives in summary form a list of the more important interactions involving antimicrobial agents. Those included are either well documented or of such potential importance that they deserve mention even if uncommon. More detailed accounts of drug interaction in general, all of which include extensive discussion of interactions involving antibacterial agents, may be found in monographs by Griffin & D'Arcy (1979), Bint & Reeves (1978), Hansten (1979) and Stockley (1974).

S.I. units

In view of the possibility that anti-bacterial drug levels may eventually be reported in S.I. units, we give in Table 26.7 the conversion factors required for some of the more important agents.

Table 26.7 Conversion factors for changing μg/ml to SI Units (μmol/l)

		Molecular Weight	*Conversion Factor*
Penicillins	Benzyl	372.5	2.68
	Phenoxymethyl	350.4	2.85
	Cloxacillin	475.9	2.10
	Flucloxacillin	493.9	2.02
	Oxacillin	441.4	2.26
	Methicillin	420.4	2.38
	Ampicillin	349.4	2.86
	Amoxycillin	365.4	2.74
	Carbenicillin	422.4	2.37
	Ticarcillin	428.4	2.33
	Mezlocillin	539.6	1.85
	Mecillinam	325.4	3.07
Cephalosporins	Cephaloridine	415.5	2.40
	Cephalothin	418.4	2.39
	Cephalexin	347.4	2.88
	Cephradine	349.4	2.86
	Cephalexin	347.4	2.88
	Cephradine	349.4	2.86
	Cefamandole	462.5	2.16
	Cefazolin	476.5	2.10
	Cefuroxime	446.4	2.24
	Cefoxitin	427.4	2.34

Table 26.7 (*continued*)

		Molecular Weight	*Conversion Factor*
Aminoglycosides	Amikacin	585.7	1.71
	Gentamicin	449–477	2.16
	Kanamycin	651.2	1.54
	Tobramycin	467	2.14
	Streptomycin	581.6	1.72
	Spectinomycin	332.4	3.01
Tetracyclines	Tetracycline	444.4	2.25
	Oxytetracycline	496.9	2.01
	Doxycycline	512.9	1.95
	Minocycline	457.5	2.19
Miscellaneous	Chloramphenicol	323.1	3.10
	Thiamphenicol	356.2	2.81
	Erythromycin	733.9	1.36
	Clindamycin	461.5	2.17
	Fusidic acid	516.7	1.94
	Rifampicin	823.0	1.22
Synthetic Agents	Sulphadimidine	278.3	3.59
	Sulphamethoxazole	253.3	3.95
	Trimethoprim	290.3	3.44
	Metronidazole	171.2	5.84
Anti-fungal Agents	Amphotericin B	924.1	1.08
	Clotrimazole	344.8	2.90
	Flucytosine	129.1	7.75
	Miconazole	479.1	2.09

References

Acocella G 1978 Clin Pharmacokinetics 3: 108
Adam W R, Dawborn J K 1971 Aust NZ J Med 1: 126
Appel G B, Neu H C 1977 New Engl J Med 296: 663, 722, 784
Barza M, Weinstein L 1976 Clin Pharmacokinetics 1: 297
Barza M, Lauermann M 1978 Clin Pharmacokinetics 3: 202
Bennett W M, Singer I, Golper T, Feig P, Coggins C J 1977 Ann Intern Med 86: 754
Bint A J, Reeves D S 1978 Antibiotics Chemother, 25: 289
Bowersox D W, Winterbauer R H, Stewart G L et al 1973 New Engl J Med 289: 84
Catzel P 1974 The Paediatric Prescriber, 4th edition. Blackwell, Oxford
Christopher T G, Korn D, Blair A D et al 1974 Kidney International 6: 38
Curtis J R, Eastwood J B 1968 Brit Med J 1: 484
Cutler R E, Christopher T G, Forrey A W, Blair A D 1975 Kidney International 7: Suppl 2, 16
Cutler R E, Orme B M 1969 J Amer Med Ass 209: 539
Czerwinski A W, Pederson J A 1979 Antimicrob Ag Chemother 15: 161
Davies P A 1975 Brit J Hosp Med 14: 517
Dawborn J K, Page M D, Schiavone D J 1973 Brit Med J 4: 382
Drouhet E 1978 Antibiotics Chemother, 25: 253
Editorial 1980 Brit Med J 1: 349
Eichenwald H F, McCracken G H Jr 1978 J Pediat 93: 93, 337, 357
Eykyn S, Phillips I, Evans J 1970 Brit Med J 3: 80
Fillastre J P, Leroy A, Godin M et al 1978 J Antimicrob Chemother 4: Suppl B, 79
Fischer E 1972 Lancet 2: 210
Gingell J C, Waterworth P M 1968 Brit Med J 2: 19
Goodwin N J, Friedman E A 1968 Ann Intern Med 68: 984
Griffin J P, D'Arcy P F A 1979 Manual of adverse drug reactions, 2nd edn. Wright, Bristol

Hansen I 1978 Antibiotics Chemother 25: 217
Hansten P D 1979 Drug interactions, 4th edn. Lea & Febiger, Philadelphia
Hewitt W L, McHenry M C 1978 Med Clin N Amer 62: 1119
Kalowski S, Nanra R S, Mathew T H, Kincaid-Smith P 1973 Lancet 1: 394
Leroy A, Humbert G, Oksenhendler G, Fillastre J P 1978 Antibiotics Chemother 25: 163
McCracken G H, Nelson J D 1977 Antimicrobial therapy for newborns. Grune and Stratton Inc, New York
McGeachie J, Girdwood R W A, Burton J A, Kennedy A C 1970 Scottish Med J 15: 257
McHenry M C, Gavan T L, Gifford R W J R et al 1971 Ann Intern Med 74: 192
McLaughlin J E, Reeves D S 1971 Lancet 1: 261
Madhavan T, Yaremchuk K, Levin N et al 1976 Antimicrob Ag Chemother 10: 464
Martindale [W] 1977 The Extra Pharmacopoeia, Wade A (ed) 27th edn. London Pharmaceutical Press
Mawer G E, Ahmad R, Dobbs S M et al 1974 Brit J Clin Pharmacol 1: 45
Noone P, Beale D F, Pollock S S, Perera M R et al 1978 Brit Med J 2: 470
Noone P, Pattison J R 1971 Lancet 2: 575
O'Grady F 1971 Brit Med Bull 27: 142
Pechere J-C, Dugal R 1979 Clin Pharmacokinetics 4: 170
Phillips M E, Eastwood J B, Curtis J R et al 1974 Brit Med J 2: 149
Price D J E, Graham D I 1970 Brit Med J 4: 525
Rhodes K H 1977 Mayo Clin Proc 52: 707
Sharpstone P 1969 Postgrad Med J 45: Suppl p. 38
Simberkoff M S, Thomas L, McGregor D, Shenkein I, Levine B B 1970 New Engl J Med 283: 116
Stamey T A, Nemoy N J, Higgins M 1969 Invest Urol 6: 582
Stockley I 1974 Drug Interactions and their Mechanisms. Pharmaceutical Press, London
Tasker P R W, MacGregor G A, de Wardener H E et al 1975 Lancet 1: 1216
Van Scoy R E, Wilson W R 1977 Mayo Clin Proc 52: 704
Whelton A 1974 Antibiotics Chemother 18: 1
Williams D M, Wimpenny J, Asscher A W 1968 Lancet 2 1058
Winchester J F, Gelfand M C, Knepshield J H, Schreiner G E 1977 Trans Amer Soc Artificial Internal Organs 23: 762

27

Laboratory control

The need for skilled laboratory control for antibacterial chemotherapy in hospital patients has never been greater than in the present day. Resistance patterns of common bacteria vary in different hospitals usually in response to varying drug usage, and are made more complex by the introduction of semi-synthetic derivatives of an increasing number of antibiotics, among some of which cross-resistance is no longer a foregone conclusion.

Advances in surgery and the widespread use of immunosuppressive drugs, and above all, the constant use of antibiotics have led to great changes in the causes of bacterial infections, and species little heard of twenty years ago may now present great problems. On the other hand these same species may be little more than commensals and skilled judgment may be required to assess their significance.

Sensitivity tests cannot be considered in isolation; they are entirely dependent upon good basic bacteriology and this in turn depends upon the receipt of a suitable specimen. It may well be necessary to start treatment at once but if so it is essential that appropriate specimens are collected first or the bacteriological diagnosis will be made more difficult or even impossible. The causative organism must be distinguished from commensals and contaminants, which usually grow more readily both in transit and in culture. If no pathogen is isolated from sputum, no sensitivity tests should be performed: to report such tests on mouth bacteria is only to mislead.

The laboratory influences drug usage greatly by the sensitivity tests it reports and it therefore has a responsibility to see that these tests are applied to appropriate organisms and suitable drugs.

In previous editions of this book we have endeavoured to cover all aspects of laboratory control, but the continuing growth of the subject makes this aim no longer feasible and this chapter is now based largely on methods used by the authors. For information about other methods readers are referred to Reeves et al (1978).

TESTS OF BACTERIAL SENSITIVITY

Diffusion tests

Although fashions in sensitivity testing may now be changing, some form of disc diffusion test remains the most widely used method throughout the world. The method was exhaustively studied over a period of 10 years by an International Collaborative Study Group and their final conclusions were reported in 1971

(Ericsson & Sherris, 1971). They did not find it possible to recommend a single method for routine use, but the Report proposed a slightly modified version (ICS method) of the method originally recommended by Ericsson (1960) employing regression lines, as a standard reference method.

In fact the ICS method has not been widely adopted outside Sweden; the Kirby-Bauer (KB) method is used throughout the United States, and in the United Kingdom the majority of laboratories continue to use the method in which the zone given by the unknown organism is compared to that given by a control organism of known sensitivity (comparative method). The WHO has now accepted the impossibility of standardizing these tests and is recommending that the choice of method should be left to the individual, but that there should be greater control of medium and discs and that results should be checked by quality control (WHO, 1977).

Basically, the ICS, KB and comparative methods are the same; they differ mainly in the method of interpretation and in some details of technique. When properly performed they all give the correct answer and likewise all are subject, to a greater or lesser degree, to the same sources of error. Similarly they are all open to abuse.

Comparison with a control

In this method the zone given by the test organism is compared to that given by a suitable control organism. The control may be on a separate plate, in which case it is essential that it is on the same medium and includes all the discs used, or both the control and the test organism can be on the same plate (Stokes method, page 472). This greatly facilitates the reading of the test and of course also controls each disc. Any sensitivity test medium can be used but low content discs are essential, except for testing organisms from urine. Three grades of sensitivity are recognized, sensitive, moderately sensitive and resistant.

Kirby-Bauer method

This method is now the official method of the Food and Drug Administration in the U.S.A. (Federal Register, 1972). The method defines three degrees of sensitivity according to zone diameter, and makes no exception for organisms from the urine. Zone diameters are interpreted by reference to published tables and the performance of the test must therefore be strictly standardized. Mueller-Hinton agar is specified with a single, usually high content, disc for each drug. Plates are inoculated with a swab dipped into a bacterial suspension adjusted to the same density as a barium sulphate standard: this should result in just confluent growth.

The ICS method (Ericsson & Sherris, 1971)

This method also interprets zone diameters by reference to published tables or charts and requires careful standardization. Plates are inoculated by flooding with a bacterial suspension adjusted to give dense but not confluent growth, and a single high content disc is used for each drug. The charts are based on regression lines prepared for each disc by plotting the minimum inhibitory concentration (MIC) of 100 strains of widely varying sensitivity against the log of the diameter of the zone produced by a high content disc. Whilst any sensitivity test medium can be used, the resulting chart applies only to tests performed on the same medium. Four categories of sensitivity are recognized, one applying only to organisms isolated from the urine and drugs excreted by the kidneys.

Only the comparative methods will be considered in detail in this chapter. Further information concerning the KB and ICS methods can be found in Brown & Blowers (1978).

Factors affecting the results of diffusion tests

Medium: Some constituents of laboratory media affect certain antibiotics. The addition of blood will reduce the inhibition zones of antibiotics which are heavily protein-bound, e.g. fusidate. Electrolytes affect many antibiotics: the activity of all aminoglycosides is depressed but others may be enhanced, e.g. bacitracin, fusidate and penicillins against Proteus spp. The activity of amingoglycosides against Pseudomonas, but not other species, varies with the amount of free Ca^{++} and Mg^{++} in the medium, and this may be substantially altered by the amount of both present in the agar used to solidify the medium (Fig. 27.1). The addition of dextrose

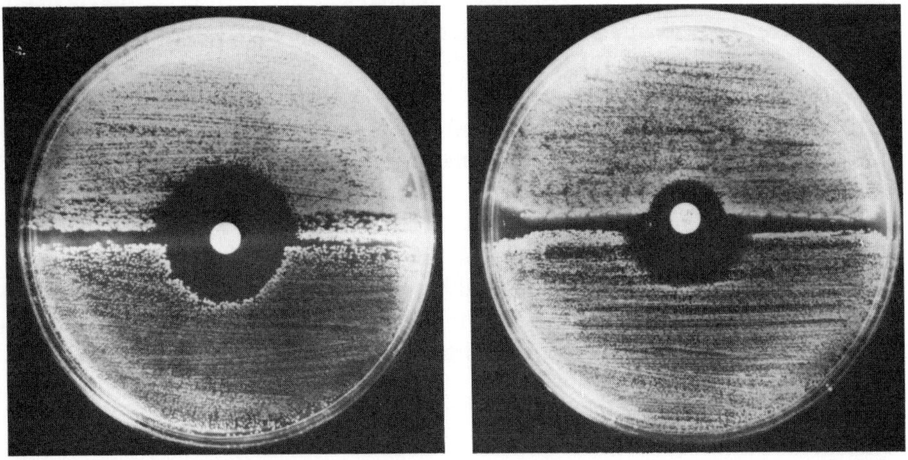

Fig. 27.1 Effect of agar on the relative sensitivity of *Ps. aeruginosa* (top half of plate) and *E. coli* (lower half of plate) to gentamicin. Discs contain 10 μg. Left – Oxoid nutrient broth No 2 solidified with Oxoid agar No 1. Right – Oxoid nutrient broth No 2 solidified with Oxoid agar No 3. Both the broth itself and agar No 1 have a very low magnesium content so that *Ps. aeruginosa* appears highly sensitive to gentamicin. Agar No 3 contains a considerable amount of magnesium and other minerals and its addition to the broth reduces the sensitivity of *Pseudomonas aeruginosa* although that of *E. coli* is unaffected (Garrod & Waterworth, 1969)

enlarges zones of inhibition produced by nitrofurantoin and by ampicillin and penicillin against some organisms (Garrod & Waterworth, 1971). This effect is seen only in diffusion tests and MIC are not altered. The action of sulphonamides and trimethoprim is reversed by thymidine and to a lesser degree by thymine. Penicillin and aminoglycosides are depressed by reducing agents such as thioglycollate and cysteine.

There is no doubt that more consistent and reliable results are obtained if a specially formulated sensitivity test medium is used, and this is essential for methods such as the Kirby-Bauer in which the zones are interpreted by reference to published tables. Those most commonly used (Mueller-Hinton, Oxoid DST and Isosensitest agars, Wellcotest agar), all have low NaCl contents but the amount of Mg^{++} and

Ca^{++} varies and in Mueller-Hinton broth may be very low: attempts are being made to standardize this. Mueller-Hinton agar may also contain significant amounts of thymidine, but this varies with different manufacturers.

Sensitivity tests should not be performed on selective media but if MacConkey agar is used for screening specimens for resistant organisms, it should be remembered that the activity of some antibiotics, particularly aminoglycosides, will be considerably reduced.

pH of medium: Streptomycin is about 500 times more active at pH 8.5 than at 5.5: all other aminoglycosides are affected similarly but to a lesser degree (see Table 27.1). The macrolides are also favoured by alkalinity but tetracyclines and fusidate are more active in an acid medium. The pH of the medium should not be altered to favour an antibiotic, but it should be remembered that circumstances which do alter it may affect the result. Thus incubation in CO_2, which lowers the pH of the medium, may make organisms appear considerably more resistant to erythromycin and lincomycin than if incubated without CO_2. Growth of most species raises the pH of nutrient agar in the surrounding area and if a drug is favoured by acidity, such as fusidate, this change may account for the 'satellitism' sometimes seen round resistant colonies. Similarly if the medium contains dextrose, any organism fermenting this will lower the pH, to the disadvantage of drugs favoured by alkalinity. Nitrofurantoin is much less active in alkaline medium and this should be borne in mind when interpreting tests with Proteus spp. which produce highly alkaline urine.

Table 27.1 The fold increase (+) or decrease (−) in the MIC of different aminoglycosides for *Staph. aureus* in broth at different pH. (Reproduced from Waterworth 1978a, with the Editors' permission)

	pH			
	5.5	6.5	7.5	8.5
Streptomycin	+64	+16	1	−8
Gentamicin	+16	+4	1	−2
Tobramycin	+16	+8	1	−2
Kanamycin	+16	+4	1	1
Amikacin	+32	+4	1	−2
Sissomicin	+16	+4	1	−2

Inoculum: The activity of many antibiotics is little affected by the number of bacteria present, but nevertheless, all zones of inhibition are reduced if the inoculum increases (Fig. 27.2). Part of the explanation of this contradiction is that visible growth appears more quickly if the inoculum is heavy, thus allowing less time for the diffusion of the antibiotic. The inoculum should be such as will produce 'dense but not confluent growth' (Fig. 27.3) and it is essential that it is uniformly distributed; Figure 27.4 illustrates the distortion of the zones often seen when sensitivity plates are inadequately spread with a wire loop. The most beautiful results are obtained by flooding with a suspension of the organism, but the preparation of dilutions is time-consuming and this method is not without risk to the operator and should never be used with highly pathogenic organisms. The Kirby-Bauer method inoculates plates with a swab dipped in diluted broth culture; this too is dependent on careful standardization and dilution. Highly satisfactory results can be achieved with the comparative method if a loopful of broth culture or bacterial suspension is applied to

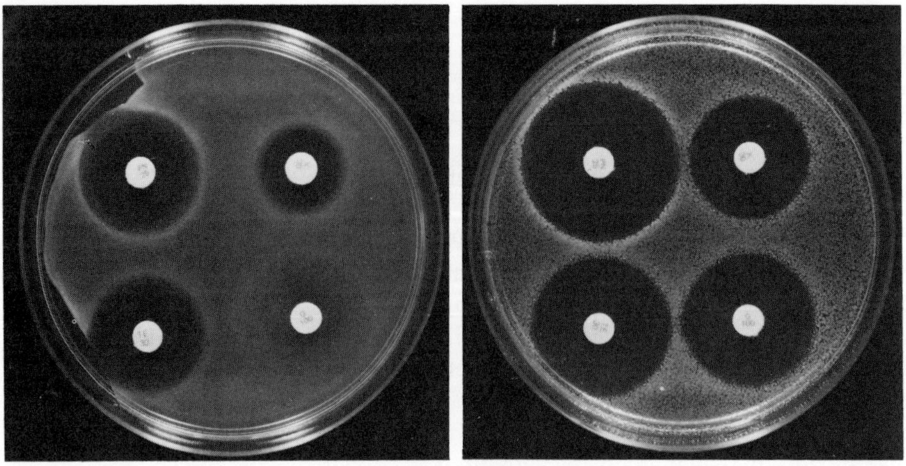

Fig. 27.2 Effect of the size of inoculum on disc sensitivity tests. Discs contain: (top left) ampicillin 25 μg, (top right) kanamycin 30 μg, (lower left) tetracycline 30 μg, (lower right) sulphafurazole 100 μg. Left – Plate flooded with overnight broth culture of *E. coli*. Right – Plate flooded with the same culture of *E. coli* diluted 1 in 5000

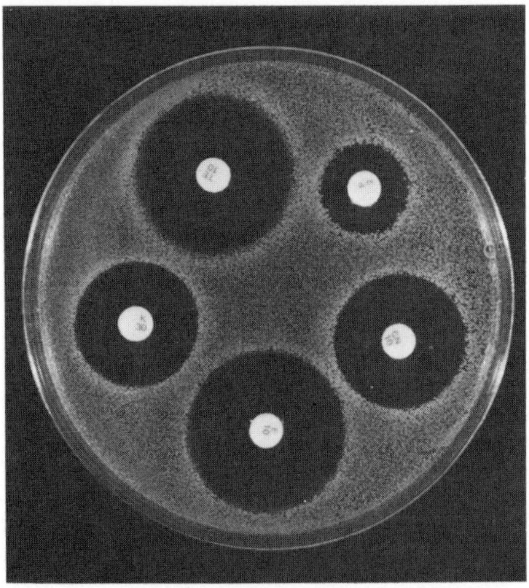

Fig. 27.3 Disc sensitivity test on a strain of *Staph. aureus* inoculated to give 'dense but not confluent growth'. Colonies at the edge of the zone round the penicillin disc (P2) are full-size, making an irregular edge and indicating that the strain produces penicillinase

the plate and spead uniformly over the plate with a dry swab (Felmingham & Stokes, 1972), preferably using a rotary plater (Pearson & Whitehead, 1974). Such a culture is illustrated in Figure 27.5.

Discs: The choice of disc content must be governed by the method of interpretation being used. The Kirby-Bauer method uses mainly high content discs and the zones are interpreted by reference to published tables. On the other hand, if zones are being interpreted by comparison with a control, the exclusive use of high content discs may give dangerously misleading results. It must be remembered that the *concentration per ml* of the drug in the immediately surrounding medium will

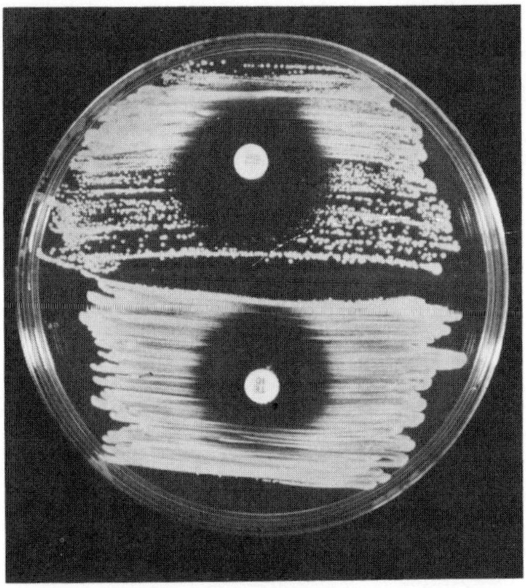

Fig. 27.4 Effect on inhibition zones of uneven distribution of the inoculum. (Top) Broth culture of *Staph. aureus* spread with a wire loop. Note the difference in the width of the zone above and below the disc. (Bottom) Colony of *Staph. aureus* taken from a primary culture and spread with a wire loop. Note the jagged edge to the zone as well as variations in its width

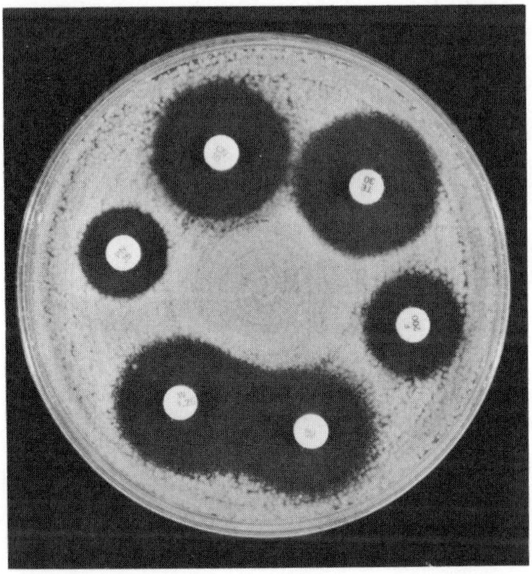

Fig. 27.5 Plate inoculated with a loopful of an overnight broth culture of *Kl. aerogenes* and spread with a dry swab using a rotary plater. Note the coalescence of the zones produced by the trimethoprim and sulphafurazole discs, indicating synergy (see page 476)

exceed the stated disc *content*. Thus *Ps. aeruginosa* may appear moderately sensitive to tetracycline if tested with a 30 μg disc, even though it requires 16 μg/ml to inhibit its growth.

Discs must be spaced far enough apart to prevent the resulting inhibition zones from overlapping. The maximum number of discs which can be tested adequately round the periphery of an 85 mm plate is six and multiple devices carrying eight discs are unsatisfactory.

Suitable discs for use with the comparative methods are given in Table 27.2. Discs must be kept dry at all times and stored in tightly sealed bottles in the cold. On removal from the refrigerator they should be allowed to attain room temperature before being opened to avoid condensation. Metronidazole discs are inactivated by light (Jones & Scott, 1977) and must therefore be protected from light at all times.

Table 27.2 Suitable disc contents (μg)

	Organisms from sites other than urine	Organisms from urine
Amikacin	10	10
Ampicillin	10	25
Carbenicillin	100	100
Cefoxitin	30	30
Cefuroxime	10	30
Cephaloridine	10	30
Chloramphenicol	10	30
Clindamycin	2	—
Colistin	50	50
Erythromycin	10	—
Fusidate	10	—
Gentamicin	10	10
Kanamycin	10	30
Lincomycin	2	—
Methicillin	5	—
Metronidazole	2.5	—
Novobiocin	5	—
Penicillin	1*	10*
Polymyxin	300*	300*
Streptomycin	10	25
Sulphonamide	100	100
Tetracycline	10	30
Tobramycin	10	10
Trimethoprim	1.25	1.25

* units

Pre-diffusion

Although a 3-hour period of pre-diffusion has been recommended, satisfactory results can be obtained without it and in clinical work the difficulties involved outweigh any possible advantages.

Length of incubation

This should be the minimum required for the normal growth of the test organism. If it is prolonged, loss of activity of the drug may permit growth of sensitive organisms which have been inhibited but not killed. This method is suitable only for fast-growing organisms and it should be remembered that anything which reduces the rate of growth (e.g. poor or selective medium or lower temperature of incubation) will enlarge the inhibition zones.

Control cultures

Control cultures are obviously essential for the comparative methods and if the Stokes method is not used, every worker reading plates should have their own control plates for comparison. Four organisms are necessary and they should be organisms known to respond to treatment with normal doses of the drug concerned; the Oxford *Staph. aureus* (NCTC 6571) is commonly used to control all drugs except polymyxins. Many drugs are excreted by the kidneys and attain high concentrations in the urine; a more resistant control with higher content discs is then permissible and a sensitive strain of *E. coli* (e.g. NCTC 10418) is generally used.

The apparent sensitivity of *Ps. aeruginosa* (but not of other species) to gentamicin and other aminoglycosides varies greatly with the Mg^{++} and Ca^{++} content of the medium. It is therefore essential that the zones given by strains of *Ps. aeruginosa* are compared to those given by a strain of known sensitivity, when the exact size of the zone will not matter. A suitable strain is NCTC 10662.

Metronidazole discs are known to deteriorate (Jones & Scott, 1977) and Milne et al (1978) have shown that incomplete anaerobiosis, which permits the growth of some Clostridia, will substantially reduce the zones produced by metronidazole discs. It is therefore desirable that each disc should be controlled and Milne et al recommend the use of *Cl. welchii* (e.g. NCTC 11229) for this purpose as this can also be used to control the other drugs likely to be tested, whereas *B. fragilis* (NCTC 9343) which is sometimes recommended, is resistant to penicillin.

Control cultures should be maintained at room temperature on agar slopes and sub-cultivated as infrequently as possible. Broth cultures should be made from these once a week and either stored in the refrigerator or subcultivated daily. The *Cl. welchii* can be maintained in Robertson's cooked meat medium.

Time can be saved and the risk of contamination greatly reduced if control plates are inoculated with swabs impregnated in bulk with diluted broth culture (Felmingham & Stokes, 1972):

Add about 15 drops of overnight broth culture of the Oxford *Staph. aureus* to 20 ml nutrient broth. (For *E. coli* NCTC 10418 and *Ps. aeruginosa* NCTC 10662 about 10 drops of culture are usually sufficient). Shake well and pipette into a jar containing sterile 3 in swabs (the quantity of broth is sufficient to impregnate about 90 swabs). Store in a screw cap glass or plastic jar at 4°C and use one swab per plate. They should keep at least one week.

Cl. welchii controls can be used in the same way. Swabs on wooden sticks are cut down to 2.5 cm in length and sterilized in the autoclave. Broth from a cooked meat culture is diluted about 1 in 10 in fresh broth and the swabs are dipped into this and placed individually in Stuart's transport medium. These too will keep for a week or more at 4°C.

Technique

Comparative method

Transfer a loopful of a well grown broth culture of the test organism to an 85 mm plate of suitable sensitivity medium (blood should be added for fastidious organisms). Using a dry swab (not the loop) first streak the inoculum across the plate and then spread uniformly over the whole area, either with a rotary plater, or by spreading at right angles to the original streak. In the absence of a broth culture a suspension can be made in a small volume of broth or water. The precise density of this and the size of the loop used do not matter greatly, presumably because a large proportion of the organisms adhere to the swab. Up to six discs may be placed round the plate, using a needle or forceps to press each firmly onto the medium. Plates should then be incubated without delay. Control cultures must be set up daily using the same medium and every disc which has been used.

If plates are to be inoculated by flooding, overnight broth cultures require diluting approximately 1/100 for streptococci, 1/1000 for staphylococci and 1/5000 for coliforms. Suitable dilutions can be prepared by adding a 2 mm loopful to 1 ml saline (streptococci) to 4 ml saline (staphylococci) and 10 ml saline (coliforms), the loop being held vertically. Using a sterile pasteur pipette, flood the plate with a well shaken suspension diluted as described, drain the excess to the side by tilting and remove with the same pipette. If only plate cultures are available, suspend portions of several colonies in a small volume of broth to give a similar density to that of an overnight broth culture and proceed as above.

Stokes method (Stokes & Ridgway, 1980)
A plate of suitable sensitivity medium is divided into three areas horizontally and the control culture is spread evenly over the upper and lower segments, using a pre-inoculated swab (see page 471). A loopful of broth culture or suspension of the test organism is then applied to the central segment and spread uniformly over the whole area with a dry sterile swab, leaving about 2 mm between this culture and the control. Two discs are then placed in each space, each about 2 cm from the edge of the plate.

If a rotary plater is used, the control is first applied to the outer area of the plate using a pre-inoculated swab. A loopful of broth culture or suspension of the test organism is then placed in the centre of the plate, this is first streaked across the area with a dry swab, which is then returned to the centre of the plate and drawn slowly outwards whilst the plate revolves, leaving about 2 mm between the two organisms (Fig. 27.6). Not more than six discs should be placed on the space between the cultures; suitable multiple devices such as the Mastring S can be used but care must be taken to ensure that the space is in the exact position required by the discs.

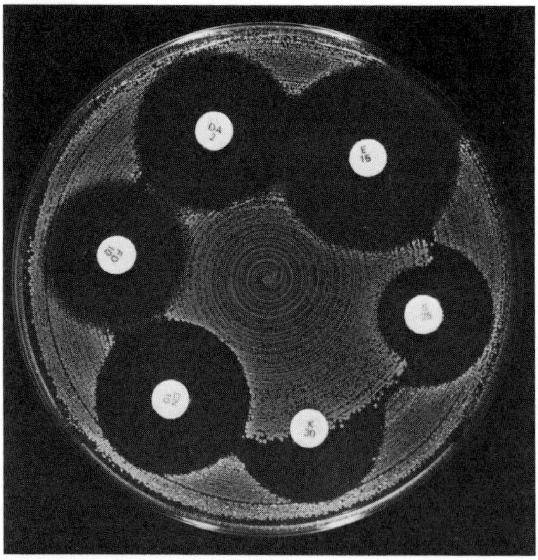

Fig. 27.6 Stokes test on a strain of *Staph. aureus* using a rotary plater. The zones produced by the unknown strain in the centre of the plate can be directly compared to those given by the control strain, round the outer area of the plate

Interpretation of results

When the control is on a separate plate these zones should be measured, using calipers or a mm rule, and recorded. The zones given by the test organism are then measured and compared to those of the control: it is essential that both measurements are made by the same worker.

Three categories of sensitivity are recognized:

1. *Sensitive:* Zone diameter not more than 6 mm smaller than that of the control. This infers that the infection should respond to treatment with normal doses.

2. *Moderately resistant.* Zone diameter of at least 12 mm but more than 6 mm smaller than that of the control, indicating that high doses will be required.
3. *Resistant:* Zone diameter of 12 mm or less (the disc being 6 mm) inferring that clinical response is unlikely.

Tests on organisms isolated from the urine are interpreted in the same way, the higher concentration of drugs in this site being allowed for by the use of higher content discs and a more resistant control organism.

In the Stokes method no measuring is necessary if the zone given by the test organism is as large or larger than that of the control. If the zone is clearly smaller the 'radius' is measured from the edge of the disc and if this measures at least 3 mm, but is more than 3 mm smaller than that of the control, the organism is classed as moderately resistant. An organism giving a zone of less than 3 mm is resistant.

The main advantages of these methods are that any variations in the composition of the medium will make little, if any, difference, and secondly, that differences in the inoculum size are obvious (particularly in the Stokes method) and can be taken into consideration when interpreting the result.

Common sources of error

Penicillinase-producing staphylococci

These are resistant to penicillin by virtue of their ability to destroy the drug, but they may show quite large inhibition zones round a penicillin disc. These organisms can be identified by their appearance at the edge of the inhibition zone. Colonies are full-sized, giving a heaped-up edge (Fig. 27.3) in contrast to the smooth edge produced by colonies of diminishing size in the control culture. The same effect is seen with ampicillin. Such organisms should be reported as penicillinase-producing or resistant.

Various Gram-negative bacilli sometimes produce similar large colonies round an ampicillin zone of inhibition; no explanation has been offered for this phenomenon which in these species does not signify β-lactamase production.

H. influenzae

Some strains are resistant to ampicillin because they produce β-lactamase. Sensitivity test media often fail to support adequate growth of this species and as a result zones may not be significantly reduced, particularly if 10 μg discs are used. These organisms can be identified more reliably by testing for β-lactamase production. Papers impregnated with penicillin and an indicator are commercially available (Oxoid, Mast Laboratories); solid growth is applied to these with a loop or swab stick and if β-lactamase is present this splits the penicillin to give penicilloic acid, which lowers the pH and changes the indicator (Slack et al 1977; Wheldon and Slack 1979).

N. gonorrhoeae

Some strains produce β-lactamase and it is essential that these are recognized. Any strains giving reduced zones with a penicillin disc should be tested for β-lactamase as above.

Methicillin-resistant staphylococci

Cultures of most of these organisms contain only a small proportion of cells capable of appearing resistant if grown on normal medium and incubated at 37°C for 18 hours, and resistance is often not obvious unless a heavy inoculum is used and incubation continued for 48 hours. The addition of 5 per cent NaCl to the medium enables the entire population of such cultures to grow on higher concentrations of methicillin; disc tests on this medium usually give satisfactory results but the medium cannot be used for tests with other drugs. Enhanced and nearly uniform resistance is seen with ordinary medium if cultures are incubated at 30°C for 18 hours, though this makes little or no difference to sensitive strains. Drew et al (1972) found that reliable results were obtained when cultures were incubated at 35°C, and as there are no recognized contraindications to maintaining diagnostic laboratory incubators at this temperature, it would seem that this is the easiest way of overcoming this problem. It is essential that the temperature is adequately controlled and does not rise above 35°C. Only methicillin should be tested. Although there is cross-resistance between methicillin, cloxacillin and flucloxacillin when tests are done by a dilution method, disc tests with cloxacillin and flucloxacillin do not always reveal resistance and should not be relied upon (Fig. 27.7).

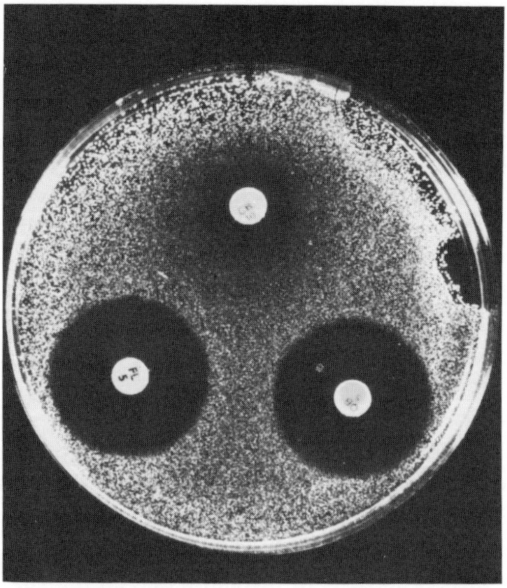

Fig. 27.7 Disc sensitivity on a methicillin-resistant strain of *Staph. aureus* incubated at 30°C. Discs contain: (top) methicillin 10 μg, (lower left) flucloxacillin 5 μg, (lower right) cloxacillin 5 μg (Garrod & Waterworth, 1971)

Cephaloridine resistance in staphylococci

Although cephaloridine is much more resistant to staphylococcal penicillinase than is benzyl penicillin, many strains of staphylococci can partially inactivate it and if tested with a heavy inoculum will appear resistant because of this. There is always cross-resistance between methicillin and other penicillinase-resistant penicillins and, though the extent of this may be variable, to cephalosporins; staphylococci resistant to methicillin may be assumed to be resistant to other penicillins and to cephalosporins.

Proteus spp.

Much confusion arises from the ability of some strains to swarm into inhibition zones (Fig. 27.8). Organisms taken from inside these zones and re-tested are no more resistant than the parent culture and as long as there is a clear edge to the zone, measurements may be taken from this and swarming disregarded.

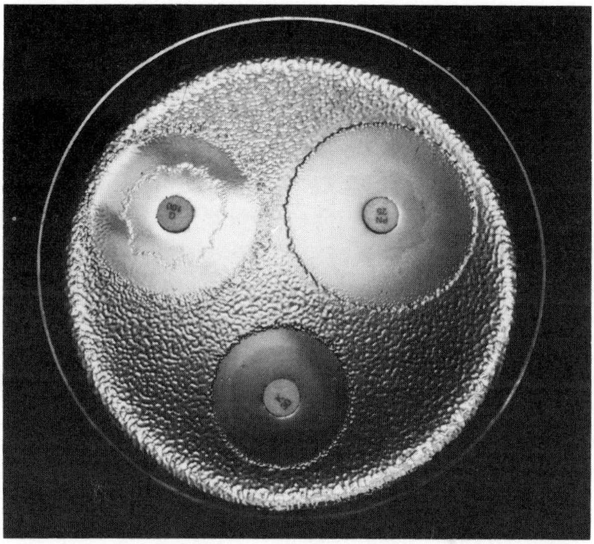

Fig. 27.8 Sensitivity test on *P. mirabilis*. Discs contain: (top left) sulphafurazole 100 μg (top right) ampicillin 25 μg (bottom) kanamycin 30 μg. Note swarming into the zones. So long as there is a clear shoulder to the zone, swarming within it can be disregarded

Polymyxins

These drugs diffuse very poorly and though growth up to the disc can safely be taken to indicate resistance, a zone of inhibition is only a very rough indication of sensitivity. Determinations of MIC are much affected by the composition of the medium and the size of the inoculum; we have obtained the most consistent results by using nutrient agar or peptone water and a light inoculum.

Sulphonamides and trimethoprim

These are much affected by the composition of the medium. Many laboratory media contain substances which inhibit the action of sulphonamides but these can be neutralized by the addition of lysed horse blood. Trimethoprim is similarly affected and Koch & Burchall (1971) have shown that this is due to the presence of thymidine or other products of folate metabolism which enable bacteria to by-pass the action of these drugs. The neutralizing effect of lysed horse blood has now been explained by Ferone et al (1975), who found that this contains an enzyme, thymidine phosphorylase, which splits thymidine into thymine and 2-

deoxyribose-1-phosphate. Thymine may also reverse the action of these drugs but much larger amounts are required.

Media containing thymidine do not simply reduce the size of the inhibition zone produced by discs containing sulphonamide or trimethoprim, they permit growth throughout the area, though the colonies may be of reduced size. Many commercially available sensitivity media are now apparently thymidine-free, probably because uridine has been added (Amyes & Smith, 1978); those which are not should be cleared by the addition of 4 per cent lysed horse blood or thymidine phosphorylase.

Sulphonamides are inactivated by *p*-aminobenzoic acid and sensitivity tests are invalidated by a heavy inoculum, which may contain enough *p*-aminobenzoic acid to inactivate the drug. If these tests are over-inoculated zones are not simply reduced, they disappear completely (Fig. 27.2): resistance cannot then be assumed; the test must be repeated. Among the more active sulphonamides it matters little which is used: results obtained with one apply to others with the possible exception of some strains of *Ps. aeruginosa* against which sulphadiazine has rather greater activity than most other sulphonamides. Thus a zone of inhibition is sometimes seen round a 300 μg sulphatriad disc (which contains sulphadiazine) though none is seen round discs containing co-trimoxazole or sulphamethoxazole. We do not believe this difference to be clinically significant.

It is preferable to test sulphonamides and trimethoprim on separate discs and if these are placed about 2 cm apart the zones may coalesce by extension, indicating synergy (see Fig. 27.5). However, synergy will only be seen if the two drugs are present in the ratio appropriate for the organism being tested and failure to demonstrate it does not mean that it will not occur. There is much discussion as to what constitutes sensitivity to co-trimoxazole. We recommend that any organism showing full sensitivity to trimethoprim, whether or not it is sensitive to sulphonamide, and any showing a zone of at least 12 mm (disc 6 mm) round both discs should be reported as sensitive to co-trimoxazole.

The choice of drugs to be tested

One of the main problems of sensitivity testing today is that of selecting which of the continually increasing number of antibacterial drugs now available should be tested. It is far better to test a small number well than a large number unreliably. In previous editions of this book we have recommended that only a single representative of each family of drugs should be tested. Unfortunately some exceptions to this rule are now necessary as cross-resistance between some of the newer semi-synthetic derivatives and their parent substances is no longer a foregone conclusion. This is particularly true among cephalosporins; cefuroxime, cefotaxime and cefoxitin (a cefamycin) may all be active against organisms resistant to earlier cephalosporins, and each of these new ones must be tested separately. Similarly cross-resistance cannot be assumed among aminoglycosides. On the other hand we see little reason to test minocycline separately; it is true that this is sometimes active against organisms resistant to tetracycline, but there seems to be too little indication for its clinical use to justify routine testing. Either carbenicillin or ticarcillin can be tested but both are not required. There is no need to test mezlocillin separately except possibly with strains of *Ps. aeruginosa* with some resistance to carbenicillin. Suitable drugs for first and second line testing are given in Table 27.3.

Table 27.3 Choice of drugs for sensitivity tests

	First line	Second line
Gram + organisms	Penicillin Methicillin Erythromycin	Fusidate Gentamicin Tetracycline Clindamycin
Gram-bacilli	Ampicillin Gentamicin Trimethoprim Sulphonamide	Amikacin Cefuroxime Chloramphenicol Tobramycin Carbenicillin Mecillinam
Urinary organisms	Ampicillin Trimethoprim Sulphonamide Nitrofurantoin Nalidixic Acid	Cephalexin Cefuroxime Mecillinam Gentamicin Amikacin Carbenicillin
Anaerobes	Penicillin Clindamycin Metronidazole	Erythromycin
Ps. aeruginosa	Carbenicillin Gentamicin Tobramycin Amikacin	Polymyxin Mezlocillin

The indiscriminate use of new drugs, which may well lead to the rapid development of bacterial resistance, can be discouraged by not reporting sensitivity to these unless there is no alternative treatment. Similarly drugs inapplicable to the specimen (e.g. nitrofurantoin for organisms from any source but urine) or to the method should not be tested. Tests with methenamine mandelate (Mandelamine) are misleading because its activity is dependent on the liberation of formaldehyde in an acid medium, and is therefore dependent on the pH of the urine (Waterworth, 1962).

Sensitivity tests in primary cultures

Diffusion tests can be incorporated in primary culture. These tests have advantages, of which the foremost are speed and simplicity; they also reveal the presence of small numbers of resistant organisms and often facilitate the identification of organisms present in mixed cultures because of the selective action on different species.

The method is particularly suitable for testing specimens of urine. Waterworth & del Piano (1976) were able to report the sensitivity on 92 per cent from their primary tests, but they point out that it is essential to have some means of first recognizing which specimens are infected or much time and medium will be wasted. These authors also recommend primary tests on swabs of pus taken from acute infections, particularly in Casualty Departments.

The main objection raised against the method is the difficulty of controlling the size of the inoculum. In practice this is seldom a problem. If the Stokes method (page 472) is used and the centre area of the plate inoculated with a loopful of urine and spread with a dry swab, the inoculum is usually very similar to that of the control applied with a swab (page 471). Similarly, swabs bearing pus applied directly to the plate almost always yield a suitable inoculum.

It must be borne in mind that penicillinase-producing staphylococci destroy penicillin and may thus make a sensitive organism also present in mixed culture appear resistant. Similarly, chloramphenicol may be inactivated by organisms which are resistant to it and other organisms may then grow on a concentration which is normally inhibitory. In either case the test should be repeated.

Antifungal drugs

As more antifungal drugs become available there is an increasing demand for sensitivity tests with fungi. These are particularly important with flucytosine (5-fluorocytosine) to which resistance develops quite frequently during treatment and may even be present before treatment starts. Yeasts may be tested by either the disc or the dilution method and with the exception of flucytosine either Sabouraud's medium or glucose broth or agar may be used. The action of flucytosine is reversed by cytosine and pyrimidine bases, which are normally present in laboratory media and a synthetic medium must therefore be used for all tests with this drug. The medium given for assays on page 501 is also suitable for sensitivity tests with all anti-fungal drugs. Alternatively Bacto-yeast-nitrogen base (Difco) with 0.15 per cent asparagine and 1 per cent dextrose added may be used; this solution can be prepared as a concentrated solution and stored in the refrigerator until required, when it is diluted 10-fold to normal strength in water or an aqueous solution of agar (2 per cent). API include flucytosine in their 10M range for MIC determination (see page 493) and supply ampoules of suitable medium for use with this drug. All sensitivity tests with flucytosine must be incubated for 48 hours as resistance may not be apparent after 24 hours' incubation.

A sensitive strain of *C. albicans* can be used as a control for all drugs except griseofulvin and the inoculum of both this and the test organism must be kept light.

Dilution methods

In the past these methods have been considered too time consuming for general use and they have been used mainly where the disc method was inapplicable, e.g. for testing slow-growing organisms such as *Myco. tuberculosis*. Another important use was the determination of the MIC or more usually the minimum bactericidal concentration (MBC) for organisms isolated from the blood of patients with endocarditis, though these tests were done less frequently than was desirable. This situation is now changing, the availability of MIC 'kits' and various forms of replicating inoculators now not only make it possible for any laboratory to perform MIC and MBC determinations where required, but also raise the possibility of using some form of dilution method for routine tests.

Determination of minimum inhibitory concentration

These tests can be done in either liquid or solid medium; if only one strain is to be tested it is easier to use broth, but if there are many strains, the dilutions can be prepared in agar plates and these inoculated with a replicator. Dilution tests are as much affected by the composition and pH of the medium as are disc tests (see page 466): serum or blood can be added for fastidious organisms. The size of the inoculum is much less critical except with sulphonamides when, as with the disc method, tests will be invalidated if it is too heavy. It must also be remembered that organisms producing β-lactamases owe their resistance to penicillins and cephalosporins to these enzymes, and the result of an MIC determination will depend largely on the size of the inoculum; this should normally be about 10^5 organisms.

It is essential that a control organism of known sensitivity be included in all such tests, and if the dilutions are prepared in broth, a second identical set must be prepared at the same time and inoculated with the control. Guidance for preparing stock solutions of antibiotics is given on page 491.

Methods

Broth dilutions. Prepare two sets of two-fold dilutions of the antibiotic in 1 ml volumes of broth. The range should start about 8-fold higher than the normal MIC for the species being tested and extend to at least one dilution below that of the control organism (see Table 14.1): a drug-free control tube must be included. Inoculate one set of tubes with 1 drop of a well-grown broth culture of the test organisms diluted 1 in 100 and the other with the control organism similarly diluted. Incubate overnight.

Agar dilution. Prepare a suitable range of two-fold dilutions of the antibiotic in water at 20 times the required concentrations. Label one sterile Petri dish for each and place 1 ml of the appropriate dilution in each. Add 19 ml melted agar cooled to 50°C and mix well (5 per cent blood should be added to the agar if required for growth). When set, incubate at 37°C with the lids tipped for about 30 min before inoculating with broth cultures diluted 1 in 100, using either a loop or a multiple replicator.

The lowest concentration inhibiting growth is taken as the MIC. An advantage of the plate dilution method is that it reveals the presence of small numbers of resistant mutants, whilst in broth these would appear simply as uniform growth.

Determination of minimum bactericidal concentration

The broth dilution method for the determination of an MIC (see above) can be converted into a bactericidal test. After the tubes have been inoculated with the test organism, a loopful of the drug-free control tube is immediately uniformly spread over one quarter of a plate of suitable medium. The resulting growth represents the original inoculum. The tubes are then incubated at 37°C for six hours or overnight, after which any showing no growth are sub-cultivated in the same way and the resulting growth compared to that from the control tube before incubation. These tests are much affected by the size of the inoculum; if this is too light the number of survivors will be very small, giving an unduly favourable result. Satisfactory results have been obtained using an inoculum of 10^6 organisms, i.e. one drop of a well grown broth culture diluted 1 in 10.

Results are interpreted as follows:

Number of colonies similar to that from the control tube before incubation—bacteristatic action only.

Reduced number of colonies—partial or slow bactericidal action.

Small numbers of colonies—incomplete bactericidal action ('persisters').

No growth—complete killing.

There is no reason to sub-cultivate tubes with the control organism which show no growth. The purpose of the control is to confirm that the drug concentrations are correct and it is immaterial whether this organism is killed.

Results can be invalidated by 'carry-over' if high concentrations are used with very sensitive organisms. This can be partially overcome by placing the loopful of the test mixture on the plate and allowing the fluid to be absorbed before spreading over the whole area (Fig. 27.9). However, there is no advantage in using high concentrations

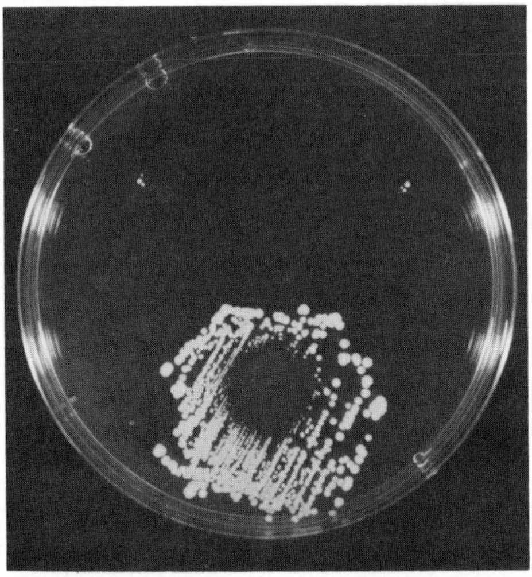

Fig. 27.9 Inhibition by carry-over in bactericidal tests. A loopful of broth containing 2 μg/ml rifampicin and inoculated with *Staph. aureus* was (a) streaked horizontally across the top half of the plate, when it yielded only one or two colonies at the ends of the streak, and (b) placed in the centre of the lower half of the plate and left until the fluid had been absorbed, when it was spread over the surrounding area

Cysteine-dependent streptococci.

These organisms, which usually grow only in the blood culture bottle containing thioglycollate, will not grow in serum broth or on blood agar, except as satellites

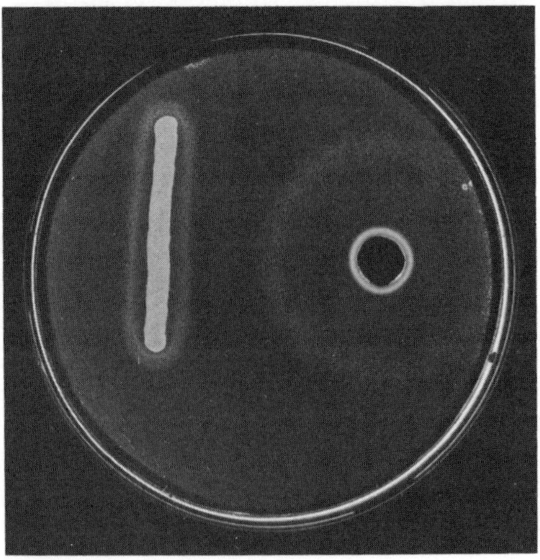

Fig. 27.10 Cysteine-dependent *Str. viridans* growing only beside a streak of *Staph. aureus* (left) and a cup containing 0.2 per cent L-cysteine (right)

of penicillin; if this is not bactericidal at, or just above the MIC, higher concentrations will not kill either.

around contaminating colonies (Fig. 27.10). Satisfactory growth can be obtained if 0.01 per cent cysteine is added to serum broth, but the activity of penicillin and the aminoglycosides will be depressed (see page 466). The MIC of the control organism will therefore be higher than usual and this must be taken into account when interpreting the result with the test organism: 0.01 per cent of cysteine must also be added to the blood agar used for sub-cultivating bactericidal tests.

Dilution methods in routine sensitivity testing

Although it appears that the determination of the MIC of multiple antibiotics is becoming increasingly common in routine work in the U.S.A., we see little likelihood of this becoming standard practice in the United Kingdom. On the other hand, the use of 'break points' (concentrations which inhibit sensitive but not resistant organisms) is certainly becoming more widespread throughout the world. The main advantages of a dilution method are that it is much less affected by the size of the inoculum than is the disc test and also, it is easier to read the presence or absence of growth than to interpret a zone of inhibition. A machine which facilitates the reading of these plates and also prints out the results is discussed on page 493.

Organisms are sub-cultivated from primary cultures to broth or peptone water in the morning, and in the evening these are replicated onto plates containing antibiotics. Usually two concentrations are used for each antibiotic, probably with a four-fold difference, and an organism is considered to be sensitive if it is inhibited by both, moderately sensitive if by only one and resistant if not inhibited by either (Fig. 27.11). Proteus must be prevented from swarming and the addition of 0.8 per cent Oxoid agar No. 1 to Isosensitest agar has been found satisfactory if the plates are adequately dried before use. As it has been shown that antibiotics remain stable in agar for at least 1 week (Ryan et al, 1970) plates can be prepared in bulk and the drugs added to agar in bottles before pouring, which facilitates mixing. Nevertheless the preparation of the antibiotic solutions and the correct labelling of the plates will present problems for many departments; the use of Adapads (Mast Laboratories, see page 493) can provide a satisfactory solution.

Inevitably there is some disagreement over the choice of the break-point concentrations. In Table 27.4 we give those which we have found satisfactory; where more than two concentrations are given the top two are recommended for urinary tract infections and the bottom two for organisms from other sites. It is essential that a reliable sensitivity test medium is used; variations in its composition or pH will alter the results obtained with some drugs and unless the Mg^{++} and Ca^{++} content is adequate (see page 466), strains of *Ps aeruginosa* which have considerable resistance to aminoglycosides will appear sensitive. The inclusion of a control strain will not overcome this problem. In general the size of the inoculum is not critical; however, most organisms which produce β-lactamases owe their resistance to penicillins and cephalosporins to this and thus if the inoculum is very light they may appear to be sensitive. If it is very heavy this may invalidate the results with sulphonamides, but if necessary this is preferable to reporting false sensitivity to penicillin, particularly with staphylococci. We have found the addition of a 2 mm loopful of a well-grown broth culture (or equivalent bacterial suspension) to 5 ml peptone water to be

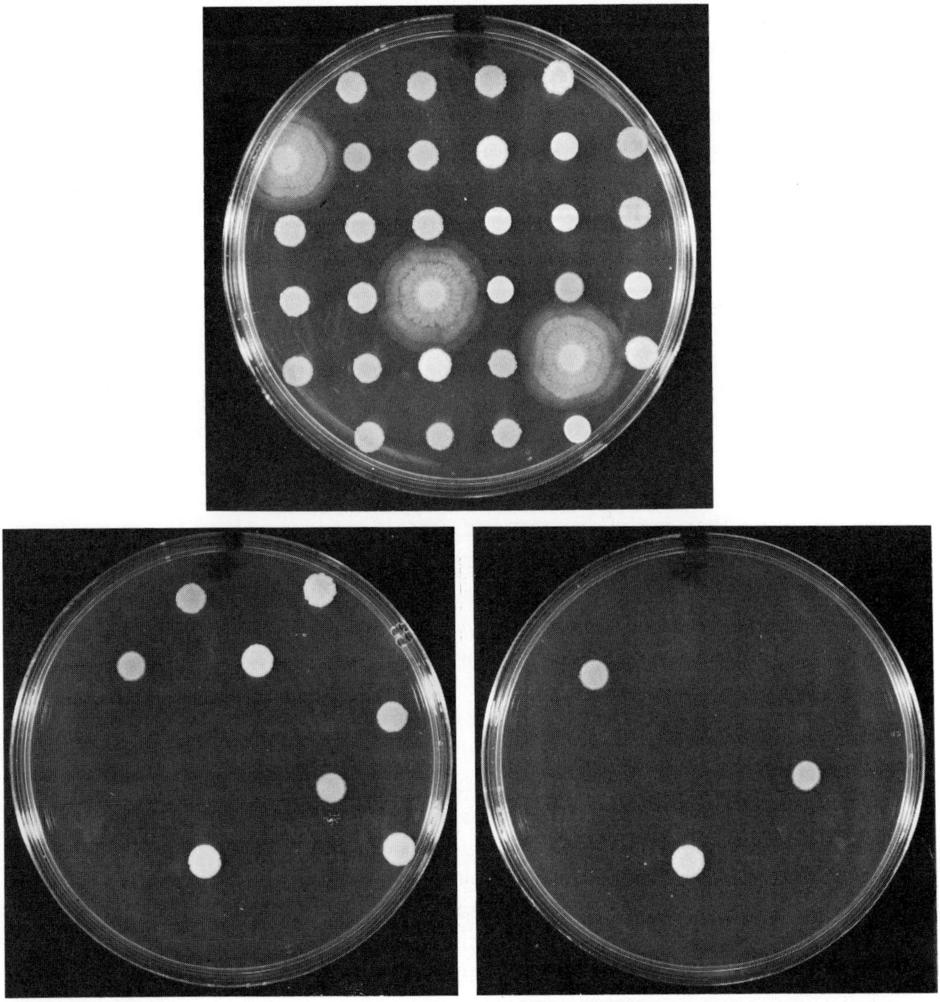

Fig. 27.11 Break-point sensitivity testing on agar plates, using a multiple inoculator. A – control plate. Note the restriction of the swarming of *P. mirabilis* by the use of double strength agar. B and C – plates containing 8 and 64 μg/ml ampicillin respectively. Strains inhibited on both plates are sensitive and those only by 64 μg/ml are moderately sensitive

satisfactory for inoculating these plates.

'Break points' in broth. One of the disadvantages of the use of 'break points' in agar is that all sensitivity tests must be set up together and will then all be read by one worker rather than by the individual reporting the specimen. Similar tests in broth would overcome this problem and have been made possible by the commercial availability of plastic trays containing dried antibiotics to which 50 or 100 μl inoculated broth is added. These are discussed on page 492. They have advantages that every worker can set up his own sensitivity tests and also do this very rapidly; on the other hand it will be more difficult to tell that the culture is mixed than when these tests are done on solid medium.

Waterworth (1981) has recently compared the results obtained by various break-point methods with those given by the disc test.

Table 27.4 Suitable concentrations of antibacterial drugs for break-point sensitivity tests in agar or broth. Where more than two concentrations are given, the first two are recommended for organisms from urine and the second two for other infections

	Concentrations μg/ml
Amikacin	16, 4
Ampicillin	32, 8, 1
Carbenicillin	256, 64
Cefoxitin	32, 8, 2
Cefuroxime	32, 8, 2
Cephaloridine	32, 8, 2
Chloramphenicol	16, 4
Clindamycin	1, 0.25
Erythromycin	1, 0.25
Fusidate	2
Gentamicin	8, 2
Kanamycin	16, 4
Methicillin	8
Nalidixic acid	32
Nitrofurantoin	32
Penicillin	0.25
Sulphamethoxazole	128, 32, 8
Tetracycline	64, 16 : 4, 1
Ticarcillin	128, 32
Tobramycin	8, 2
Trimethoprim	8, 2, 0.5

Sensitivity tests for Myco. tuberculosis

The laboratory control of the treatment of tuberculosis is a highly specialized subject beyond the scope of this chapter. In an excellent comprehensive article on this subject Collins & Yates (1978) draw attention to some of the problems facing small laboratories performing their own sensitivity tests. For example, the short shelf-life of drug-containing medium and the need to have control strains replaced with fresh wild strains at very frequent intervals. It therefore seems preferable that strains of *Myco. tuberculosis* should be sent to regional centres specializing in these tests, but those seeking further information should refer to the article by Collins & Yates.

TESTS OF COMBINED ACTION

When the combined action of two drugs is tested *in vitro* the results may show one of three effects:

1. *Indifference:* when the action of the two drugs together is no greater than that of the more active alone.
2. *Antagonism:* when the activity of one drug is diminished in the presence of the second.
3. *Synergy:* when the activity of the two drugs acting together significantly exceeds that of either acting alone in the same concentration. Small increases in activity are considered additive.

These effects may apply to either the bacteristatic or the bactericidal action of the drugs.

Combined bacteristatic action

This can be studied most revealingly by the chessboard method. In this a range of dilutions of both drugs in broth (or agar) is mixed together so that every concentration of each is present alone and in every possible combination with the other. The results of four such tests are given in Table 27.5 and Figure 27.12. If these tests are being performed to demonstrate synergy, it is important that the concentrations used include, or are close to, the MIC of each drug.

Table 27.5 Results of three tests of combined bacteristatic action by the chequerboard method
All concentrations in μg/ml += growth −= no growth

		Tetracycline					
		0.5	0.25	0.12	0.06	0.03	nil
Novobiocin	0.5	−	−	−	−	−	−
	0.25	−	−	−	−	−	−
	0.12	−	−	+	+	+	+
	0.06	−	−	+	+	+	+
	0.03	−	−	+	+	+	+
	nil	−	−	+	+	+	+
				A			

		Trimethoprim					
		16	8	4	2	1	nil
Sulphafurazole	4	−	−	−	−	−	+
	2	−	−	−	−	−	+
	1	−	−	−	−	−	+
	0.5	−	−	−	−	+	+
	0.25	−	−	−	−	+	+
	nil	−	+	+	+	+	+
				B			

		Nalidixic acid						
		32	16	8	4	2	1	nil
Nitrofurantoin	128	−	−	−	−	−	−	−
	64	−	+	+	+	+	+	+
	32	−	−	+	+	+	+	+
	16	−	−	+	+	+	+	+
	8	−	−	−	+	+	+	+
	4	−	−	−	+	+	+	+
	2	−	−	−	−	+	+	+
	1	−	−	−	−	+	+	+
	nil	−	−	−	−	−	+	+
				C				

A—Indifferent. Tetracycline and novobiocin *v Staph. aureus*. (see p. 227)
B—Synergic. Trimethoprim and sulphafurazole *v N. gonorrhoeae*.
C—Antagonistic. Nitrofurantoin and nalidixic acid *v. Proteus mirabilis*.

Method. Prepare a range of six or eight two-fold dilutions in broth at twice the required concentrations with each drug. Set up sufficient sterile tubes in the form of a square. Take each dilution of drug A in turn and place 1 ml in each tube of a horizontal row, placing 1 ml of drug-free broth across the last row. 1 ml of each dilution of drug B is then placed in each tube of a vertical row: 1 ml broth only is added to the last row. Inoculate each tube with approximately 10^5 organisms (i.e. one drop of a 1 in 100 dilution of a well grown broth culture). The MIC of each drug alone is read first. The degree of combined effect is sometimes expressed as the fractional inhibitory concentration (FIC); this is the inhibitory concentration of a drug when in combination, expressed as a fraction of the MIC when acting alone, and the sum of the FICs of both drugs gives a numerical value for combined effect. A figure of >0.25 indicates synergy.

Combined bacteristatic action can also be demonstrated by disc test and the present day practice of placing many discs on a single plate often reveals strange interactions. That most frequently seen—and of most significance— is the synergy between sulphonamides and trimethoprim which is discussed on page 27. Synergy is also seen between polymyxins and sulphonamides or trimethoprim against Proteus spp. The antagonism between nalidixic (or oxolinic) acid and nitrofurantoin may also be seen in routine testing but is unlikely to have any clinical significance. On the other hand the marked antagonism seen between erythromycin and clindamycin or lincomycin against staphylococci or streptococci resistant to the former is highly significant, as such strains usually fail to respond to treatment with clindamycin and rapidly acquire resistance to this too (see page 192 and Fig. 8.2).

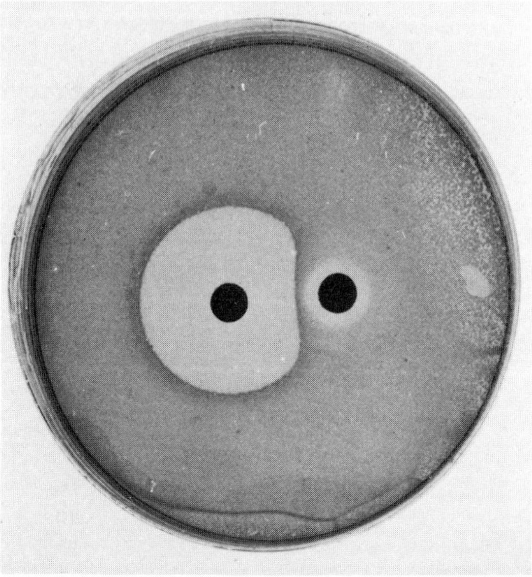

Fig. 27.12 Bacteristatic antagonism between nitrofurantoin (Rt) and nalidixic acid (Lt) against *Pr. rettgeri*

Tests of combined bactericidal action

These are chiefly of interest for the purpose of identifying a synergic combination for the treatment of endocarditis. Totally bactericidal effect must be the aim of such treatment and anything short of this may fail, no matter how sensitive the organism is to the bacteristatic action of the drug. Tests of bactericidal action are therefore required. It may also be necessary to test these combinations against staphylococci, some of which may be 'tolerant' to penicillins (see page 59).

Bactericidal synergy is only seen between drugs which singly are incompletely bactericidal. An inhibitory concentration of one drug will always be required (e.g. penicillin) but a subinhibitory concentration of the second (e.g. gentamicin) may render the mixture fully bactericidal.

Bactericidal synergy is most frequently seen between penicillins or cephalosporins and aminoglycosides against streptococci, particularly enterococci and other strains having some degree of resistance to penicillin. The MBC of penicillin should first be determined (see page 479) and if the strain is incompletely killed, combined tests should be done. Some workers prefer to save time by preparing an extra set of penicillin dilutions and adding a fixed concentration of gentamicin (e.g. 1 μg/ml) to each tube in this. In fact this is illogical as either all the concentrations of penicillin which inhibit growth will then kill, or none of them will. What is much more revealing is to determine the MBC of gentamicin in duplicate, adding an inhibitory concentration of penicillin (e.g. 2 μg/ml) to one set of the dilutions. It may then be found that the amount of gentamicin required to kill the whole inoculum is quite low, despite the relative resistance of streptococci to aminoglycosides; this is illustrated in Table 27.6.

The introduction of Sensititre and API 10M MIC trays (see page 492) has made these tests possible for any laboratory. Combined effect may be tested by setting up the MIC of one antibiotic in duplicate, adding the second antibiotic to the ampoule of broth used for one; the second antibiotic can, if necessary, be provided by discs (see page 493).

Table 27.6 Minimum bactericidal concentration of penicillin and gentamicin, singly and together, for *Str. faecalis* in 10 per cent serum broth.
Results of sub-cultures from tubes showing no growth after overnight incubation.

	Concentration—μg/ml							
	16	8	4	2	1	0.5	0.25	nil
Penicillin	+	+	+	+	*	*	*	*
+ gentamicin 1 μg/ml	−	−	−	−	*	*	*	*†
Gentamicin	−	−	+	+	*	*	*	*
+ penicillin 2 μg/ml	−	−	−	−	−	+	+	+‡

* = growth in tube
\+ = small numbers of survivors
− = no growth
† = containing 1 μg/ml gentamicin
‡ = containing 2 μg/ml penicillin

The half chess board

If it is necessary to test more than two drugs, it is generally sufficient to use only a single concentration of each and to test these alone and in every possible combination. This can be done most conveniently if the tubes are arranged as a half chess board.

Method. To prepare the test given in Table 27.7, first set up and label sterile tubes as indicated in the table. Inoculate 100 ml broth containing 10 per cent serum with 10 drops of well grown broth culture and shake well. Using this, prepare 10 ml volumes of each drug at twice the required concentration. Place 1 ml of each in the appropriately labelled tubes and finally add 1 ml of drug-free broth to all tubes on the diagonal border, which contain each drug singly, and to an empty tube for the control. Immediately

Table 27.7 Result of sub-cultures of a half chess board test on a strain of *Staph. aureus* isolated from a patient with endocarditis.

		Cloxacillin	Fusidate	Rifampicin	Vancomycin	Gentamicin	Erythromycin	Clindamycin	Cefuroxime
Cloxacillin	5 μg/ml	+	++	–	+	–	++	++	+
Fusidate	5 μg/ml		*	–	++	+	++	++	++
Rifampicin	5 μg/ml			–	–	–	–	–	–
Vancomycin	5 μg/ml				+	–	+	++	+
Gentamicin	2.5 μg/ml					(+)	–	–	–
Erythromycin	2.5 μg/ml						++	+	++
Clindamycin	2.5 μg/ml							+	++
Cefuroxime	5 μg/ml								+

* Growth in tube after overnight incubation.
Results of sub-cultures indicated as follows:
++ growth similar to original inoculum (static effect only).
+ some reduction in number of colonies but many survivors.
(+) <10 colonies.
– no growth (complete cidal effect)

sub-cultivate a loopful of the control onto a blood agar plate and spread uniformly over a quarter of the surface. After six hours' incubation (or overnight) sub-cultivate all tubes showing no growth onto blood agar as above and compare the resulting growth to that from the control tube before incubation (i.e. the original inoculum), see page 479.

Results should be recorded as in Table 27.7. Combined action can then be assessed by comparing the growth from tubes containing two drugs to that from each drug singly: if the former yields more colonies than the latter (e.g. cloxacillin plus erythromycin in Table 27.7) the mixture is antagonistic, but if fewer (e.g. cloxacillin plus gentamicin) it is synergic.

This test is particularly useful for staphylococci when a wide variety of drugs may need to be tested. The drug concentrations used should not be too high, both because of the risk of invalidating the results by carry-over (see page 480) and also because they should be levels which are attainable in the blood: suitable concentrations are given in Table 27.8.

Table 27.8 Suitable drug concentration for the half chess board bactericidal test

	Final concentration in broth
Amikacin	10
*Ampicillin	2 or 10
Carbenicillin	100
*Cefuroxime	10
*Cephaloridine	2 or 10
Chloramphenicol	10
Clindamycin	2
Cloxacillin	5
Erythromycin	2
Fusidate	5
Gentamicin	2
Kanamycin	10
*Penicillin	2 or 10
Rifampicin	2
Streptomycin	10
Tetracycline	2
Tobramycin	2
Trimethoprim	2
Vancomycin	10

* The higher concentration should not be used with highly sensitive organisms or the results may be invalidated by carry-over.

Choice of antibiotics to test

These tests are made unnecessarily laborious if unsuitable drugs are tested. Table 27.9 gives the drug combinations which are most likely to have bactericidal activity. Tetracyclines and chloramphenicol always antagonize penicillins, but in contrast they may show synergy with rifampicin. Synergy is usually seen between penicillin and any aminoglycoside against streptococci and may still occur despite considerable reistance to the latter (see page 120); if the strain is highly resistant and shows no synergy, a different aminoglycoside should be tested.

Diffusion methods for combined bactericidal activity

The two disadvantages of the half chess board method are first, that only a single concentration of each drug is used and second, that only a minute proportion of the

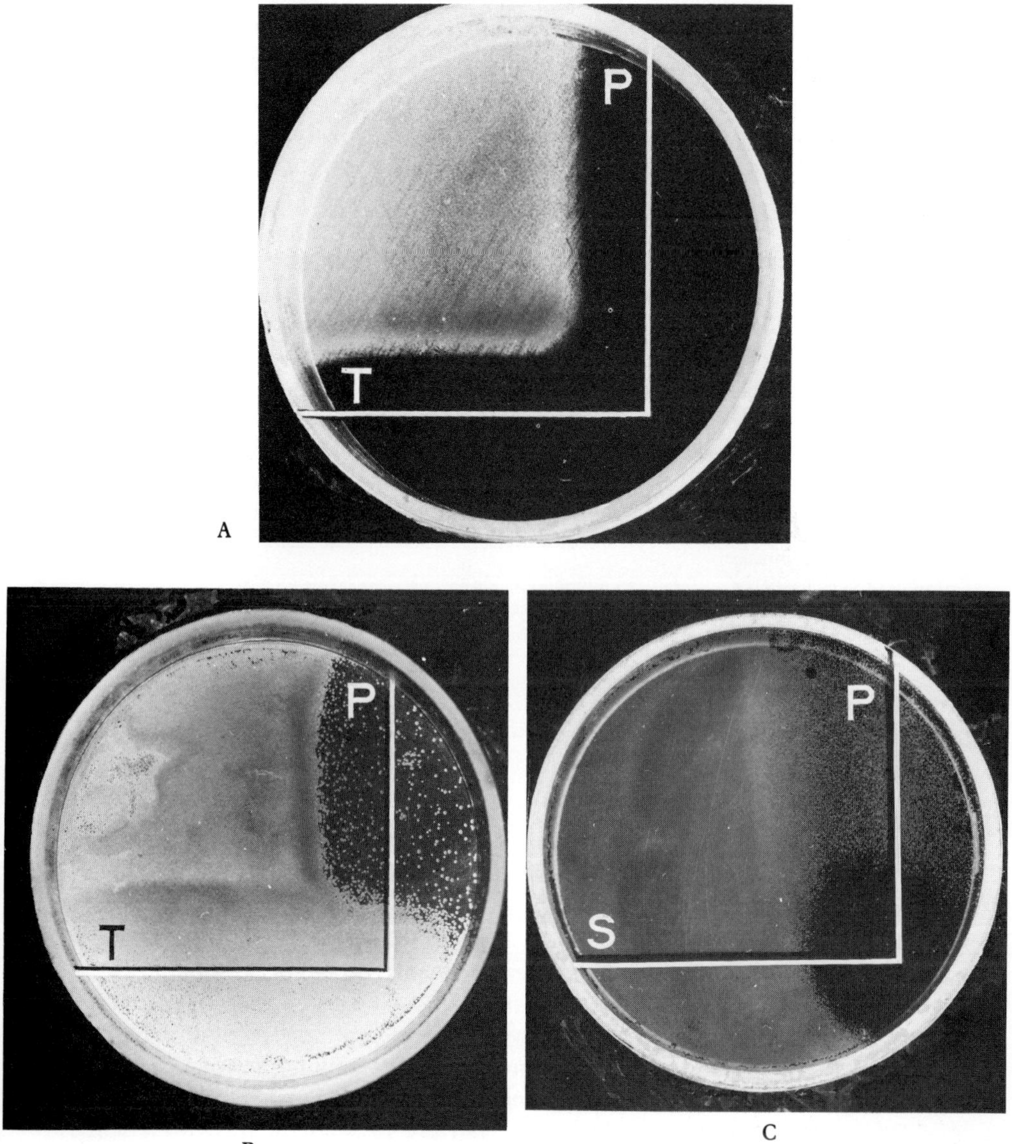

Fig. 27.13 Tests by the cellophane transfer method on a strain of *Str. faecalis* isolated from a patient with bacterial endocarditis. A. Tambour after overnight incubation on a plate into which penicillin and tetracycline had been pre-diffused from blotting paper strips. This shows bacteristatic sensitivity. B. The same tambour after a further 24 hours' incubation on antibiotic-free medium. Tetracycline alone was purely bacteristatic. Penicillin alone killed most of the inoculum but left some survivors. Where both drugs are present in the area round the angle formed by the strips, the tetracycline has eliminated the bactericidal effect of the penicillin (antagonism). C. Tambour after incubation on antibiotic-free medium following exposure to penicillin and streptomycin. Penicillin alone left survivors, streptomycin alone was barely inhibitory. The presence of both drugs sterilized the inoculum (synergy)

original inoculum is sub-cultivated. Both these disadvantages are overcome by the cellophane transfer technique. In this a cellophane tambour is inoculated on the inside with the test organism and placed on a plate into which antibiotics have been pre-diffused from blotting paper strips placed at a right angle. Nutrients and antibiotics diffuse through the cellophane to permit growth on the inside of the tambour, the plate remaining sterile. After a period of incubation the tambour is transferred to a plate of drug-free medium and any bacteria surviving in the inhibition zones will then be able to grow. After further incubation the tambour will show the bactericidal effect of each drug alone at the ends of the strips and their combined action in the area surrounding the angle where the strips meet.

This method was used most successfully for testing penicillin and aminoglycosides against streptococci and has now been replaced, to a large extent, by the β-lactamase method of Anand & Paull (1976) given below. Technical details of the cellophane transfer method are given in earlier editions of this book and may also be found in Waterworth (1978b). The tambours are illustrated in Figure 27.13.

Table 27.9 Combinations of drugs which may show bactericidal synergy, in order of probability

Streptococci		
Penicillin or cephalosporin	+	an aminoglycoside
Erythromycin	+	an aminoglycoside
Rifampicin	+	erythromycin or clindamycin
Staphylococci		
Cloxacillin or cephalosporin	+	an aminoglycoside
Rifampicin	+	erythromycin, fusidate, clindamycin
Erythromycin or clindamycin	+	an aminoglycoside
Gram-negative bacilli		
Ampicillin, carbenicillin, cefuroxime, cefoxitin, trimethoprim	+	an aminoglycoside
Rifampicin	+	chloramphenicol, tetracycline

β-lactamase method

In this method blotting paper strips impregnated with penicillin and gentamicin are applied at a right angle on a plate uniformly inoculated with the test streptococcus. After incubation the plate is sprayed with β-lactamase and re-incubated. The penicillin is thus inactivated and any organisms which were inhibited by this but not killed will grow. The aminoglycoside remains present and the method is therefore only applicable to organisms which are relatively resistant to this; bactericidal synergy can only be assumed if the sterile area on the final culture extends beyond any zone of inhibition produced by the aminoglycoside. This is illustrated in Figure 27.14.

We have found these tests easier to read if the blotting paper strips are pre-diffused into the agar and removed before the plate is inoculated.

Technique. Immerse 0.5 × 5 cm strips of sterile blotting paper (shortened dipstrips will suffice) in antibiotic solutions, remove any excess by lightly blotting on sterile blotting paper and place at a right angle on a plate of suitable medium. Allow to diffuse at 37°C for 3 hours. (Suitable antibiotic concentrations are penicillin 50 μg/ml, gentamicin 100 μg/ml).

Remove the blotting paper strips and uniformly inoculate the plate with the test organism: the inoculum should be heavy enough to give just confluent growth. Incubate for 6 hours or overnight. Spray the surface of the plate with a commercial β-lactamase. This can be done most economically by placing about 1 ml of diluted β-lactamase in a sterile bijou bottle and using a Shandon Laboratory Spray Gun to produce an aerosol. The plate should be held about 10 ins away. Re-incubate the plate for a further 24 hours. Synergy is assumed if there is growth around the ends of both strips and a sterile area in the angle between them (Figure 27.14).

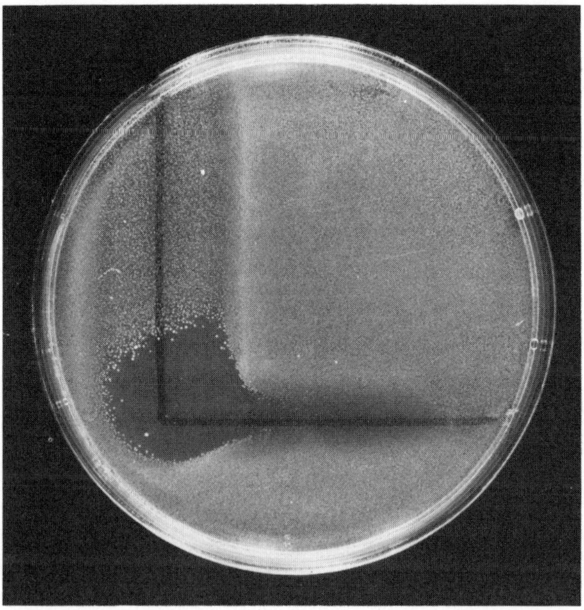

Fig. 27.14 Bactericidal test of the combined action of penicillin and gentamicin against *Str. faecalis*. The antibiotics were pre-diffused from blotting paper strips (penicillin vertical, gentamicin horizontal) and the plate flooded with diluted culture. After 6 hours' incubation the plate was sprayed with beta-lactamase and re-incubated

Preparation of stock solutions

Tablets and capsules should not be used to prepare solutions: they contain binding materials, 'fillers' and other materials as well as the antibiotic. The pure substance should be obtained, and is available for many antibiotics in preparations supplied for injections, and although these tend to be over-filled they are usually sufficiently accurate for clinical work and preferable to inaccurate weighing on inadequate balances. If the drugs are to be weighed out from samples received from the manufacturers, the purity should be noted and taken into account in the dilution. Many antibiotics are highly soluble: for those which are not there are usually special preparations for injection some of which are not suitable for laboratory purposes:

Chloramphenicol. Chloramphenicol succinate has little activity *in vitro*. Pure chloramphenicol powder is available from the manufacturers and should be used. This has a solubility of only 2.5 mg/ml in water but can be dissolved to give 10 mg/ml in ethanol.

Fusidate is now available as an injection preparation but this is relatively insoluble in water, and should be dissolved in the first instance in the buffer provided with it.

Erythromycin lactobionate (injection preparation) may be used, but if erythromycin base is obtained from the manufacturers, this must first be dissolved in a small amount of ethanol, after which it may be diluted in water.

Clindamycin phosphate is inactive *in vitro*. Clindamycin hydrochloride which is soluble in water should be obtained from the manufacturers.

Nystatin is insoluble in water, but owing to its very fine particle size it can be used as a suspension. It is very unstable and must be freshly prepared.

Sulphonamides, nitrofurantoin and *nalidixic acid* all have a low solubility in water but can be brought into solution by raising the pH. A 10 mg/ml solution can be prepared by suspending the drug in the appropriate volume of water and adding 10M NaOH a drop at a time until the solution is clear. Solutions of nitrofurantoin are unstable.

Trimethoprim is available from the manufacturers. The lactate is soluble in water (1 g = 760 mg base), the base can be brought into solution by lowering the pH with lactic acid.

Polymyxins. The sulphomethyl forms of both polymyxin B and colistin are unsuitable for sensitivity testing (see page 207): the sulphate should be used.

Rifampicin has a low solubility in water but dissolves readily in 0.01M HCl or methanol.

Commercial devices for sensitivity testing

There are at present two fully automated systems available for sensitivity testing, the Autobac 1 (Pfizer) and the MS2 (Abbott). In both of these, inoculated broth is added to compartments in a plastic cuvette in each of which an antibiotic disc has been placed. Both machines compare growth in the presence of the antibiotic to growth in a control drug-free compartment and print out the result as sensitive, intermediate or resistant, corresponding to the Kirby-Bauer test. With most species the result is available in about 3 hours. The cuvettes are expensive and the running costs of the machine are therefore very high.

There are also now a number of products available which can provide substantial help in the determination of MICs, some of which are ideally suited to small laboratories performing such tests infrequently.

Dynatech MIC 2000. This machine offers considerable assistance to any laboratory wishing to perform large numbers of MICs regularly, by distributing 50 or 100 μl of previously prepared dilutions accurately and rapidly into microtitre trays. The problem of making these dilutions has now been overcome by the provision of tablets containing the appropriate amounts of antibiotic, which are then dissolved in 20 ml broth. Two weeks' supply of trays can be prepared at a time and stored frozen until required. An automatic inoculator is available which will both inoculate the trays and also sub-cultivate after incubation for bactericidal effect.

In the majority of laboratories it is the preparation of the antibiotic solutions and dilutions which presents the greatest problems. Two products are now on the market which overcome this and make the determination of MIC or MBC possible in any laboratory.

Sensititre (Seward Laboratory) are plastic trays containing dried antibiotic dilutions, and all that is required is the addition of 50 μl of inoculated broth to each well. (Phillips et al 1978; Pykett 1978). Each tray contains eight dilutions of 11 drugs and can of course be made into a bactericidal test by sub-cultivating after incubation. Three different combinations of drugs are available, for Gram-positive,

Gram-negative and urinary organisms; they have the advantage of stability at room temperature for at least 12 months.

API 10M. When originally introduced with a limited range of drugs for determining the MIC of enterobacteria, these consisted of conventional API plastic strips containing dried dilutions of antibiotics, which were then filled with pre-inoculated 'acidification' broth. A red-yellow colour change indicated growth. It is anticipated that the format of these will eventually be changed so that a sensitivity test broth can be used, thus enabling a wider range of organisms to be tested. These strips would have the advantages that only the drugs required need be tested and they can readily be made into tests of combined action by adding a second drug to the ampoule of broth used. One very welcome feature is that every well can be labelled.

Discs for dilutions. Flowers (1978) has recommended the use of sensitivity discs as a source of antibiotic for preparing dilutions. He obtained consistent results with both penicillin and gentamicin discs, by preparing two-fold dilutions in 200 μl volumes of broth in a WHO perspex haemagglutination plate.

Mast MIC Method. Shafi (1975) showed that agar plates could be prepared for the determination of MICs by applying filter papers impregnated with the appropriate amount of drug to the surface of plates and allowing these to diffuse for at least three hours. The papers were then removed and the plates inoculated with a replicator. Mast Laboratories have modified this method and the papers can now be placed in the dishes before the plates are poured. The plates must be refrigerated overnight before use; as the papers are not removed, every plate is precisely and clearly labelled. These are excellent for determining the MIC of large numbers of strains but cannot readily be made into a bactericidal test. They offer very considerable advantages if used for routine sensitivity testing by the break-point method (see page 482) and papers for this purpose (*Adapads*) are available. (Waterworth, 1980). A week's supply of plates can be poured by simply placing the papers in the Petri dishes and then feeding these into a plate-pouring machine.

Repliscan (Cathra). The reading of many agar plates inoculated with a multiple replicator is exceedingly boring and it is easy to record the results incorrectly. A machine is now available which gives help not only with the reading of sensitivity tests but also with the identification of Gram-negative bacilli. Plates containing antibiotics and media for biochemical tests are inoculated with a replicator (36 strains). After overnight incubation the result for each position on every plate is fed into a computer which will then print out the identity of the organism followed by its sensitivity pattern. The *Replireader* is a smaller model suitable for departments handling only a small number of organisms daily. These machines have been favourably reported on by Brown & Washington (1978) and Waterworth (1980a). They also have the great advantage that they do not require any other special equipment and use 85 mm Petri dishes.

Break points in broth

This method was referred to on page 482. Two products may be shortly available: 'Sensititre' (Seward Laboratory) employs the plastic tray containing dried dilutions of antibiotics used for MIC determinations but in this case four organisms can be tested in each tray. Each organism has two horizontal rows of 12 wells, containing usually two dilutions of 11 drugs: 50 μl inoculated broth is added to each. Three different drug combinations are envisaged for Gram-positive, Gram-negative and urinary organisms.

ATB (API). These plastic strips have two rows of 16 wells containing usually two dilutions of each drug dried in them and 150 μl inoculated broth is added to each. This product has the advantage that each organism is tested on a separate strip and every well is labelled individually.

ANTIBIOTIC ASSAYS IN BODY FLUIDS

Apart from studying the pharmacokinetics of new drugs, assays may be required in clinical practice for either of two purposes:

1. To verify that adequate concentrations are being achieved, for example:
   a. in treatment of relatively resistant infections when sustained high blood levels are required (e.g. carbenicillin in life-threatening infections due to *Ps. aeruginosa*).
   b. to check adequate absorption of oral penicillins in serious infections (e.g. bacterial endocarditis).
   c. to confirm adequate penetration into the cerebrospinal fluid, particularly in enterobacterial or pseudomonal meningitis.
   d. to account for the failure of theoretically adequate treatment, particularly by evidence of failure to penetrate into joints or cavities.
2. To guard against excessive blood levels. This applies particularly to antibiotics likely to cause eighth nerve damage.
   a. in patients with known impairment of renal function.
   b. in the elderly, whose clearance of antibiotics may be considerably slower than normal.
   c. in all patients who have received full doses of these drugs for more than a week, after which time blood levels frequently rise and should be checked regularly.
   d. in neonates, whose renal and hepatic handling of drugs is imperfectly developed.

The interval between the collection of the blood and the administration of the last dose must be stated and if this is not known the result is meaningless. If the level is being done to avoid toxicity, the blood should be taken shortly before the next dose is to be given (trough level). Peak levels vary greatly and do not necessarily indicate delayed excretion as does a significant level at the end of the interval between doses (Line et al, 1970). Significant trough levels are given in Table 27.10. If peak levels are required, it is customary to take blood one hour after intramuscular injection and Reeves & Wise (1978) suggest that this is also the most satisfactory time following bolus intravenous injection. If the drug is given orally the interval should be two hours. Bactericidal assays against the patient's own organism (see page 502) can with advantage be done as a peak level and immediately before the next dose is given.

It is obviously essential to know whether any other antibacterial drug is being given and it should be remembered that blood from a patient with impaired renal function may still contain an antibiotic last given 48 hours or more before.

For many years all antibiotics were assayed by the tube dilution or an agar diffusion method. It is now generally accepted that the dilution method is only

Table 27.10 Suggested maximum serum levels to avoid the risk of toxicity from antibacterial drugs

	Concentration μg/ml Trough	Peak
*Gentamicin	2	
*Tobramycin	2	
Amikacin	5	
Streptomycin	3	
Vancomycin	5	
Penicillin		100
Chloramphenicol		50
Flucytosine		80

* It may be necessary to have higher levels in life-endangering Pseudomonas infections.

suitable for bactericidal assays(see page 502). Until recently diffusion assays required overnight incubation; the great majority of assays performed in the clinical laboratory are of aminoglycosides, and the delay in obtaining the result meant that two or even more doses might have been given before it was available. Various new methods have now been developed specifically for assaying these drugs, with which a result can be obtained in two hours or less.

These are:

1. *Urease method* (Noone et al, 1971). This method is based on measurement of the increase of pH produced by *P. mirabilis* in a urea-containing medium, which is progressively inhibited by increasing concentrations of gentamicin and other aminoglycosides. Some laboratories have found it difficult to obtain reliable results with this method and it is also costly in technician time.

2. *Enzymic methods*. Smith et al (1972) showed that gentamicin is adenylated by an enzyme produced by R-factor-carrying *E. coli*, and if (^{14}C) adenosine triphosphate is added it is then possible to measure the amount of (^{14}C) adenylated gentamicin present. Broughall & Reeves (1975) have since modified this method and recommend the use of the acetyl transferase enzyme with (^{14}C) acetyl coenzyme A. Both methods are accurate and reliable but have the disadvantages of requiring expensive and hazardous materials and a liquid scintillation counter, which is seldom available in microbiology departments.

3. *Immunoassay techniques*. Both radio-immune assay and fluorescence immunoassays are coming into use, and the latter have the advantage that they do not require radioactive materials. Commercially prepared kits are available for some of these methods but they do of course, require special equipment for reading.

All these methods have the advantage of speed in obtaining a result and of lack of interference from other antibiotics. Nevertheless they all suffer from some disadvantages in the average clinical laboratory. In contrast the plate diffusion method requires no special equipment, can be set up very quickly, and if suitably modified, a result can be obtained within three hours. This method also has the advantage that it can be used for assaying any anti-bacterial drug in any type of specimen. Only diffusion assays will be described here and the reader is referred to the article by Broughall (1978) for further information concerning the other methods.

Plate diffusion methods

In these methods, standard solutions of the antibiotic, together with the fluid to be assayed, are applied to seeded agar plates. After incubation the diameter of the inhibition zones produced by the standards are measured and plotted against the log of their concentration: ideally the resulting line is straight. The diameter of the zone produced by the unknown is then measured and the concentration can then be read from the standard line.

When well done this method gives excellent results but it requires carefully standardized technique. Assays should only be done by experienced staff who perform them regularly and the preparation of the standards should never be delegated to more junior staff. All tests and standards must be set up in triplicate. Control sera of known antibiotic content should be included regularly in routine assays to check the accuracy of the results obtained which should be within ±15 per cent of the correct level.

Preparation of the plates

Assays may be performed on large square glass dishes, 25 × 25 cm or 30 × 30 cm (available from Mast Laboratories) or on plastic Petri dishes (85 mm circular or 100 mm square). The latter are easier to handle and more economical if only small numbers of assays are being performed, but it is essential that each plate carries both standards and unknown.

Various assay agars are available; in practice most sensitivity test agars are also suitable. Shanson & Hince (1977a) found Oxoid DST and Isosensitest agars the most reliable for assaying gentamicin and they also reported Difco Assay Medium No. 5 to be unsatisfactory for this antibiotic.

Many antibiotics are affected by pH (see page 467) and the sensitivity of an assay can be increased by altering the pH of the medium to favour the drug being assayed. The optimum pH for various drugs is given in Table 27.11. All aminoglycosides are more active at high pH (see Table 27.1) but in practice satisfactory results can be obtained without altering sensitivity agar (pH 7.2–7.3) except for streptomycin: for this it must be raised to 7.8 or no zone will be obtained with the recommended bottom standard.

Plates must be poured on a level surface and large glass dishes should be placed on a levelling tripod and checked with a spirit level. The depth of the medium need not be more than 2 mm, deeper plates requiring more serum to fill the wells: large glass dishes should be warmed to prevent the agar setting before it has levelled out.

Choice of test organisms

Many organisms have been recommended for assaying different antibiotics, some of which are given in Table 27.11, but in clinical assays the possible presence of a second drug and its effect on the recommended organism must always be borne in mind (see page 501). Spore suspensions are particularly convenient as these will keep almost indefinitely at 4°C. Suspensions of vegetative organisms can be kept for many months in liquid N_2 or at 70°C and will also keep at 4°C for at least four weeks. Instructions for preparing suspensions are given below.

Table 27.11 Appropriate organisms for assaying antibacterial drugs

Drug	Organism	NCTC number	Optimum pH
Penicillins, Cephalosporins	*B. subtilis*	8236	6.8
	S. lutea	8340	
	Staph. aureus	6571	
Carbenicillin, Ticarcillin	*Ps. aeruginosa*	10490	
Streptomycin	*B. subtilis*	8236	7.8
	Staph. aureus	6571	
Amikacin, Gentamicin, Kanamycin, Tobramycin	*B. subtilis*	8236	
	Kl. edwardsii	10896	
Tetracycline	*B. cereus*	10320	6.6
	Staph. aureus	6571	
Chloramphenicol	*S. lutea*	8340	
Erythromycin, Clindamycin	*B. subtilis*	8236	7.8
	Staph. aureus	6571	
Fusidate	*C. xerosis*	9755	6.6
Vancomycin	*B. subtilis*	8236	7.8
	Staph. aureus	6571	
Trimethoprim, Sulphonamides	*B. pumilis*	8241	7.3
Anti-fungal	*Sacch. cerevisiae*	10716	7.2
	C. albicans		

Preparation of spore suspensions. Grow cultures on agar, preferably in Roux Bottles, for one week at 37°C (30°C for *B. cereus*). Suspend the growth in sterile distilled water and heat for 30 minutes at 65°C. Wash the spores in water and resuspend in water. Suspensions will keep at 4°C indefinitely.

Suspensions of vegetative organisms can be prepared from broth cultures (if not granular) or by suspending growth from solid medium in broth. They will keep at 4°C for up to four weeks or may be stored indefinitely at −70°C or in liquid nitrogen.

Inoculation of plates

Plates may be inoculated either by pre-seeding the agar or by flooding plates which have first been dried. The former is quicker and ensures a uniform inoculum throughout, but care must be taken to see that the agar is cooled to 48°C before adding the inoculum unless this is a spore suspension. If for any reason deep plates are used, a thin layer of uninoculated agar should be poured first and a thin surface layer of seeded agar added when the first is set. Flooding is usually more satisfactory for rapid assays of aminoglycosides (see page 502), as storage of pre-seeded plates at 4°C lengthens the incubation period required to obtain a result.

The size of the inoculum is generally much less critical than with sensitivity tests, but obviously it must be the same throughout any one assay. Ideally growth should be just confluent for overnight assays, but very much heavier if the result is to be read within a few hours.

Application of standards and samples to plates

Various methods have been advocated for applying drug-containing solutions to seeded plates, some of which were described in earlier editions of this book. The majority of workers now use wells (or 'cups') punched out of the agar with a sterile cork-borer, usually 7–9 mm in diameter: smaller wells require less serum but are more difficult to fill. The cork-borer may be attached to a flask on a vacuum pump and the plug of agar removed by suction or the holes can be cut and the agar plug removed with a wire loop or small scalpel. In either case great care must be taken not to disturb the surrounding medium or leakage will occur, resulting in a distorted zone.

Cups may either be filled with a Pasteur pipette or a measured volume may be placed in each. The former has the advantage that any slight variations in the depth of the medium will be cancelled out, but it requires more technical expertise. It is essential that the cups are *filled* and this can only be done by placing the tip of the pipette in the cup and adding the fluid until the meniscus has disappeared and the fluid is level with the surface of the plate. Bennett et al (1966) give an excellent description of this method.

Blotting paper discs may be used for very small specimens. The plates should then be as thin as possible, but even so the test will be much less sensitive than the agar cup method. A measured volume of the drug standards and test fluid must be placed on the discs before these are applied to the seeded plates and the discs must be large enough to absorb the fluid completely.

Pre-diffusion or pre-incubation of plates

The sensitivity of an assay can be increased by allowing the antibiotic to pre-diffuse into the agar for a period before incubation, thus increasing the size of the zone. In contrast, a result may be obtained more rapidly if plates are inoculated and incubated for one hour before the arrival of the specimen; zones will then be smaller but accurate results are still obtained (Shanson & Hince, 1977b).

Standard solutions

Protein binding. All anti-bacterial drugs are bound to plasma proteins but the extent of this varies from <20 per cent (e.g. ampicillin) to >95 per cent (e.g. cloxacillin). Bound drugs are microbiologically inactive and standards for serum assays must therefore be prepared in serum. Pooled human serum is ideal, but if obtained from samples sent to the laboratory for serology, these must first be tested to ensure that they do not contain inhibitory drugs. There may be considerable difference in the extent of binding by human and horse serum, for example, cloxacillin is respectively 94.5 per cent and 70 per cent bound (Rolinson & Sutherland, 1965), so that only human serum should be used for standards. However, with drugs with low binding capacities (including the aminoglycosides) the difference is small and horse serum can be used if desired (Shanson & Daniels, 1975). Cerebrospinal fluid should be assayed against standards prepared in normal saline.

Preparation of drug solutions. Ideally assay standards should be prepared from drugs obtained from the manufacturers for this purpose. The potency should be stated (gentamicin, for example, is usually only about 60 per cent pure) and this must be allowed for in the original dilution. If pharmaceutical preparations are used there may be some loss of accuracy due to overfilling of the ampoules; unless the purity of these powders is stated, the whole ampoule should be dissolved. Some workers recommend that antibiotics should be dissolved in phosphate buffer. This should not be used for aminoglycosides and is not essential for other drugs, sterile glass distilled water is satisfactory. Some drugs, particularly penicillins, and cephalosporins, are unstable; concentrated solutions (e.g. 100 μg/ml) may be kept for one week at 4°C, or for several weeks at −20°C, in the latter case they should be dispensed in aliquots and never re-frozen. These antibiotics are particularly unstable in serum and if specimens cannot be assayed on the day of receipt, the appropriate standards should be prepared in serum and stored with the specimen at at least −20°C. Problems concerning the preparation of stock solutions of certain drugs are discussed on page

Concentration of standards for assays. The bottom standard should contain the lowest concentration of the drug which will give a measurable zone of inhibition. What this will be will depend on the sensitivity of the test organism, the diffusibility of the drug and the extent of protein-binding. Serum samples should not be diluted, so the top standard should be rather higher than the highest level anticipated, together with two intermediate levels. Suitable concentrations for use with some drugs are given in Table 27.12.

Table 27.12 Suitable standard solutions, in serum, for serum assays

Drug	Concentrations, μg/ml	Test organism
Gentamicin	30, 10, 3, 1	*B. subtilis*
Tobramycin	30, 10, 3, 1	*Kl. edwardsii*
Kanamycin	100, 30, 10, 3	*Staph. aureus*
Amikacin	100, 30, 10, 3	
*Streptomycin	100, 30, 10, 3	*B. subtilis*
Vancomycin	100, 30, 10, 3	*Staph. aureus*
Penicillin	40, 8, 1.6, 0.3	*B. subtilis*
Ampicillin	1, 0.25, 0.06, 0.015	*S. lutea*
Chloramphenicol	50, 25, 12.5, 6.25	*S. lutea*
Carbenicillin	50, 25, 12.5, 6.25	*Ps. aeruginosa* NCTC 10490
Flucytosine	30, 10, 3, 1	*C. albicans* *Sacch. cerevisiae*

* pH of the medium must be raised to 7.8.

Incubation. The period of incubation required and its temperature will depend on the test organism. *S. lutea* usually grows better at 30°C and overnight incubation is required, as it is for carbenicillin assays using *Ps. aeruginosa.* If a heavy inoculum of *Kl. edwardsii* (NCTC 10896) is used, there will usually be adequate growth after 3½ to 4 hours' incubation at 37°C, 1 hour of which may have been before the antibiotic solutions were applied (see page 502). Shanson & Hince (1977a) found that incubation at 40°C made early reading rather easier, but the temperature must not rise above this. Most other test organisms will grow fast enough for zones to be measured after 5–6 hours' incubation, particularly if the inoculum is heavy, but unless specimens are received early in the day it is usually easier to incubate overnight.

Table 27.13 Methods of assaying various antibiotics in specimens containing other antibacterial agents

Drug to be assayed	Other drugs present	Method
Amikacin Gentamicin Tobramycin	Penicillins Ampicillins Carbenicillins Sulphonamides Trimethoprim Chloramphenicol Tetracyclines Erythromycin Clindamycin Fusidate	Use *Kl. edwardsii* NCTC 10896 as test organism
	Cephalosporins	Add β-lactamase to serum
Streptomycin	Rifampicin	Use resistant *Staph. aureus* NCTC 11150
All	Aminoglycoside	Treat with cellulose phosphate Add 1% sodium polyanethol sulphonate to medium
	Sulphonamides	Add 0.005% *p*-amino-benzoic acid to medium
	Trimethoprim	Add 0.01% thymidine to medium

Reading of assays. The accuracy of the method is greatly improved if a zone reader which magnifies the zones is used. Several are now available, of which we prefer the Dynatech Zone Diffusion Reader.

Specific problems

Penicillin. Modern dosage often results in very high blood levels and several dilutions of the serum will be required if *S. lutea* or *Staph. aureus* is used as the test organism. Serum specimens should generally be assayed against *B. subtilis,* but if low levels are anticipated in other specimens, such as cerebrospinal fluid, *S. lutea* should be used. Suitable standards for both are given in Table 27.12.

Carbenicillin and ticarcillin. The strain of *Ps. aeruginosa* normally used for sensitivity control is not suitable. The Elsworth strain, NCTC 10490, which is much more sensitive to carbenicillin should be used. Plates should be inoculated by flooding and the resulting growth no heavier than just confluent. *Staph. aureus* should not be used as carbenicillin may contain small quantities of penicillin which might invalidate the assay.

Sulphonamide and trimethoprim. These should both be assayed against *B. pumilis*, with an inoculum giving no more than just confluent growth in a thymidine-free medium (see page 475). If both drugs are being administered the trimethoprim level can be determined by inactivating the sulphonamide by the addition of 5 μg/ml *p*-aminobenzoic acid to the medium. It is not possible to assay the combined drugs other than by simply determining the dilution of the patient's serum which inhibits growth.

Metronidazole. This can be assayed using either the *Cl. welchii* (NCTC 11229) recommended as the control for sensitivity tests or a sensitive strain of *Bacteroides fragilis* such as NCTC 9343. The inoculum should be no heavier than that required to give just confluent growth and the plates must be well dried before being incubated anaerobically: anaerobiosis must be checked with an indicator (see page 471). Suitable standard solutions may contain 50, 25, 12.5 and 6.25 μg/ml. If *Cl. hystolyticum* (NCTC 503) is used as test organism, standards can be taken down to 0.12 μg/ml, but the less sensitive assay is usually satisfactory.

Flucytosine. Serum levels of this drug should not be allowed to rise above 80 μg/ml and regular assays will be required in patients with renal impairment. Flucytosine is inactivated by cytosine and pyrimidine bases and a special medium is therefore required. We find that recommended by Proctor (1976) the most satisfactory; it also has the advantage of not requiring filtration and it keeps well in the refrigerator.

Proctor's assay agar (Proctor, 1976)

Dextrose	10 g
Casamino acids (Difco)	10 g
Sodium B glycerophosphate	2.5 g
Yeast extract (Difco)	0.5 g
Agar	3 g
Water	100 ml

The pH should be 6.8–7.0 without adjustment. Sterilize at 115°C for 10 minutes.

Either *Saccharomyces cerevisiae* (NCTC 10716) or a sensitive strain of *C. albicans* can be used as the test organism. This should be grown overnight on the assay agar and the growth suspended in sterile water. Plates can be inoculated by pre-seeding the agar or by flooding the surface of well-dried plates: in either case the resulting growth must be only just confluent. Suitable standards, in serum, contain 30, 10, 3 and 1 μg/ml flucytosine.

Assays during combined treatment

Assays of one drug are frequently requested on patients receiving other anti-bacterial agents, the presence of which may invalidate the assay if unsuspected. Whilst this problem may sometimes be insurmountable in microbiological assays, there are two possible approaches to the problem.

1. By inactivation of the second drug. All penicillins and cephalosporins can be inactivated by the addition of Whatman's broad-spectrum beta-lactamase to the serum before assay (Waterworth, 1973). Cefoxitin (a cephamycin) is more resistant but the addition of an equal volume of the β-lactamase and incubation at 37°C for one hour before assay may suffice.

Sulphonamides can be inactivated by the addition of 5 μg/ml of *p*-aminobenzoic acid to the medium, and trimethoprim by 10 μg/ml thymidine: both should be added when the patient is receiving co-trimoxazole. Despite the addition of thymidine, colonies of the test organism in the zone containing trimethoprim may be smaller than normal, giving the effect of a double zone. This difference in growth should be disregarded and only the clear zone measured.

All aminoglycosides are selectively bound by cellulose phosphate powder (Stevens and Young, 1977). 0.5 ml serum should be added to about 50 mg of the powder in a narrow tube and vortexed: it can be centrifuged immediately and the supernatant serum assayed. Alternatively if the specimen is very small the activity of all aminoglycosides can be significantly reduced by lowering pH of the medium to 6.0 (see Table 27.1, page 467). Low concentrations are also inactivated by the addition of 1 per cent sodium polyanethol sulphonate to the medium, which has no effect on other antibiotics except polymyxins (Edberg et al, 1976).

2. Alternatively a test organism may be chosen which is sensitive to the drug to be assayed but resistant to any other drugs present, as is generally done for the clinical assay of aminoglycosides. *Kl. edwardsii* NCTC 10896 is resistant to all the commonly used antibacterial drugs except nalidixic acid and the newer cephalosporins, and its use largely overcomes the hazard of the presence of undisclosed antibiotics; β-lactamase must be added for cephalosporins. This organism is only slightly sensitive to streptomycin and if this has to be assayed in the presence of rifampicin, a rifampicin-resistant strain of *Staph. aureus* (such as NCTC 11150) should be used.

It is always preferable to use an organism which is naturally resistant to the drug not being assayed, but this is seldom possible. Resistance in naturally sensitive species is often unstable and may be lost on storage or frequent sub-cultures. These organisms should be maintained on medium containing a stable drug to which they are resistant or preferably kept frozen.

Isoniazid, PAS, ethionamide, ethambutol, pyrazinamide, and thiacetazone do not interfere with the assay of other antibacterial drugs.

These methods for selective assays are summarized in Table 27.13 but they should only be undertaken by workers with considerable experience. The method used must be well controlled and the edge of the zone of inhibition examined carefully; if this is not like that round the standards, the validity of the test should be questioned.

Rapid assay method for aminoglycosides

Test organism: *Kl. edwardsii* NCTC 10896. Plates, in either large square glass dishes or plastic Petri dishes, should be poured in advance; Oxoid DST or Isosensitest agar is recommended. Plates should not be refrigerated but can be kept at room temperature for up to three days: they should be well dried at 37°C before use, the time required depending upon how long they have been poured.

The stock suspension of *Kl. edwardsii* (NCTC 10896) (see page 497) should be diluted to contain 10^9–10^{10} organisms per ml before flooding the surface of the plates and removing any excess fluid with a Pasteur pipette. Incubate at 37°C or 40°C for one hour.

Cut the required number of wells and fill with the standard sera and specimens, all in triplicate. Continue incubation until the zones are clearly defined, probably 2½–3 hours.

Measure the zones produced by the standard solutions and prepare a graph by plotting the zone diameter against the log of the concentration, using semi-log paper. Measure the zones given by the unknown sera and read the concentrations from the standard graph.

Bactericidal Assays

Test organism: an overnight broth culture of the patient's infecting organism. Serum should be added if enrichment is required but glucose broth should not be used as overnight cultures in this may be dead (Waterworth, 1972).

Medium. This must support the growth of the test organism; simple nutrient broth, Mueller-Hinton broth or Oxoid Isosensitest broth are suitable. At least 10 per cent of serum must be added.

Inoculate 20 ml medium with two drops of well shaken culture: shake well. Pipette 1 ml volumes into a row of sterile tubes. Add 1 ml of the patient's serum to the first tube, mix well and transfer 1 ml to the second tube. Repeat, thus producing a row of doubled dilutions of the patient's serum all inoculated with his own organism. The number of dilutions required will depend on the sensitivity of the organism, the antibiotic dosage and the time at which the blood was taken.

One tube of inoculated broth alone is included as the control: this should immediately be sub-cultivated by spreading a loopful uniformly over half a blood agar plate.

Incubate the tubes overnight at 37°C. Record the highest dilution inhibiting growth (minimum inhibitory dilution) and then sub-cultivate all tubes showing no growth, as above. Incubate overnight.

Interpretation. The cultures from the tubes showing no growth are compared to that from the control tube before incubation. A similar number of colonies indicates bacteristatic action only, the presence of only a very small number of colonies suggests incomplete bactericidal action. Sterile sub-cultures, indicating complete killing, from dilutions of 1 in 4 upwards is usually considered satisfactory.

If the organism is completely killed only by the combined action of penicillin and gentamicin, there may be a wide difference between the minimum inhibitory dilution and that which kills. If penicillin dosage is high, the serum may inhibit at 1/100 or more, but the organism will be completely killed only in very much lower dilutions which contain the necessary amounts of gentamicin.

References

Amyes S G B, Smith J T 1978 J Antimicrob Chemother 4: 421
Anand C M, Paull A 1976 J Clin Path 29: 1130
Bennett J V, Brodie J L, Benner E J, Kirby W M M 1966 Appl Microbiol 14: 170
Broughall J M 1978 In: Laboratory methods in antimicrobial chemotherapy. Ed Reeves D S, Phillips I, Williams J D, Wise R. Churchill-Livingstone, Edinburgh, p 194
Broughall J M, Reeves D S 1975 J Clin Path 28: 140
Brown D, Blowers R 1978 In: Laboratory methods in antimicrobial chemotherapy. Ed Reeves D S, Phillips I, Williams J D, Wise R. Churchill-Livingstone, Edinburgh, p. 8
Brown S D, Washington J A II 1978 J Clin Microbiol 8: 695
Collins C H, Yates M D 1978 In: Laboratory methods in antimicrobial chemotherapy. Ed Reeves D S, Phillips I, Williams J D, Wise R. Churchill-Livingstone, Edinburgh, p 115
Drew W L, Barry A L, O'Toole R, Sherris J C 1972 Appl Microbiol 24: 240
Edberg S C, Bottenbley C J, Gam K 1976 Antimicrob Agents Chemother 9: 414
Ericsson H M 1960 Scand J Clin Lab Invest 12: Suppl 50
Ericsson H M, Sherris J C 1971 Acta Path Microbiol Scand Section B Suppl 217
Federal Register 1972 37: 20525
Felmingham D, Stokes E J 1972 Med Lab Technol 29: 198
Ferone R, Bushby S R M, Burchall J J, Moore W D, Smith D 1975 Antimicrob Agents Chemother 7: 91
Flowers D J 1978 J Clin Path 31: 855
Garrod L P, Waterworth P M 1969 J Clin Path 22: 534
Garrod L P, Waterworth P M 1971 J Clin Path 24: 779
Jones P H, Scott A P 1977 J Clin Path 30: 1028
Koch A E, Burchall J J 1971 Appl Microbiol 22: 812
Line D H, Poole G W, Waterworth P M 1970 Tubercle 51: 76
Milne S E, Stokes E J, Waterworth P M 1978 J Clin Path 31: 933
Noone P, Pattison J R, Samson D 1971 Lancet 2: 16
Pearson C H, Whitehead J E M 1974 J Clin Path 27: 430
Phillips I, Warren C, Waterworth P M 1978 J Clin Path 31: 531
Proctor A G 1976 In: Microbiological methods. Collins C H, Lyne P M, 4th ed. Butterworths, London, p 142
Pykett A H 1978 J Clin Path 31: 536
Reeves D S, Phillips I, Williams J D, Wise R 1978 Laboratory methods in antimicrobial chemotherapy. Churchill-Livingstone, Edinburgh
Reeves D S, Wise R 1978 In: Laboratory methods in antimicrobial chemotherapy. Ed Reeves D S, Phillips I, Williams J D, Wise R. Churchill-Livingstone, Edinburgh, p 137

Rolinson G N, Sutherland R 1965 Brit J Pharmacol 25: 638
Ryan K J, Needham G M, Dunsmoor C L, Sherris J C 1970 Appl Microbiol 20: 447
Shafi M S 1975 J Clin Path 28: 989
Shanson D C, Daniels J V 1975 J Antimicrob Chemother 1: 219
Shanson D C, Hince C J 1977a J Antimicrob Chemother 3: 17
Shanson D C, Hince C 1977b J Clin Path 30: 521
Slack M P E, Wheldon D B, Turk D C 1977 Lancet 2: 906
Smith D H, van Otto B, Smith A L 1972 New Engl J Med 286: 583
Stevens P, Young L S 1977 Antimicrob Agents Chemother 12: 286
Stokes E J, Ridgway G L 1980 Clinical bacteriology, 5th edn. p 215 Arnold, London
Waterworth P M 1962 J Med Lab Technol 19: 163
Waterworth P M 1972 J Clin Path 25: 227
Waterworth P M 1973 J Clin Path 26: 596
Waterworth P M 1978a In: Reeves D S, Phillips I, Williams J D, Wise R (eds) Laboratory methods in chemotherapy, Churchill Livingstone, Edinburgh, p 85
Waterworth P M 1978b In: Reeves D S, Phillips I, Williams J D, Wise R (eds) Laboratory methods in chemotherapy, Churchill Livingstone, Edinburgh, p 4
Waterworth P M 1980 J Clin Path In press
Waterworth P M 1981 J Antimicrob Chemother In press
Waterworth P M, del Piano M 1976 J Clin Path 29: 179
Wheldon D B, Slack M P E 1979 J Clin Path 32: 738
WHO Expert Committee on Biological Standardization 1977 Technical report series 610, p 98

Index